RHINOLOGY AND SINUS DISEASE

A Problem-Oriented Approach

RHINOLOGY AND SINUS DISEASE

A Problem-Oriented Approach

Steven D. Schaefer, MD
Professor and Chairman
Department of Otolaryngology
New York Eye and Ear Infirmary
New York, New York

with 293 illustrations

Mosby

St. Louis Baltimore Boston Carlsbad Chicago Minneapolis New York Philadelphia Portland
London Milan Sydney Tokyo Toronto

Mosby
Dedicated to Publishing Excellence

A Times Mirror
Company

Publisher: Geoff Greenwood
Editor: Robert A. Hurley
Editorial Assistant: Jori Matison
Project Manager: Linda Clarke
Production Editor: Jennifer Harper
Composition Specialist: Christine Boles
Designer: Carolyn O'Brien
Manufacturing Manager: William A. Winneberger, Jr.
Cover Design: Hyperdesign, Inc.

Printed in the United States of America
Composition by Mosby Electronic Production, Philadelphia
Printing/binding by Maple-Vail Book Manufacturing Group

Mosby, Inc.
11830 Westline Industrial Drive
St. Louis, Missouri 63146

Library of Congress Cataloging-in-Publication Data

Rhinology and sinus disease : a problem-oriented approach / [edited by] Steven D. Schaefer.—1st ed.
p. cm.
Includes bibliographical references and index.
ISBN 0-8016-7800-5 (alk. paper)
1. Nose—Diseases. 2. Paranasal sinuses—Diseases. I. Schaefer, Steven D., 1945- .
[DNLM: 1. Nose Diseases—therapy. 2. Paranasal Sinus Diseases—therapy. 3. Otorhinolaryngologic Surgical Procedures. WV 300 R473s 1998]
RF341.R48 1998
616.2' 12—dc21
DNLM/DLC
for Library of Congress

97-50427
CIP

98 99 00 01 02 / 9 8 7 6 5 4 3 2 1

CONTRIBUTORS

Tom I. Abelson, MD
Ear, Nose, and Throat Surgeon
Cleveland Clinic
Solon, Ohio

Daniel G. Becker, MD
Instructor
Department of Otolaryngology
University of Pennsylvania
Philadelphia, Pennsylvania

Andrew Blitzer, MD
Professor of Clinical Otolaryngology
Columbia University College of Physicians and Surgeons
Director, New York Center for Voice and Swallowing Disorders
New York, New York

Orval E. Brown, MD
Associate Professor
University of Texas Southwestern Medical Center
Active Staff
Children's Medical Center of Dallas
Dallas, Texas

Peter A. R. Clement, MD, Ph.D.
Professor in Otorhinolaryngology
Free University of Brussels
Chairman, E.N.T. Department
University Hospital
Laarbeeklaan 101-1090
Brussels, Belgium

Robert Della Rocca, MD
Clinical Professor
New York Medical College
Surgeon Director
New York Eye and Ear Infirmary
New York, New York

Jay N. Dolitsky, MD
Assistant Professor
Department of Otolaryngology-Head and Neck
The New York Eye and Ear
Affiliated Hospitals of New York Medical College
New York, New York

Paul J. Donald, MD, FRCS(C)
Professor
Department of Otolarynology-Head and Neck Surgery
University of California, Davis
Director, UCDMC Center for Skull Base Surgery
U.C. Davis Medical Center
Sacramento, California

Wolfgang Draf, MD, D Med Sci, FRCS Ed.
Professor
Mainz University
Marburg University
Director
Department of ENT, Head, Neck and Facial Plastic Surgery, Communications Disorders
Hospital Fulda
Fulda, Germany

Willard E. Fee, Jr., MD
Professor and Chair
Division of Otolaryngology-Head and Neck Surgery
Stanford University Medical Center
Stanford, California

Wolfgang Freysinger, Ph.D.
University ENT Department
University of Innsbruck/Austria
Laudeskraukenhaus, Innsbruck
Austria

William H. Friedman, MD, FACS
Chief, Department of Otolaryngology
Deaconess/Incarnate World Health Systems
St. Louis, Missouri

Charles W. Gross, MD
Professor
Department of Otolaryngology-Head and Neck Surgery
Department of Pediatrics
University of Virginia
University of Virginia Health Sciences Center
Charlottesville, Virginia

William E. Gross, MD
Assistant Clinical Professor
Department of Otolaryngology
Vanderbilt University
Private Practice
Middle Tennessee Medical Center
Munfreesboro, Tennessee

Andreas R. Gunkel, MD
University ENT Department
University of Innsbruck/Austria
Laudeskraukenhaus, Innsbruck
Austria

Peter H. Hwang, MD
Assistant Professor
Department of Otolaryngology-Head and Neck Surgery
Oregon Health Sciences University
Portland, Oregon

Gary D. Josephson, MD
Assistant Professor of Otolaryngology and Pediatrics
Chief, Division of Pediatric Otolaryngology-Head and Neck Surgery
University of Miami School of Medicine
Miami, Florida

George P. Katsantonis, MD, FACS
Clinical Professor of Otolaryngology
St. Louis University
Park Central Institute
St. Louis, Missouri

Rainer Keerl, MD
Department of ENT, Head, Neck and Facial Plastic Surgery, Communication Disorders
Hospital Fulda
Fulda, Germany

David W. Kennedy, MD
Professor and Chairman
Department of Otolaryngology-Head and Neck Surgery
University of Pennsylvania School of Medicine
Hospital of the University of Pennsylvania
Philadelphia, Pennsylvania

Hueston C. King, MD, FACS, FACAI
Clinical Professor
Department of Otolaryngology
University of Texas Southwestern Medical Center
Dallas, Texas

William Lawson, MD, DDS
Professor of Otolaryngology
Mt. Sinai School of Medicine
Attending in Otolaryngology
Chief of Otolaryngology
Bronx Veterans Hospital
New York, New York

Howard L. Levine, MD
Director, The Mt. Sinai Nasal-Sinus Center
Cleveland Ear, Nose, Throat and Facial Surgery
Cleveland, Ohio

Richard L. Mabry, MD
Professor
Department of Otolaryngology
University of Texas Southwestern Medical Center
Dallas, Texas

Elizabeth Maher, MD
Clinical Assistant Professor
New York Medical College
Adjunct Surgeon
New York Eye and Ear Infirmary
New York, New York

Scott C. Manning, MD
Associate Professor
Department of Otolaryngology-Head and Neck Surgery
University of Washington School of Medicine
Chief, Pediatric Otolaryngology-Head and Neck Surgery
Children's Hospital and Medical Center
Seattle, Washington

Bradley F. Marple, MD
Assistant Professor
Department of Otolaryngology
University of Texas Southwestern
Chief, Department of Otolaryngology
Dallas Veterans Administration Hospital
Dallas, Texas

Sam J. Marzo, MD
Senior Resident
Department of Otolaryngology
Loyola University Medical School
Maywood, Illinois

David S. Mazza, MD
Assistant Clinical Professor of Pediatric Allergy
Columbia University College of Physicians and Surgeons
R.A. Cooke Institute of Allergy
St. Luke's/Roosevelt Hospital
New York, New York

Thomas V. McCaffrey, MD, Ph.D.
Professor, Otorhinolaryngology
Mayo Medical School
Consultant, Otorhinolaryngology
Mayo Clinic
St. Mary's Hospital/Rochester Methodist Hospital
Rochester, Minnesota

James P. Milite, MD
Assistant Professor of Ophthalmology
New York Medical College
Coordinator of Medical Education
New York Eye and Ear Infirmary
New York, New York

Raj Murali, MD
Professor
Department of Neurosurgery
New York Medical College
Director of Neurosurgery
St. Vincent's Medical Center
New York, New York

H. Bryan Neel, III, MD, Ph.D.
Professor and Past Chairman of Otolaryngology-Head and Neck Surgery
Mayo Medical School
Consultant
Mayo Clinic
Rochester, Minnesota

Anthony J. Reino, MD, M.Sc.
Assistant Clinical Professor
Mt. Sinai School of Medicine
Assistant Attending
Mt. Sinai Hospital
Associate Director ENT
Bronx VA Medical Center
New York, New York

Dale H. Rice, MD
Tiber/Alpert Professor and Chair
Department of Otolaryngology-Head and Neck Surgery
USC School of Medicine
University Hospital
Los Angeles, California

Stephen J. Salzer, MD
Clinical Instructor in Surgery-Otolaryngology
Yale-New Haven Hospital
Attending Staff
Greenwich Hospital
Greenwich, Connecticut

Gillian M. Shepherd, MD
Clinical Associate Professor of Medicine
Cornell University Medical College
Associate Attending Physician
The New York Hospital
Consultant, Memorial Sloan Kettering Cancer Center
New York, New York

James A. Stankiewicz, MD
Professor and Vice Chairman
Loyola University Medical School
Loyola University Medical Center
Maywood, Illinois

Jordan Stern, MD
Assistant Professor
New York Medical College
Director, Head and Neck Service
Department of Otolaryngology
The New York Eye and Ear Infirmary
New York, New York

Walter F. Thumfart, MD, Ph.D.
University Professor
University of Innsbruck/Austria
Chairman & Head of the ORL Department
Laudeskraukenhaus, Innsbruck
Austria

Paul H. Toffel, MD
Clinical Professor
Department of Otolaryngology-Head and Neck Surgery
University of Southern California School of Medicine
Chief of Department of Otolaryngology-Head and Neck Surgery
Daniel Freeman Memorial Hospital
Inglewood, California

Rainer Weber, MD
Department of ENT, Head, Neck and Facial Plastic Surgery, Communication Disorders
Hospital Fulda
Fulda, Germany

Barbara Zeifer, MD
Assistant Professor, Radiology
Albert Einstein College of Medicine
Director of Radiology
New York Eye and Ear Infirmary
Section Director, Head and Neck Imaging
Beth Israel Medical Center
New York, New York

This book is dedicated to Drs. Edward Delafield and John Rodgers

These two relatively unknown young physicians returned from London to New York City in 1818 with the intent of caring for diseases of the eye. With the modest help of the citizens of New York, they founded in 1820, the first institution in the western hemisphere for the care of eye diseases, the New York Eye Infirmary. As many of their patients were recent immigrants and also had various diseases of the ear, an act of the New York Legislature would later officially change the institution's name to The New York Eye and Ear Infirmary. This heretofore unknown concept of specializing in disease of the eye and ear was so successful, that in 1824, a friend and fellow student of these physicians, Dr. Edward Reynolds, would begin a sister hospital, The Massachusetts Eye and Ear Infirmary. It is from this humble beginning that the modern specialties of ophthalmology and otolaryngology began in the United States.

PREFACE

Rhinology and the management of sinus disease have undergone significant changes in the past two decades. The interest in these areas has been partly driven by the convergence of such technologies as computed tomography and surgical endoscope, and refinement of surgical procedures ranging from endonasal to craniofacial operations.

This book utilizes a case-oriented approach to the diagnosis and management of nasal and sinus disease. Some topics, such as ethmoidectomy, have been deliberately covered by multiple authors to illustrate a range of opinions. The authors were selected based on their expertise in their assigned topic as demonstrated by reputation, experience, and related publications. It is with deep appreciation that I acknowledge their contributions as several of the authors are themselves the source of many fine textbooks.

Steven D. Schaefer, MD

CONTENTS

RHINOLOGY AND SINUS DISEASE

A Problem-Oriented Approach

SECTION

ONE

DIAGNOSTIC TECHNIQUES

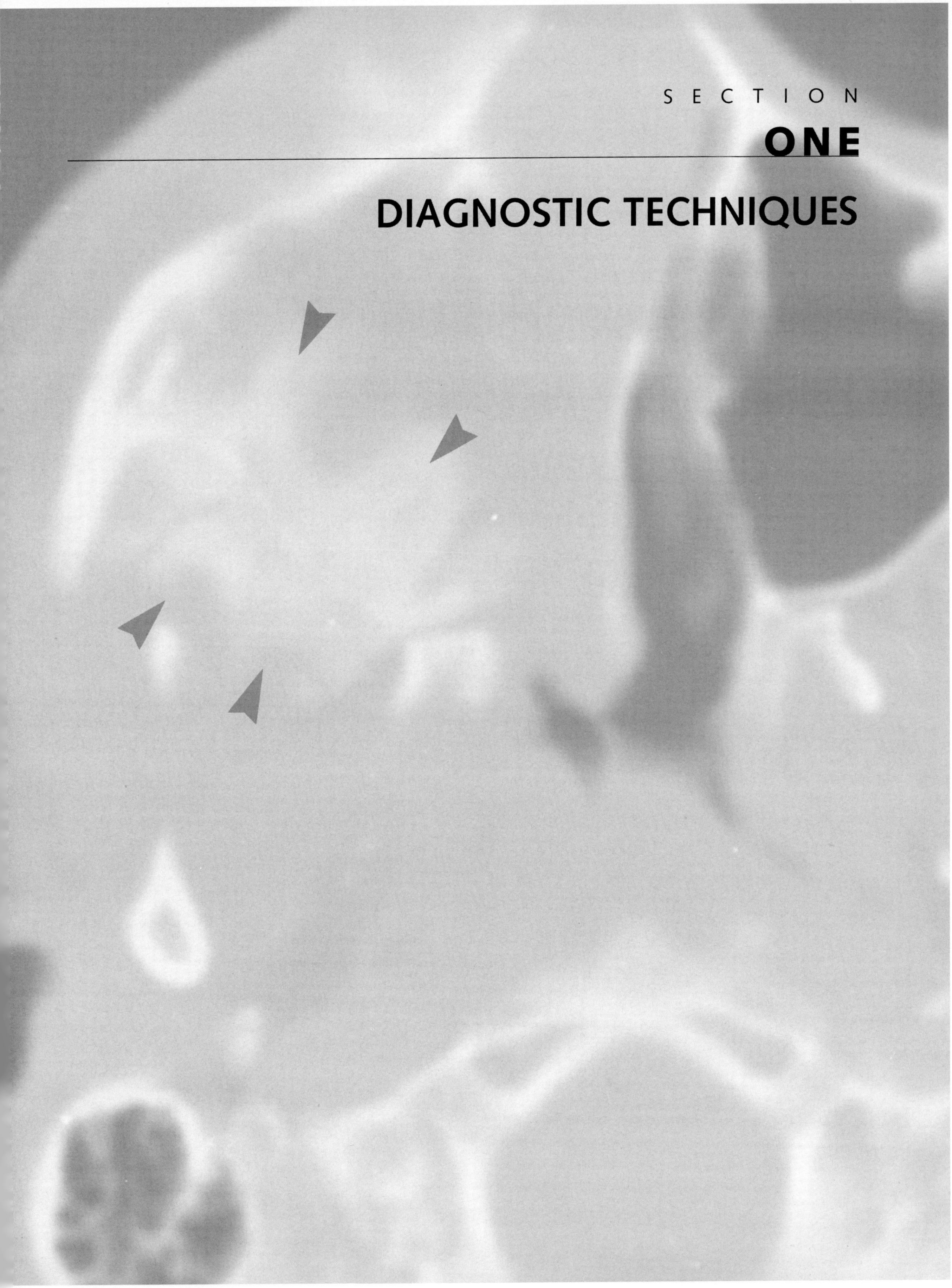

CHAPTER 1

Imaging of the Nose and Paranasal Sinuses

Barbara A. Zeifer

The advancement of sinonasal imaging has paralleled our expanding knowledge of surgical anatomy and sinonasal physiology. Computed tomography (CT) provides high-resolution images at high speeds and low radiation doses. Computer-generated reformations can produce an image in any spatial plane, adjusted in real time by the operator. Three-dimensional CT reconstructions can provide bony and surface anatomy in seconds. Image sharpness and resolution in magnetic resonance imaging (MRI) have vastly improved also. A significant reduction in scan time has occurred with the development of fast spin echo, and most recently, echo planar imaging.

Current CT and MRI techniques promise sharp and accurate visualization of the paranasal sinus (PNS) and nasal cavity. Close communication between the otolaryngologist and radiologist maximizes the information obtained from the examination.

IMAGING TECHNIQUES

Plain radiography

Plain radiography plays a limited role in the evaluation of the PNS. The anatomic detail produced by this technique is extremely limited, particularly in the evaluation of the ethmoidal labyrinth. However, plain films of the sinuses quickly determine whether a frontal sinus or maxillary antrum contains a fluid collection. This is a simple and fast technique with immediate results that can determine appropriate therapy. Plain film evaluation of mucosal disease is otherwise fraught with both false-negative and false-positive results (Fig. 1-1). Plain radiography may be convenient but is not generally recommended.

Computed tomography

CT is the imaging modality of choice for the evaluation of the nose and PNS and should be the first cross-sectional examination ordered. The anatomy of the PNS is defined by complex bony plates, and the differential diagnosis of sinonasal pathology is dependent on the extent and character of bony distortion. CT best demonstrates this bony detail.

Experience has shown that direct coronal imaging best delineates the anatomy of the PNS, particularly the structures composing the ostiomeatal unit (OMU).[1] Axial scans are useful in the evaluation of sinus neoplasm; the walls of the sphenoid and frontal sinuses; and the soft tissues of the pharynx, orbits, and midface. Indirect sagittal imaging (see further discussion) is useful to evaluate frontal sinus drainage and occasionally the sphenoethmoid recess.

Technologic advances have produced not only extremely fast conventional scans but also the helical or spiral CT scan. In helical scanning, "slip-ring" technology allows the x-ray tube to move continuously in the same direction without stopping or resetting. During tube motion, the table moves continuously also. This results in the production of a single continuous image analogous to a telephone cord, with diagonal orientation of the slices. Reconstruction of these data results in production of images in the orthogonal, X-Y plane. Although this type of scan is extremely fast, it may result in significant loss of image sharpness, depending on technical factors. It is extremely useful for production of 1-mm incremental scans for both two- and three-dimensional reconstructions.

Intravenous contrast is occasionally required for CT of the PNS. Any pathologic process that extends beyond the confines of the sinonasal cavity, either inflammatory or neoplastic, should be evaluated with iodinated contrast material to determine the extent of disease. Tumor mapping requires contrast injection to help distinguish neoplastic tissue from retained secretions. Finally, contrast administration may help determine the vascularity of a lesion and help confirm or exclude diagnoses such as juvenile nasopharyngeal angiofibroma (JNA) and hemangioma.

Iodinated contrast material should not be used indiscriminately owing to the potential for adverse reactions and side effects. These range from mild (nausea, vomiting, warmth, flushing, nasal congestion, rash, hives) to moder-

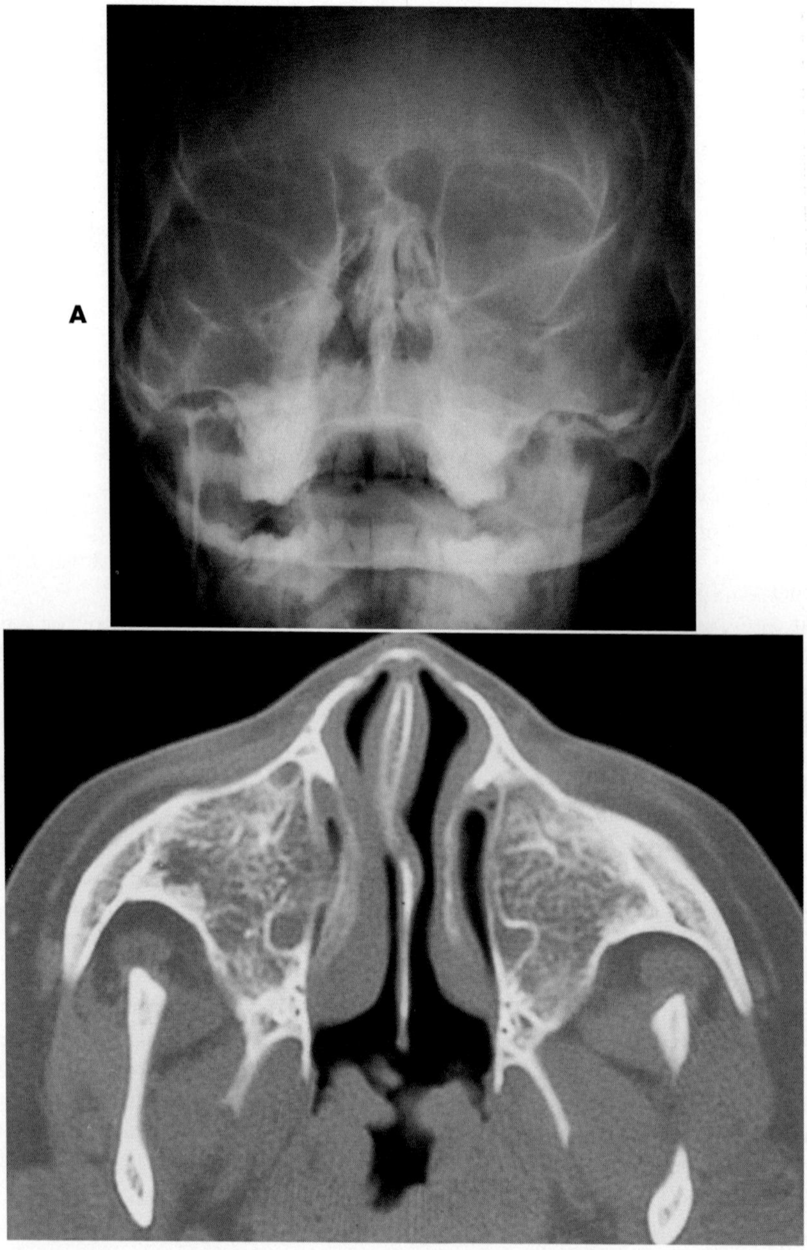

Fig. 1-1. Severe maxillary hypoplasia. **A,** Waters view. **B,** Axial computed tomography (CT). This 14-year-old patient with renal failure was given several courses of antibiotics for maxillary sinusitis based on the complete opacification of the maxillary antra seen on plain radiography. CT examination eventually demonstrated the maxillary antra to be severely underpneumatized. Note the trabecular bone within the antral cavities.

ate (hypotension, pulse changes, wheezing, mild laryngospasm) to severe (severe laryngospasm, anaphylaxis, arrhythmia, cardiopulmonary arrest). Death is reported to occur in 0.009% of injections.[2] The incidence of reactions is higher in patients with a history of allergy, asthma, previous reaction to contrast media, and cardiovascular disease and in those receiving β-blockers.[3,4] Low osmolar, nonionic contrast produces fewer adverse effects, including the most severe ones.[5] Nonionic contrast agents are currently 10 to 15 times more expensive than their ionic counterparts. As a result, many institutions tend to limit the use of nonionic contrast material to those patients at increased risk for developing adverse reactions. Guidelines for nonionic contrast use have been published by the American College of Radiology and are widely accepted.[2]

Magnetic resonance imaging

MRI has the advantage of improved soft tissue characterization with multiplanar capabilities. It is therefore an excellent tool for the evaluation of the brain, pharynx, parapharyngeal space, masticator space, and temporal fossa. For sinus imaging, MRI is particularly useful in distinguishing inflammatory disease from tumor and is essential for accurate tumor mapping. MRI is less valuable in routine imaging of the PNS where sharp delineation of bony anatomy is of paramount importance. Cortical bone generates no signal on an MR scan, so the bony plates of the midface are seen only indirectly by visualization of their investing mucosa. Furthermore, MRI is extremely sensitive in detecting any increased tissue water content. As a result, even slight mucosal edema is detected. This sensitivity has not proved useful in clinical practice.

Injection of gadolinium-DTPA, the MRI contrast agent, is required for the diagnosis and mapping of sinonasal tumor. Gadolinium is widely used and is extremely safe, with only rare adverse reactions reported in the literature.[6] On T1-weighted sequences performed after gadolinium injection, smooth intense enhancement of inflammatory tissue and varying degrees of tumoral enhancement are seen. The high signal of fatty tissue on T1-weighted sequences can potentially obscure contrast enhancement, so fat saturation or fat suppression techniques are routinely performed. This eliminates the high signal emanating from fatty tissues and allows contrast enhancement to become conspicuous. Comparison of the T1-weighted fat-suppressed image after gadolinium injection with the corresponding T2-weighted image is extremely sensitive and accurate for tumor delineation.

MRI is generally considered a safe, noninvasive imaging modality. However, high-strength magnetic fields and radiofrequency pulsations are used, and in some patients MRI involves potential risks and hazards. Patients with embedded metallic foreign bodies and various biomedical implants and devices must be thoroughly screened before an MR examination.

The most common contraindication to MR scanning is the presence of a cardiac pacemaker. Electrical interference from the radiofrequency fields can severely alter pacer function.[7] External pacing wires, temporary pacer wires, and Swan-Ganz thermodilution catheters are likewise contraindicated.[7] An intraocular foreign body can cause vitreal hemorrhage and blindness because of movement of the metallic fragment.[8] Plain radiography of the orbits is considered an adequate screening examination for demonstration of metallic foreign bodies. Particles too small to be detected by this method are considered unlikely to pose any risk of injury.[9] Metallic fragments in the spinal canal are also potentially dangerous. Intracranial aneurysm clips are of concern because many are ferromagnetic and will deflect in the magnetic field. Death has been reported from subsequent intracranial hemorrhage.[10] Therefore, any patient with an aneurysm clip should not undergo an MR examination unless the type of clip is known to the physician and the manufacturer states that it is nonferromagnetic.[11] All hemodynamic clips, heart valve prostheses, and orthopedic implants are safe in a magnetic field. Intravascular implants become incorporated into the vessel wall after 6 weeks and can be scanned after the appropriate waiting period.[12] Cochlear implants will be inactivated by the magnetic field, and patients with these devices should not undergo MRI.

Angiography

Diagnostic angiography of the nose and PNS is rarely indicated. Both conventional x-ray and digital angiography are used primarily for preoperative embolization of extremely vascular lesions such as JNA, or for intra-arterial chemotherapy. Magnetic resonance angiography (MRA) is excellent for delineation of large vessels but is not considered reliable enough to accurately map abnormal arterial structures. Although CT angiography is available, it is technically limited when the vascular structures are surrounded by bone, as is the case with the higher branches of the external carotid artery.

RADIOGRAPHIC ANATOMY

It is useful to consider the nose and PNS as three discrete, functional, anatomic regions: the ostiomeatal unit (OMU), the frontal recess (FR), and the sphenoethmoid recess (SER).

Ostiomeatal unit

The OMU is the central convergence pathway for drainage of the maxillary sinus, anterior ethmoidal labyrinth, and frontal sinus. It is best visualized in the coronal plane and is composed of the uncinate plate, inner maxillary sinus ostium, infundibulum, semilunar hiatus, ethmoidal bulla, middle turbinate, and middle nasal meatus (Fig. 1-2). The uncinate plate should be identified first and is seen on coronal CT as a free bony projection off the lateral nasal wall. As a result of this anatomy, one can identify a continuous air channel from the maxillary antrum up through the infundibulum and semilunar hiatus into the nasal cavity. The infundibulum is the air channel lateral to the uncinate plate and medial to the orbital plate or the Haller cell, if present. The ethmoidal bulla is the anterior ethmoidal air cell that directly contributes to the OMU. It forms the roof of the semilunar hiatus and often the infundibulum.

The anatomy of the anterior skull base is also best visualized in the direct coronal plane and is well seen at the level of the OMU. The crista galli provides the anterior attachment of the falx cerebri and is frequently pneumatized. In virtually every individual, there is a height differential between the ethmoid roof and the cribriform plate. The latter structure is lower and thereby forms the olfactory groove. A thin intervening plate, the lateral lamella, connects the cribriform plate with the ethmoid roof and is a point of structural weakness (Fig. 1-3). The anterior ethmoidal artery runs along the lateral lamella as it courses anteriorly along the intracranial surface of the cribriform plate.[13] The anterior ethmoidal foramen can often be seen,

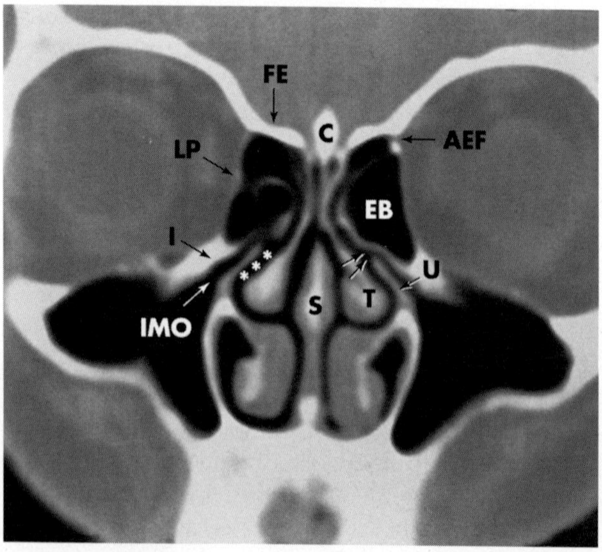

Fig. 1-2. Ostiomeatal unit (OMU). Coronal CT. *I,* infundibulum; *U,* uncinate plate; *EB,* ethmoidal bulla; *T,* middle turbinate; *IMO,* inner maxillary sinus ostium; *LP,* lamina papyracea; *FE,* fovea ethmoidalis; *C,* crista galli; *AEF,* anterior ethmoidal foramen; *S,* nasal septum; *small arrows,* semilunar hiatus; *asterisk,* middle nasal meatus.

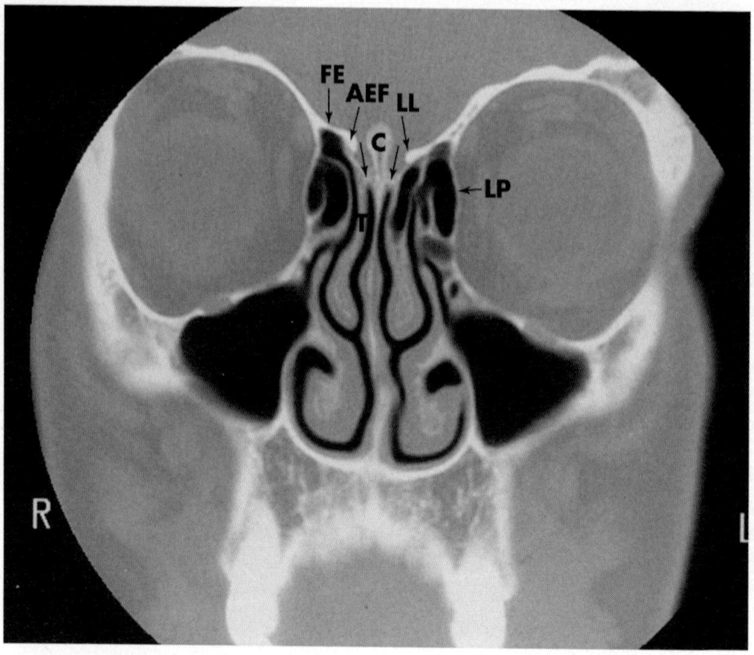

Fig. 1-3. Anterior skull base. Coronal CT. *C,* crista galli; *FE,* fovea ethmoidalis; *AEF,* anterior ethmoidal foramen; *LL,* lateral lamella; *LP,* lamina papyracea; *T,* neck of middle turbinate attaching to skull base at the junction of cribriform plate and lateral lamella; *small arrows,* cribriform plates forming floor of olfactory fossae.

both laterally at the orbital plate and medially at the lateral lamella (Figs. 1-2 and 1-3). Anteriorly, the neck of the middle turbinate extends superiorly up to the skull base, attaching to the junction of the cribriform plate and lateral lamella. The lateral attachment of the middle turbinate extends to the lamina papyracea and forms the basal lamella. This oblique coronal plate is high anteriorly and low posteriorly. It divides the anterior group of ethmoidal air cells (below and anterior) from the posterior ethmoid air cells (above and posterior) (Fig. 1-4).

Frontal recess

The anatomy of the FR is often poorly delineated on routine coronal and axial scans. This region is instead best seen in the sagittal plane. Obviously, direct sagittal scanning is not possible in adult patients. A separate series can be performed, acquiring 1-mm thick axial images from the base of the frontal sinus to the center of the ethmoidal labyrinth. Sagittal images are produced on the computer console by manipulation of these scan data. The configuration of the FR depends on the development of the agger nasi and suprabullar ethmoidal air cell or frontal bulla cell. These cells can bulge into the FR, creating narrowing and distortion of this critical outlet (Fig. 1-5).[14] Anatomic variability of this region is the rule rather than the exception, and there is no true "normal" appearance.

Sphenoethmoid recess

The spatial orientation of the SER is also best suited for sagittal imaging. The sphenoid ostium is frequently identified high along the anterior sphenoid wall, but variations in its location are seen. Pneumatization of the sphenoid bone by extramural extension of the posterior ethmoid produces the Onodi cell. This air cell, directly contiguous with the posterior ethmoid, abuts the optic canal, often separated from it by a thin or dehiscent bony rim (Fig. 1-6).

INFLAMMATORY DISEASE

Sinusitis: evaluation

Normal sinus mucosa is thin and not identifiable on CT examination. It can be visualized on T-2 weighted MRI as a thin, linear hyperintensity paralleling the sinus wall. Inflammatory disease is identified as peripheral soft tissue thickening in the sinus cavity. It is extremely important that mucosal abnormalities be interpreted within a clinical context, as areas of thickening are frequent incidental findings on both CT and MRI.[15,16] Conversely, an occasional patient is encountered with clinical symptoms of sinusitis and is found to have normal or near-normal CT examination results. Irritation of sinonasal mucosa without significant swelling most likely accounts for this apparent discrepancy.

Thickening of the mucosal lining is specific for neither acute nor chronic inflammation. The presence of a sharp air-fluid level indicates outflow obstruction with or without superimposed infection, provided that the patient has not had a recent antral lavage. Chronic sinusitis can be associated with accumulation of thick, tenacious secretions in a sinus cavity. This type of fluid is seen as bubbly or even spongelike material. Occasionally a thick mucoid droplet can be seen along the medial maxillary wall as it is propelled toward the inner sinus ostium.

Long-standing chronic mucosal inflammation may incite an osteitic reaction of the sinus wall that results in varying degrees of bony thickening. This can be seen either with or without associated mechanical obstruction. The degree of bony thickening is often more pronounced in the absence of ostial obstruction.[17] While this type of bony change is almost diagnostic of inflammatory disease, other causes of dense bone must be excluded. The differential diagnosis includes radiation therapy, Paget's disease, fibrous dysplasia, and osteoblastic metastases.

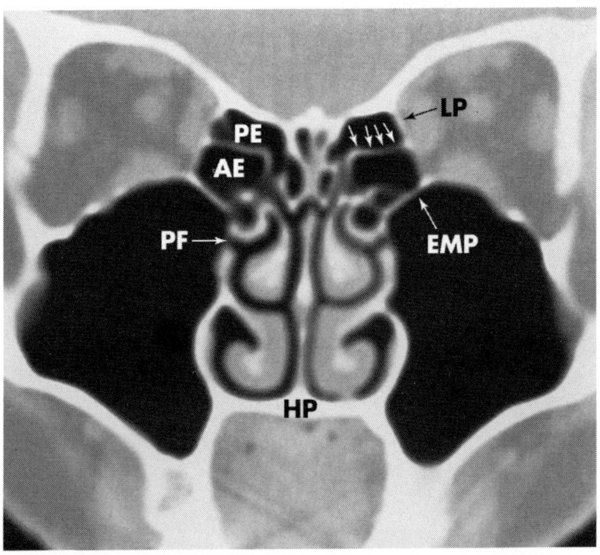

Fig. 1-4. Basal lamella. Coronal CT. *PE*, posterior ethmoid; *AE*, anterior ethmoid; *LP*, lamina papyracea; *EMP*, ethmoidomaxillary plate; *PF*, posterior nasal fontanelle; *HP*, hard palate; *arrows*, basal lamella.

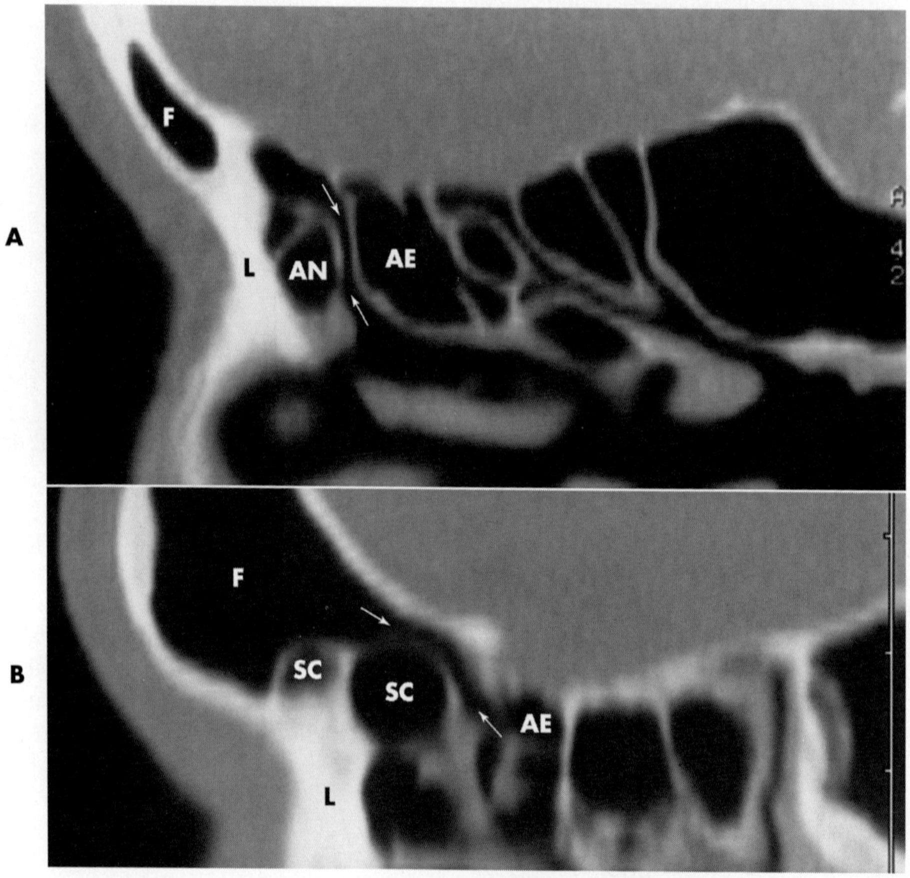

Fig. 1-5. Frontal recess. Sagittal reconstructions. **A,** Prominent agger nasi cell. **B,** Prominent suprabullar cell, different patient. *F,* frontal sinus; *L,* lacrimal bone; *AN,* agger nasi; *AE,* anterior ethmoid; *SC,* suprabullar cell, *arrows,* superior and inferior extent of frontal recesses.

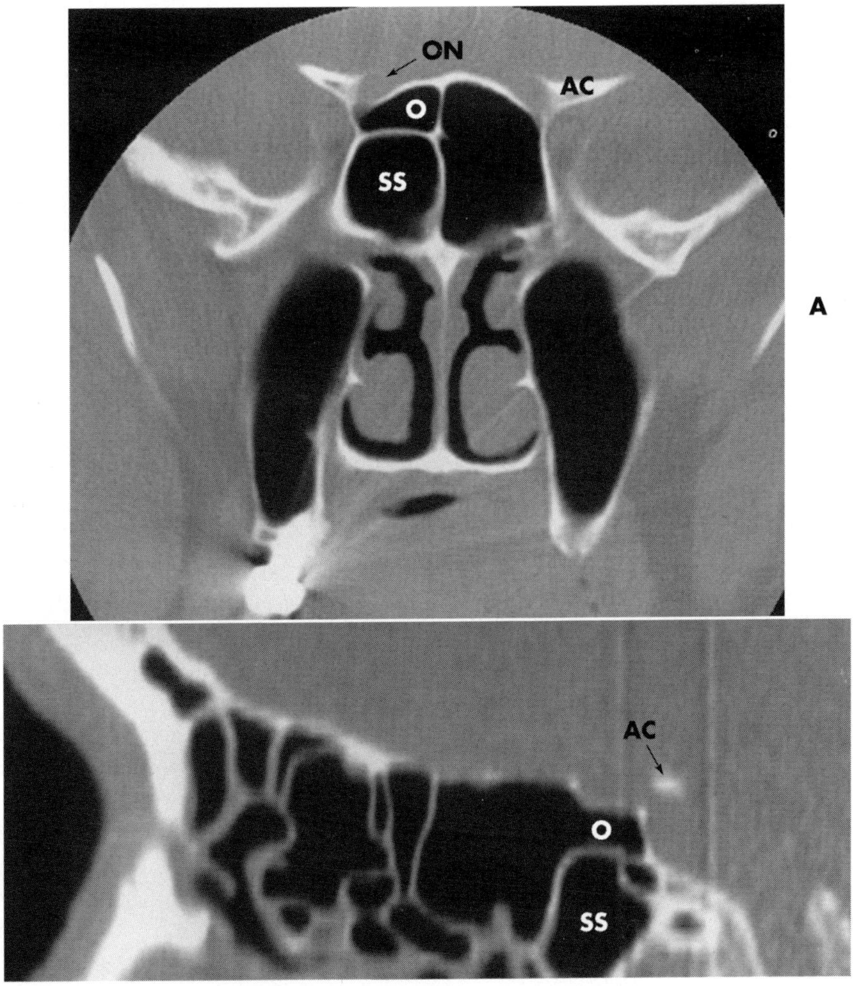

A

B

Fig. 1-6. Onodi cell. **A,** Coronal CT. **B,** Sagittal reformation. The right sphenoid sinus is small and inferior in location. The posterior ethmoid has pneumatized the sphenoid bone, lying above the sphenoid sinus. The sagittal reformation confirms the posterior ethmoid origin of this air cell that lies in direct apposition to the optic canal. *O,* Onodi cell; *ON,* optic nerve; *SS,* sphenoid sinus; *AC,* anterior clinoid process.

Rarely, chronic inflammatory disease can produce bony erosion even in the absence of polyps or mucocele.

Retention cysts are frequent findings both in patients with sinusitis and in those without symptoms.[18] Mucous and serous cysts are indistinguishable but are usually found inferiorly within the maxillary antrum, broad based against the alveolar ridge. They are not distinguishable from isolated polyps, unless the polyp is clearly pedunculated. A retention cyst can fill an antral cavity but never causes bony expansion.

Dental disease may coexist with maxillary sinusitis and can act as a nidus for continual reinfection of the treated antrum. It is possible to recognize significant dental infection on CT examination of the PNS. Most dental infections begin as infection of the root canal and pulp. This can spread to the periodontal membrane space and eventually the bone of the adjacent alveolar ridge. In the chronic stage, a periapical granuloma forms, eventually liquefying to produce a radicular cyst that may become dehiscent and form an oroantral fistula. These are identified as sharply defined, rounded lytic lesions in the alveolar bone immediately adjacent to the root of a tooth that is clinically nonviable[19] (Fig. 1-7). Granulomats are typically 1 cm or less in diameter, while radicular cysts can become larger, occasionally expanding into the maxillary antrum (Fig. 1-8).

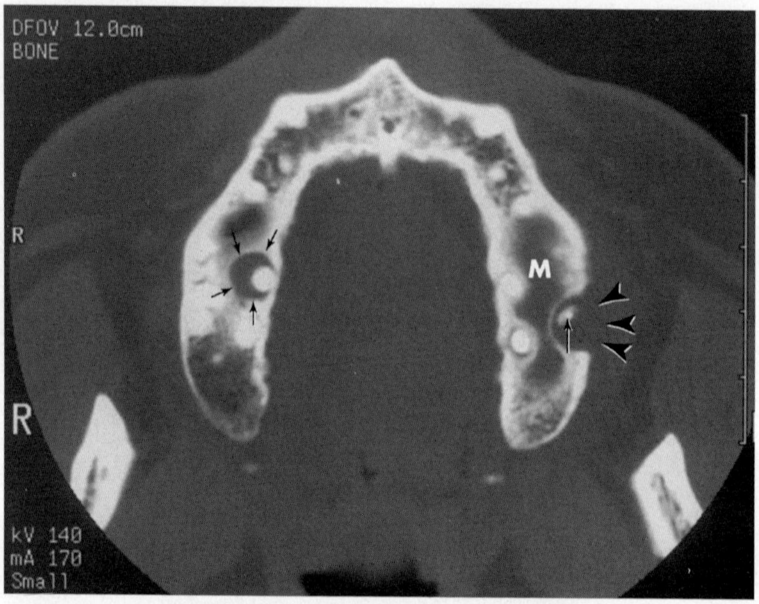

Fig. 1-7. Dental disease and maxillary sinusitis. Axial CT through the maxilla. This 56-year-old man had undergone a recent root canal of the left maxillary second molar. He developed an oroantral fistula with drainage of infected material. There is a 1-cm, well-defined cystic lesion surrounding the buccal root of the involved tooth that is widely dehiscent *(arrowheads).* The root canal is identified as a metallic density within the partially destroyed root *(arrow).* Note the periapical lucency surrounding the lingual root of the right maxillary first molar *(small arrows),* representing either a radicular cyst or a periapical granuloma. This patient had complete opacification of the left maxillary sinus and refractory maxillary sinusitis. *M,* opacified alveolar recess of maxillary sinus.

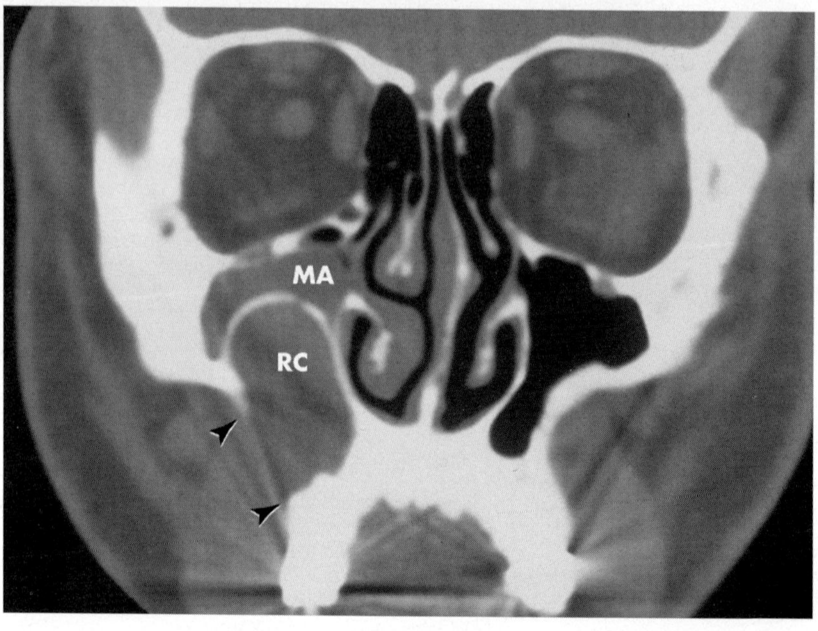

Fig. 1-8. Radicular cyst. Coronal CT showing an expansile lesion originating from the maxillary alveolar ridge, with a well-defined bony rim. There is a large dehiscence producing an oroantral fistula *(arrowheads).* There was secondary maxillary sinusitis with antral opacification. *RC,* radicular cyst; *MA,* maxillary antrum.

Sinusitis: preoperative assessment

The coronal CT scan is an absolute requirement for the preoperative evaluation of a patient with chronic or recurrent acute sinusitis. Today, most of these patients are being considered for functional endoscopic sinus surgery (FESS), and interpretation of the CT scan must be tailored to this specific situation. The goal of imaging is to first identify, describe, and emphasize any variations of normal anatomic development (Box 1-1). The effect of these anomalies on sinonasal architecture must be determined, as any distortion of the OMU may predispose a patient toward developing recurrent sinus infections[20,21] (Fig. 1-9). Second, the location and extent of sinus disease must be noted. It is of particular importance from a surgical standpoint to define a pattern of involvement that suggests obstruction of or interference with the normal mucociliary clearance mechanism. This directs the surgeon toward the functional areas of the PNS (OMU, FR, SER) that are the focus of an endoscopic procedure (Fig. 1-10). Congenital problems such as unilateral choanal atresia are occasionally discovered as the etiology for recurrent sinus infections (Fig. 1-11). Finally, it is critical to identify potential anatomic pitfalls that may require special care or attention during an endoscopic procedure. These include areas of bony thinning or dehiscence of the lamina papyracea, carotid canals, and optic canals (Fig. 1-12), where critical neurovascular structures could be injured. Rarely, the anterior ethmoidal artery can be seen as a thin, soft tissue density hanging down on a mesentery from the ethmoid roof. Unusual septations, Onodi cells, sinus hypoplasia, and low anterior cranial fossa must be noted preoperatively. Any previous surgical changes must be described. Clearly, the preoperative CT scan not only aids in patient selection but is indispensable in planning the surgical procedure.

BOX 1-1

Variations of Sinonasal Anatomy

Nasal cavity
Septal deviation and spur
Paradoxically curved middle turbinate
Concha bullosa cell
Inferior/superior turbinate pneumatization
Choanal atresia

Anterior ethmoid
Supraorbital ethmoid
Agger nasi
Prominent ethmoidal bulla
Haller cell

Uncinate
Pneumatized
Hook-shaped/inverted
Duplicated
Dehiscent, fibrous inferior attachment

Maxillary
Hypoplasia
Septation
Alveolar recess

Posterior Ethmoid
Palatine cell
Onodi cell

Sphenoid
Thin/dehiscent walls
Dehiscent optic canal
Carotid grooves
Septal recess
Multiseptated

Granulomatous sinusitis

Granulomatous diseases affecting the nose and paranasal sinuses are of both infectious and noninfectious etiologies. Infectious diseases include actinomycosis, norcardiosis, blastomycosis, tuberculosis, syphilis, rhinoscleroma, and leprosy. Noninfectious entities include Wegener's granulomatosis and sarcoidosis, as well as foreign body reaction from beryllium, chromate salts, and cocaine.[22] Lethal midline granuloma is now classified as either a prelymphomatous condition or a true lymphoma. All these granulomatous diseases are destructive in nature and have similar characteristic features. They typically originate in the nasal cavity with secondary spread to the paranasal sinuses. Initially, nonspecific soft tissue nodules are found along the nasal septum with mucosal thickening and retained secretions. Perforation of the cartilaginous nasal septum is the hallmark of this group of disorders. Destruction of the bony septum and sinus walls occurs later in the disease course (Fig. 1-13).

Fungal sinusitis

Nongranulomatous fungal sinusitis is categorized into four distinct forms based on the status of the host immune system: invasive fungal sinusitis in the immunocompromised host, chronic indolent sinusitis in the immunocompetent host, mycetoma in the immunocompetent host, and allergic fungal sinusitis (AFS) in the immunologically "hypercompetent" or atopic host.[23] Saprophytic growth of fungal organisms can be seen in the diseased sinus and is of no clinical significance.

Invasive fungal sinusitis is an acute fulminant disease marked by vascular invasion that leads to necrosis of bone and mucosa, producing a destructive pattern of disease. Early on, there is nonspecific opacification of sinus cavities with subsequent development of bony destruction. Orbital, cavernous sinus, and intracranial extension frequently complicates the course of this disease. Chronic invasive fungal disease is seen in the United States in mildly immunosuppressed patients such as those with diabetes, in whom mucormycosis typically develops. These patients manifest a more prolonged course, their disease is responding to treatment favorably to surgical debridement and antifungal medication.

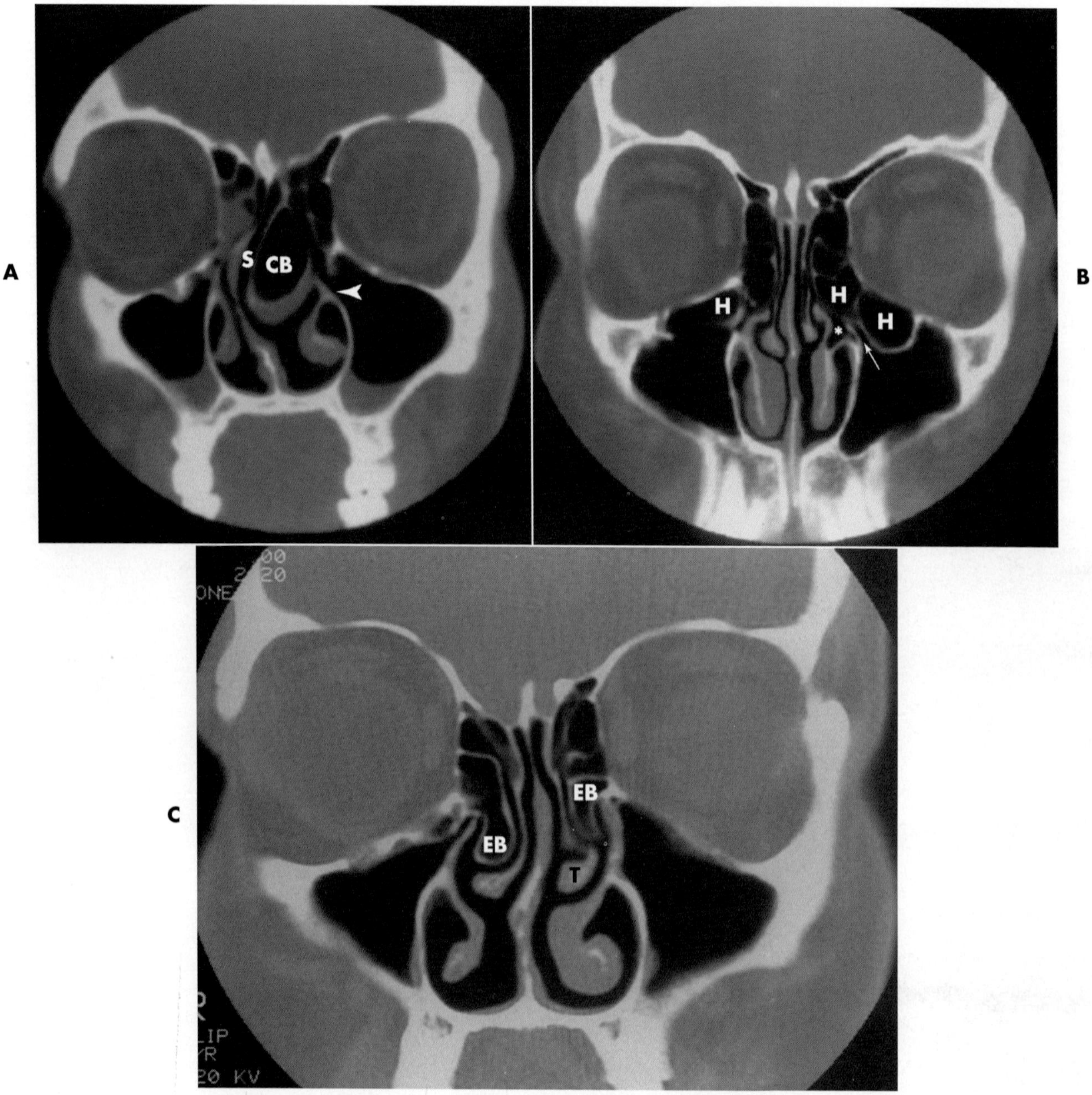

Fig. 1-9. Variants of sinonasal anatomy. Coronal CT. **A**, This huge concha bullosa *(CB)* is associated with a septal deviation *(S)* and marked crowding of both OMUs. The left uncinate plate *(arrowhead)* nearly abuts the lateral border of the conchal cell. **B**, Prominent Haller cells *(H)* create elongation and narrowing of the infundibulum. The left uncinate plate is duplicated, creating a diverticulum of the infundibulum *(asterisk); arrow,* inner maxillary sinus ostium. **C**, Huge ethmoidal bulla *(EB)* bulge inferiorly into the middle meati, between the middle turbinates and uncinate plates. Note the paradoxical curvature of the left middle turbinate *(T)*.

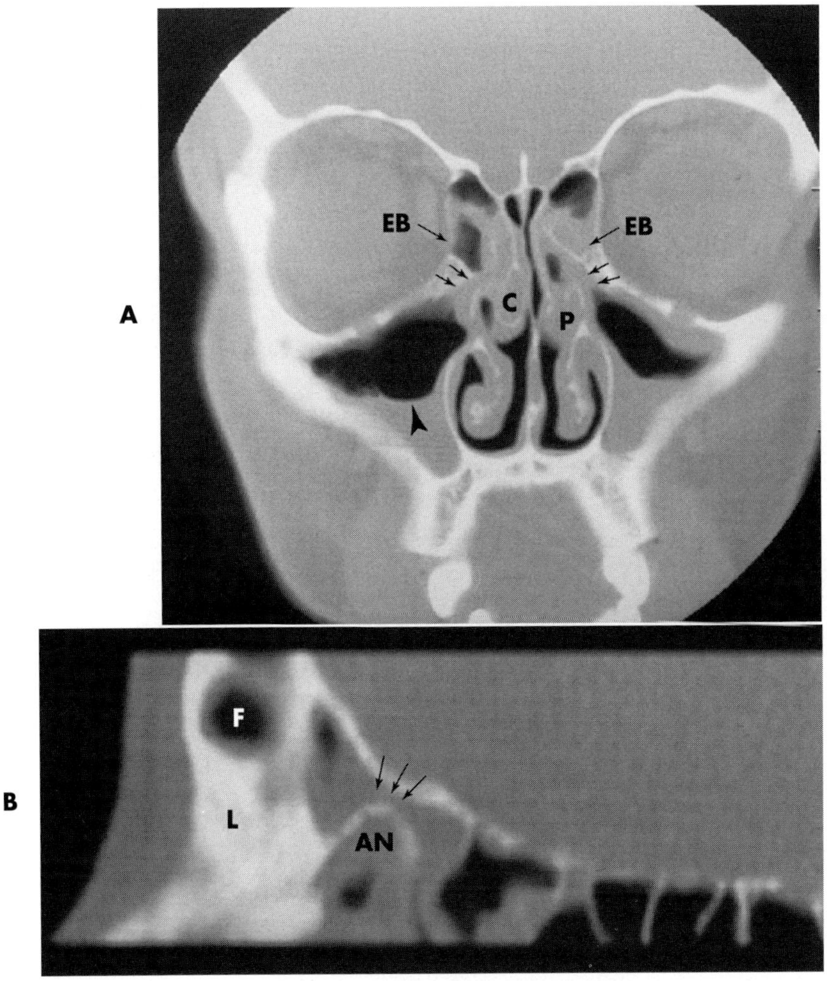

Fig. 1-10. Sinusitis. **A,** Coronal CT showing OMU disease. There is an opacified concha bullosa cell *(C)* on the right that compromises the nasal cavity. The right inner sinus ostium, infundibulum, and semilunar hiatus are all diseased. There is moderate ethmoidal and maxillary sinusitis with an antral fluid collection *(arrowhead).* On the left, the uncinate plate is inverted and a discrete nasal polyp obstructs the meatus. There is opacification of the inner sinus ostium and infundibulum with moderate maxillary and ethmoidal disease. *EB,* ethmoidal bulla; *P,* left meatal polyp, *arrows,* infundibulum. **B,** Sagittal CT reformat, different patient. A large agger nasi bulges superiorly to cause narrowing and horizontal deviation of the frontal recess. *F,* frontal sinus; *AN,* agger nasi cell; *L,* lacrimal bone; *arrows,* frontal recess.

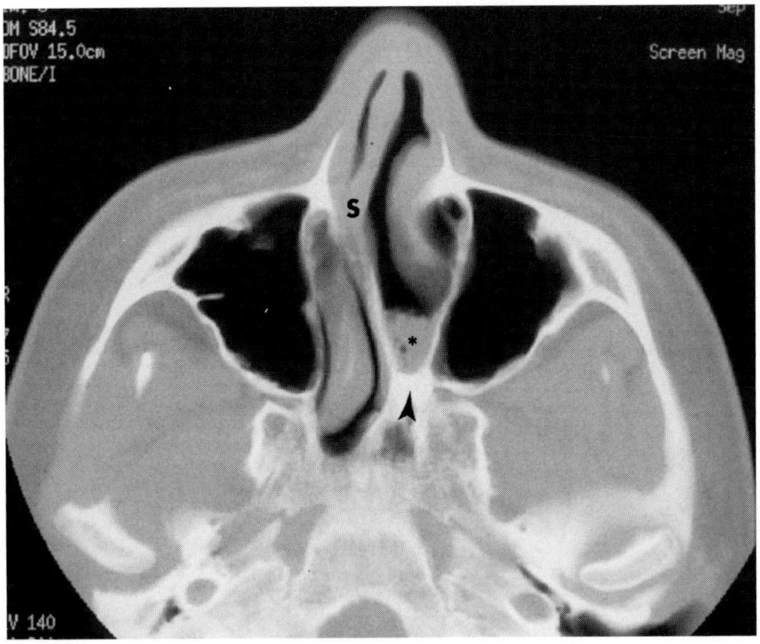

Fig. 1-11. Choanal atresia. Axial CT. This 14-year-old girl had been treated throughout childhood for recurrent sinusitis and nasal stuffiness. There is a well-defined bony atresia plate on the left with retained secretions, and a pronounced right septal deviation compromising the right nasal cavity. *S,* nasal septum; *arrowhead,* bony atresia plate; *asterisk,* retained secretions.

Chronic indolent fungal disease is extremely rare in the United States. It is a slowly progressive, invasive, granulomatous infection that eventually leads to bone destruction. It initially causes nonspecific mucosal thickening that is typically unilateral and not responsive to standard medical treatment. Fluid collections are rare, and when present should raise the suspicion of bacterial infection.

Mycetoma is a noninvasive fungal ball. It causes complete or near-complete opacification of a sinus cavity and is often associated with thickening of the sinus walls. Mycetoma is usually hyperdense on CT and contains dense floc-

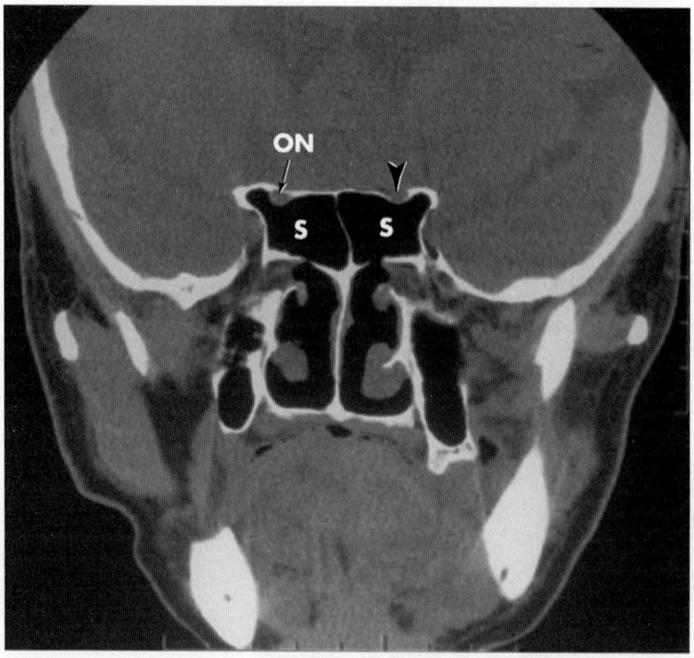

Fig. 1-12. Dehiscent optic canal. Coronal CT. The right optic canal is thin and partially dehiscent. The optic nerve *(ON)* bulges inferiorly into the sphenoid sinus *(S)*. Notice the normal optic canal on the left *(arrowhead)*.

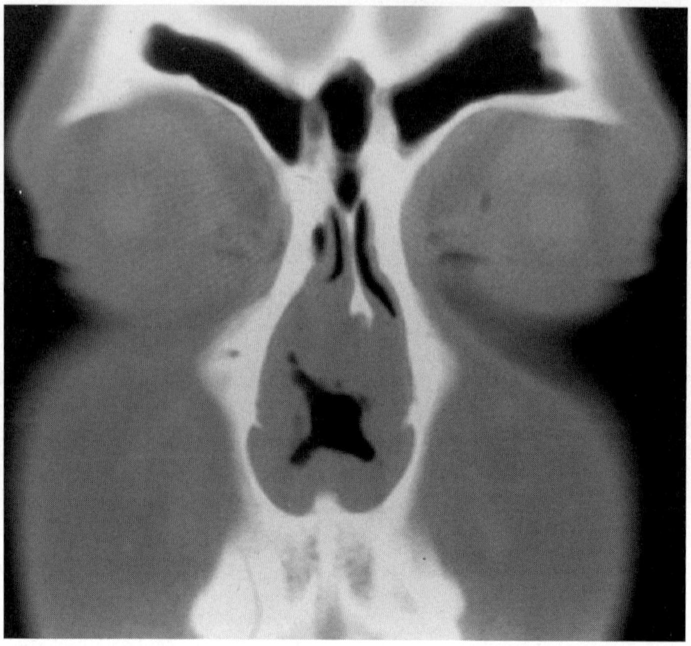

Fig. 1-13. Wegener's granulomatosis. Coronal CT through the anterior nasal cavity showing marked thickening of the nasal mucosa. Tiny bubbles indicate the presence of thick secretions. The septal perforation is diagnostic of granulomatous rhinitis.

culent calcifications in 25% of cases)[24] (Fig. 1-14). Mycetoma is markedly hypointense on all MRI sequences.

AFS typically occurs in atopic patients with nasal polyposis. It is a hypersensitivity reaction to fungal antigens, most belonging to the Dematiaceae family.[23] This entity is a unilateral or bilateral process. The involved sinus contains a peripheral rim of low-density, edematous mucosa, with complete opacification of the central cavity by homogeneous high-attenuation material corresponding to thick, allergic mucin. The sinus walls may be surprisingly expanded and destroyed. The high-attenuation contents enable the radiologist to exclude neoplasm. Low-density nasal polyps are almost always identified. On MRI, the thick, allergic mucin is extremely hypointense, mimicking an aerated sinus cavity. This is due to pronounced desiccation. Polyps and associated mucosal inflammation typically remain hyperintense on T2-weighted sequence (Fig. 1-15).

Mucocele

Obstruction of a sinus ostium may result in the development of a mucocele. The obstructive pathology may be neoplasm, polyp, trauma, or chronic mucosal inflamma-

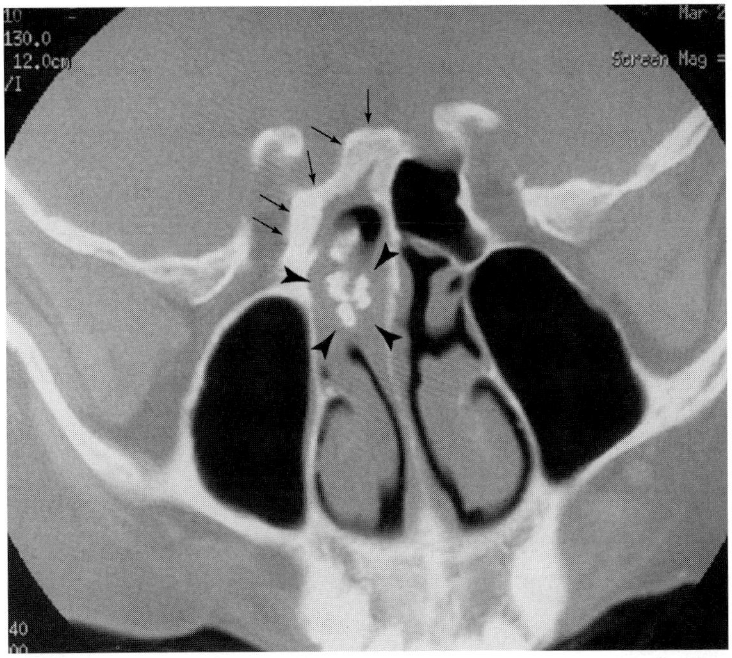

Fig. 1-14. Mycetoma. Coronal CT showing a calcified mass in the nasal cavity and sphenoid sinus *(arrowheads)* associated with sclerosis of the sinus walls *(arrows)*. The mycetoma was easily shelled out endoscopically.

A

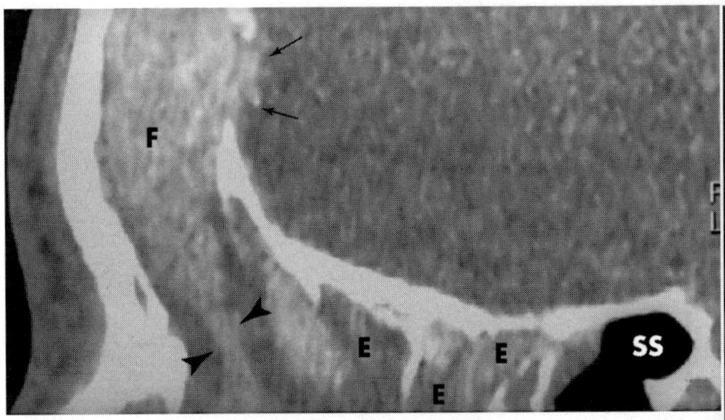

B

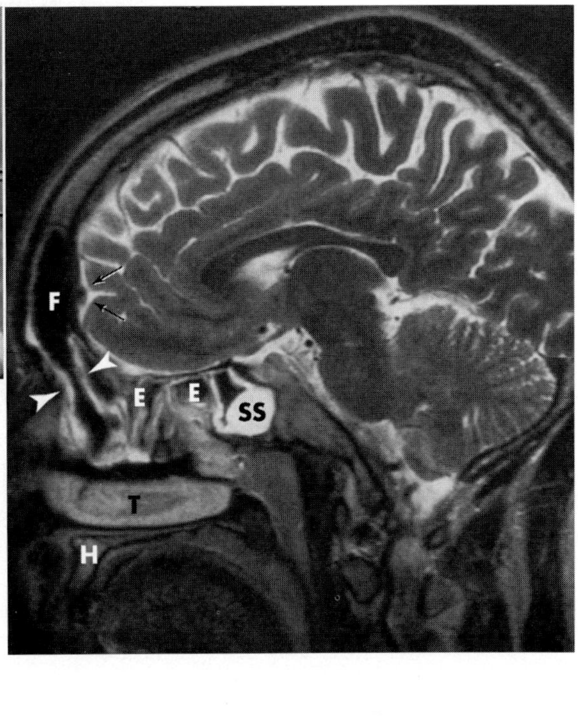

Fig. 1-15. Allergic fungal sinusitis. **A,** Sagittal CT reformat. **B,** Sagittal T2 magnetic resonance imaging (MRI) obtained on the same day. The frontal sinus *(F)*, frontal recess *(arrowheads)*, and many ethmoidal air cells are filled with high-density material corresponding to allergic mucin. This material is signal void on the MRI. Without the accompanying CT, this could have been misread as an aerated sinus cavity. Mucosal edema is hypodense on CT and hyperintense on T2 MRI. Note the expansion of the posterior frontal table *(arrows)*. *E*, anterior ethmoidal air cells; *SS*, sphenoid sinus with inflammatory disease; *T*, inferior turbinate; *H*, hard palate.

tion. The frontal sinus is the most common one to produce a mucocele, followed by the ethmoid and maxillary sinuses. Sphenoid sinus mucoceles are rare. On CT examination, the sinus cavity is completely opacified. Early on, the sinus walls are intact and the differential diagnosis includes sinusitis with fluid, a large retention cyst, and a polyp. As pressure builds, the sinus walls thin and expand, eventually developing areas of dehiscence. In the maxillary sinus, mucocele formation is associated with chronic inflammatory change with osteitic thickening of the antral wall; this bony thickening, along with other areas of more typical expansile thinning, is highly suggestive of antral mucocele. On MRI, the signal intensity characteristics of mucoceles can vary tremendously, depending on the relative protein concentration and the degree of hydration.[25] Most frequently, however, the mucocele is at least partially hydrated and is therefore hyperintense on the T2-weighted MRI sequence. Occasionally, when the mucocele is of long standing and dehydrated, it is hypointense on the T2-weighted sequence and isointense or hyperintense on T1. Other combinations of high and low signal intensity on T1 and T2 can also occur.[25] Frequently, concretions of debris and thick mucous are seen as rounded collections within the mucocele itself. In almost every patient with a mucocele, there is evidence of significant inflammatory disease elsewhere in the sinonasal cavity (Fig. 1-16).

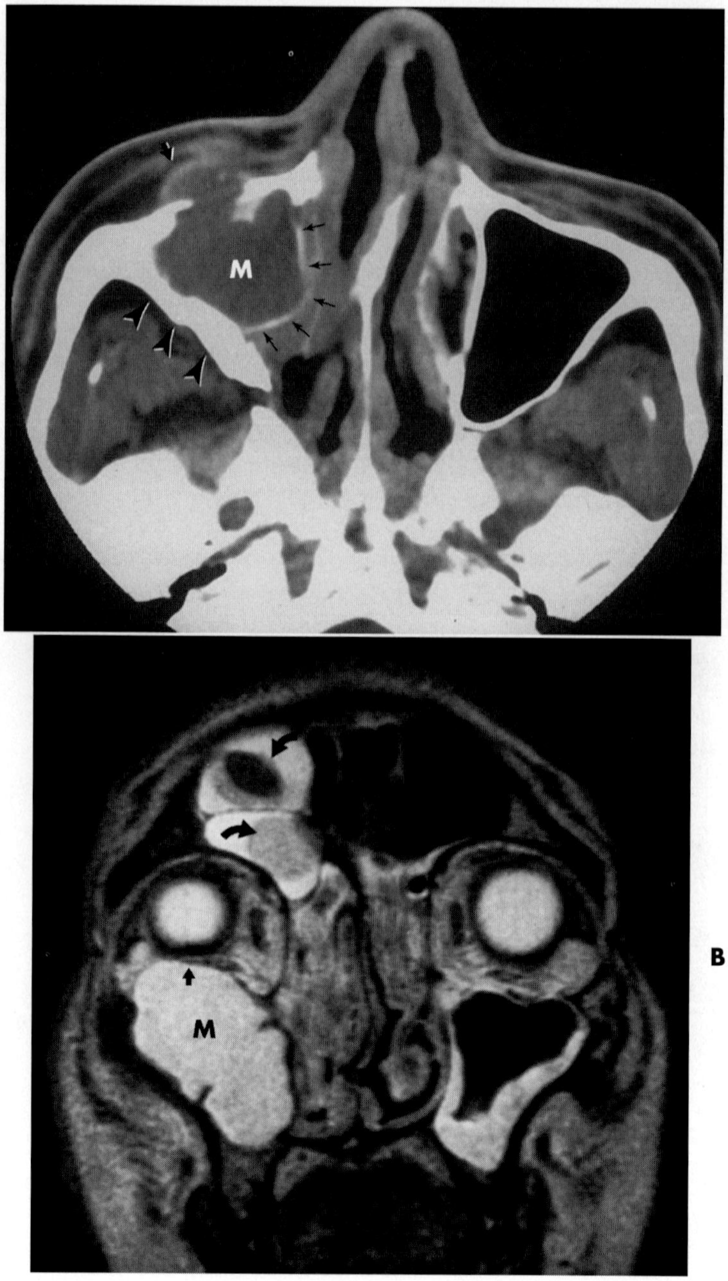

A

B

Fig. 1-16. Maxillary mucocele. **A**, Axial CT. **B**, Coronal T2 MRI. There is an expanding mass in the right maxillary antrum that is hypodense on CT and hyperintense on T2 MRI *(M)*. The lesion was hyperintense on the T1 sequence (not shown). There is marked thickening of the lateral antral wall *(arrowheads)*, thinning of the medial antral wall *(small arrows)*, and expansion into the orbit and cheek *(thick arrows)*. On the MRI, note the hyperintense mucosal disease in the left antrum as well as mucosal disease and lower intensity debris in the right frontal sinus *(curved arrows)*.

POLYPS

Individual polyps are seen as smoothly rounded or pedunculated soft tissue masses in the nose and PNS. When strategically located within one of the three functional areas, they can obstruct sinus drainage. Acute sinusitis, chronic sinusitis, or even mucocele can occur as complications. Diffuse sinonasal polyposis produces more pronounced opacification of the PNS (Fig. 1-17). The multiple packed polyps may exert a pressure effect on adjacent bony structures, with resultant enlargement of the nasal cavity or sinus. This expansile process is slow and gradual, so that the bone has time to remodel around the mass effect. As a result, expansion and distortion occur with preservation of the bony plates. Infundibular polyposis can cause inferior displacement of the uncinate plate, which then assumes an inverted U configuration. Nasal polyps frequently cause expansion of the superior nasal fossa and sphenoethmoid recess that can be easily identified on a coronal CT. Polyposis is often associated with accumulation of highly proteinaceous and mucoid secretions. These secretions are hyperdense on CT, hyperintense on T1-weighted MRI, and hypointense on T2.

Antrochoanal polyps have a distinct radiographic appearance. Both the maxillary sinus and middle meatus are completely opacified by hypodense material on CT. The antral contents extrude through the medial maxillary wall into the middle nasal meatus and then extend posteriorly into the nasopharynx. The polyp most frequently expands through the lateral nasal wall at the posterior nasal fontanelle, behind the posterior attachment of the uncinate plate. Normal lack of bone at this point provides a path of least resistance. There is usually some radiographic evidence of a slowly expansile process with identification of a partially intact, medialized lateral nasal wall and inferomedial displacement of the ipsilateral inferior turbinate. Less commonly, all or part of the polyp exits through the infundibulum. CT in this case demonstrates marked widening of the infundibular space with distortion or poor visualization of the uncinate plate (Fig. 1-18).

CEREBROSPINAL FLUID RHINORRHEA

Leakage of cerebrospinal fluid (CSF) into the nose and PNS is most frequently associated with severe head injury and skull base fractures. Approximately 80% of CSF leaks are produced by this mechanism, while 16% are found to be complications of sinonasal and skull base surgery[26]; CSF rhinorrhea is a known complication of FESS.[27] The remaining 3% to 4% are considered to be spontaneous CSF fistulas, further categorized as high pressure, due to tumor and/or hydrocephalus, and low pressure, for which no cause can be determined.[26] The latter is rare.

Imaging studies play a central role in the evaluation of known or suspected CSF rhinorrhea. For patients with known trauma or who have undergone previous surgery, noncontrast CT will delineate the bony defect. When a posttraumatic encephalocele is suspected, MRI is useful to demonstrate the degree of dural herniation and the location of neural tissue (Fig. 1-19). For patients with spontaneous CSF rhinorrhea, CT should be performed first. Close attention is paid to anatomic regions known to be associated with spontaneous CSF leakage: the anterior skull base, sella turcica, sphenoid sinus, parasellar

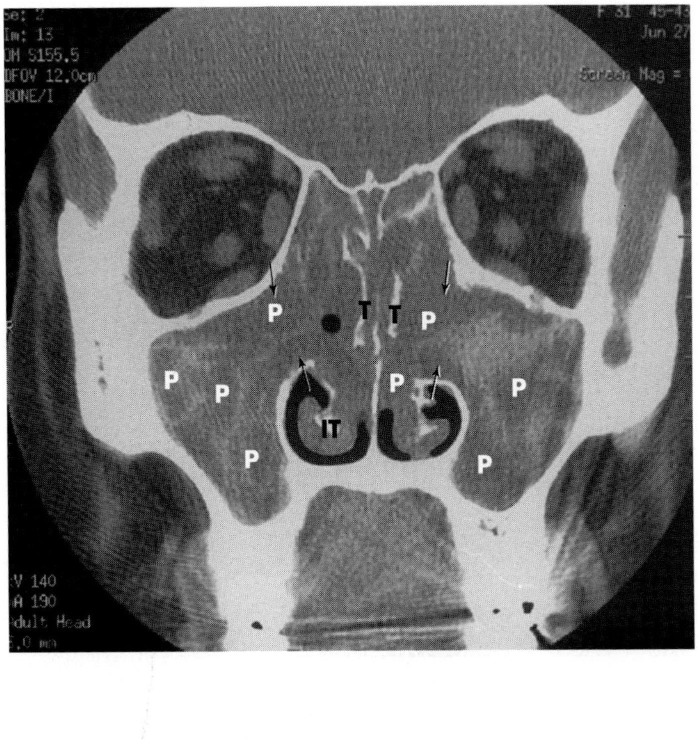

Fig. 1-17. Diffuse polyposis. Coronal CT. This 31-year-old woman had a long history of polyposis requiring multiple surgical procedures including partial middle turbinectomies, subtotal ethmoidectomies, and middle meatal antrostomies. The sinus contents are that of nodular peripheral polyps and central proteinaceous, hyperdense secretions. *P,* polyp; *T,* middle turbinates; *IT,* inferior turbinate; arrows delineate antrostomy margins;

A

B

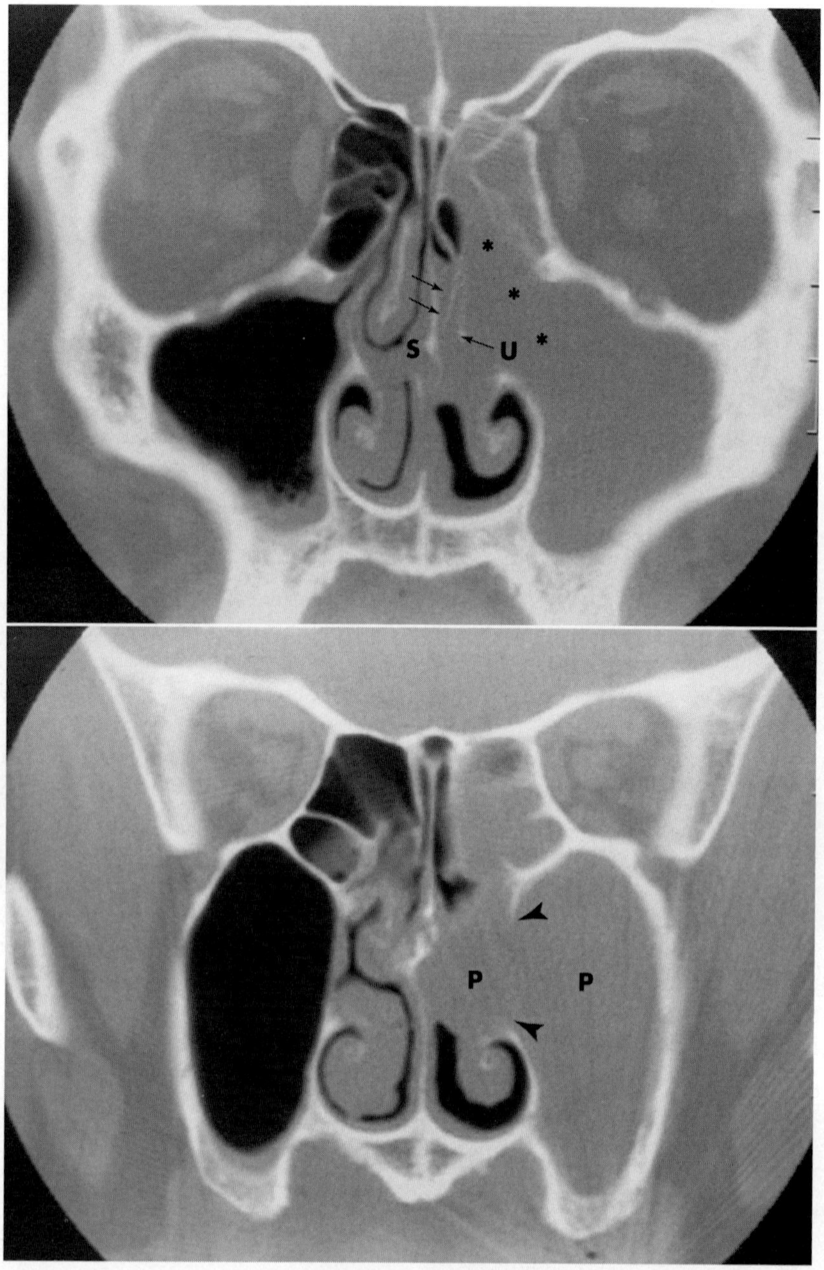

Fig. 1-18. Antrochoanal polyp. **A,** Coronal CT at the level of the OMU. **B,** Coronal CT at the center of the nasal cavity. There is complete opacification of the left maxillary antrum with gross widening of the inner sinus ostium and infundibulum due to the polyp *(asterisks)*. The uncinate plate *(U)* is straightened and medialized, as is the neck of the middle turbinate *(small arrows)*. The posterior nasal fontanelle is expanded and the polyp extends through it into the nasal cavity, obstructing the OMU. *S,* nasal septum; *P,* polyp; arrowheads delineate margins of fontanelle and defect.

region, middle cranial fossa, and petrous temporal bone (via the eustachian tube).[22, 28] Contrast-enhanced CT or MRI of the brain should be performed at the same time to assess for tumor and increased intracranial pressure. If the origin of the rhinorrhea cannot be identified on CT and if the patient is actively leaking, a CT cisternogram should be performed. This is a safe, minimally invasive study that requires a lumbar puncture followed by intrathecal injection of 5 to 10 ml of nonionic iodinated contrast material. The patient is then placed in a position that enhances CSF leakage and is brought back to the CT scanner. The coronal scan with 3-mm thick slices is repeated, followed by 1-mm thick slices through any area of subtle dehiscence. Although irregular mineralization of the anterior skull base is a frequent incidental finding, the CT cisternogram may reveal actual CSF leakage through one of these regions (Fig. 1-20).

For patients in whom the clinical diagnosis of CSF rhinorrhea is suspected but uncertain, a radionuclide CSF study may be chosen as the initial screening examination.[29] For this study, the nasal cavity is packed with pledgets, and a lumbar puncture is followed by intrathecal injection of indium-111 DTPA. Gamma camera imaging is performed over the subsequent 24 hours, after which time the radioactivity accumulation in the nasal packing is compared with serum counts. A pledget count

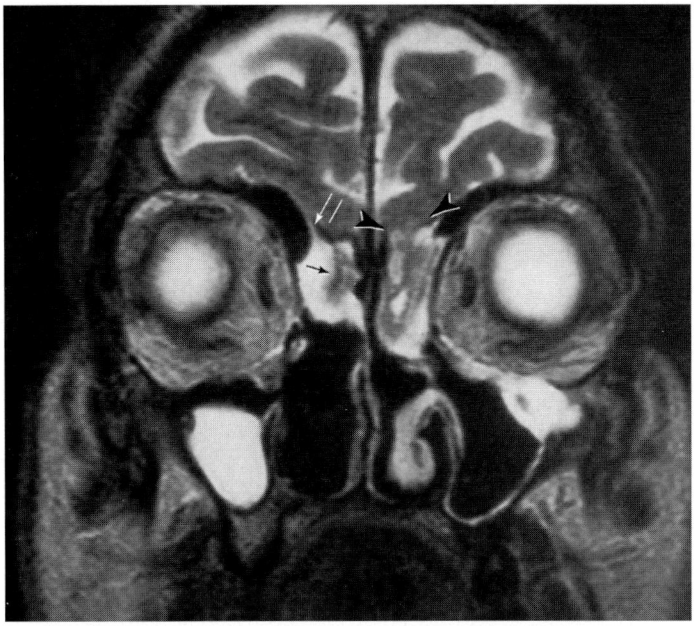

Fig. 1-19. Postoperative encephalocele. Coronal T2 MRI. Following endoscopic sinus surgery, this patient presented with bilateral cerebrospinal fluid (CSF) rhinorrhea. There is a large defect in the left anterior skull base, including the fovea ethmoidalis and cribriform plate *(arrowheads).* Brain tissue clearly herniates through this defect into the ethmoidal cavity. MRI nicely distinguishes neural tissue from the hyperintense fluid. On this slice the right anterior skull base is identified *(double arrow),* but neural tissue is identified below *(single arrow),* protruding through a more anterior defect.

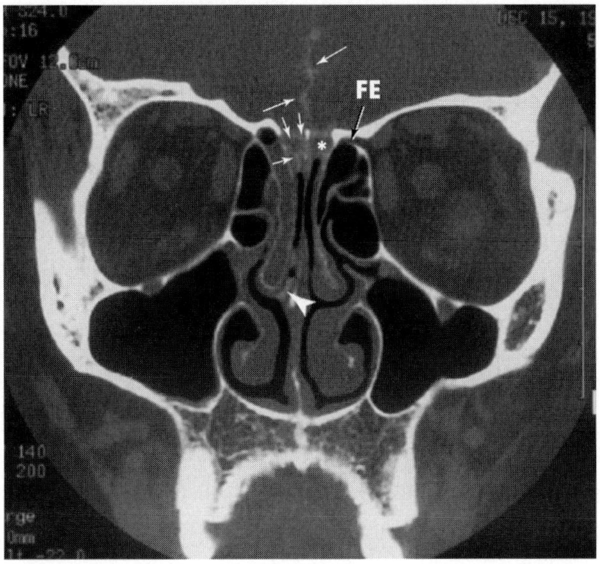

Fig. 1-20. Spontaneous CSF rhinorrhea. Coronal CT, postcontrast cisternogram. This 57-year-old woman presented with spontaneous, idiopathic CSF rhinorrhea. Precontrast CT examination demonstrated slight irregularity of the cribriform plates without a gross bony defect. After intrathecal contrast injection, hyperdense contrast is noted within the subarachnoid space of the interhemispheric fissure and olfactory fossa *(small arrows).* The olfactory bulb *(asterisk)* is seen as a soft tissue density above the cribriform plate. A trickle of contrast was noted to traverse the cribriform plate *(arrow).* A small collection of contrast was also noted within the nasal cavity *(arrowhead); FE,* fovea ethmoidalis.

1.5 times that of the serum count is considered positive for CSF rhinorrhea.[29] This is a sensitive examination that only grossly localizes the site of leakage.

NEOPLASTIC DISEASE

Tumors of the nose and PNS are encountered far less frequently than inflammatory disease and polyposis. Malignant disease of the nose and PNS account for less then 1% of all malignancies in the body and only 3% of all head and neck malignant tumors.[22] The differential diagnosis of an expansile sinonasal lesion often includes both neoplastic and inflammatory or polypoid disease. Therefore, the main goal of imaging in this setting is to distinguish benign from malignant disease and tumor from mucosal inflammation and retained secretions. Less important from a practical standpoint is the need to offer a specific histologic diagnosis, although such a diagnosis may be apparent after review of the radiographic studies. For patients diagnosed with tumor, the details of tumor location and extent provided by the imaging studies are critical in the determination of operability and in planning radiation therapy.

CT and MRI are often used together to achieve these goals in complicated clinical situations. CT is usually the first study ordered and is the most valuable in determining the integrity of bony structures, the specific character of bony changes, the presence or absence of calcifications, and the density of sinus contents. MRI is more sensitive in delineating tumor margins and in distinguishing cellular tissue from entrapped secretions. MRI is extremely useful in this regard because 95% of neoplastic disease is intermediate or slightly low in signal intensity on the T2-weighted MRI sequence.[30] Exceptions to this rule include neurogenic tumors and adenoid cystic carcinoma, both of which may have well-defined cystic or mucinous areas that are hyperintense on the T2-weighted sequence. On the other hand, most inflammatory lesions are hyperintense on T2; exceptions to this rule include the occasional mucocele, polyp, or retention cyst that is chronic and desiccated with little residual water content. These abnormalities are therefore intermediate or even low in signal on the T2-weighted sequence.

Imaging characteristics

Every expansile lesion of the nose and PNS manifests a set of specific radiographic features. Careful analysis of these imaging characteristics will enable the viewer to arrive at a clinically useful differential diagnosis.

Tissue of origin. The first step in analyzing an expansile mass is to decide whether it is arising from bone, mucosa, or dental tissues. Bone lesions will be centered on a bony plate or septation; dental lesions will arise out of the maxillary alveolar ridge. Displacement of a tooth into the maxilla or adjacent root resorption is a useful indicator of dental origin.

Site of origin. Defining the isocenter of a mass lesion is often helpful in arriving at a more specific diagnosis. Certain lesions of the PNS are site specific: these include inverted papilloma, JNA, and esthesioneuroblastoma. Antrochoanal polyps need to be distinguished from inverted papilloma by other criteria, since the site of origin is similar. Most malignant tumors occur with greatest frequency in the maxillary antrum or the nasal cavity, a nonspecific location.

Integrity of sinus walls. The effect of an expansile process on the walls of a sinus cavity is determined by the growth rate of the lesion rather than its histologic appearance. A slowly expansile mass such as a polyp, neural tumor, or minor salivary gland tumor exerts pressure on the sinus wall that causes expansion but allows the bone to remodel progressively around it. Aggressive lesions such as squamous cell carcinoma (SCC) cause gross destruction of a bony plate without any expansile characteristics. Lymphoma typically produces a permeative destructive pattern, as does the early phase of some aggressive sarcomatous lesions. The presence of sclerosis indicates chronic inflammatory disease, which of course can coexist with or be caused by an obstructing neoplasm.

Cellularity. The cellularity of a lesion is determined by observing its density on CT and its signal intensity characteristics on MRI. Tumor is isodense to muscle on CT and may enhance with intravenous contrast injection. On MRI, tumor is isointense to muscle on T1 and frequently enhances after contrast injection. Tumor tissue is mildly hyperintense to muscle on T2-weighted MRI, while inflammatory disease is clearly hyperintense. Tumor tissue with higher interstitial water content is more heterogeneous and higher in signal intensity on the T2 MRI.

Calcification. The presence of calcification is extremely useful in limiting a differential diagnosis. Periosteal new bone is diagnostic of osteogenic sarcoma. Coarse, flocculent calcifications can be seen in chondroid lesions, mycetoma, and fibroosseous lesions of both facial and dental origin. Reactive tumoral septations may be seen in inverted papilloma.

Intracranial extension/perineural invasion. Any aggressive sinonasal lesion can expand into or infiltrate the cranium. These lesions include inverted papilloma, JNA, polyposis, and all malignant lesions, particularly SCC and esthesioneuroblastoma. Perineural invasion can produce "skip lesions" with normal intervening neural channels. This is thought to represent macroscopic reappearance of the tumor with compression of the tumor and nerve in the bony canal.[31] More typically, however, cranial base foramina are widened. MRI with contrast injection has proved extremely sensitive in detecting perineural infiltration. Perineural invasion is seen in SCC, adenoid cystic carcinoma, and sarcomatous lesions.

Correlating the imaging characteristics of mass lesions and weighting them as to their relative degrees of significance requires knowledge of individual tumors. The specific radiographic features of the most frequently encountered lesions are discussed in the following sections.

Benign tumors of soft tissue origin

Nasal papillomas, making up a distinct group of benign neoplasms, arise from nasal mucosa. Fungiform or septal papillomas rarely require imaging studies, as they are localized to the nasal cavity. They can be seen as nonspecific soft tissue masses broad based against the nasal septum. Cylindrical cell papillomas are rare but have characteristics similar to those of inverted papilloma (IP), a site-specific lesion of the sinonasal cavity. These tumors arise most frequently from the lateral nasal wall. Rarely, they arise from the nasal septum or within a sinus cavity. Early on, an isolated nasal mass can be seen without bone erosion and is indistinguishable from a nasal polyp or other small neoplasm. Small inverted papillomas can be obscured clinically and radiographically by coexistent polyposis. As the tumor grows, bone involvement is the rule. The presence of a mass lesion in the maxillary antrum and nasal cavity with gross destruction of the intervening lateral nasal wall is highly suggestive of this diagnosis. Occasionally, areas of bony expansion may also occur. IP can invoke reactive changes in the posterolateral antral wall, producing an irregular scalloped contour, often with septations extending from the sinus wall toward the center of the lesion. The entire antrum is typically enlarged. It is exceedingly rare, however, to identify frank destruction of the posterolateral antral wall. This finding should raise the suspicion of malignant degeneration or a secondary mucocele (Fig. 1-21). In general, however, imaging studies do not help diagnose the presence of malignant change.

The benign nonepithelial tumors encountered include JNA and neural tumors. JNA arises from the nasal cavity in the vicinity of the sphenopalatine foramen and is another site-specific lesion of the sinonasal cavity (Fig. 1-22). JNA is a benign but aggressive tumor, extending through the sphenopalatine foramen to invade the pterygopalatine fossa in 89% of cases.[32] It then causes anterior bowing of the posterolateral antral wall, the radiographic hallmark of this tumor. This path of tumor growth results in complete detachment of the pterygoid plate, which is typically seen to be floating within tumor mass. From the sphenopalatine foramen, tumor gains access to the orbital apex, cavernous sinuses, and masticator space. There is frequent invasion of the sphenoid sinus also. JNA is a highly vascular tumor exhibiting dense enhancement after intravenous contrast injection. On MRI, multiple feeding vessels are identified as rounded and serpiginous flow voids. A characteristic dense contrast stain is seen on angiography.

Neurogenic tumors (schwannoma, neurofibroma) arising in the paranasal sinuses tend to be well-circumscribed, slow-growing lesions associated with bone expansion and remodeling. They may contain areas of cystic degeneration that produce high signal intensity on T2 MRI, atypical for sinonasal tumors. Malignant degeneration is rare and is always associated with a more destructive process.

Malignant tumors of soft tissue origin

Of the malignant mucosal tumors, SCC is the most common, accounting for nearly 80% of sinus malignancies.[22] On CT, SCC is an irregular, poorly marginated, grossly destructive soft tissue mass. On MRI, SCC is an irregular heterogeneous mass lesion, isointense to slightly hyperintense on T2-weighted images, but less intense than secretions or inflammatory disease. It enhances irregularly with contrast injection (Fig. 1-23).

The glandular tumors make up 10% of all malignant sinus tumors and are most commonly found in the antrum and nose.[22] The rare adenocarcinomas have been linked to inhaled carcinogens.[22] Radiographically, adenocarcinoma is indistinguishable from SCC. The minor salivary tumors include adenoid cystic carcinoma and the less common mucoepidermoid carcinoma. In general, these lesions tend to be slower growing than SCCs and are therefore associated with bone expansion. Minor salivary gland tumors may contain areas of cystic necrosis with serous and or mucous collections that create a heterogeneous or high signal intensity pattern on T2-weighted MRI.[30] Adenoid cystic carcinomas have a well-known propensity for perineural extension.

Malignant melanoma arising from the mucous membranes of the head and neck is rare. When involving the nose and paranasal sinuses, this tumor is most likely to arise from the nasal septum and turbinates. These lesions are generally seen as heterogeneously enhancing soft tissue masses on CT that expand, remodel, and often erode their surrounding bony plate. The more aggressive the lesion, the more destructive it will appear. The MRI characteristics are variable. Melanomas frequently have foci of hemorrhage that produce areas of high signal intensity on the T1-weighted sequence with associated low signal on T2. This tumoral hemorrhage has been found to have a greater influence on the T1 and T2 relaxation times than melanin.[33]

Esthesioneuroblastoma is an uncommon malignancy arising from olfactory epithelium found high in the nasal cavity. Therefore, this tumor is another site-specific lesion, characteristically located in the superior nasal cavity adjacent to the cribriform plate. In the early stages, a small esthesioneuroblastoma is seen as a nonspecific soft tissue mass that has expansile characteristics. Unfortunately, most of these lesions present much later on, exhibiting both smooth expansile and gross destructive changes. Extension into the ethmoidal labyrinth is the

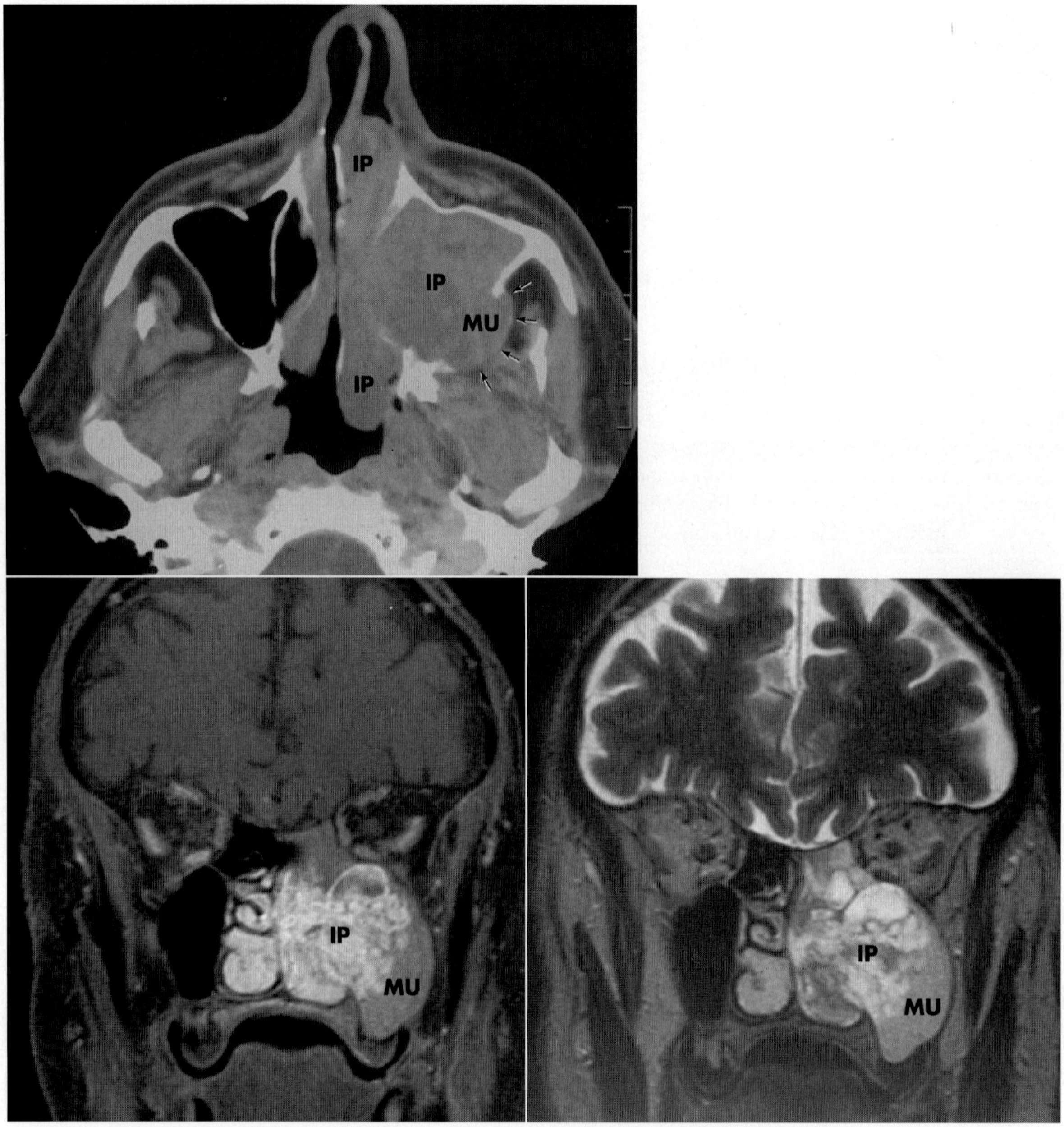

Fig. 1-21. Inverted papilloma. **A,** Axial CT, noncontrast. **B,** Coronal T1 fat-suppressed postcontrast MRI. **C,** Coronal T2 MRI, same level as **B.** This 67-year-old man presented with a nasal mass. Biopsy revealed inverted papilloma *(IP).* CT demonstrated a soft tissue mass in the nose and antrum with destruction of the lateral nasal wall. Tumor margins were not apparent. Expansion of the posterolateral antral wall was noted *(arrows),* a finding extremely rare for an uncomplicated IP, and a focus of squamous cell carcinoma was suspected. On the MRI, tumor completely obstructed antral drainage without reaching the posterior antral wall. Homogeneous nonenhancing isointense material was noted to fill the posterior antrum completely. The diagnosis of secondary mucocele was made and was confirmed at surgery. *MU,* mucocele.

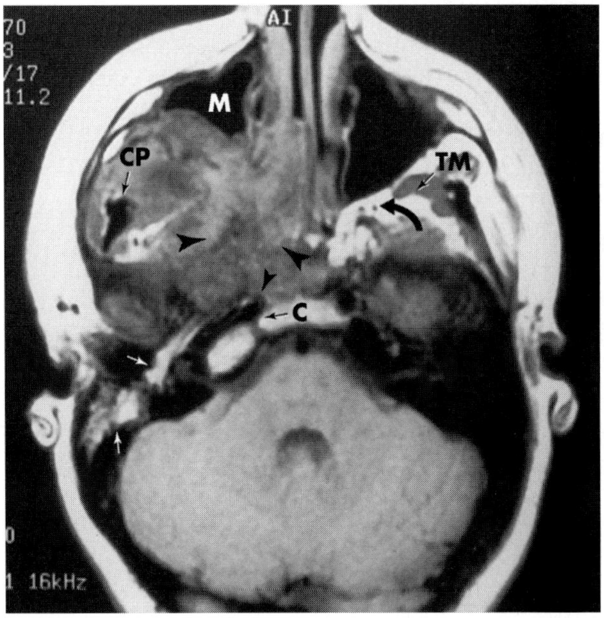

Fig. 1-22. Juvenile nasopharyngeal angiofibroma. Axial T1 MRI, noncontrast. This 15-year-old boy presented with a nasal mass. There is a bulky heterogeneous mass in the nasal cavity, destroying the lateral nasal wall posteriorly at the level of the sphenopalatine foramen. Tumor has completely replaced the pterygopalatine fossa and infratemporal fossa, producing the classic radiographic feature of anterior bowing of the posterior antral wall. The pterygoid process is faintly seen surrounded by tumor tissue *(large arrowheads).* The skull base is eroded, and tumor is seen to abut the petrous carotid artery (*small arrowhead).* Both sphenoid sinus and cavernous sinus were invaded, and other sections demonstrated several vascular structures (not shown). Note the fluid in the mastoid and middle ear cavity due to eustachian tube obstruction *(arrows). C,* petrous carotid artery; *M,* maxillary antrum; *CP,* coronoid process of mandible; *TM,* normal temporalis muscle on the left; *curved arrow,* normal hyperintense fat in the left pterygopalatine fossa. (Courtesy of Dr. Joseph Fehgali, New York.)

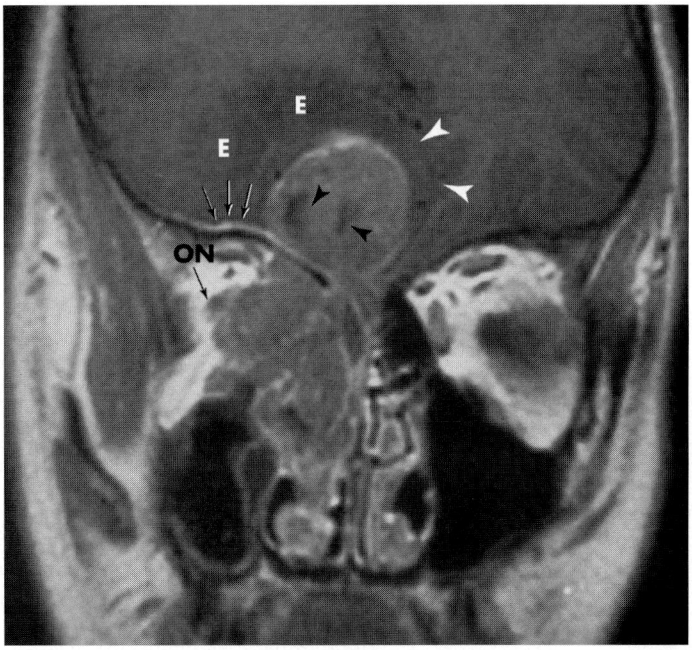

Fig. 1-23. Squamous cell carcinoma, anaplastic. Coronal T1 postgadolinium MRI. This young woman presented with rapidly progressing proptosis. MRI revealed a multilobulated irregular mass involving the nasal cavity and anterior ethmoid. There was gross destruction of the lamina papyracea and anterior skull base with obvious extension of mass into the orbit and cranium. Note the low-signal-intensity necrotic areas within enhancing tissue *(small arrowheads),* reactive dural enhancement *(arrows),* parenchymal edema *(E),* and the midline shift of the interhemispheric fissure (*large arrowheads).* Esthesioneuroblastoma could have an identical appearance. *ON,* optic nerve.

rule; maxillary sinus, orbital, and intracranial extension are also common.[34] Before MRI, it was unusual to diagnose intracranial extension preoperatively. Today, high-resolution MRI with gadolinium is extremely sensitive in delineating intracranial involvement and should be performed in all cases of suspected esthesioneuroblastoma. The CT appearance of esthesioneuroblastoma is that of a homogeneous soft tissue mass; both tumoral calcification and hyperostosis of the anterior skull base have been reported. On MRI, this tumor has variable signal intensity patterns and can be either heterogeneous or homogeneous.[22] Intracranial extension of esthesioneuroblastoma has been associated with adjacent parenchymal cyst formation.[35]

Non-Hodgkin's lymphoma is the most common malignant nonepithelial tumor to occur in the PNS. It accounts for 8% of PNS malignancies.[36] Lymphoma is seen as a heterogeneous soft tissue mass, isointense on CT, typically producing a permeative destructive pattern of bone involvement. Lymphoma infiltrates across bony plates of the PNS, leaving a washed-out "ghost" of bone in place (Fig. 1-24). On MRI, lymphoma is isointense on all sequences, because of dense cellularity with little interstitial water.

Soft tissue sarcoma is occasionally found in the nose and PNS. On CT, these bulky, homogeneous tumors do not enhance. Sarcomas are low to intermediate in signal intensity on MRI, with irregular enhancement. Their effect on adjacent bone ranges from expansion to gross destruction, depending on their growth rate.

Benign tumors of bone origin

Osteoma is a common lesion representing benign proliferation of mature bone. It occurs almost exclusively in the head and neck. Compact or ivory osteomas are seen as extremely dense, sharply defined masses within the paranasal sinuses, usually broad based against a septation (Fig. 1-25). The cancellous osteomas are variable in density on imaging studies owing to a fibrous component and may even appear as a soft tissue density on plain films. CT demonstrates their osseous character. Osteomas vary tremendously in size: they may be extremely small or may entirely fill a sinus cavity, producing a cast of the lumen. They may extend beyond the confines of the sinus walls.

The rare osteoblastoma is a well-circumscribed expansile lesion. It may be composed predominantly of ossified tissue or may present as a more mixed fibrous and osseous lesion.[22] Osteoblastoma is generally larger and more lobulated than osteoma.

Fibrous dysplasia has a wide range of radiographic appearances, depending on the relative content of fibrous and osseous tissue. Head and neck involvement is common, occurring in 50% of cases of polyostotic and 30% of cases of monostotic fibrous dysplasia.[37] Fibrous dysplasia causes diffuse enlargement of the involved bone, a finding that must be distinguished from true expansion. Three radiographic subtypes have been described: cystic, mixed, and sclerotic.[38] The mixed form is the most common and is seen as a hazy "ground-glass" appearance on plain film and CT (Fig. 1-26). On T1-weighted MRI, the lesions are homogeneous and vary from mildly hy-

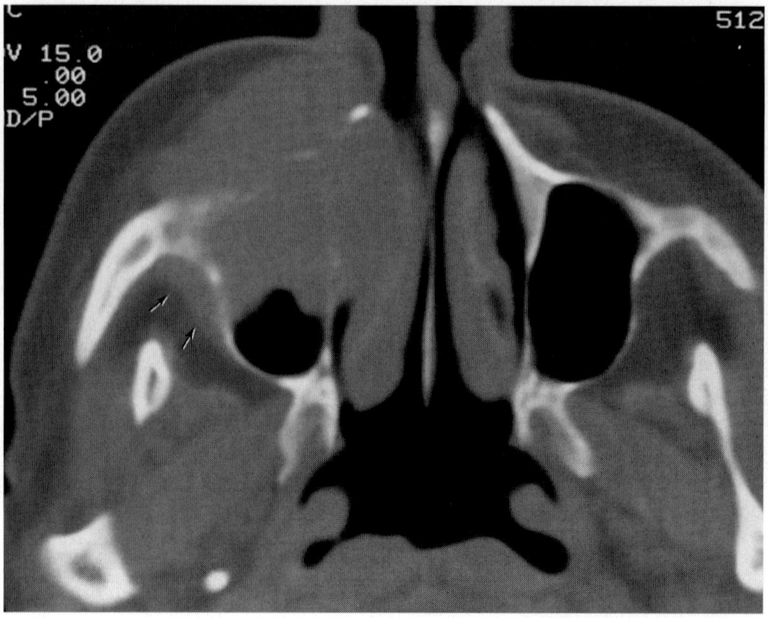

Fig. 1-24. Lymphoma. Axial CT bone window. There is a mass lesion involving the right maxillary antrum. It has infiltrated through the anterior and posterior antral walls without displacing the bony plates. Arrows indicate tumor in the retromaxillary space.

perintense to markedly hypointense, which may be confusing to the observer. On the T2-weighted sequence, however, marked hypointensity predominates, which, along with the diffuse enlargement of the bone, produces the hallmark of this lesion on MRI (Fig. 1-27).

The ossifying fibroma is a lesion most frequently found within the facial bones. It tends to have a greater soft tissue component and a more aggressive appearance than fibrous dysplasia, but the two may be indistinguishable. These lesions are well-circumscribed, expansile masses that may be of homogeneous soft tissue density, densely sclerotic, or mixed.[38]

The brown tumor of hyperparathyroidism is the most common giant cell lesion of the facial bones. These lesions consist of unilocular or multilocular lytic, expansile masses that have well-defined margins. After treatment and healing, brown tumors can fill in with new bone formation and become radiodense.[39] The giant cell granuloma may be indistinguishable from brown tumor. These are often aggressive lesions, at times mimicking malignant tumors. Giant cell granulomas are usually in the anterior aspect of the mandible and maxilla. They may contain calcific, ossific, or osteoid components.[40]

Malignant tumors of bone origin

The plasma cell dyscrasias are most commonly associated with the generalized bone disease of multiple myeloma. Solitary plasmacytoma of bone or extraosseous plas-

A

B

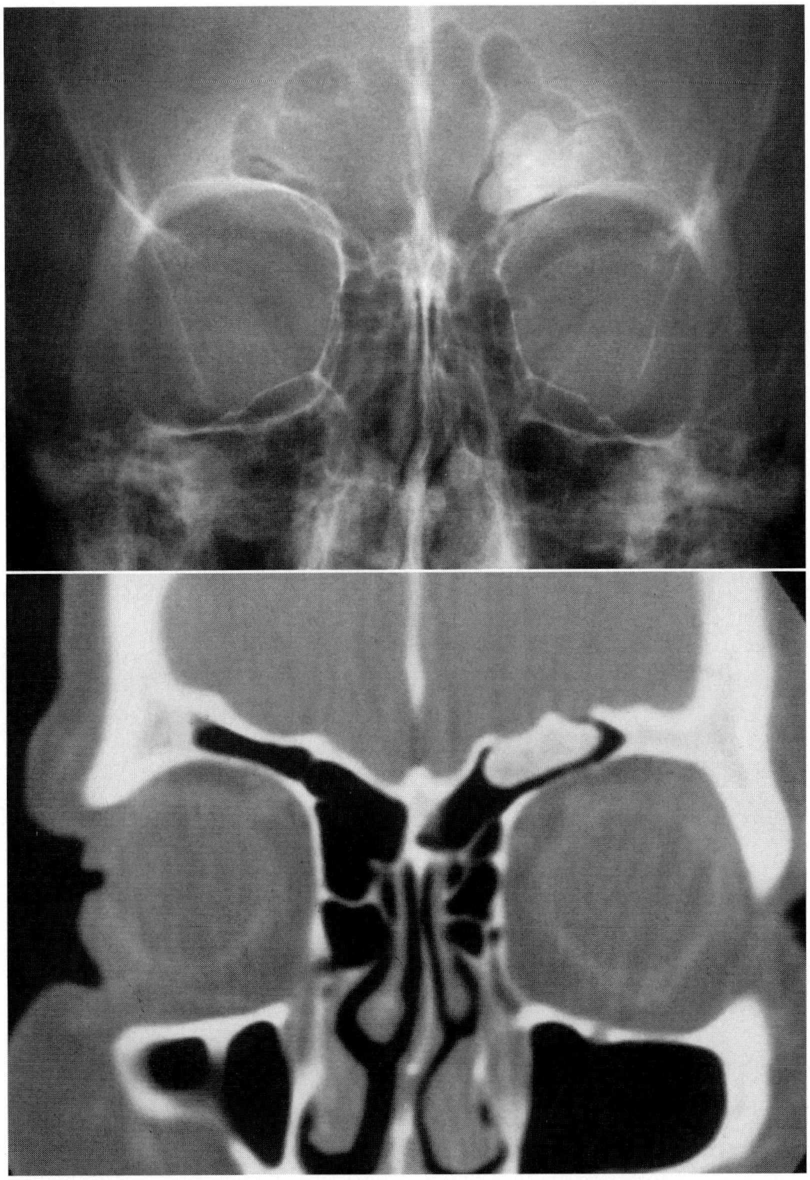

Fig. 1-25. Frontal sinus osteoma. **A,** Caldwell view. **B,** Coronal CT. There is a gently lobulated osteoma in the left frontal sinus, broad based against the frontal roof.

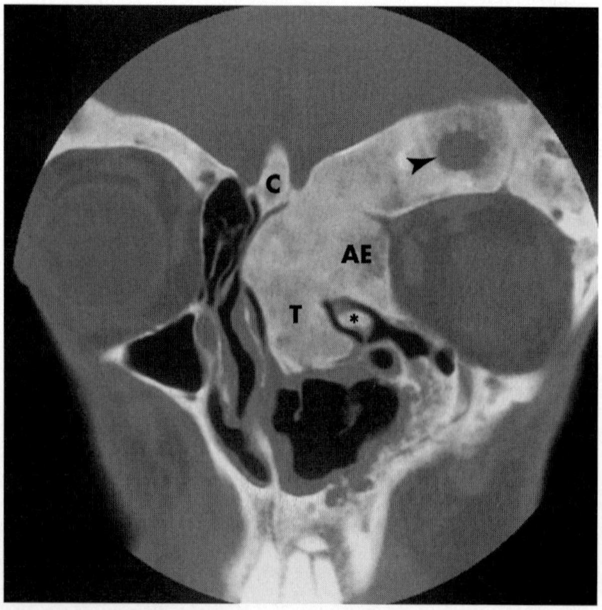

Fig. 1-26. Fibrous dysplasia, polyostotic. Coronal CT showing gross enlargement of the frontal and ethmoid bones, crista galli *(C)* middle turbinate *(T)*, maxilla, and uncinate plate *(asterisk)* by homogeneous dysplastic bone. Note the cystic lesion in the left frontal bone (arrowhead). AE, anterior ethmoid.

A

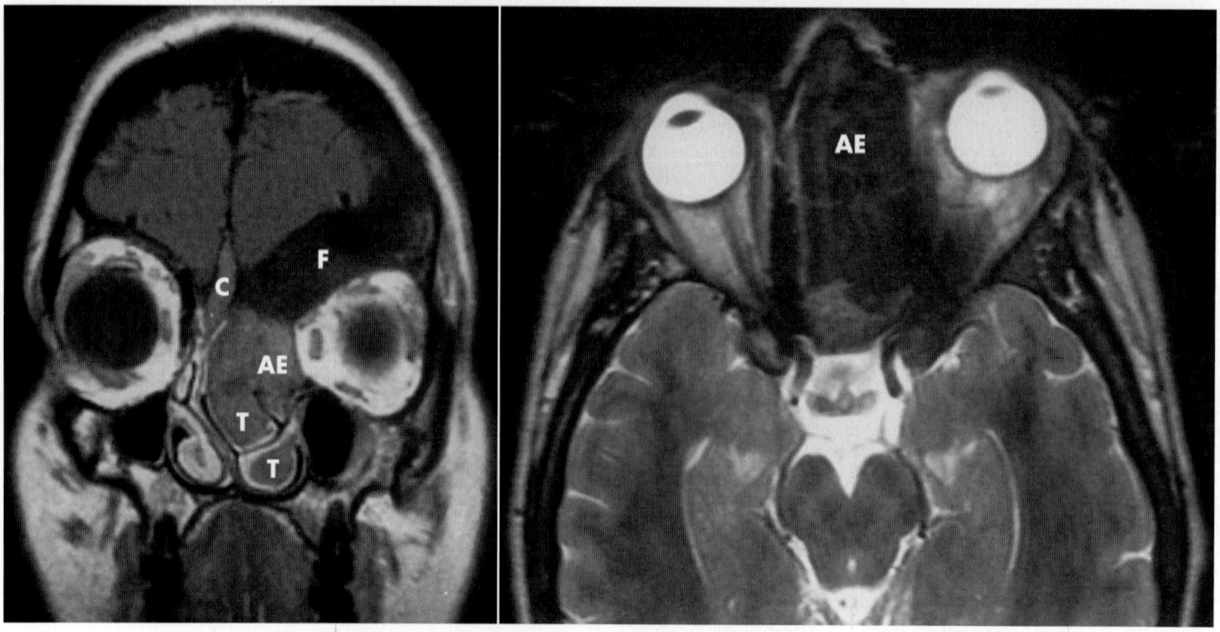

B

Fig. 1-27. Fibrous dysplasia, polyostotic. **A,** Coronal T1 postgadolinium MRI. **B,** Axial T2 MRI through the ethmoidal labyrinth. There is involvement of the crista galli *(C)*, left frontal bone, and ethmoid and both middle and inferior turbinates *(T)*. On the T1 sequence, mild enhancement in some areas is due to the presence of vascular fibrous tissue. The frontal bone remains dark owing to the predominant osseous component. The T2 sequence demonstrates low signal intensity, confirming the diagnosis of fibrous dysplasia. *AE,* anterior ethmoid; *F,* frontal bone.

macytoma may also occur. Involvement of the paranasal sinuses is seen as soft tissue masses that are expansile and destroy the sinus walls. These tumors are associated with lytic skeletal lesions in 85% of cases.[22] Osteogenic sarcoma occasionally occurs in the paranasal sinuses. Seven percent of osteosarcomas are said to occur in the jaw[41] (Fig. 1-28). These destructive lesions are often purely lytic but may be associated with amorphous calcifications or a typical sunburst appearance of radiating periosteal new bone. In the absence of new bone formation, the specific diagnosis of osteogenic sarcoma will not be suggested. Chondrosarcoma of the paranasal sinuses is encountered uncommonly. Chondrosarcoma is an aggressive soft tissue mass that may contain amorphous, mottled, or reactive calcifications within the tumor matrix. Periosteal reaction is not typically seen.[22] The better-differentiated lesion is more sharply defined on imaging studies and may appear benign.

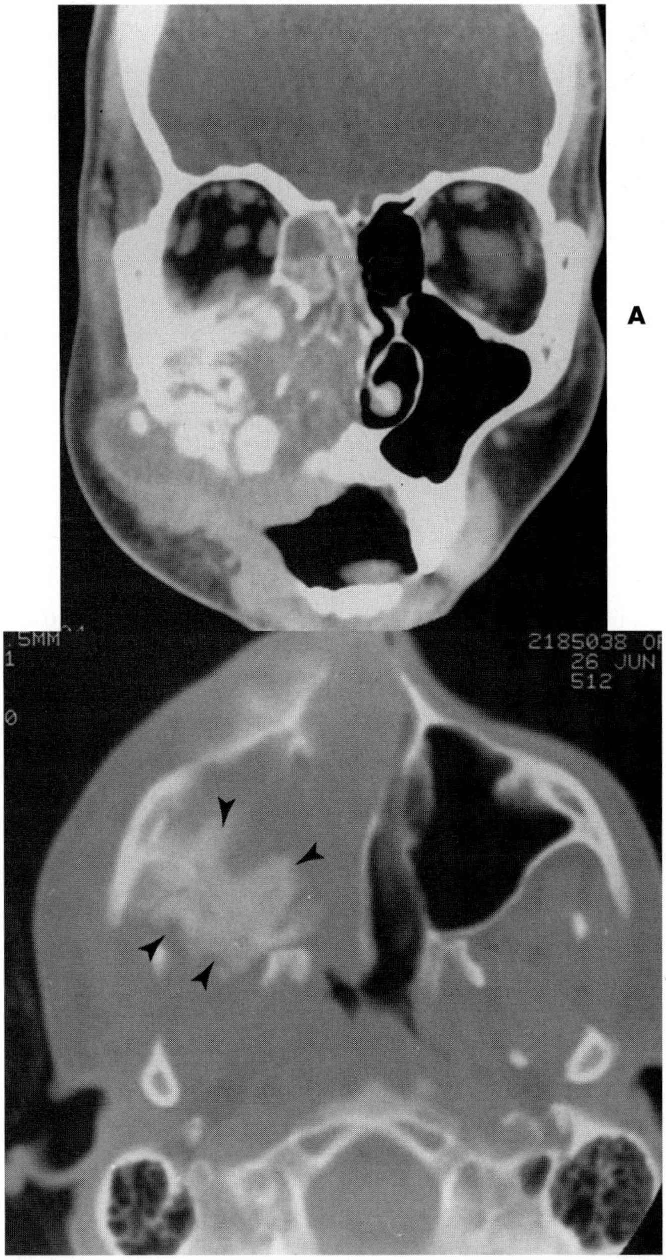

A

B

Fig. 1-28. Osteogenic sarcoma. **A,** Coronal CT, soft tissue window. **B,** Axial CT, bone window. There is an aggressive, destructive mass lesion involving the nose and maxillary antrum, extending into the buccal soft tissues. The orbital floor has been infiltrated. Opacification of ethmoid air cells is due to retained secretions. Irregular, amorphous tumoral bone is seen on the coronal image; a sunburst pattern of periosteal reaction is seen on the axial image *(arrowheads).*

ACKNOWLEDGMENTS

My sincere thanks to Ms. Olga Paredes for her assistance in preparation of the manuscript.

REFERENCES

1. Zeifer B: *Radiographic evaluation of the paranasal sinuses*. In Mehta D, editor: *Atlas of endoscopic sinonasal surgery*, Philadelphia, 1993, Lea & Febiger, pp 53-60.
2. American College of Radiology: *Manual on iodinated contrast media*, 1991, American College of Radiology.
3. Moore RD, Steinberg EP, Powe NR, et al: Frequency and determinants of adverse reactions induced by high-osmolality contrast media, *Radiology* 170:727-732, 1989.
4. Lang DM, Alpern MB, Visintainer PF, Smith ST: Increased risk for anaphylactoid reaction from contrast media in patients on β-adrenergic blockers or with asthma, *Ann Intern Med* 115:270-276, 1991.
5. Wolf GL, Arenson RL, Cross AP: A prospective trial of ionic vs nonionic contrast agents in routine clinical practice: comparison of adverse effects, *AJR* 152:939-944, 1989.
6. Niendorf HP, Brasch RC: *Gd-DTPA tolerance and clinical safety*. In Brasch RC, editor: *MRI contrast enhancement in the central nervous system*, New York, 1993, Raven Press, pp 11-21.
7. Shellock FG, Kanal E: *MR procedures and patients with electrically, magnetically, and mechanically activated implants and devices*. In *Magnetic resonance bioeffects, safety, and patient management*, New York, 1994, Raven Press, pp 123-132.
8. Kelly WM, Paglen PG, Pearson A, et al: Ferromagnetism of intraocular foreign body causes unilateral blindness after MR study, *AJNR* 7:243-245, 1986.
9. Shellock FG, Kanal E: *Screening patients before MR procedures*. In *Magnetic resonance bioeffects, safety, and patient management*, New York, 1994, Raven Press, pp 91-99.
10. Klucznik RP, Carrier DA, Pyka R, Haid RW: Placement of a ferromagnetic intracerebral aneurysm clip in a magnetic field with a fatal outcome, *Radiology* 187:855-856, 1993.
11. Shellock FG, Kanal E: *MR procedures and patients with biomedical implants, materials, and devices*. In *Magnetic resonance bioeffects, safety, and patient management*, New York, 1994, Raven Press, pp 101-131.
12. Teitelbaum GP, Bradley WG, Klein BD: MR imaging artifacts, ferromagnetism, and magnetic torque of intravascular filters, stents, and coils, *Radiology* 166:657-664, 1988.
13. Kainz J, Stammberger H: The roof of the anterior ethmoid: a place of least resistance in the skull base, *Am J Rhinol* 4:191-194, 1989.
14. Kuhn FA, Bolger WE, Tisdal RG: The agger nasi cell in frontal recess obstruction: an anatomic, radiologic and clinical correlation, *Op Tech Otolaryngol Head Neck Surg* 2:226-231, 1991.
15. Duvoisin B, Agrifoglio A: Prevalence of ethmoid sinus abnormalities on brain CT of asymptomatic adults, *AJNR* 10:599-601, 1989.
16. Rak KM, Newell JDII, Yakes WK, et al: Paranasal sinus on MR images of the brain: significance of mucosal thickening, *AJR* 156:381-384, 1991.
17. Silver JA, Baredes S, Bello JA, et al: The opacified maxillary sinus. CT findings in chronic sinusitis and malignant tumors, *Radiology* 163:205-210, 1987.
18. Fascenelli FW: Maxillary sinus abnormalities, *Arch Otolaryngol* 90:98-101, 1969.
19. Goaz PW, White SC: *Infections and inflammations of the jaws and facial bones*. In *Oral radiology*, St. Louis, 1987, Mosby-Year Book, pp 465-483.
20. Messerklinger W: *Endoscopy of the nose*. Baltimore, 1978, Urban & Schwarzenberg.
21. Stammberger H: Endoscopic endonasal surgery—concepts in treatment of recurring rhinosinusitis. Part I. Anatomic and pathophysiologic considerations, *Otolaryngol Head Neck Surg* 94:143-156, 1986.
22. Som PM, Brandwein M: *Sinonasal cavities: tumors and tumorlike conditions*. In Som PM, Curtin HD, editors: *Head and neck imaging*, St. Louis, 1996, Mosby-Year Book, pp 185-262.
23. Corey JP, Delsupehe KG, Ferguson BJ: Allergic fungal sinusitis: allergic, infectious, or both?, *Otolaryngol Head Neck Surg* 113:110-119, 1995.
24. Zinreich SJ, Kennedy DW, Malat J, et al: Fungal sinusitis: diagnosis with CT and MR imaging, *Radiology* 169:439-444, 1988.
25. Som PM, Dillon WP, Fullerton GD, et al: Chronically obstructed sinonasal secretions: observations on T1 and T2 shortening, *Radiology* 172:515-520, 1989.
26. Beckhardt RN, Setzen M, Carras R: Primary spontaneous cerebrospinal fluid rhinorrhea, *Otolaryngol Head Neck Surg* 104:425-432, 1991.
27. Hudgins PA, Browning DG, Gallups J, et al: Endoscopic paranasal sinus surgery: radiographic evaluation of severe complications, *AJNR* 13:1161-1167, 1992.
28. Yeates AE, Blumenkopf B, Drayer BP, et al: Spontaneous CSF rhinorrhea arising from the middle cranial fossa: CT demonstration, *AJNR* 5:820-821, 1984.
29. Zinreich SJ, Benson ML, Oliverio PJ: *Sinonasal cavities: CT normal anatomy, imaging of the osteomeatal complex, and functional endoscopic surgery*. In Som PM, Curtin HD, editors: *Head and neck imaging*, St. Louis: 1996, Mosby-Year Book, pp 97-125.
30. Som PM, Shapiro MD, Biller HF, et al: Sinonasal tumors and inflammatory tissues: differentiation with MR imaging, *Radiology* 167:803-808, 1988.
31. Parker GD, Harnsberger HR: Clinical-radiologic issues in perineural tumor spread of malignant diseases of the extracranial head and neck, *RadioGraphics* 11:383-399, 1991.
32. Som PM, Cohen BA, Sacher M, et al: The angiomatous polyp and the angiofibroma: two different lesions, *Radiology* 144:329-334, 1982.
33. Hammersmith SM, Terk MR, Jeffery PB, et al: Magnetic resonance imaging of nasopharyngeal and paranasal sinus melanoma, *Magn Reson Imaging* 8:245-253, 1990.
34. Schuster JJ, Phillips CD, Levine PA: MR of esthesioneuroblastoma (olfactory neuroblastoma) and appearance after craniofacial resection, *AJNR* 15:1169-1177, 1994.
35. Som PM, Lidov M, Brandwein M, et al: Sinonasal esthesioneuroblastoma with intracranial extension: marginal tumor cysts as a diagnostic MR finding, *AJNR* 15:1259-1262, 1994.
36. DePena CA, van Tassel P, Lee Y: Lymphoma of the head and neck, *Radiol Clin North Am* 28:723-743, 1990.
37. Mirra JM, Gold RH: *Fibrous dysplasia*. In Mirra JM, Piero P, Gold RH, editors: *Bone tumors*, Philadelphia, 1989, Lea & Febiger, pp 191-226.
38. Kumar R, Madewell JE, Lindell MM, Swischuk LE: Fibrous lesions of bone, *RadioGraphics* 10:237-256, 1990.
39. Som PM, Lawson W, Cohen BA: Giant-cell lesions of the facial bones, *Radiology* 147:129-134, 1983.
40. Rhea JT, Weber AL: Giant-cell granuloma of the sinuses, *Radiology* 147:135-137, 1983.
41. Oot RF, Parizel PM, Weber AL: Computed tomography of osteogenic sarcoma of nasal cavity and paranasal sinuses, *J Comput Assist Tomogr* 10:409-414, 1986.

CHAPTER

2

Nasal Endoscopy

Wolfgang Draf
Rainer Weber
Rainer Keerl

PROBLEM
A 62-year-old woman presents with a 6-month history of nasal stuffiness on both sides and recurrent bleeding.

BOX 2-1

Local problem

Angiofibroma (child, juvenile, adult)
Malignant tumor (carcinoma, sarcoma)
Foreign body

Unspecific infection with or without nasal polyps
Complications after nasal or sinus surgery or trauma
Atrophic rhinitis
Combination of two local problems such as nasal polyps and bleeding from the anterior nasal septum due to digital manipulation

Systemic disease

Wegener's disease
Lymphoma
Combination of a local problem causing nasal stuffiness and a systemic disease predisposing to nasal bleeding e.g., hypertonus

The combination of nasal stuffiness and bleeding may be a localized problem or a manifestation of a systemic disease. Nasal endoscopy plays a major role in differentiating the underlying cause (see Box 2-1).

MEDICAL HISTORY

Other symptoms of local disease should be sought, such as recurrent sinus or nasal infections, hyposmia, and headache. Allergic rhinitis must be ruled out. Previous operations or traumas should be considered, along with coagulation disorders, hypertonus, and immunologic or renal diseases.

Our patient had no history of nasal problems up to now. There was no previous nasal or sinus surgery. She was otherwise healthy and took no drugs.

PHYSICAL (EAR, NOSE, AND THROAT) EXAMINATION

Endoscopy of the nose and paranasal sinuses is essential for proper diagnosis of nasal and paranasal sinus diseases.[1-12] It is well established as a therapeutic tool in endonasal surgery.[9,10,12,13-25]Furthermore, it can be used as a documentation device by means of videoendoscopy or a special photocamera.

Advances in fiberoptic technology have led to the development of flexible and rigid nasal endoscopes, which provide excellent intranasal illumination and permit detailed examination of the nasal cavity. The entire cavity, including the accessible components of the ostiomeatal complex, can now be closely inspected in the office setting. Headlight and nasal speculum examination permits visualization of only the anterior part of the nasal cavity and offers a limited view of the middle nasal meatus.

Instrumentation

Both rigid and flexible endoscopic systems are available, each with special advantages and disadvantages (Table 2-1). Both instrumentations should be available in order to choose the best in individual cases.

We recommend the following systems (Fig. 2-1):

1. Rigid endoscope: As a routine device, a forward-oblique 30-degree wide-angle telescope, 4 mm in outside diameter, autoclavable (Fig. 2-2). In special cases, 0- or 70-degree angle telescope, 4 mm in outside diameter, or 30-degree telescope 2.7 mm in outer diameter, are necessary.
2. Flexible rhinolaryngoscope (Fig. 2-3).
3. Xenon light source (see Fig. 2-1) to achieve natural light conditions as far as possible.
4. CCD videocamera (see Fig. 2-2) for documentation, presentation, and more comfortable working using monitors. Modern cameras with digital signal processing allow individual programming. Once programming is made, operation of the cam-

Table 2-1. Comparison of rigid and flexible nasal endoscopic systems (+ marks the superior system regarding this quality)

	RIGID SYSTEM	FLEXIBLE SYSTEM
Optical quality	+	
Documentation	+	
Mobilization of turbinates	+	
Difficult-to-reach passageways	+	+
Postoperative control		+
Versatility		+
Use in children		+
Comfort		+
Usefulness as a therapeutic tool	++	

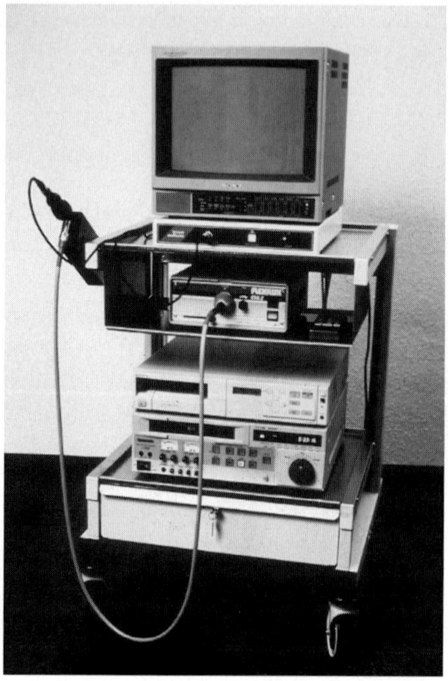

Fig. 2-1. Equipment for videoendoscopy on a special trolley *From top to bottom*: monitor; camera control unit with programming board in aluminum case and—on the left side—CCD camera with endoscope in a telescope holder with heating system; Xenon Video Cold Light Fountain; color video printer; videorecorder. (Courtesy of Stuemer, Würzburg, Germany.)

era can be started with one button only. Integrated self-adapting systems prevent fading or dissolving and provide brilliant video pictures at any time during the examination. A second monitor allows patients to follow the examination "on-line," which increases their compliance significantly. The videocamera can be adapted to be put up on both rigid and flexible endoscopes.

In the patient in Fig. 2-4, *A*, nasal endoscopy revealed a diffuse swelling of both inferior turbinates and the nasal septum with a granulomatous mucosa. There was no other pathologic finding in the nose, nasopharynx, ear, mouth, throat, or larynx.

RADIOGRAPHIC EXAMINATION

For radiologic examination of the nose and paranasal sinuses, computed tomography (CT) and magnetic resonance imaging (MRI) are standard. CT gives a better presentation of bony structures and plays a major role in preoperative imaging of chronic sinusitis. MRT is better in differentiating soft tissues and early signs of infiltration into the area. In the patient in Fig. 2-4, CT showed enlarged inferior turbinates but no opacification of the sinuses. Chest radiography demonstrated a widened mediastinum with enlarged bilateral hilar lymph nodes (Fig. 2-4, *B*).

HISTOLOGIC EXAMINATION

Abnormal swelling or appearance of the mucosa should lead to diagnostic endoscopy and carefully directed endoscopic biopsy to secure the diagnosis. In the patient in Fig. 2-4, noncaseating epitheloid granulomas were found in the biopsies of both inferior turbinates and the nasal septum, and sarcoidosis was diagnosed.

TREATMENT

Treatment with corticosteroids was performed by a specialist in internal diseases.

A

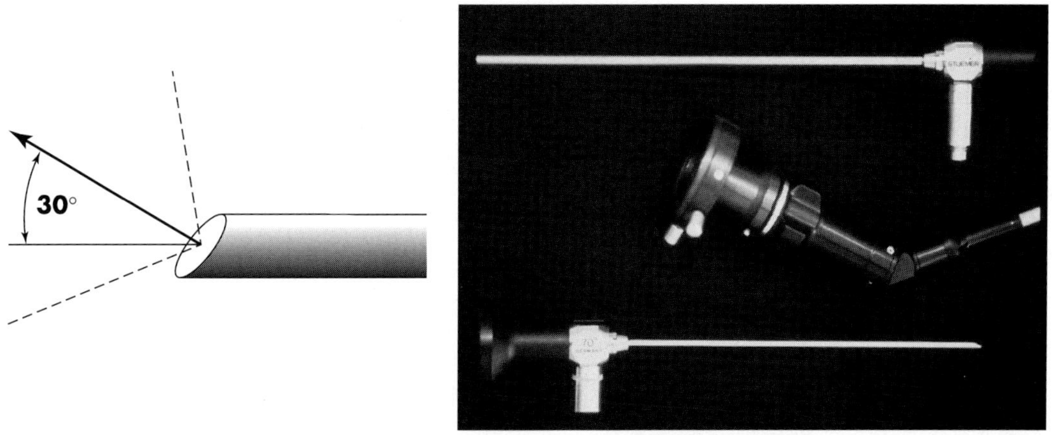

B

Fig. 2-2. **A**, Straightforward 0-degree wide-angle telescope, forward-oblique 30-degree wide-angle telescope; CCD videocamera 606000. **B**, Visual angle of forward-oblique 30-degree wide-angle telescope (Courtesy of Stuemer, Würzburg, Germany).

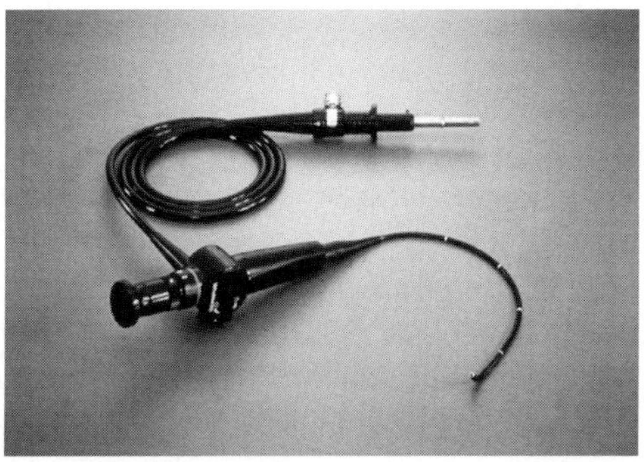

Fig. 2-3. Flexible rhinolaryngoscope ENF P3 (outside diameter 3.6 mm, bending upward and downward 130 degrees) (Courtesy of Olympus, Hamburg, Germany).

A

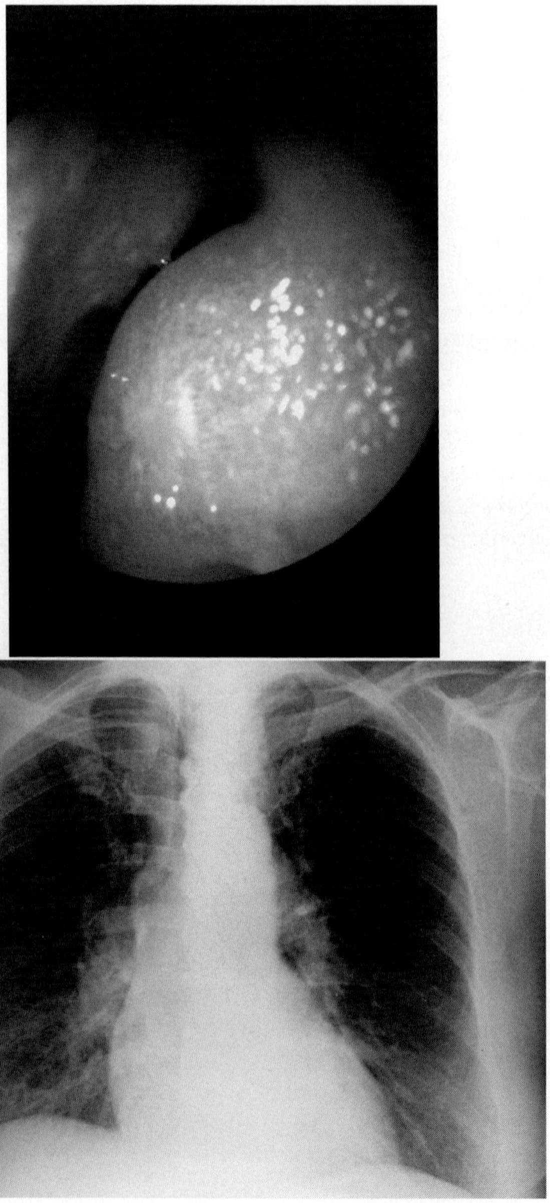

B

Fig. 2-4. **A,** Endoscopic view of the enlarged left inferior turbinate with a granulomatous mucosa due to sarcoidosis. **B,** Chest radiograph with bilateral enlargement of hilar lymph nodes due to sarcoidosis.

DISCUSSION

Endoscopy is performed with the patient in the supine position if possible. The patient is more relaxed and the head is well supported in two planes. For on-line demonstration, a prone position is preferable. In diagnostic clinical routine, the prone position using the flexible endoscope is also preferred. Endoscopy requires only topical nasal anesthesia, if any at all, and is well tolerated by the awake, unsedated patient. Children may have an overall fear of any manipulations, painful or not; the flexible system is preferable for them. It is advisable to speak calmly and frankly with children and to explain that the examination is very important and may cause some discomfort or pain that will not last very long. This approach is successful in most cases without any anesthesia. One should not lie to a child and say that endoscopy does not cause pain; the patient will lose faith in the examiner and in other future physicians.

Whichever instrument is used, the technique performed should be methodical.

We differentiate therapeutic from diagnostic endoscopy. Although therapeutic endoscopy (endoscopic endonasal sinus surgery) is not the topic of this chapter, the indications for it are listed in Table 2-2.[10,15,19]

In many cases, both microscope and endoscope are used to combine their advantages.[13,14,17] Especially in cases of more severe bleeding, the operation could be continued using the microscope being outside of the surgical sight. Furthermore, various magnifications can be chosen, depending on the individual problem. A self-restraining speculum enables the examiner to work with both hands.

Table 2-2 Indications for therapeutic nasal endoscopy (endoscopic endonasal sinus surgery)

Chronic or persistent acute infection of all paranasal sinuses
Mucoceles of ethmoid and sphenoid sinus
Mucoceles of maxillary and frontal sinus if localized medially
Orbital complications of acute and chronic sinusitis if there is no abscess localized laterally
Selected foreign bodies
Selected benign and malignant tumors (great experience mandatory)
CSF leak (sphenoid sinus, ethmoid roof, cribriform plate, basal posterior wall of frontal sinus)
Dacryocystorhinostomy
Decompression of orbit (endocrine ophthalmopathy)
Decompression of optic nerve
Selected cases of angiofibroma
Tornwaldt's cyst
Postoperative care after sinus surgery

CSF, Cerebrospinal fluid.

DIAGNOSTIC ENDOSCOPY

The following anatomic structures should be evaluated with regard to size, shape, and topographic relation to other structures: nasal septum; inferior, middle, and upper nasal meatuses and turbinates; olfactory cleft; uncinate process; agger nasi; and natural or accessory ostium of the maxillary sinus (if visible). Pathologic findings such as secretions (Fig. 2-5, *A*) inflammatory mucosal reactions, foreign bodies (Fig. 2-5, *B* and *C*), polyps, and tumors (Fig. 2-5, *D* to *F*) should be described precisely.

The findings should be compared with normal anatomy and its variations,[6,26,27] physiology, and the complaints of the patient. It is then essential to make a synopsis of all data and look for congruency of patient complaints, endoscopic findings and results of other examinations (CT, MRT, microbiology, allergology). This provides proper diagnosis and leads to optimized individual therapy. Anatomic variations such as septal deviation or septal spurs, concha bullosa, and inverted uncinate process are found in asymptomatic patients. Their appearance does not predict the necessity of surgery. In evaluating the turbinates, it is necessary to consider their changing size due to the nasal cycle, along with physical and pharmacologic influences.[28,29]

Nasal endoscopy is indispensable for the objective assessment of response to treatment.[7] It may eliminate the need for repeated radiographic follow-up examinations. Documentation by video clip is the best way to compare pretherapeutic and posttherapeutic findings, such as reduction of nasal polyps by the topical steroid budesonide (Pulmicort Topinasal)[30] (Fig. 2-6).

Another important role for nasal endoscopy is in postoperative care. One has to keep in mind the physiology of wound healing[29,31-34] with the four phases of blood crusts, obstructive (lymph)edema, mesenchymal reorganization, and scarring. Therapeutic intervention should correspond to the time-dependent individual physiologic or pathologic findings, as analyzed by nasal endoscopy.

In the first 7 to 12 days after functional endoscopic sinus surgery (FESS), hard-to-remove blood crusts cover the whole wound (Fig. 2-7, *A*). These should not be removed, to prevent major damage to the underlying healing tissue. Only in cases of severe obstruction of the nose and sinus ostia with subsequent bacterial infection is intervention necessary. Less traumatic is rinsing with saline solution (Ems brine, Rhinocare), to moisten the wound and lyse adhesive crusts. While crusts consist of blood originating from surgery, they are formed by dehydrated secretions later on and continue to decrease in shape for

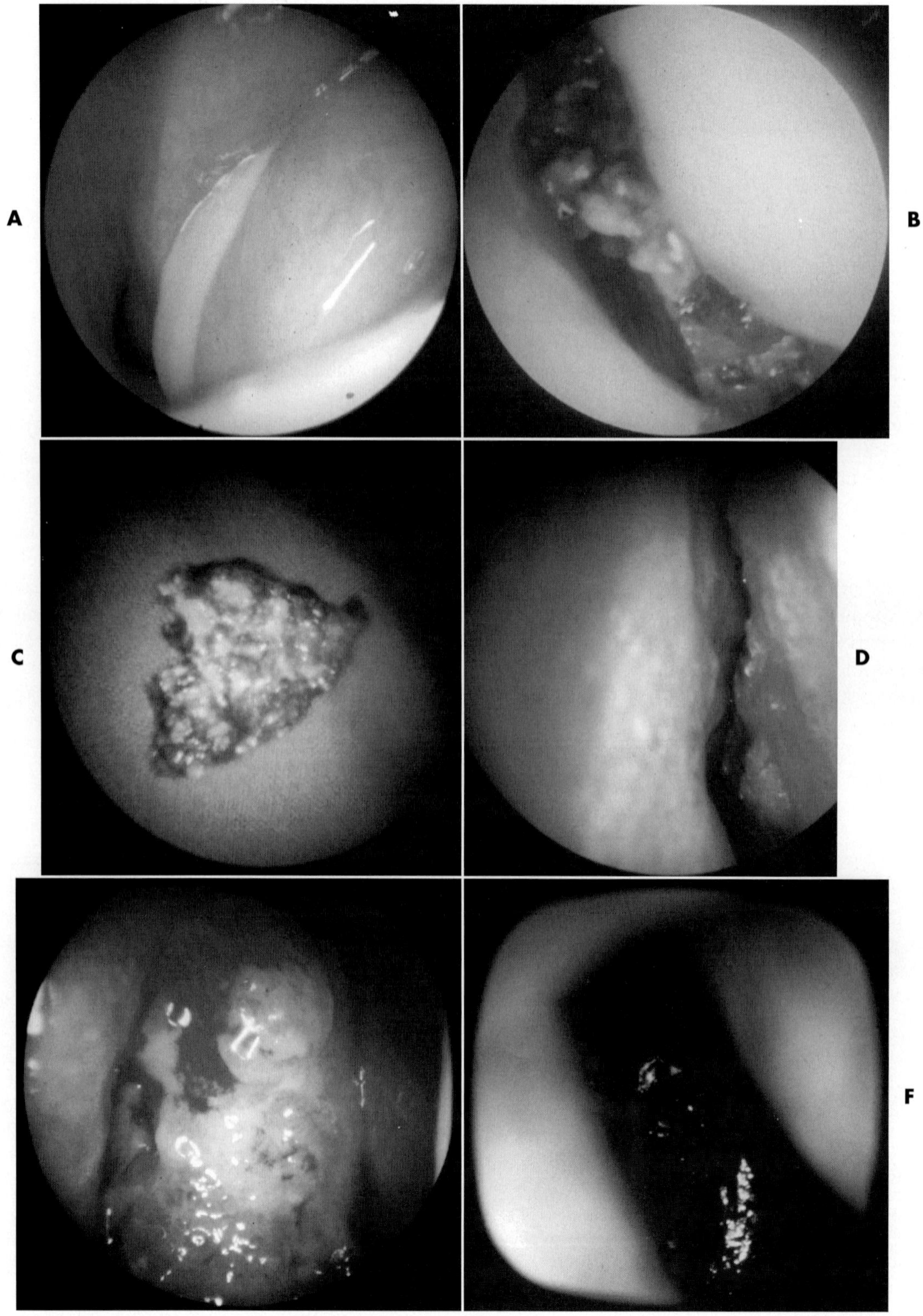

Fig. 2-5. Pathologic intranasal findings (endoscopic view). **A,** Acute exacerbation of chronic polypoid sinusitis of the left side, with a polyp and pus in the middle meatus. **B,** Foreign body in the left nasal cavity. **C,** Foreign body after endoscopic removal (incrusted, irregular-formed piece of rubber). **D,** Adenocarcinoma of the right ethmoid. **E,** Malignant melanoma of the right middle turbinate. **F,** Carcinoma of the nasopharynx (view from the left side).

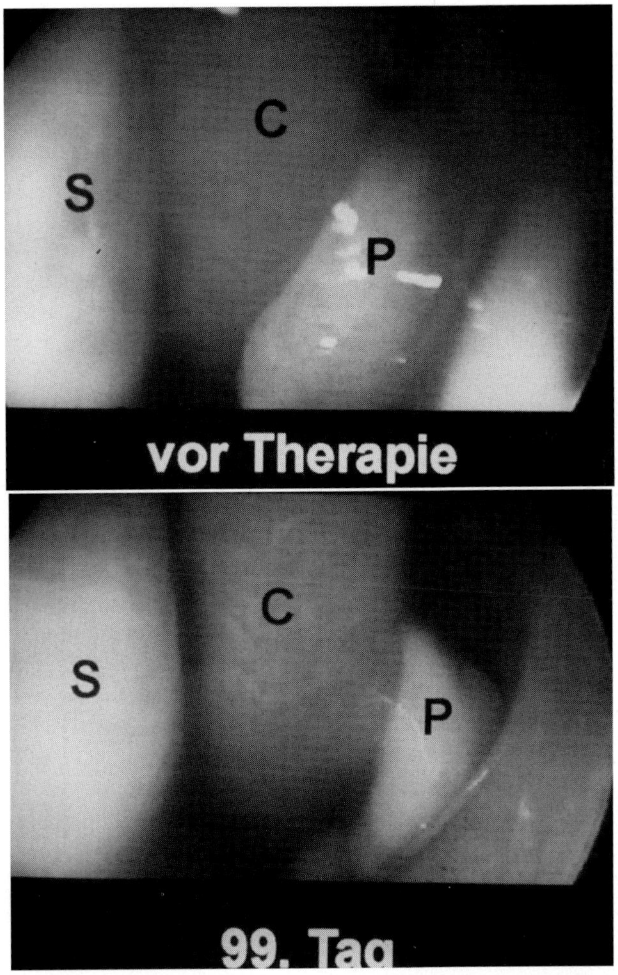

A

B

Fig. 2-6. Reduction of nasal polyps after application of topical budesonide (Pulmicort Topinasal). Endoscopic view in the left nose with a 30-degree wide-angle optic. **A,** Before therapy. **B,** 99 days after therapy. *P,* nasal polyp; *C,* middle turbinate; *S,* nasal septum.

at least 6 weeks. In some cases they persist for more than 6 months.

Under the crust, new granulation tissue is found at the end of the first week or beginning of the second week, followed by edema some days later. Granulation tissue is seen for 2 to 4 weeks, predominantly at the anterior lateral nasal wall (Fig. 2-7, *B*). It is replaced by collagenic connective tissue stepwise covered by thin layers of epithelium, and it disappears in time. If epithelial cells do not grow over these granulations or if severe inflammatory reactions occur, granulation tissue may persist, cause profound secretions, and build bridges for subsequent formation of synechia. If this is the case, granulations should be removed or treated with silver nitrate. Systemic and topical steroids clearly reduce the extent of granulations.

Two weeks after surgical lesion, increasing edema is the predominant finding (Fig. 2-7, *C*). The increasing swelling narrows the ethmoid cavity and entrance to the paranasal sinuses significantly up to the point of macroscopically complete obstruction in some cases (fourth week, Fig. 2-8, *A*). Definite decrease of edema and mucosal swelling in most cases occurs not before 7 to 12 weeks postoperatively (Fig. 2-7, *D*). This leads to widening of the ethmoid and openings to the paranasal sinuses and ultimately in a well-epithelialized cavity with some sickle-shaped scars (after 12 to 18 weeks in most cases, Fig. 2-7, *E*). Only steroids are effective in reducing diffuse edematous swelling, shown by topical application of budesonide (Fig. 2-9). Persistent localized edema can be removed surgically or cauterized. Contact zones between the healing, middle turbinate and the lateral nasal wall beyond the third or fourth week should be separated in an attempt to prevent major synechia (see Fig. 2-8, *B*). In special cases, insertion of a silicone sheet for some weeks may be necessary. All manipulations should be made with proper instruments to minimize surgical trauma with subsequent inflammatory reaction. Sharp-biting forceps

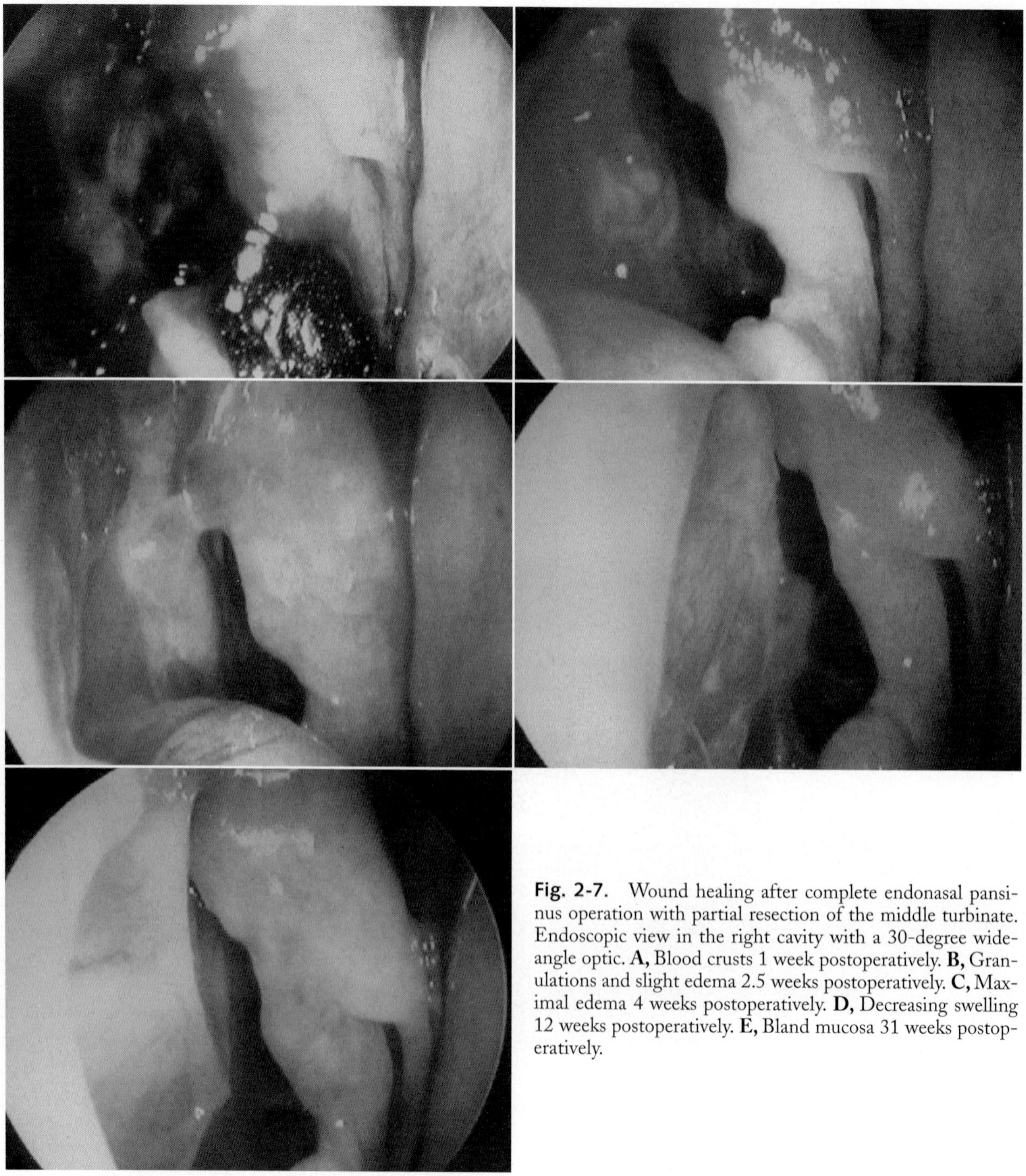

Fig. 2-7. Wound healing after complete endonasal pansinus operation with partial resection of the middle turbinate. Endoscopic view in the right cavity with a 30-degree wide-angle optic. **A,** Blood crusts 1 week postoperatively. **B,** Granulations and slight edema 2.5 weeks postoperatively. **C,** Maximal edema 4 weeks postoperatively. **D,** Decreasing swelling 12 weeks postoperatively. **E,** Bland mucosa 31 weeks postoperatively.

A
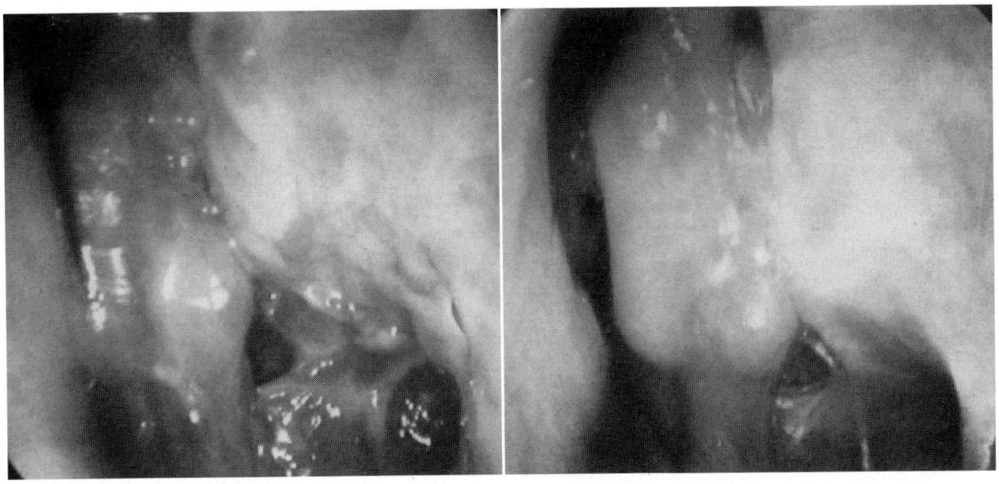
B

Fig. 2-8. Wound healing after complete endonasal pansinus operation with partial resection of the middle turbinate. Endoscopic view in the left cavity with a 30-degree wide-angle optic. **A,** Complete obstruction of the ethmoid cavity because of major swelling 4 weeks postoperatively. **B,** Subsequent development of synechia between the middle turbinate and lateral nasal wall 22 weeks postoperatively.

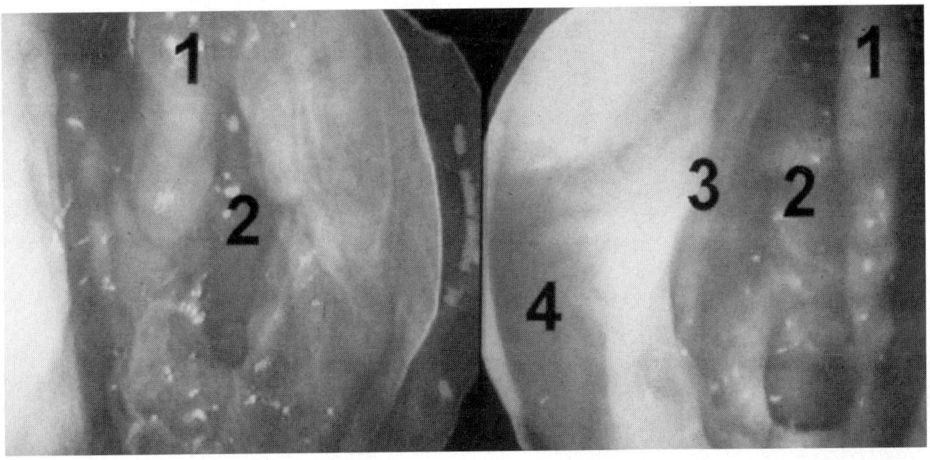

Fig. 2-9. Wound healing after complete endonasal pansinus operation with partial resection of the middle turbinate. Endoscopic view in the right and left cavity with a 30-degree wide-angle optic 25 weeks postoperatively. The right side was treated with topical budesonide (Pulmicort Topinasal) and healed in faster and more complete way than the left side. *1,* Middle turbinate; *2,* ethmoid cavity; *3,* lateral nasal wall; *4,* maxillary sinus.

are best to remove only the pathologic tissue and do not tear off healthy mucosa (Fig. 2-10).

Morphologic changes in the ethmoid cavity and other sinuses can be seen, although these are epithelialized and appear bland because of subepithelial scar remodeling, which continues beyond the sixth month. Healing time can be reduced by application of topical steroids (Fig. 2-9). Wide-open pathways to the maxillary and frontal sinus 6 months postoperatively with a normal mucosa inside the sinuses will remain open most probably because scar remodeling has finished comprehensively (Fig. 2-11). Flexible endoscopy (Fig. 2-12) enables inspection of the maxillary and frontal sinus around adhesions in the anterior ethmoid and is of utmost importance for postoperative evaluation. With a flexible endoscope with working channel (ENF T3, Olympus, Hamburg, Fig. 2-12), small polyps or scars and persistent granulations can be removed particularly in the critical region of the frontal recess or within the maxillary sinus. This minimizes the trauma and achieves a better outcome of sinus surgery than with rigid endoscopes and normal nasal forceps.

DOCUMENTATION AND DATA PROCESSING[35]

A special camera enables endoscopic photographs to be made. Using videoendoscopy, the data can be stored as videotape. Modern computer technology makes it possible to capture single frames or video clips from this tape (hardware: video machine light with digital player recorder, Fast, Munich, Germany). These digitalized frames or clips can be labeled or changed in any manner with image processing software (CorelDRAW). After-

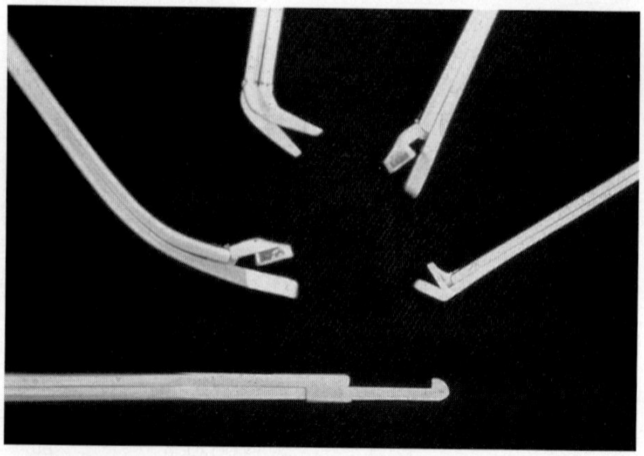

Fig. 2-10. Cutting forceps straight and upcutting in various sizes and bends, and a through-cutting punch (Courtesy of Stuemer, Würzburg, Germany).

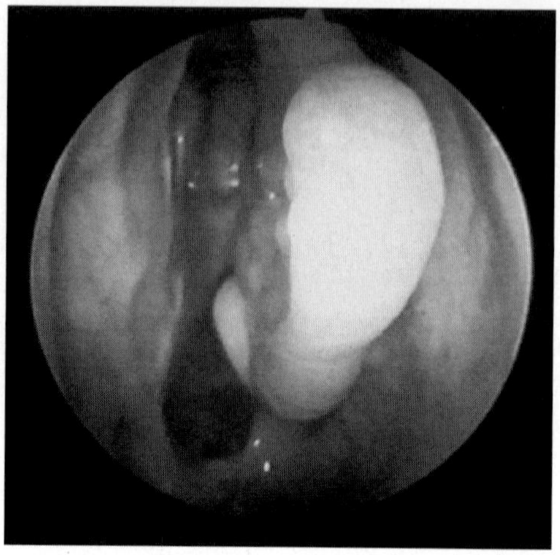

Fig. 2-11. Well-healed sinus cavity 6 months after endonasal pansinus operation (right side).

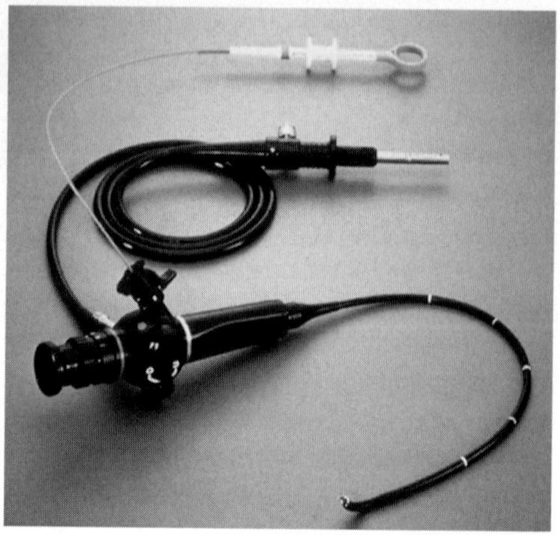

Fig. 2-12. Flexible rhinolaryngoscope ENF T3 with working channel (outside diameter 5.0 mm, bending upward and downward 130 degrees; diameter of working channel, 2.2 mm, Olympus, Hamburg, Germany).

ward, printing by an image laser printer or playing back on videotape is possible.

REFERENCES

1. Bolger WE, Kennedy DW: Changing concepts in chronic sinusitis, *Hosp Pract (Off Ed)* 27 (91) 20-22, 26-28, 1992.
2. Bolger WE, Kennedy DW: Nasal endoscopy in the outpatient clinic, *Otolaryngol Clin North Am* 25:791-802, 1992.
3. Draf W: *Endoscopy of the paranasal sinuses*, New York, 1983, Springer.
4. Kennedy DW: The role and techniques of nasal endoscopy, *Rhinol Suppl* 14:191-193, 1992.
5. Kennedy DW, Zinreich SJ, Rosenbaum AE, Johns ME: Functional endoscopic sinus surgery. Theory and diagnostic evaluation, *Arch Otolaryngol* 111:576-582, 1985.
6. Lanza DC, Kennedy DW: *Nasal endoscopy and its surgical applications.* In Lee KJ, editor: *Essential otolaryngology, head & neck surgery*, ed 6, Norwalk, Conn, 1995, Lange, pp 409-425.
7. Lanza DC, Kennedy DW: Current concepts in the surgical management of nasal polyps, *J Allergy Clin Immunol* 87:543-546, 1992.
8. Messerklinger W: Endoscopy of the nose, Baltimore, 1978, Urban & Schwarzenberg.
9. Stammberger H: Endoscopic endonasal surgery—concepts in treatment of recurring rhinosinusitis. Part II. Surgical technique. *Otolaryngol Head Neck Surg* 94:147-156, 1986.
10. Stammberger H: *Functional endoscopic sinus surgery*, Philadelphia, 1991, BC Decker.
11. Stammberger H: The role of nasal endoscopy, *Rhinol Suppl* 14:193-194, 1992.
12. Wigand ME: *Endoscopic surgery of paranasal sinuses and anterior skull base*, New York, 1990, Thieme.
13. Draf W, Weber R: *Endonasale Chirurgie der Nasennebenhöhlen—das Fuldaer mikro-endoskopische Konzept.* In Ganz H, Schätzle W, editors: *HNO Praxis Heute 12*, Berlin, 1992, Springer, pp 59-80.
14. Draf W, Weber R: Endonasal pansinusoperation in chronic sinusitis. I. Indications and operation technique, *Am J Otolaryngol Head Neck Med Surg* 14:394-398, 1993.
15. Hosemann W, Göde U, Wagner W: Epidemiology, pathophysiology of nasal polyposis, and spectrum of endonasal sinus surgery, *Am J Otolaryngol* 15:85-98, 1994.
16. Hosemann W, Göde U, Wigand ME: Indications, technique and results of endonasal endoscopic ethmoidectomy, *Acta Otorhinolaryngol Belg* 47:73-83, 1993.
17. Keerl R, Weber R, Draf W: *The endonasal pansinusoperation.* CD-ROM, St. Louis, 1996, Ullstein-Mosby.
18. Kennedy DW: Functional endoscopic sinus surgery. Technique, *Arch Otolaryngol* 111:643-649, 1985.
19. Rice DH, Schaefer SD: *Endoscopic paranasal sinus surgery*, New York, 1988, Raven Press.
20. Schaefer SD: Endoscopic total sphenoethmoidectomy, *Otolaryngol Clin North Am* 22:727-732, 1989.
21. Schaefer SD: Endoscopic frontal sinusotomy, *Op Tech Otolaryngol Head Neck Surg* 1:128-130, 1990.
22. Schaefer SD: Endoscopic sinus surgery: posterior approach, *Op Tech Otolaryngol Head Neck Surg* 1:104-107, 1990.
23. Schaefer SD, Close LG: Endoscopic management of frontal sinus disease, *Laryngoscope* 100:155-160, 1990.
24. Schaefer SD, Manning S, Close LG: Endoscopic paranasal sinus surgery: indications and considerations, *Laryngoscope* 99:1-5, 1989.
25. Stammberger H: Endoscopic endonasal surgery—concepts in treatment of recurring rhinosinusitis. Part I. Anatomic and pathophysiologic considerations, *Otolaryngol Head Neck Surg* 94:143-147, 1986.
26. Lang J: *Clinical anatomy of the nose, nasal cavity and paranasal sinuses*, New York, 1993, Thieme.
27. Becker SP: Applied anatomy of the paranasal sinuses with emphasis on endoscopic surgery, *Ann Otol Rhinol Laryngol* 103:3-32, 1994.
28. Keerl R, Weber R, Huppmann A: Darstellung zeitabhängiger Veränderungen der Nasenschleimhaut unter Einsatz modernster Morphsoftware, *Laryngorhinootologie* 74:413-418, 1995.
29. Weber R, Keerl R: Einsatz moderner Bild-Datenverarbeitung in der klinisch rhinologischen Forschung, *Eur Arch Otorhinolaryngol Suppl* I:271-296, 1996.
30. Weber R, Keerl R, Huppmann A, Schick B: Nasenpolypen und topische Kortikoidtherapie, *HNO* 3:224-228, 1995.
31. Hosemann W, Wigand ME, Goede U: Normal wound healing of the paranasal sinuses: clinical and experimental investigations, *Eur Arch Otorhinolaryngol* 248:390-394, 1991.
32. Weber R, Keerl R, Huppmann A, et al: Investigation of wound healing after paranasal sinus surgery with time lapse video—first results, *Am J Rhinol* 10:235-238, 1996.
33. Weber R, Keerl R, Huppmann A, et al: Wound healing after paranasal sinus surgery by video time lapse sequences, *Op Tech Otolaryngol Head Neck Surg* 6:237-240, 1995.
34. Weber R, Keerl R, Huppmann A, et al: The influence of after care on wound healing after endonasal sinus surgery, *Laryngorhinotologie* 75:208-212, 1996.
35. Keerl R, Weber R: Einsatz moderner Bild-Datenverarbeitung in der rhinologischen Aus- und Weiterbildung, *Eur Arch Otorhinolaryngol* Suppl I:297-315, 1996.

SECTION

TWO

RHINOLOGY

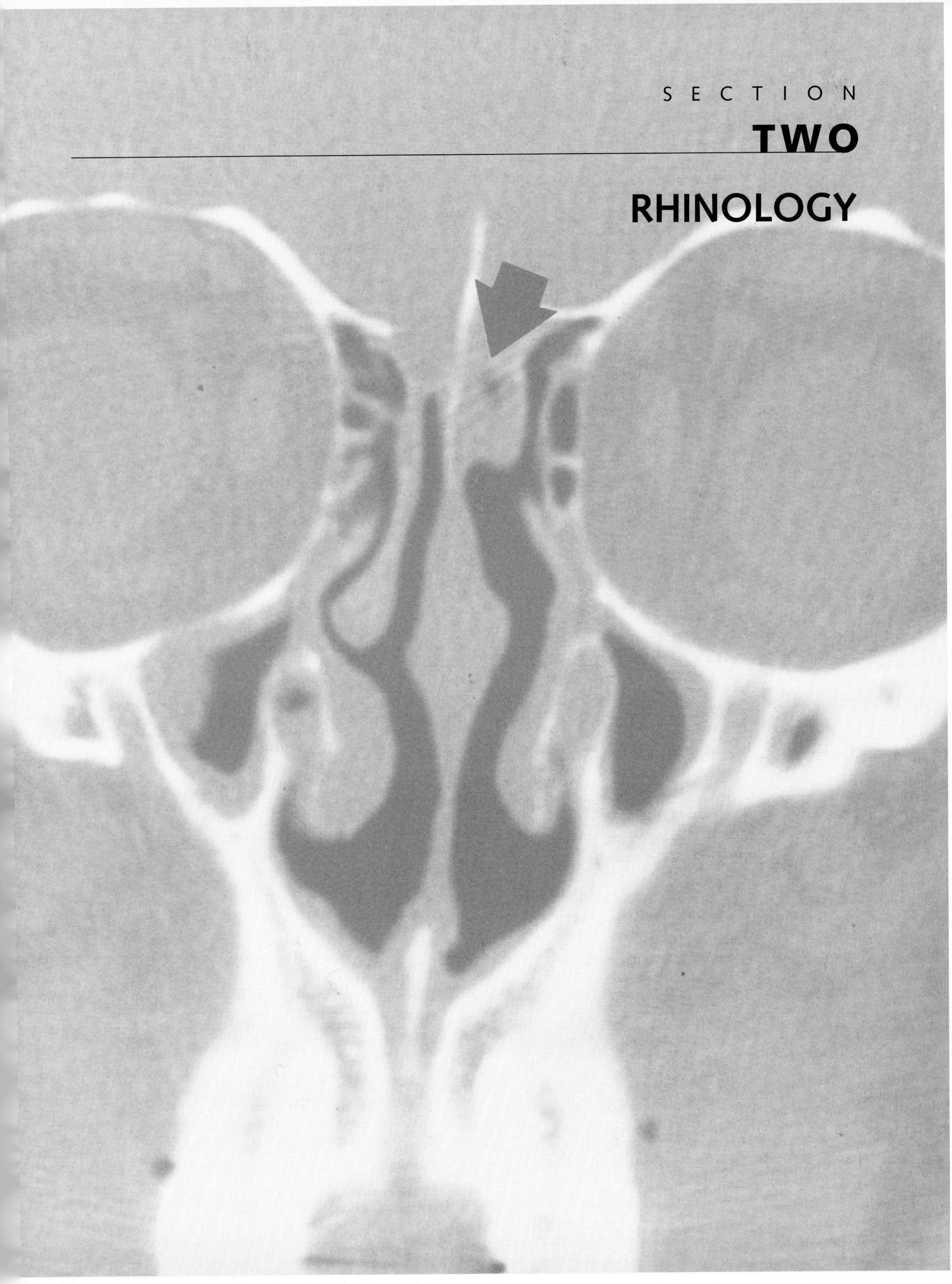

CHAPTER

3

Epistaxis

Tom I. Abelson

PROBLEM

A 67-year-old man with medication-controlled hypertension and a previous myocardial infarction presents with a long history of intermittent brief left epistaxis and a 3-day history of three episodes of right epistaxis. These episodes consist of gushing epistaxis lasting 5 to 20 minutes and are associated with expectoration of blood clots.

The scenario described above is a common presentation for patients with posterior epistaxis. This patient had been to the emergency room twice. The first time nothing was done therapeutically because the bleeding had stopped. The second time an anterior pack was placed on the right, and the left septum was cauterized. The third bleed lasted 5 minutes, and the patient's visit to the otolaryngologist's office occurred 4 hours later.

There are an endless variety of presentations of epistaxis and a plethora of ways to approach the problem. This chapter presents a common approach, a discussion of options, and the results of an informal survey of otolaryngologists.

Epistaxis is common and usually self-limited. The most common presentation is similar to the bleeding our patient has had on the left side. If seen within a few days, a site can usually be found in Little's area on the anterior septum. Topical anesthesia, vasoconstriction, cautery with silver nitrate, and instruction in nasal hygiene usually solve the problem.

At the other extreme, the patient with intractable posterior epistaxis usually presents to the emergency room. The patient is admitted with a posterior pack in place, and the subsequent course of action is determined by the success of the pack, the preference of the consulting otolaryngologist, the general medical condition of the patient, and the facilities available in the hospital.

Our patient introduces a different set of decisions, since the bleeding is severe but brief, and not active on presentation. In addition, he is in the otolaryngologist's office rather than the hospital. Thorough evaluation is indicated if for no other reason than that the recurrences are likely to continue.

MEDICAL HISTORY

A general medical history must be taken. The physician inquires about previous bleeding or bruising (at any site); the use of medications that could affect coagulation (including over-the-counter antiinflammatory drugs); hypertension; and trauma. Information about smoking and drinking habits is elicited. Specific questions are asked to try to localize the site of bleeding. For example, many patients treat epistaxis by putting their heads back or lying down. Even anterior epistaxis will flow posteriorly in this position. Ask the patient whether the blood came out of the nose or down the throat when the bleeding first began. Ask where he thinks it would have gone had he held his head in a level, upright position and not pinched the nose.

PHYSICAL EXAMINATION

Previously placed packs, if present, are removed. Topical anesthetic (4% topical lidocaine) and vasoconstrictors such as oxymetazoline (Afrin) 0.05% or phenylephrine (Neo-Synephrine) 0.5% to 1% are applied with cotton pledgets (repeatedly, if necessary) to prepare the nose for examination. Physical examination is accomplished using a headlight (or head mirror) with a nasal speculum and, if necessary, rigid (preferred) or flexible nasal endoscopes.

If the bleeding is not immediately life threatening, time should be spent obtaining adequate topical anesthesia. A comfortable patient is dramatically easier to evaluate and treat. Many patients are terrified by the idea of blood coming from within the head, since they do not understand the anatomy of the nose. The nasopharynx must be included in the examination. Hemotympanum is not uncommon in posterior epistaxis. Other signs of bruising or pale mucosa can be a sign of systemic coagulopathy, anemia, or some other hematologic abnormality. If there is any possibility of a systemic problem, a complete blood count and coagulation studies should be obtained.

RADIOLOGIC EXAMINATION

Radiology does not play a role in the evaluation of most cases of epistaxis. Sinusal, nasal, or nasopharyngeal malignancy occasionally presents with epistaxis, and appropriate radiologic evaluation is helpful. Angiography is discussed later in the context of the evaluation of posterior epistaxis and the surgical treatment or embolization of difficult sites.

The evolution of endoscopes and their presence in the office has dramatically changed our ability to identify specific sites of epistaxis and to treat them more directly. In our patient, if no site can be identified, hypertension is under control, and coagulation studies are normal, I advise him about nasal hygiene, discontinue antiinflammatory medication, and tell him to call immediately should bleeding recur. An ill or infirm patient may be admitted to the hospital for observation for 24 hours to allow prompt reevaluation and treatment if the bleeding recurs.

Our patient had a normal examination and nasal endoscopy. He was advised about nasal hygiene. He returned within 2 hours with an active bleed. Nasal endoscopy with a rigid endoscope identified an arterial bleeder under the posterior end of the inferior turbinate. This area could be suctioned and then cauterized directly with silver nitrate. Packing was not placed. The bleeding did not recur. Before the days of nasal endoscopes, this patient would most likely have been admitted for 4 days with a posterior nasal pack in place.

BLOOD SUPPLY OF THE NOSE

To serve its purpose of humidification and warming of inspired air, the mucosa of the nose has a copious blood supply. This includes branches originating with the internal and external carotid systems. The various terminal branches of both systems, including the sphenopalatine, greater palatine, superior labial, anterior ethmoid, and posterior ethmoid arteries anastomose (Kiesselbach's plexus) in the area of cartilaginous nasal septum known as Little's area, which is the most common site of epistaxis.

External carotid system

The external carotid supply consists of the external maxillary (facial) artery and the internal maxillary artery, which provide the major blood supply to the nose through the sphenopalatine artery and descending palatine artery. The internal maxillary artery is divided into three divisions (maxillary, pterygoid, and pterygopalatine) as it passes the lateral pterygoid muscle. It is in the pterygopalatine fossa, posterior to the maxillary sinus, where the terminal branches can be ligated. The six terminal branches are the posterior superior alveolar artery, infraorbital artery, artery to the foramen rotundum and pterygoid canal, pharyngeal artery, descending palatine artery, and sphenopalatine artery (Fig. 3-1).

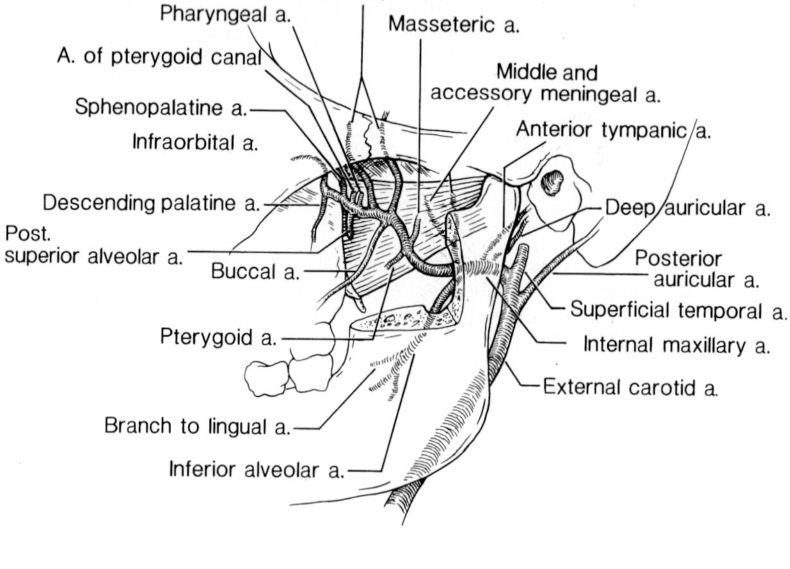

Fig. 3-1. Branches of the internal maxillary artery.

The sphenopalatine artery enters the nose through the sphenopalatine foramen at the posterior middle turbinate. It divides and supplies both the medial and lateral walls of the nasal cavity. The descending palatine artery leaves the nasal cavity through the pterygopalatine canal, supplies the palate, and returns to the nose through the incisive foramen (Figs. 3-2 and 3-3).

Internal carotid system

The internal carotid artery supplies the ethmoid arteries, which branch from the ophthalmic artery. The ophthalmic artery exits the cranial fossa, enters the orbit, and divides into several branches, including the anterior and posterior ethmoid arteries, which exit the orbit by means of canals through the frontoethmoidal suture line (Fig. 3-4). Each ethmoidal artery also divides to supply both the medial and lateral walls of the nose.

More detailed descriptions of the anatomy of the nose and blood supply are available.

ETIOLOGY OF EPISTAXIS

Local and systemic disease can cause epistaxis. Trauma can be external (e.g., fracture, surgery, foreign body), self-induced (digital), or environmental (dry heated air, allergy). Allergy and infections (viral or bacterial), septal deformity, and septal perforation can predispose to epistaxis. Tumors and granulomatous disease must be considered, even though they are unusual.

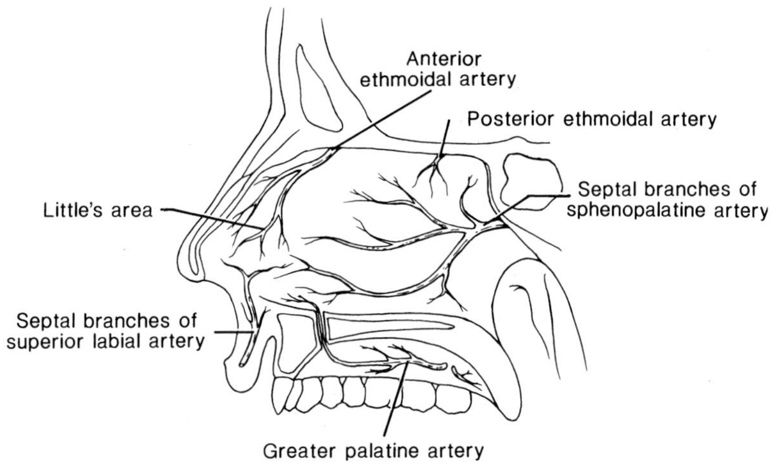

Fig. 3-2. Blood supply of the nasal septum.

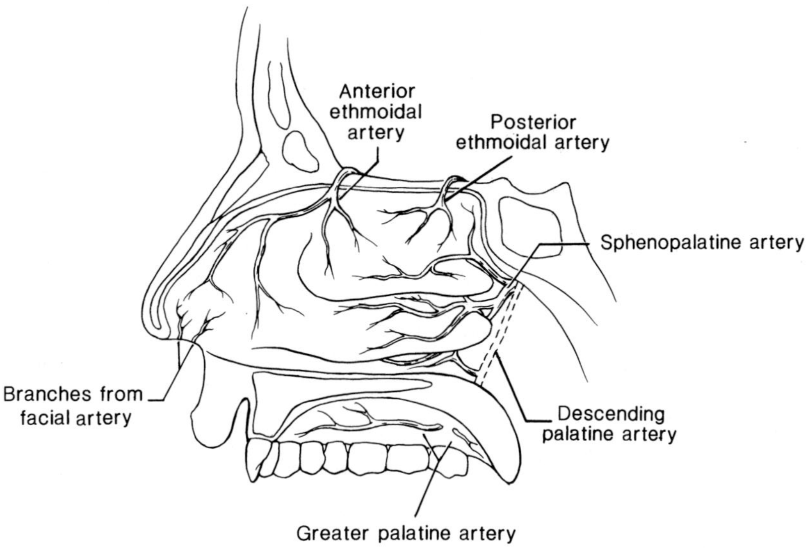

Fig. 3-3. Blood supply of the lateral wall of the nose.

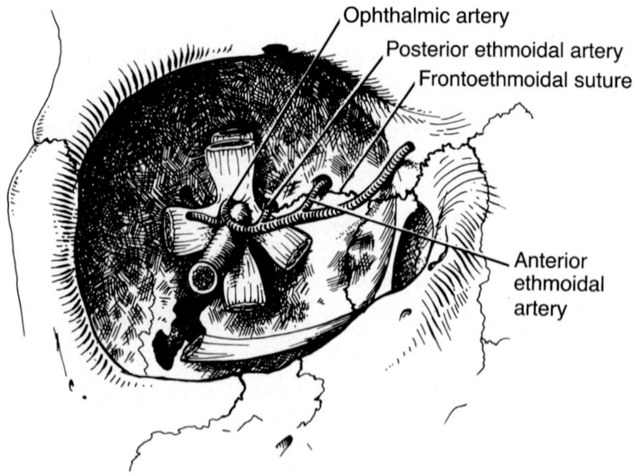

Fig. 3-4. Intraorbital view of the anterior and posterior ethmoid arteries from the ophthalmic artery.

Systemic diseases such as blood dyscrasias, hematologic malignancies, thrombocytopenia, hereditary hemorrhagic telangiectasia, leukemia, alcoholism, liver disease, and arteriosclerosis can predispose to epistaxis, as can medication-induced coagulation abnormalities such as those caused by chemotherapy, anticoagulation therapy, antiinflammatory medication, intranasal medication use, and toxin exposures. Neoplasm is unusual but should always be considered. Many cases of epistaxis fall into the idiopathic group.

TREATMENT

After the examiner has taken a complete history, assessed the general medical status of the patient, and performed a thorough head and neck examination with special attention to the nose and nasopharynx, with topical medication applied and endoscopy performed as needed, the location of the bleeding is often apparent.

Cautery

Anterior bleeding is controlled with silver nitrate cauterization. This can be accomplished comfortably only after the nose is thoroughly anesthetized topically and vasoconstricted, as described previously for nasal endoscopy. Indiscriminate use of silver nitrate is to be avoided. Some physicians use suction cautery for anterior epistaxis. Patients are told that the nose will be somewhat runny and partially obstructed for a period after the cauterization. They are advised to avoid blowing the nose—gentle sniffing is less traumatic. The mouth should be open during sneezing (some patients, especially children, sneeze fairly actively for a short time after cautery). Patients are advised to avoid physical strain for 1 week, and digital manipulation of the nose should cease. Several days after cautery, one brief period of bleeding may occur with dislocation of the eschar. Several periods of bleeding or a very active bleeding episode warrants a call to the physician. If no bleeding has occurred for 1 week, the area is probably healed.

Anterior packing

Recurrent or difficult-to-control anterior bleeding can be treated with nasal packing. It is again stressed that aggressive and thorough placement of topical anesthesia and vasoconstriction is critical to the positioning of an effective pack of any kind. The patient should be continuously reassured, and each step should be explained so that there are no surprises. It is the job of the treating physician to earn the patient's trust and cooperation.

Quarter-inch ribbon gauze impregnated with antibiotic ointment is the traditional packing material. Merocel nasal packs have the advantage of ease of insertion and can be customized so as to put pressure on a specific bleeding site. Removal of this packing material can be traumatic, however. Occasionally, absorbable packing material such as Gelfoam (gelatin), Surgicel (oxidized cellulose), and Avitene (microfibrillar collagen) can be used. This is especially useful if nasal endoscopy has localized the bleeding under the inferior turbinate. Placement of absorbable material between the bleeding site and a Merocel pack can lessen the chance of bleeding on removal of the pack. Nonabsorbable packing is left in place for 3 or 4 days. Patients with nasal packing are usually placed on a broad-spectrum antibiotic. Absorbable packing or porcine strip packing (frozen salt pork) are especially useful in patients with blood dyscrasias or on chemotherapy in whom removal of packing can reactivate the bleeding.

Posterior packing

Posterior epistaxis for which a site cannot be localized endoscopically, or bleeding that cannot be controlled by

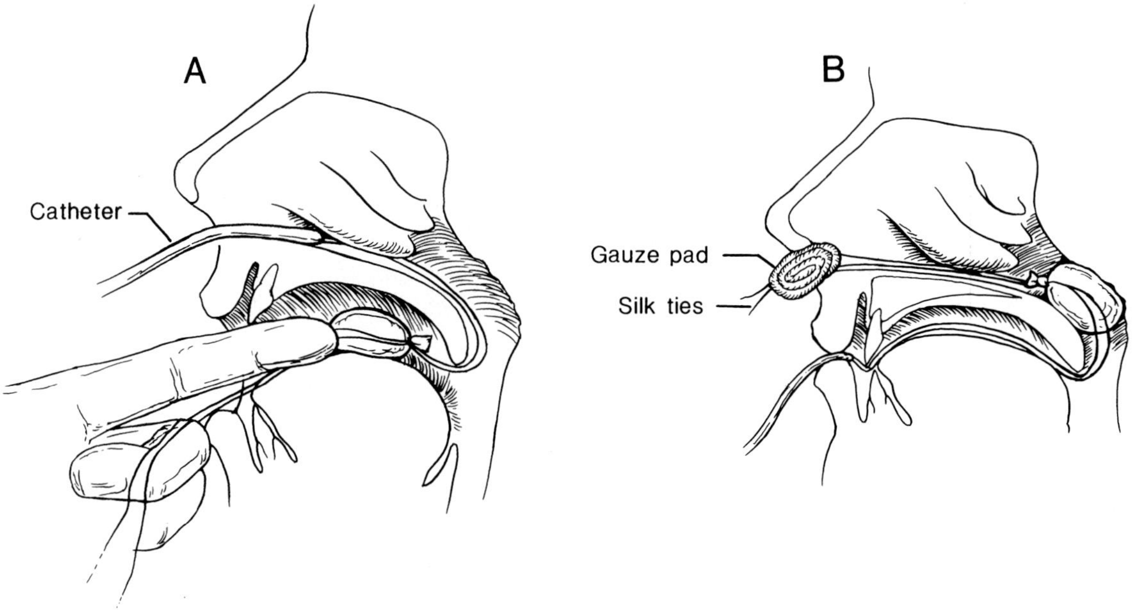

Fig. 3-5. Placement **A** and **B,** and positioning and securing of a gauze posterior nasal pack.

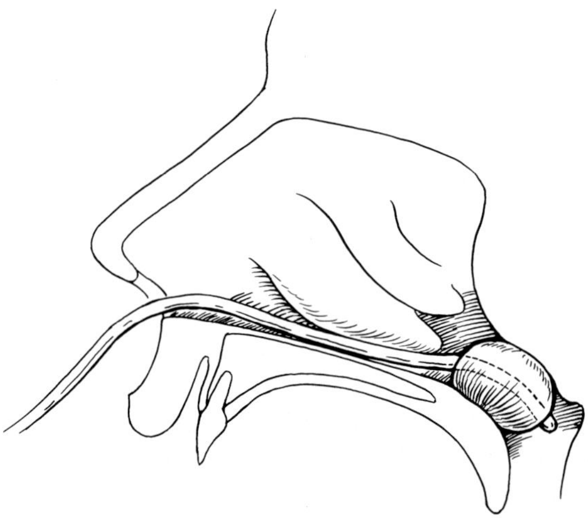

Fig. 3-6. Positioning of a balloon (Foley catheter) posterior pack.

anterior packing, can be treated with a posterior nasal pack. This may be a "classic" pack consisting of a gauze tampon placed through the mouth into the nasopharynx and held in place by a silk suture or umbilical tape brought out through the nostril (Fig. 3-5) or an inflatable balloon (Fig. 3-6). Balloon devices have become increasingly popular owing to ease of placement and are therefore the posterior pack of choice in many emergency rooms. It is stressed that the purpose of the nasopharyngeal portion of a posterior pack is usually not to put pressure on the bleeding site itself. Rather, this pack serves as a buttress to prevent anterior packing material from falling into the nasopharynx, providing more pressure on the posterior bleeding sites. Many otolaryngologists use a Foley catheter balloon as the posterior buttress, with gauze packing as the anterior portion of the pack.

Posterior packs are very uncomfortable for the patient. They have also been associated with hypoventilation and sudden death. Hospitalization is indicated for all patients with posterior packs. Many otolaryngologists admit all such patients to intensive care units for careful monitoring with oxygen by face tent or mask, continuous oxymetry, and cardiac monitoring. With the availability of oxymetry units, many patients are now admitted to step-down units or specialty care units on otolaryngologic floors. Wherever the patient is admitted, careful monitoring of general status, fluid balance, nutrition, and oxygenation is critical to his or her care.

Posterior packing is left in place for 3 to 5 days and antibiotic prophylaxis is used. The use of analgesia and sedation must be judicious because of potential side effects and hypoventilation. Other complications of posterior packing include pain, dysphagia (the pack should be large enough to fill the choana while not distorting the soft palate), eustachian tube dysfunction, infection, synechia formation, scarring of the lip or nasal ala, and recurrent bleeding. The expense of hospitalization and monitoring is also an important consideration. For these reasons some physicians consider arterial ligation the treatment of choice for posterior epistaxis; others reserve ligation for failure of packing to control epistaxis.

Examination under anesthesia

Failure of packing to control epistaxis can be caused by several factors, including inadequate placement of the pack, lack of cooperation by the patient, the severity of the bleed, and anatomic factors such as deviated septum. Under anesthesia, the septum can be straightened, endoscopy performed, and packing placed meticulously. One of the more experienced attending physicians during my residency told me he had never ligated a vessel for epistaxis, but he had not infrequently packed noses with the patients under anesthesia in order to control persistent epistaxis. Others may believe that if the patient is under anesthesia and epistaxis has not responded to previous packing, arterial ligation should be performed.

Arterial ligation

The most effective treatment for any type of bleeding is to clip or ligate the ruptured vessel immediately proximal to the bleeding site. Unfortunately, it is often difficult to identify the exact site of bleeding in severe or persistent epistaxis. There are several approaches to the ligation of arteries supplying the nasal mucosa.

Ligation of the external carotid artery. Ligation of the external carotid artery can be effective in controlling epistaxis. The anatomy is well known to head and neck surgeons, and ligation is usually performed just distal to the superior thyroid artery, both to protect the blood supply to the thyroid and to ensure ligation of the external rather than the internal carotid. The procedure can be performed quickly and, if necessary, under monitored local anesthesia. Since this ligation is far from the bleeding site, and since there is copious contralateral and internal carotid flow to the nose, this technique is not always effective. It may be combined with ligation of the ethmoidal arteries as described later.

Transantral ligation of the internal maxillary artery. Local or general anesthesia can be used for this procedure, which was popularized by Chandler and Serrins.[1] The posterior wall of the maxillary sinus is exposed through a Caldwell-Luc approach. The mucosa and bone of the posterior wall of the maxillary sinus are removed. Under microscopic control the posterior periosteum is incised, and the internal maxillary artery and its branches are identified in the surrounding fat pad. Ideally the internal maxillary artery and three of its terminal branches (the sphenopalatine, pharyngeal, and descending palatine) are interrupted with locking vascular clips.[2] This procedure ligates the vessels close to their entrance into the nasal cavity and is therefore very effective.

Transoral ligation of the internal maxillary artery. Maceri and Makielskish[3] described an approach to the internal maxillary artery through the buccal fat pad. This technique is helpful in cases of sinus trauma or chronic sinusitis. The vessel is ligated more proximately than in the transantral technique, and postoperative trismus can be troublesome.

Ligation of the ethmoidal arteries. If the epistaxis is high in the nose in areas supplied by the ethmoidal system, ligation must include clipping of the anterior, and sometimes the posterior, ethmoidal arteries. These arteries are approached through an external ethmoidectomy or Lynch incision. The anterior ethmoid artery is identified in the frontoethmoidal suture line approximately 1.5 to 2.5 cm posterior to the lacrimal crest. The orbit is retracted and the artery is cut between vascular clips. If bleeding persists, the suture line is followed posteriorly until the posterior ethmoid artery is identified. It is clipped but not ligated because it is only 4 to 7 mm anterior to the optic nerve.

Embolization

Epistaxis from the external carotid system can be localized with angiography and treated with embolization of foreign material into the vasculature. This technique is very effective when the bleeding is from areas supplied by the internal maxillary artery and when the experienced angiographer can embolize distally in the system. Facial pain and trismus are brief but frequent side effects. Serious complications include facial paralysis and stroke (from leak of material into the internal carotid system). Elden and colleagues[4] reported 82% control of epistaxis by means of embolization.

The areas of the nasal cavity supplied by the ethmoidal arteries (internal carotid supply) cannot be embolized. Although there is controversy about the timing of embolization, posterior packing, and arterial ligation, embolization is clearly the treatment of choice when other therapies fail and when there are contraindications to surgery. As will be seen in later discussion, acceptance of embolization is directly related to the experience of the treating otolaryngologist and the interventional radiologist.

TREATMENT OF HEREDITARY HEMORRHAGIC TELANGIECTASIA

Hereditary hemorrhagic telangiectasia can lead to frequent epistaxis. Treatment options include septal dermoplasty and laser surgery. Septal dermoplasty was described by Saunders.[5,6] Skin grafts are used to replace the septal, floor of nose, and turbinate mucosa. Parkin and Dixon[7,8] discussed the use of first the Nd:YAG laser and then the argon laser for treatment of the telangiectasias. Improvement, if not cure, is the rule. Retreatment is frequently necessary.

COMMUNITY SURVEY

In preparation for this chapter, I sent a survey to the members of the Northeastern Ohio Otolaryngology and Head and Neck Surgery Society. My goal was to ascertain the order in which different modes of treatment are instituted by physicians in the community, some of whom are full-time members of two academic departments and others of whom are in private community practice. I was particularly interested in the attitudes toward posterior packing versus ligation and/or embolization in intractable posterior epistaxis. Although the survey does not lend itself to scientific or statistical analysis, it does point out the variety of treatments used, and it highlights the importance of experience and the availability of ancillary support in the treatment planning for epistaxis patients.

Of 101 surveys sent out, 54 were returned. In one question, physicians were asked to list the order in which they would institute various therapeutic techniques in the case of posterior epistaxis in which they did or did not suspect involvement with the ethmoidal systems.

Balloon devices are used by more respondents than any other types of posterior packing. The next most common technique involves the use of a Foley catheter as the posterior buttress with traditional anterior packing. Fewer physicians employed the traditional gauze posterior pack as their first choice.

Given the failure of a posterior pack, unilateral ligation of the internal maxillary artery is most commonly used as the next step, with almost as many using embolization at this point. It is most interesting that of those who are comfortable with both ligation and embolization, 19 would embolize first and 17 would ligate first. A number of respondents noted in the "comments" section that they practice in institutions in which embolization is not performed by the radiologists.

At the end of the survey, comments were solicited. A number of these comments related to the unavailability of embolization in some institutions, or conversely to the ease of embolization in institutions that do not have otolaryngology residents to assist in surgery and in the postoperative care of these difficult cases.

A number of physicians specifically commented on the efficacy of the nasal endoscope in the care of epistaxis, consistent with the case presented in this chapter. Vaseline gauze and Merocel were vastly preferred to Surgicel, Telfa, cotton roll, Gelfoam, and Oxycel as packing material. In anterior epistaxis requiring packing, 11% of respondents leave the packing in place for 1 day, 27% for 2 days, 46% for 3 days, 10% for 4 days, and 5% for 5 days. Most use antibiotics in patients with packing in place; cephalosporins or amoxicillin are the most popular antibiotic choices.

ARTERIAL LIGATION VERSUS POSTERIOR PACKING VERSUS EMBOLIZATION

Whenever there are multiple techniques for treatment of a disease entity, there is controversy over the best technique.[9,10] Those who consider that posterior packing is preferable to ligation cite the avoidance of anesthesia, the cost of anesthesia and surgery, the effectiveness of packing in most cases, and the possibility of surgical complications as reasons to start with packing. Others believe that the discomfort of posterior packs, their possible complications, the cost of hospitalization, and possible failure of control suggest that ligation should be performed early.

In their retrospective review of embolization versus transantral ligation, Strong and colleagues conclude that the efficacy and cost of the two procedures are comparable and that "the choice of treatment modality should be based on the benefits of each procedure as it pertains to the specific needs of the individual patient." I would add the obvious comment that the experience of the otolaryngologist and interventional radiologist also play a key role in decision making.

SUMMARY

Epistaxis can be minimal and a nuisance ("a hassle and a mess," as I tell patients who need some reassurance for the usual anterior bleed). It can also be dramatic and life threatening. The treatment can range from simply holding the nose for 10 minutes to ligation of the ethmoid vessels after failed posterior packs and embolization of the internal maxillary artery. The protocol for treatment is dictated by the site and severity of the bleeding, as well as the experience and comfort level of the treating otolaryngologist and consultants (including anesthesiologists and radiologists). The broader the experience of the physician, the greater his or her ability to tailor the treatment to the individual needs of particular patients and or their medical conditions.

REFERENCES

1. Chandler JR, Serrins AJ: Transantral ligation of the internal maxillary artery for epistaxis, *Laryngoscope* 75:1151-1159, 1965.
2. Pearson GW, MacKenzie RG, Goodman WS: The anatomical basis of transantral ligation of the maxillary artery in severe epistaxis, *Laryngoscope* 79:969-984, 1969.
3. Maceri DR, Makielskish KH: Intraoral ligation of the maxillary artery for posterior epistaxis, *Laryngoscope* 94:737-741, 1984.
4. Elden I, Montanera W, Terbrugge K, et al: Angiographic embolization for the treatment of epistaxis: a review of 108 cases, *Otolaryngol Head Neck Surg* 111:44-50, 1994.
5. Saunders WH: Septal dermoplasty for control of nosebleeds caused by hereditary hemorrhagic telangiectasia or septal perforations, *Trans Am Acad Ophthalmol Otolaryngol* 64:500-506, 1960.

6. Saunders WH: Septal dermoplasty: ten years experience, *Trans Am Acad Ophthalmol Otolaryngol* 723:153-160, 1968.
7. Parkin JL, Dixon JA: Laser photocoagulation in hereditary hemorrhagic telangiectasia, *Otolaryngol Head Neck Surg* 89:204-208, 1981.
8. Parkin JL, Dixon JA: Argon laser treatment of head and neck vascular lesions, *Otolaryngol Head Neck Surg* 93:211-216, 1985.
9. Strong EB, Bell A, Johnson LP, Jacobs JM: Intractable epistaxis: transantral ligation vs. embolization: efficacy review and cost analysis, *Otolaryngol Head Neck Surg* 113:674-678, 1995.
10. Collie BS, Wax MK, Wetmore SJ: Epistaxis: a comparison of treatment, *Otolaryngol Head Neck Surg* 109:60-65, 1993.

CHAPTER

4

Allergic Management of Nasal Polyps

Richard L. Mabry
Hueston C. King

PROBLEM

The patient is a 42-year-old businessman who presents with a complaint of bilateral nasal congestion that has lasted about 1 year and is increasing in severity.

Nasal polyposis has been recognized for 3000 years, yet today the etiology remains a matter of conjecture. For decades, allergy was considered the primary cause of nasal polyps, based largely on the histologic picture of eosinophilic infiltration within a myxoid stroma.[1] Currently it is thought that only a small portion of nasal polyps have an allergic origin.[2-6] However, in patients with allergy, treatment of the polyps without identification and treatment of the allergic problem results in a higher incidence or recurrence.[7] Therefore it behooves the rhinologist treating a patient with polyp disease to consider allergy, both to inhalants and foods, as a contributory factor. The work-up for this may be as simple as an appropriate allergic history or as complex as skin tests or in vitro tests for inhalants and withdrawal-challenge or similar diagnostic tests for foods. Other than this the standard medical management of polyps generally follows the same lines in both allergic and nonallergic patients.

MEDICAL HISTORY

The patient is unaware of any precipitating cause for his nasal obstruction, which has been progressive and most recently constant. He denies a seasonal or diurnal fluctuation. He has experienced a loss of taste and smell and has developed snoring. He also has related slight dyspnea on exertion, without wheezing or coughing. He denies sneezing or having itchy mucous membranes but has noted progressive clear rhinorrhea. Some facial fullness has been present. He is unaware of any family history of allergy.

Patients with polyposis often develop symptoms so gradually that they are unaware of the actual time of onset, and although either infection or severe allergic challenges can act as triggers, it is unusual to obtain such a history. Patients with inhalant allergy generally have a history of typical symptoms, which may be seasonal or perennial, depending on the antigens to which they are sensitive. These symptoms include rhinorrhea, pruritus, sneezing, and nasal congestion. If asthma is a part of the symptom complex, wheezing will also be a complaint. It has been shown that a family history of allergy in both parents indicates about a 50% likelihood of allergy in the child, while one allergic parent suggests about a 25% chance.[8] However, a negative family history does not make allergy totally unlikely, and the presence of allergy in one's family is not always accurately known.

PHYSICAL EXAMINATION

The patient is mildly overweight, appears to be the stated age, and is in no distress. He is observed to be breathing through the mouth. Slight infraorbital edema is present. Pale gray polyps appear to issue from the middle meatus bilaterally, reaching the level of the insertion of the inferior turbinates. The nasal mucosa appears pale and boggy. Application of topical vasoconstrictors produces no change in the polyps and only slight shrinkage of the turbinates. The septum does not appear to be obstructing either airway. Profuse clear mucus is present in the nose. Polyps are visible in the superior portion of the choanae on mirror examination of the nasopharynx, but no true choanal polyps are present. The remainder of the ear, nose, and throat examination is unremarkable.

Depending on their size, nasal polyps may hinder respiration minimally or may totally obstruct nasal breathing, resulting in obligate mouth breathing. The patient with polyps and associated allergy may also have other allergic stigmata, such as "allergic shiners" (discolored and puffy lower eyelids), Dennie's lines (horizontal wrinkles below the lower eyelashes), and a typical "allergic salute" (rubbing the palm of the hand upward over the nasal tip). Clear rhinorrhea has more to do with polyps obstructing the normal posterior route of nasal mucus than does the presence of nasal allergy.

RADIOGRAPHIC EXAMINATION

Plain films of the patient's paranasal sinuses demonstrated bilateral antral mucosal thickening and a suggestion of ethmoid clouding, with intranasal masses corresponding to the polyps. Computed tomography (CT) confirmed disease involving the anterior ethmoids, ostiomeatal complex, and antra. The frontal and sphenoid sinuses were clear.

Patients with polyp disease may demonstrate minimal or extensive disease of the paranasal sinuses in radiographs, either plain films or CT scans. The latter are preferable because of their ability to demonstrate more accurately changes in all the sinuses; plain films are primarily helpful in diagnosis of antral and frontal disease. Magnetic resonance imaging (MRI) is rarely useful in the diagnosis of sinus and polyp disease because of a tendency to "overcall" pathology.

No radiographic finding is pathognomonic of nasal polyps associated with allergy. Extensive unilateral disease, with varying densities within the involved sinuses, often expanding to remodel or erode bony partitions, suggests allergic fungal sinusitis. This is a different entity from other types of nasal polyposis and allergy and is not a part of this discussion.

LABORATORY EXAMINATION

A nasal smear demonstrated a predominance of eosinophils. Radioallergosorbent testing (RAST) for 12 index inhalant antigens (grasses, weeds, trees, molds, dust mites) showed class V reactions for Bermuda and timothy grass, class III for ragweed and marsh elder, and class II for oak and *Dermatophagoides farinae* (dust mites).

Patients with allergic rhinitis typically are said to demonstrate a predominance (greater than 20%) of eosinophils on nasal smear.[9,10] Unfortunately, if the patient has been treated with nasal steroids, the proportion of eosinophils in the nasal secretions may be diminished, and certain forms of nonallergic rhinitis (nonallergic rhinitis–eosinophilia syndrome [NARES]) may show large numbers of eosinophils intermittently in nasal smears. As a practical matter, it is often more appropriate to simply perform specific testing for allergy.

The presence of allergen-specific immunoglobulin E (IgE) can be determined by skin testing (skin-prick test, intradermal testing) or by in vitro methods using a marker that is radioactive (RAST) or fluorometric or colorimetric (enzyme-linked immunosorbent assay [ELISA]). The skin testing method is said to be more sensitive, the in vitro method more specific; both have their proponents and detractors. It has been shown that the use of a screening panel of up to about 12 antigens provides significant information on sensitivity and specificity for inhalant allergy evaluation.[11,12]

A factor that has not been considered in the potentially allergic etiology of nasal polyps is food hypersensitivity. This may result from the lack of agreement over what constitutes food "allergy". If the definition of food allergy most widely used in the United States is accepted, the condition is limited to IgE-mediated offenders, which may be identified by RAST or skin testing. If indeed such tests have been used for foods in any of the studies reported, they have not been mentioned. Because IgE-mediated food sensitivity represents a very small percentage of adverse food reactions, such testing would not be likely to add much to the statistical picture. If, however, the definition of food allergy most commonly used in Europe (adverse reactions to food involving any aspect of the immune system) is accepted, the relationship to nasal polyps might be considerably higher.[13]

The evaluation of hypersensitivity to non–IgE-mediated foods is considerably more difficult. There is no simple test for non–IgE-mediated food reactions, and elimination and challenge, the only definitive test, is a major challenge in the case of nasal polyps. The erratic growth pattern of nasal polyps makes a cause-and-effect relationship difficult. A potentially large factor in nasal polyp production may therefore be overlooked, and there is at present no simple way to evaluate its importance. Should a simple test identifying food hypersensitivity become available, this format will be much more applicable to the average patient with nasal polyps.

Polyp formation in susceptible people in response to acetylsalicylic acid stimulation is a well-documented phenomenon, and many foods, including fresh fruits, contain significant amounts of salicylates that may induce the same reaction. The importance of these substances in naturally occurring form has not as yet been well evaluated.

TREATMENT

The patient was instructed in appropriate environmental control to avoid inciting allergens. Immunotherapy was begun for relevant antigens. Symptomatic control was sought through the use of a nonsedating antihistamine, combined with intraturbinal/intrapolyp injection of a repository corticosteroid. When the response to these measures was less than desired, dietary manipulation was instituted to avoid food classes that cross-react with grasses and weeds (cereal grains, melons, and members of the gourd family). The continued presence of symptomatic polyps necessitated surgical intervention in the form of polypectomy and functional endoscopic sinus surgery. The patient was maintained on topical nasal steroid sprays from the second to twelfth weeks after surgery, at that time they were discontinued. Allergy immunotherapy has been continued and polyps have not recurred.

It seems evident that nasal polyps have a multifactorial etiology, and therefore no single form of treatment may be expected to be uniformly effective. It does not now appear that inhalant allergy is a primary factor in many cases of nasal polyposis, but the condition may coexist and add to the patient's discomfort as well as impeding any other form of treatment. A limited form of inhalant allergy screening may therefore be considered. The physician may be guided by the patient's history in this decision. If treatment specific for IgE-mediated disease is elected, patients should be warned that the therapy will probably not affect the polyps per se but may provide ancillary help in improving their overall condition.

Control of food hypersensitivity may offer the best form of allergic management, if the patient is strongly enough motivated to cooperate. Such an approach requires a careful diary of everything eaten over a period of 14 days. Humans are habit eaters, and over this long a period of time most basic foods in the patient's diet will become evident. A new diet must then be devised containing none of the foods eaten frequently enough to be likely to affect the immune system, and the patient must agree to adhere to this diet long enough to determine whether or not any of the foods in his or her usual diet are affecting the growth of the nasal polyps. This may be a matter of a few weeks. By this time, some effect on the polyps should be visible if any is to occur, although the condition may not be fully resolved. This is a long and involved process, but considering the recurrent nature of nasal polyps and the frequent need for surgical removal, it may be worthwhile for the patient who is persistent enough to follow through. One of the authors had a patient who was able to totally clear his nose of polyps by undergoing a spring-water-only fast of several days. This sequence was repeated by the patient as needed and was uniformly effective. Several other patients have improved on similar dietary regimens, although less dramatically. A generalization from this small sample would be inappropriate, however.

The medical management of polyps involves primarily the use of corticosteroids, which may be administered orally for systemic effect, topically, or by intranasal injection. Systemic corticosteroids may be given orally, either as a predetermined tapered-dose pack or in a dosage and duration individualized by the physician. The latter is preferable, as the commercial packs often provide therapeutic levels for only a few days, while therapy for 1 or 2 weeks may be necessary to achieve adequate results. Adrenal suppression is minimized by administering the corticosteroid as a single morning dose, generally 20 to 40 mg prednisone or the equivalent to begin, and tapering this dosage gradually after the effect has been achieved. Some physicians choose to administer a single intramuscular injection or a repository steroid, but these may result in suppression of endogenous cortisol production for up to 4 weeks or more.[14] Even low doses of systemic corticosteroids, administered over long periods of time, may produce adverse systemic effects.[15]

Topical steroids are helpful to prevent recurrence of nasal polyps. However, because large polyp masses generally prevent the sprays from gaining access to the involved mucosa, they are much less helpful than systemic administration or intranasal injection in such situations. One exception is seen in the work of Lildholdt and colleagues,[16] who used budesonide drops applied in the head-down, Moffat position to achieve polyp regression over a period of 2 to 3 months.

Intraturbinal and intrapolyp injections are extremely technique sensitive, and temporary or permanent visual loss has been reported in rare instances as a result of retinal vessel vasospasm or embolization related to the injected material. Although the reader is strongly encouraged to study the published technique for performing injections before attempting the maneuver, it has been extremely effective in the hands of one of the authors.[17] After application of a topical vasoconstrictor/anesthetic, the injection must be placed just beneath the mucosa of the inferior turbinates at their anterior tip, using only gentle pressure. Direct intrapolyp injection is also possible, but frequently the material rapidly leaks out of the injection site. Therefore, it has been preferable to place about 0.3 ml of injected material into each turbinate, and the balance into the depth of the largest polyp mass.

The definitive treatment of inhalant allergy by appropriate immunotherapy does not usually yield immediately recognizable beneficial results. However, such treatment, in patients in whom atopy is a contributory factor to polyp disease, definitely diminishes the likelihood of polyp reformation.[18]

DISCUSSION

Statistically there is minimal, if any, correlation between systemic allergy and nasal polyposis. This is not to indicate that the two cannot be related in any way. The nasal polyp is an edematous protuberance of the nasal mucosa, usually occurring initially in the ethmoid labyrinth and being propelled mechanically into the nasal cavity. Although the initiating factors are still obscure, it is not unreasonable to consider any source of insult affecting the nasal mucosa, be it allergy, infection, or mechanical, as capable of aggravating the condition. On the basis of current studies, however, allergy cannot be considered the primary cause of most nasal polyps.

Alternative hypotheses include mucosal allergy,[19] in which the allergic reaction is confined to the mucosa of the structure involved; a divergent pattern of T-cell production and activity[20]; and an altered cytokine production.[21] All have good supporting studies, based strongly on the fact that laboratory analysis of the cells and fluid directly related to the nasal polyps differs markedly from studies made on the patient's blood. This finding, although conducive to inspiring further investigation, offers little guidance to the clinician concerned with assessing current approaches to treatment.

CONCLUSION

Only a few patients with nasal polyps have significant contributory allergy. However, in these cases, appropriate management of the hypersensitivity, whether to inhaled allergens or ingested substances, generally lessens the likelihood of recurrent polyps. In a few situations, appropriate allergy therapy actually results in resolution of symptomatic polyps. In either instance, definitive therapy should be continued even after symptomatic improvement.

REFERENCES

1. Hansel FK: *Allergy of the nose and paranasal sinuses,* St. Louis, 1936, Mosby, pp. 131-135.
2. Mygind N: *Essential allergy*, Oxford, 1986, Blackwell Scientific Publications, pp 324-325.
3. Drake-Lee AB, Pitcher-Wilmott RW: A clinical profile and recurrence of nasal polyps, *J Laryngol Otol* 98:783-787, 1984.
4. Settipane GA, Chaffee FH: *Nasal polyps in asthma with rhinitis: a review of 6037 patients,* J Allergy Clin Immunol 59:17-21, 1977.
5. Caplin I, Haynes TJ, Spahn J: Are nasal polyps an allergic phenomenon?, *Ann Allergy* 29:631-634, 1971.
6. Slavin RG: Allergy is not a significant cause of nasal polyps, *Arch Otolaryngol Head Neck Surg* 118:343, 1992.
7. Mabry RL: Does allergy play a role in nasal polyposis?, *Allergies Otolaryngol* 1:2-6, 1993.
8. Mygind N: *Essential allergy*, Oxford, 1986, Blackwell Scientific Publications, pp 51-53.
9. Krause HF: *Otolaryngic allergy and immunology*, Philadelphia, 1989, WB Saunders, pp 116-121.
10. Mullarkey MF, Hills JS, Well DR: Allergic and non-allergic rhinitis: their characterization with attention to the meaning of nasal eosinophils, *J Allergy Clin Immunol* 63:122-126, 1980.
11. King WP: Efficacy of a screening radioallergosorbent test, *Arch Otolaryngol* 108:781-786, 1982.
12. Lehr AJ, Mabry RL, Mabry CS: The screening RAST: is it a valid concept?, *Otolaryngol Head Neck Surg* 117:54-55, 1997.
13. King HC: Exploring the maze of adverse reactions to foods, *Ear Nose Throat J* 73:237-241, 1994.
14. Mikhail GR, Livingood CS, Mellinger RC, et al: Effect of long-acting parenteral corticosteroids on adrenal function, *Arch Dermatol* 100:263-268, 1969.
15. Saag KG, Koehnke R, Caldwell JR, et al: Low dose long-term corticosteroid therapy in rheumatoid arthritis: an analysis of serious adverse effects, *Am J Med* 96:115-123, 1994.
16. Lildholdt T, Fogstrup J, Gammelgaard N, et al: Management of nasal polyps by steroid nose drops, *Am J Rhinol* 5:25-27, 1991.
17. Mabry RL: Corticosteroids in otolaryngology: intraturbinal injection, *Otolaryngol Head Neck Surg* 91:717-720, 1983.
18. Mabry RL: Does nasal allergy play a role in nasal polyposis? *Allergies Otolaryngol*, 1:2-6, 1993.
19. Shatkin JS, Delsupehe KG, Thisted RA, Corey JP: Mucosal allergy in the absence of systemic allergy in nasal polyposis and rhinitis: a meta-analysis, *Otolaryngol Head Neck Surg* 111:553-556, 1994.
20. Liu CH, Shun CT, Hsu MM: Lymphocyte subsets and antigen-specific IgE antibody in nasal polyps, *Ann Allergy* 72:19-24, 1994.
21. Miller CH, Pudiak DR, Hatem F, Looney RJ: Accumulation of interferon gamma-producing TH1 helper T cells in nasal polyps, *Otolaryngol Head Neck Surg* 111:51-58, 1994.

CHAPTER

5

Septoplasty: Its Place in Modern Management of Chronic Nasal and Sinus Obstructive Disease

Paul H. Toffel

PROBLEM

A 32-year-old Caucasian male presents with a several-year history of unrelenting chronic nasal obstruction associated with intermittent long and progressive bouts of rhinosinusitis. He has associated purulent postnasal discharge and marked episodes of central facial cephalgia. He also has a history of sports-related nasal trauma as a youth, and his nasal pyramid is crooked to the right. Nasal examination and endoscopy reveal a markedly bowed nasal septum to the right, huge middle turbinates filling the superior nasal vault, and a nasal pyramid deflected markedly to the right. There is purulent drainage and some inflammatory polyposis egressing from the right ostiomeatal complex. Coronal nasal/sinus computed tomography (CT) confirms the nasal physical findings and reveals right polypoid ethmoidal mucosal disease.

This case presents the multifaceted analysis required of the modern rhinologic and endoscopic nasal surgeon to determine the elements contributing to the patient's pathologic condition. Septal deformity may be a substantial portion of the problem, but by no means would it be the only element.[1] The place of septal deformity correction in the management of complex nasal obstruction cases such as this is the theme of this chapter.

Surgical rhinology has undergone substantial technical advances worldwide over the past two decades. This is primarily the result of the splendid diagnostic and management techniques proposed by our European endoscopic colleagues.[2-5] The management of all aspects of functional rhinology and sinusology has evolved toward anatomically specific diagnosis of obstructive pathologic conditions by the introduction of direct coronal CT imaging and the concurrent development of precision endoscopic, diagnostic, and surgical techniques.[1, 7-10] Thanks to integration of methods pioneered by Messerklinger in Austria[3,4] and Wigand in Germany[5] during the 1970s, all modern nasal surgeons can now analyze nasal and sinus anatomic defects with road-map clarity by means of CT scans and then combine the best of endoscopic techniques with traditional rhinologic surgery to correct pathologic conditions with a specificity, precision, and security never before achievable.

My method of management of the septal deformity as an element of the total picture of chronic anatomic nasal obstruction represents a distillation of traditional rhinologic, endoscopic, and (when appropriate) open rhinoplastic techniques.

INITIAL EVALUATION OF CHRONIC NASAL AND SINUS OBSTRUCTIVE DISEASE

Medical history

When a patient presents with a chief complaint of unrelenting chronic nasal obstruction, a thorough history is taken to determine whether the problem is related to allergies or is truly mechanical and chronic and has failed to respond to previous medical and allergy therapies.

It is important to seek out symptoms of central facial pain or pressure and chronic purulent postnasal discharge, since these are key indicators of both ostiomeatal complex (OMC) and nasal obstruction. It is also important to determine whether the patient has experienced any episodes of smoldering or recurrent purulent rhinosinusitis. A history of nasal trauma is always pertinent.

Physical examination

Thorough anterior rhinoscopy and nasal endoscopy are accomplished in concert with the remainder of the otorhinolaryngologic examination. It is important to perform anterior rhinoscopy and endoscopy after application of a shrinking agent, to allow the best possible inspection of anatomic structures. One should not forget, however, to note the anatomic appearances *before* shrinkage, since this is the patient's physiologic state and should be given due consideration. I look for the degrees of nasal pyramid abnormalities, septal deviation and spurs, nasal valve encroachment, inferior and middle turbinate hypertrophy, and potential encroachment of the key ostiomeatal outflow tract area between the anterior middle turbinate and lateral wall of the nose. Also noted are any purulent discharge, polyposis, or tumefaction within the nasal cavity. The septal deformity may represent only a portion of the anatomic problems that can chronically obstruct the nose and sinuses.

Limited ostiomeatal coronal nasal and sinus CT scans

The coronal nasal and sinus CT scan is essential for precise identification of anatomic variants that obstruct the nose and sinuses and their interface, the ostiomeatal tract.[6] Advances in CT imaging clearly demonstrate previously hidden and unappreciated nasal and sinus pathology.[7] A limited (approximately 15-slice) CT scan can be done at a markedly reduced cost while still providing detailed information regarding nasal and sinus anatomy and pathology. Radiologists provide these films at only slightly more than the cost of regular sinus x-rays and with no greater radiation exposure. Regular sinus x-rays may be considered nearly obsolete compared with value of these cost-effective CT studies.

Confirmation of substantial nasal pyramid or valve, septal, turbinate, ostiomeatal tract, or sinus pathology warrants consideration of anatomy-specific traditional and/or endoscopic nasal and sinus surgery. Contributing septal deformities are usually corrected as part of this protocol.[1,10]

Medical treatment

Even in the face of substantial mechanical obstructive nasal and sinus factors, an attempt at therapeutic medical control should be made in all patients. This must also be continued after new surgical or endoscopic mechanical therapy in an attempt to prevent recurrent disease.[1]

Medical management usually combines topical and systemic corticosteroids, antihistamines, decongestants, periodic antibiotics, and (in some cases) allergy desensitization and immune analysis and therapy in order to shrink hypertrophic membranes contributing to mechanical obstruction. When (1) all possible medical management fails to help the patient and (2) the combination of history, physical examination, and CT evaluation indicates persistent and significant obstructive factors involving the septum, nasal pyramid, nasal valve, turbinates, or ostiomeatal tract or sinus hypertrophy, combined rhinologic and/or endoscopic anatomy-specific surgery is warranted. Typically, many of these factors contribute to the disease process, and correction of the septum will be carried out in conjunction with other necessary anatomic corrections. The septal deformity is rarely an isolated cause of chronic unrelenting nasal obstruction.[1]

Surgical and endoscopic technique for chronic nasal and sinus obstructive disease

The combination of history, physical examination (including diagnostic endoscopy), and limited OMC coronal CT will identify those patients who might benefit from surgical correction of anatomic functional deformities. In any given patient, the obstruction anatomy may vary from simple septal deviation to turbinate hypertrophy, polyposis, nasal pyramid deflection, OMC obstruction, sinus polyposis, or any combination thereof. The specific abnormalities determine the logical order for the correction.[1,7-10]

The technical aspects of simultaneous endoscopic and rhinologic surgery are facilitated by the wearing of a narrow-beam fiberoptic headlight throughout the endoscopic aspects of the procedure. This single feature allows easy flow back and forth between endoscopic and normal rhinologic surgery at any time necessary during the overall procedure, allowing surgeons to easily use all tools in their armamentarium.[7,9]

Septoplasty is usually performed first, but if hypertrophied turbinates do not allow space for a repositioned septum, these should be corrected first on the more obstructed side. Often if a concha bullosa exists with a huge middle turbinate also obstructing the ostiomeatal tracts, it is easier to conclude the endoscopic sinus surgery in conjunction with middle turbinate correction before proceeding to the septal work; sinus endoscopy can then be performed on the opposite side after septal repositioning has opened that ethmoid cleft for better access. Nasal polyposis requires excision before anything can be accomplished, and usually the nasal pyramid work is saved for last.

The main point of the concept of secure endoscopic sinus surgery as an adjunct to functional nasal surgery is that whatever is required can be done in the hands of a competent rhinologic and endoscopic surgeon, at one setting, and in whatever order indicated by the specific anatomy and pathologic condition. Appropriate technique also allows rhinoplasty to be comfortably performed in conjunction with endoscopic surgery if indicated or requested.[10]

SEPTOPLASTY

The surgical anatomy of the nasal septum is beautifully illustrated in two outstanding contemporary atlases: *Clinical anatomy of the nose, nasal cavity* and *paranasal sinuses* by Professor Dr. Johannes Lang of the University of Wurzburg, Germany; and *Surgical anatomy of the nose* by Dr. M. Eugene Tardy, Jr, and colleagues of the University of Illinois.[11,12] I have had the honor of meeting and observing both of these outstanding scholars and have found my surgical career shaped by the clear and precise understanding of complex anatomy that they convey. The nasal and sinus surgeon should have both these atlases readily available for reference regarding septal surgery.

Septal anatomy

Drawing upon Dr. Tardy's atlas, we find that the septum divides the nasal chambers into two cavities, lends critical support to the bony and cartilaginous vault, forms a wall on which the all-important functioning mucous membrane is draped, and aids in air flow through the nose.[12]

The septum is dealt with in the most obstructive nasal and sinus operations, with correction ranging from a simple repositioning of moderate, caudal, or cephalic deflection to a major total septal reconstruction. Furthermore, because the septum represents the central keystone of nasal support, a thorough understanding of its anatomy, physiology, and relationship to the surrounding interconnected nasal anatomy is critical. The most functional endoscopic sinus result is not successful if a satisfactory nasal airway is not preserved or created by appropriate septal surgery.[13]

The anatomic components of the septum include the nasal process of the frontal bone, the perpendicular plate of the ethmoid, a portion of the medial segments of the nasal bones, the vomer and crest of the sphenoid, the nasal crest of the palatine bone, the nasal crest and spine of the maxilla, the quadrangular cartilage, the medial upper lateral cartilages, and the membranous septum (Fig. 5-1).[11,12]

The vomer and ethmoid plates, along with the maxillary crest, are the segments of bony septum that are of principal interest to the nasal surgeon. Lying between the cribriform plate above and the vomer below, the perpendicular plate of the ethmoid is also in contact with the undersurface of the nasal bones and the posterior surface of the sphenoid crest. Significant deviations or widening of the perpendicular plate of the ethmoid contribute to posterior superior airway obstruction, which may encroach into the ethmoid clefts. This deviated condition, if unrecognized, can also be responsible for postoperative airway obstruction where none existed previously after nasal pyramid reduction, as in rhinoplasty. Segmental excision of the offending perpendicular plate during septoplasty prevents these potential complications. Patients are also encountered in whom the ethmoid perpendicular plate is inordinately wide (up to 5 to 6 mm) and even pneumatized; adequate resection again is necessary to prevent potential postoperative airway blockage with endoscopic sinus procedures.

The vomer forms the basis of the bony septum, articulating above to the perpendicular plate of the ethmoid, below with the nasal crest of the maxilla and palantine bone, behind with the crest of the sphenoid, and in front with the quadrangular cartilage. The vomer is often deviated or projected into the nasal airway as spurs, existing independent of, or in concert with, enlarged deviated crests of the maxilla. A tongue of quadrangular cartilage is insinuated between the vomer and perpendicular plate

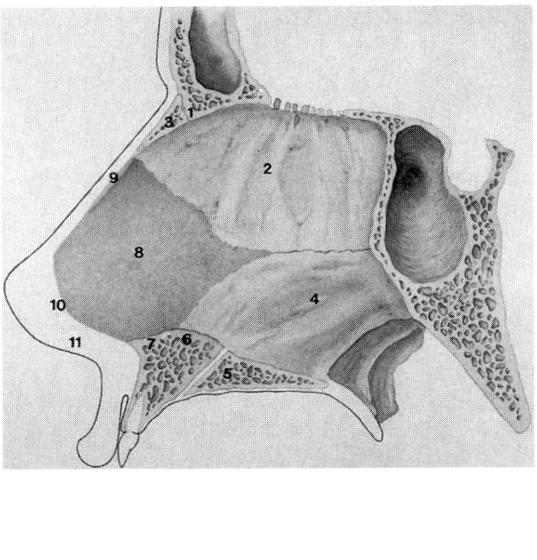

Fig. 5-1. *1,* Nasal process of frontal bone. *2,* Perpendicular plate of ethmoid bone. *3,* Nasal bone. *4,* Vomer bone. *5,* Palatine bone. *6,* Maxillary crest. *7,* Nasal spine. *8,* Quadrangular cartilage. *9,* Upper lateral cartilage. *10,* Caudal margin quadrangular cartilage. *11,* Membranous septum. (From Tardy ME Jr., et al: *Surgical anatomy of the nose,* New York, 1990; Raven Press.)

of the ethmoid posteriorly for a variable distance. Nasal bone grafts are occasionally derived from vomerine segments harvested during septoplasty.[11,12]

The quadrangular cartilage is the most important surgical component of the septum providing midline support to the nose; when significantly deformed, it requires reconstruction and realignment to preserve as much of its integrity as possible. It is preferable to perform as conservative a dissection and realignment of the septal cartilage as possible, to avoid a major sacrifice of nasal cartilage, which may conceivably be invaluable later in life if needed for further reconstruction.

The mucoperichondrium enveloping the quadrangular cartilage is inserted into the bony-cartilaginous articulation with the maxillary crest at the base of the septum, into which the mucoperiosteum covering the bony nasal floor is also inserted. Gaining access to the bony septal floor for reconstruction may necessitate the elevation and bringing into continuity of two subperichondrial and mucoperiosteal flaps by sharp or semisharp dissection ("superior and inferior tunnels"), the so-called *maxillary-premaxillary approach* to the nasal septum. Most reconstructive septal operations may be performed with adequate access by elevating only a single mucoperichondrial flap alongside the quadrangular cartilage, brought into continuity with both mucoperiosteal flaps flanking the perpendicular plate of the ethmoid and vomer by blunt disarticulation of the osseocartilaginous junction of the cartilage and bony septum (Fig. 5-2).[12]

Of practical surgical consequence is the fact that the portion of the septum anterior to the piriform aperture represents the significant supportive function of the nose; a vertical line drawn from the dorsal junction of the nasal bones and quadrangular cartilage through the nasal spine will delineate that anterior portion of the nasal septum that provides principal support from that portion posteriorly that does not (Fig. 5-3).[11,12] Structures posterior to this line participate minimally in nasal support and, can therefore, be sacrificed with less concern than cartilaginous structures anterior to it.

Surgical septal method

In my personal method of septoplasty, I may vary from minimal endoscopic resection of localized spurs or deflections adjacent to the middle turbinates and OMC, in functional sinus cases; to traditional full, but gentle, headlight dissection for greater deformities; to open rhinoplastic approach to the septum for grossly deformed and twisted cases.

Usually I place a hemitransfixation incision on the side of the greater septal pathology and elevate only one mucoperichondrial flap. After removing an inferior strip of quadrilateral cartilage and any deviated portion of the maxillary crest, I separate the cartilaginous and bony septum, using bilateral mucoperiosteal flaps posterior to the junction area (Fig. 5-2). I remove deflections along the vomerine-ethmoid suture line and reduce the thickened keystone area of septum near the bony-cartilaginous confluence with biting forceps or micro-osteotomes (2-mm, 3-mm, unguarded), being careful to eliminate the buckling torque commonly found at the junction area (Fig. 5-4).

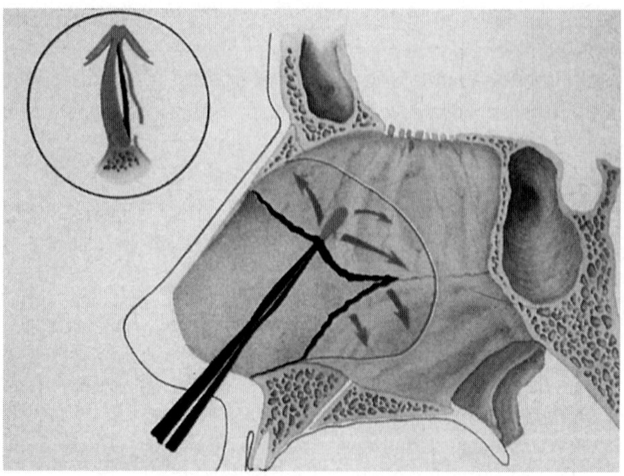

Fig. 5-2. Disarticulation of the quadrangular cartilage–perpendicular plate junction by blunt dissection: a fundamental preliminary exercise in realignment of most deviated septums. (From Tardy ME Jr., et al: Reconstructive surgery of the deviated nasal septum and nose. Monograph, Instruction Course of the American Academy of Otolaryngology–Head and Neck Surgery, New Orleans, 1982.)

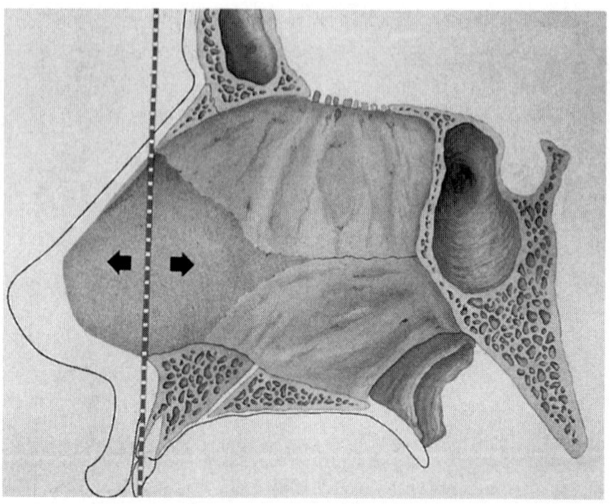

Fig. 5-3. The septal skeleton, posterior to the dotted line dropped from the dorsal osseocartilaginous junction to the spine, contributes very little to support of the external nose, in contradistinction to that portion distal to the line. (From Tardy ME Jr.: *Surgical anatomy of the nose,* New York, 1990, Raven Press.)

I work deeply on the septum in the posterior region, removing spurs and infracturing the ethmoid plate carefully, if necessary. Correction of posterior septal pathology is greatly aided by using an intense fiberoptic headlight placed between the eyes and/or endoscopic visualization. I manage deflected septal cartilage by additional maneuvers of shaving, scoring, and excising alternating strips. I close the hemitransfixion incision with through-and-through 4-0 chromic sutures on a small straightened needle, and I quilt the mucoperichondrial flaps to prevent septal hematoma. I do not place extra incisions in the flaps for drainage; rather, I use a light dressing system of Merocel sponges for several days, with silicon-flanged airway tubes for postoperative respiration. This is done under cover of postoperative cephalosporin antibiotics. This gives excellent septal results without postoperative widening, and negligible synechiae formation when septal surgery is combined with endoscopic sinus procedures.[9]

Surgical management of the case

As shown in the CT scans, this patient had severe septal deflection in conjunction with other anatomic obstructions, including enlarged middle turbinates with concha bullosae formation and secondary hyperplastic ethmoidal sinusitis (Fig. 5-5). He was managed with the following (Fig. 5-6):

- Gentle general anesthesia supplemented with local anesthesia.
- Combined one-stage endoscopic and fiberoptic headlight management of the septal, nasal pyramid, turbinate, and OMC pathology.
- Merocel sponge of the OMC and septal areas, with airway tubes, removed with brief anesthesia and careful debridement 5 to 7 days later, under cover of cephalosporin antibiotics.

Results

Of 1168 consecutive septoplasties performed between 1986 and 1996, 97% resulted in permanent correction, in conjunction with other anatomic corrections in most cases, as turbinate modification or OMC endoscopy.

I have found no difficulty in combining gentle septoplasty, whether traditional, endoscopic, or open technique, with any other indicated rhinologic or endoscopic

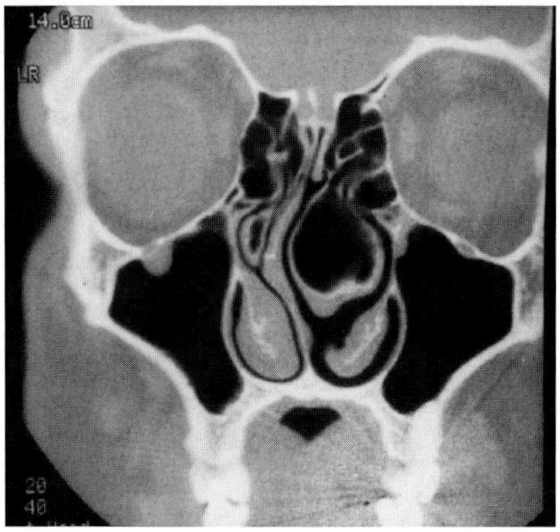

Fig. 5-5. Preoperative computed tomography (CT) of the presented patient.

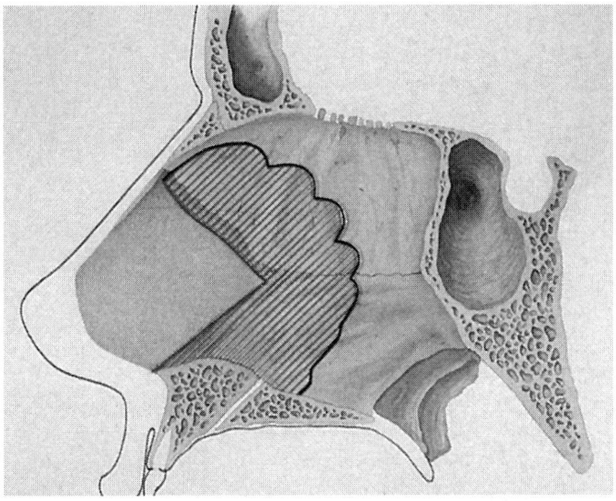

Fig. 5-4. Typical extent of bony septal vomerine and ethmoid plate resection, and cartilaginous excision along the maxillary crest, which eliminates the major buckling torque at the bony cartilaginous junction. (From Tardy ME Jr., et al: Reconstructive surgery of the deviated nasal septum and nose. Monograph, Instruction Course of the American Academy of Otolaryngology–Head and Neck Surgery, New Orleans, 1982.)

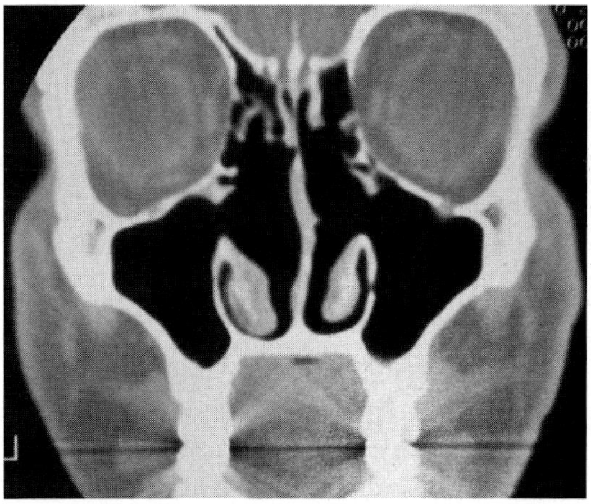

Fig. 5-6. Six-month postoperative CT of the presented patient.

procedure. Whatever technique is used, the key is always gentle handling of the tissues.

REFERENCES

1. Toffel PH: *Chronic nasal obstruction.* In Gates GA, editor: *Current therapy in otolaryngology–head and neck surgery*, vol 4, Philadelphia, 1990; BC Decker, pp 283-287.
2. Kennedy DW: Functional endoscopic sinus surgery, technique, *Arch Otolaryngol Head Neck Surg* 3:643-649, 1985.
3. Kennedy DW, et al: Functional endoscopic sinus surgery, theory and diagnostic evaluation, *Arch Otolaryngol Head Neck Surg* 3:576-582, 1985.
4. Stammberger H. Endoscopic endonasal surgery; concepts in the treatment of recurring rhinosinusitis. II. Surgical technique, *Otolaryngol Head Neck Surg* 94:147-156, 1986.
5. Wigand ME, et al: Endonasal sinus surgery with endoscopic control; from radical operation to rehabilitation of the mucosa, *Endoscopy* 10:255-260, 1978.
6. Zinreich SJ, et al: Paranasal sinuses: CT imaging requirements for endoscopic surgery, *Radiology* 163:769-775, 1987.
7. Toffel PH, et al: Secure endoscopic sinus surgery as an adjunct to functional nasal surgery, *Arch Otolaryngol Head Neck Surg* 115:822-825, 1989.
8. Toffel PH: Endoscopic surgery in chronic sinus disease, *J Respir Dis* 12:546-548, 1991.
9. Toffel PH: *Nasal polyposis.* In Gates GA, editor: *Current therapy in otolaryngology–head and neck surgery*, vol 5, Philadelphia, 1994, BC Decker, pp 383-391.
10. Toffel PH: American Academy of Otolaryngology–Head and Neck Surgery Instruction Courses. In Johnson JT, editor: vol 5, St. Louis, Mosby, 5:165-171, 1992.
11. Lang J: *Clinical anatomy of the nose, nasal cavity and paranasal sinuses*, Stuttgart, 1989, Georg Thieme Verlag.
12. Tardy ME Jr. et al: *Surgical anatomy of the nose*, New York, 1990, Raven Press.
13. Tardy ME Jr., et al: Reconstructive surgery of the deviated nasal septum and nose. Monograph, Instruction Course of the American Academy of Otolaryngology–Head and Neck Surgery, New Orleans, 1982.

CHAPTER

6

Endoscopic Management of Cerebrospinal Fluid Rhinorrhea

Steven D. Schaefer

PROBLEM

A 46-year-old man presents with a 5-month history of clear, left-sided rhinorrhea after intranasal sinus surgery.

Cerebrospinal fluid (CSF) rhinorrhea may be noted at the time of sinus surgery or after such surgery or head trauma. The diagnosis and management of CSF rhinorrhea in the acute and the chronic condition have important similarities and differences. The treatment of such patients is outlined in Fig. 6-1.

MEDICAL HISTORY

Patients with clear rhinorrhea after sinus surgery or head trauma should be evaluated for CSF rhinorrhea. The history may reveal other signs of an intracranial communication that may or may not be apparent or associated with the injury by the patient. Such signs may include a history of headache, meningismus, unexplained fever, or meningitis. The author has treated patients who were unaware of the significance of such signs after previous surgery. At revision surgery, these patients were found to have evidence of an intracranial fistula.

Further questioning of the patient cited above revealed that he had been readmitted to the hospital several days after endoscopic ethmoidectomy for CSF rhinorrhea. At that admission, a lumbar drain was placed for several days, and after discharge the patient had persistent CSF rhinorrhea. Three months postoperatively he was treated at another hospital for bacterial meningitis. Magnetic resonance (MR) imaging during this admission showed a tract from the roof of the left ethmoid sinus into the frontal lobe of the brain. The patient fully recovered from meningitis. Review of the initial surgical records revealed that during the left anterior ethmoidectomy, CSF was noted draining from the lateral aspect of the anterior third of the left middle turbinate. The surgeon had attempted to repair the fistula with a middle turbinate flap.

PHYSICAL EXAMINATION

A complete head and neck examination should be performed. Such an examination can also help identify other signs of potential injuries or complications from the previous surgery or head trauma. Examination of the nose should be performed with a rigid 0- and 30-degree endoscope. During nasal endoscopy, the current state of the nose and sinuses should be evaluated, the site of the fistula localized, and the potential mechanism of injury assessed. Physical examination of patients with presumed chronic CSF rhinorrhea should be directed toward establishing the existence and identification of the site of the fistula. In patients without obvious rhinorrhea, evidence of a fistula can be elicited by placing them in what is called the *provocative position.* This consists of having patients place the head immediately above the knees while sitting in a chair. After 5 minutes, most patients with clinical CSF rhinorrhea show evidence of drainage from the nose. Any clear fluid draining from the nose can be collected and ana-

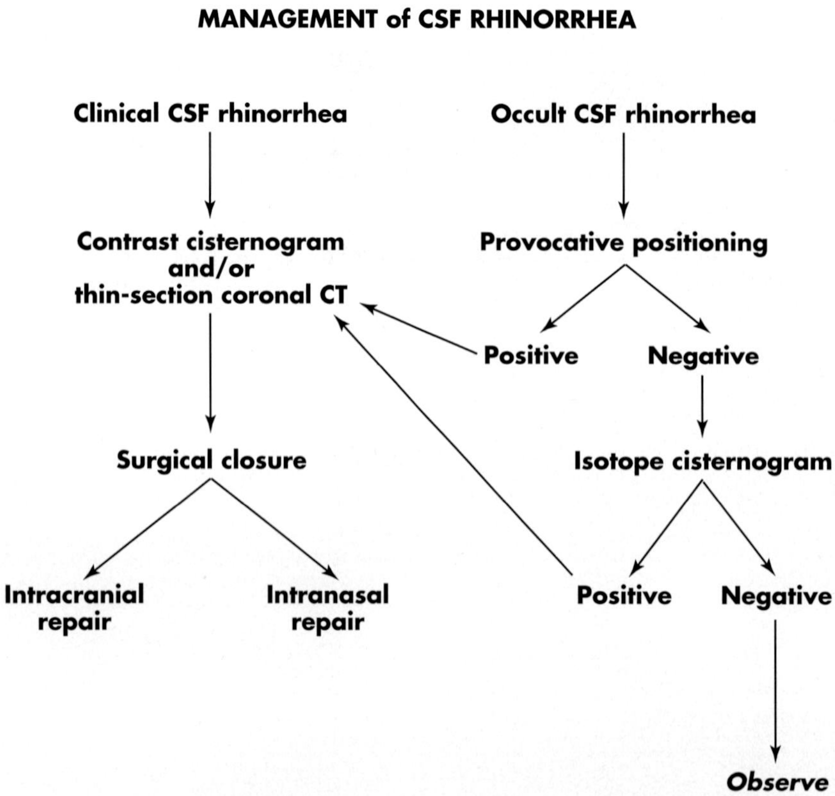

Fig. 6-1. Algorithm for management of cerebrospinal fluid (CSF) rhinorrhea.

lyzed. The simplest form of analysis is to place several drops of the fluid on filter paper or a paper tissue. Cerebrospinal fluid is relatively devoid of the protein present in blood and mucus and should leave a clear, homogeneous ring as the fluid spreads on the paper. When CSF is mixed with blood, a series of concentric rings appear as the fluid is absorbed by the paper. This "ring sign" is problematic since mucus and other body fluids mixed with blood can give a false-positive sign.[1] A much more specific test for CSF rhinorrhea is β_2-transferrin analysis; β_2-transferrin is found only in CSF, and the presence of this protein in nasal fluid is a definite confirmation of a fistula.[2] The widespread use of this test suffers from the lack of laboratories to perform the analysis and the delay in receiving the results.[3]

In our patient, significant findings included several drops of clear fluid draining from the left nostril when placed in the provocative position. Endoscopy showed the anterior third of the left middle turbinate to be partly intact and the middle third replaced by scar. Clear fluid was noted at the presumed junction of the anterior and middle thirds of this turbinate. The bulla ethmoidalis was intact and a middle meatus antrostomy was present. There was no evidence of active sinonasal infection (Fig. 6-2).

RADIOGRAPHIC EXAMINATION

The form of radiographic examination depends on the quantity of CSF rhinorrhea. When this condition is suspected, and drainage from the nose cannot be established, an isotope cisternogram is recommended. This procedure involves the placement of a radioisotope-labeled agent within the subarachnoid space, followed by scanning the head for evidence of CSF draining into the nose. Neurosurgical cottonoids or pladgets of cotton are also placed within the nasal cavity to further detect the leakage of CSF into the nose. The specitivity of this procedure in patients with a history of head trauma or an uncertain site of fistula can be improved by placing the cottonoids in the nasopharynx, beneath the middle turbinate, and between the middle turbinate and septum.[4] Detection of radioactivity on cottonoids placed within the nasopharynx suggests that the site of the fistula is at the ear by way of the eustachian tube, or that it results from an injury to the middle fossa or sphenoid sinus. Radioactivity at the middle meatus cottonoid suggests an injury to the roof of the ethmoid sinus. The presence of the radioactive agent on cottonoids placed in the superior nose is consistent with a communication from the subarachnoid space through the cribriform

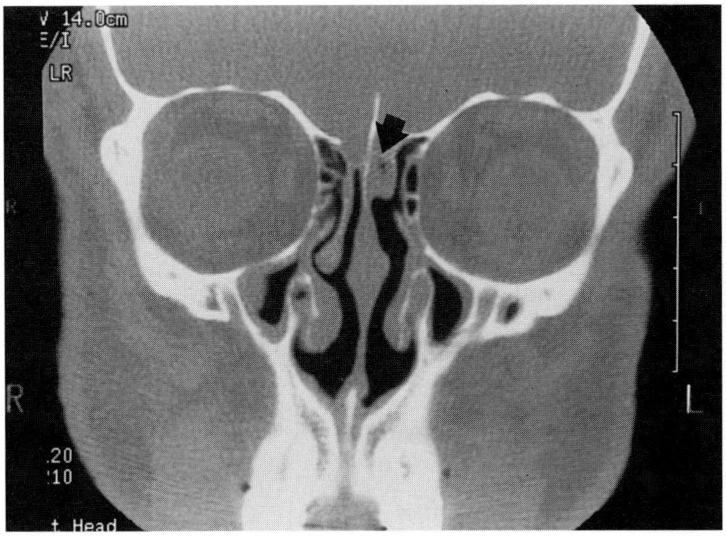

Fig. 6-2. Coronal thin-section computed tomographic (CT) scan of a patient showing a defect in the roof of the left anterior nose (lateral lamella of the cribriform plate, *arrow*).

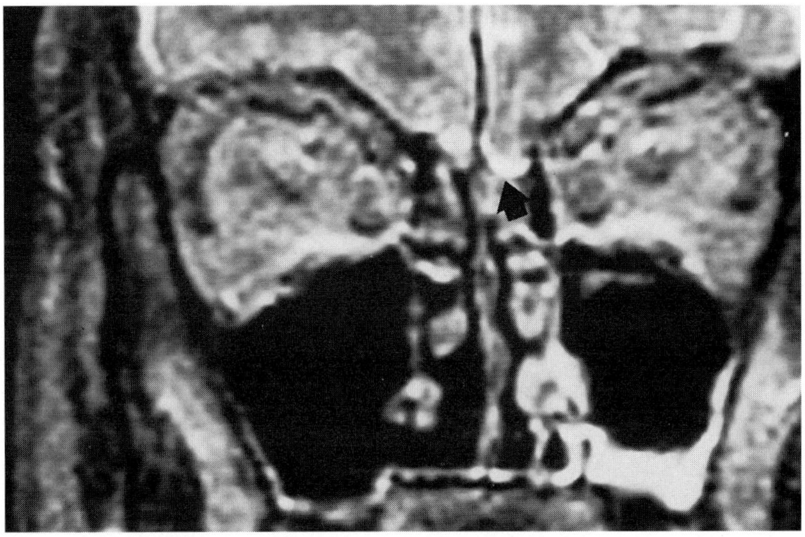

Fig. 6-3. Coronal MR scan reveals a small encephalocele protruding through the anterior cranial fossa floor defect into the left ethmoid sinus.

plate or at its articulation with the septum or middle turbinates. The presumptive site of the injury can be further localized by thin-section coronal computed tomographic imaging (CT) of the skull base. When there is obvious CSF rhinorrhea or a positive provocative test, a more specific procedure is a contrast CT cisternogram. A water-soluble iodinated contrast agent, is instilled in the subarachnoid space, and the head is placed in a dependent position. Coronal and if relevant axial, CT scans are obtained to delineate the site of the fistula. The scan is an excellent guide to localizing the fistula at the time of surgical repair and confirms the clinical impression of CSF rhinorrhea. The use of coronal thin sections at the site of injury further improves the localization of the fistula.

As our patient had a positive provocative test, thin-section coronal CT imaging of the anterior cranial fossa floor with metrizamide cisternography was performed. This study revealed a CSF fistula at the lateral crux of the cribriform plate or medial aspect of the roof of the left anterior ethmoid sinus (Fig. 6-2). The CT images also suggested a possible encephalocele. Follow-up MRI confirmed the CT suspicions of an encephalocele (Fig. 6-3).

TREATMENT

Indications

In both acute and chronic CSF fistulas, the management goals are to establish a water-tight closure and to prevent meningitis. The surgical procedure is the same in both forms of fistula. The only difference in treatment is that the closure rate of chronic fistulas can be significantly improved by spinal fluid diversion. The placement of a closed lumbar drainage system at the time of surgical repair of the chronic fistula permits both diversion of CSF and instillation of fluorescein for localization of the difficult-to-visualize fistula. Such drains should be managed by a neurosurgeon in a neurosurgery unit, in view of the potential for pneumocephalus, seizures, and brain herniation.[3] Spinal fluid diversion with fistula closure is regarded as optional in chronic CSF rhinorrhea. However, CSF diversion alone may be a successful form of management for the acute fistula.

Surgical Technique

Surgical closure can be performed under local or general anesthesia. I prefer general anesthesia because of the potentially longer length of surgery compared with sinus endoscopy and the use of spinal drainage in long-standing fistulas. The first step is identification of the fistula. In some iatrogenic fistulas, this step must be preceded by completion of the ethmoidectomy to permit inspection of the roof of the ethmoid sinus. In the patient used for this discussion the anterior ethmoid cells were relatively intact and the posterior portion of the free margin of the middle turbinate was missing (Fig. 6-4). Identification of the fistula can be assisted by placing the patient in the head-down position, while the anesthesiologist increases the intrathoracic pressure. Intrathecal fluorescein may be useful and when properly diluted with CSF can be placed in the subarachnoid space through the spinal drain. The illumination provided by a xenon light source is more than sufficient to identify the fluorescein, and avoids the need for ultraviolet light.[5]

After the location of CSF leakage is identified, the mucous membrane, fragments of bone, and arachnoid must be debrided from around and from within the fistula site. Less than meticulous debridement of the fistula results in failure of closure, because the graft cannot adhere to the roof of the sinus, or the growth of arachnoid into the fistula will preserve the fistulous track. Various ear instruments, including round knives, canal wall elevators, and dissectors, are particularly useful for debriding the fistula. These same instruments may be used to perform the next step, which is creation of a pocket between the roof of the ethmoid or nose and the anterior cranial fossa dura. This pocket may be difficult to make, but it is useful in order to anchor the graft in place. In patients with encephaloceles, bipolar cautery may be used to shrink the brain before developing the bone-dura pocket. After preparation of the fistula site, careful hemostasis should be obtained by placement of neurosurgical cottonoids while the graft is obtained.[6]

Although various forms of middle turbinate or septal flaps have been described for the closure of CSF leaks, I have come to prefer grafts. Specifically, flaps are limited by their pedicles, may be rather thick, can be difficult to inset precisely at the fistula site, and may obscure the visualization of the fistula. Grafts from such sites as the nasal septum or inferior turbinate overcome the problems with flaps. These donor sites also provide bone that can be used in larger defects (>1 cm). After harvesting and thinning of the graft, it is placed in the bone-dura pocket with the mucosal surface facing the nose. Tissue glue or Avitene paste (prepared by mixing Avitene with a small quantity of water) helps adhere the graft to the recipient site. As it is difficult to place the graft in the proximal or anterior part of the bone-dura pocket, the tissue glue helps secure the graft to the roof of the ethmoid or nose. The graft is further held in place by Gelfoam and absorbable packing, such as Sur-

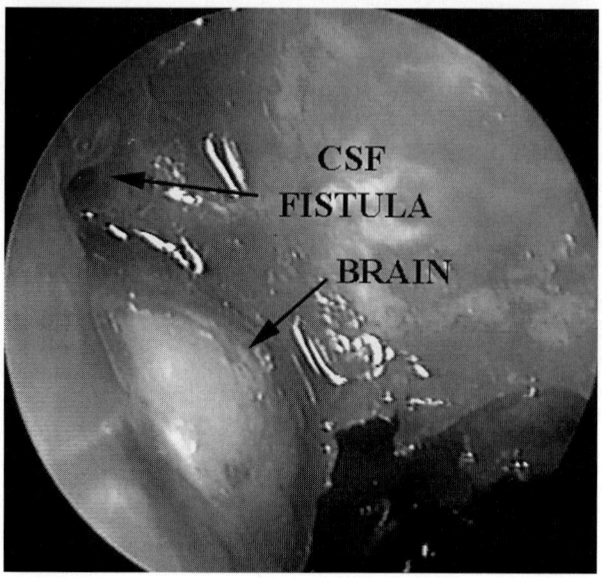

Fig. 6-4. Intraoperative photograph of the patient in Fig. 6-3 showing a CSF fistula and an encephalocele.

gicel or Oxycel. Nonabsorbable packing is avoided because of the potential for dislocating the graft during removal of the packing (Fig. 6-5).

After the operation, bed rest is prescribed for the patient for several days. Spinal fluid diversion typically lasts 5 days and requires bed rest during this period. Patients should be given stool softeners to avoid straining, which increases intracranial pressure. Nose blowing is discouraged, and opening of the mouth is recommended for sneezing, to avoid pneumocephalus.

DISCUSSION

CSF rhinorrhea may be posttraumatic, spontaneous, or iatrogenic. In my experience, posttraumatic CSF rhinorrhea may resolve after reduction of the facial fracture that lead to the rhinorrhea. However, one report noted a significantly better outcome from combined manipulation of the facial fracture and dural repair than from either form of treatment alone.[7] The preoperative evaluation of such patients is often limited to CT scanning to identify or confirm the site of the fracture. In contrast, spontaneous and iatrogenic rhinorrhea can be more difficult to confirm and localize, as illustrated in this chapter. In evaluating patients with such possible causes of rhinorrhea, the pathogenesis of the fistula is an essential element in planning and preventing such problems.[4] Spontaneous CSF rhinorrhea may be the result of various congenital defects or fistulas to the nose or sinuses. Other causes include hydrocephalus, which may be recognizable by enlargement of the cerebral ventricles on brain imaging.

Many iatrogenic injuries occur in patients with a deep olfactory fossa (Keros type 3) at the junction of the lateral lamella of the cribriform plate and frontal bone, which forms the roof of the ethmoid sinus. At this site, the bone may be dehiscent or minimal, and the likelihood of penetration of the anterior cranial fossa floor is increased. Another common site of injury is the roof of the posterior ethmoidal sinus, caused when the surgeon advances the instruments superiorly into the nose. As the anterior cranial fossa floor is sloping approximately 15 degrees posteroinferiorly, endonasal sinus surgery should be viewed as a procedure of rotation of the instruments inferiorly, rather than advancement of those instruments farther into the nose. Instruments advanced posterosuperiorly into the nose may penetrate the floor of the anterior cranial fossa. Given this consideration, I have modified the technique for the anterior-to-posterior approach (Messerklinger) to total ethmoidectomy, to include a posterior-to-anterior dissection of the most superior ethmoid cells, using a 30-degree endoscope for visualization of the skull base. Another concern is elimination of such key landmarks as the middle turbinate, which increases the likelihood of penetration of the skull base. In such cases, I agree with others that computer-guided surgery may help to minimize such injuries.[9]

Contrast cisternography is the current examination of choice for identification of CSF fistulas. A promising new imaging technology is magnetic resonance cisternography. This is a noninvasive, noncontrast, fast spin echo MR sequence with fat suppression that identifies the CSF. Projections can be obtained in both the coronal and sagittal planes, which improves identification of the fistula site. One investigation found that MR imaging correctly identified 19 of 21 surgically confirmed fistulas, whereas only seven such fistulas were noted by thin-section CT scanning.[4] However, until there is suf-

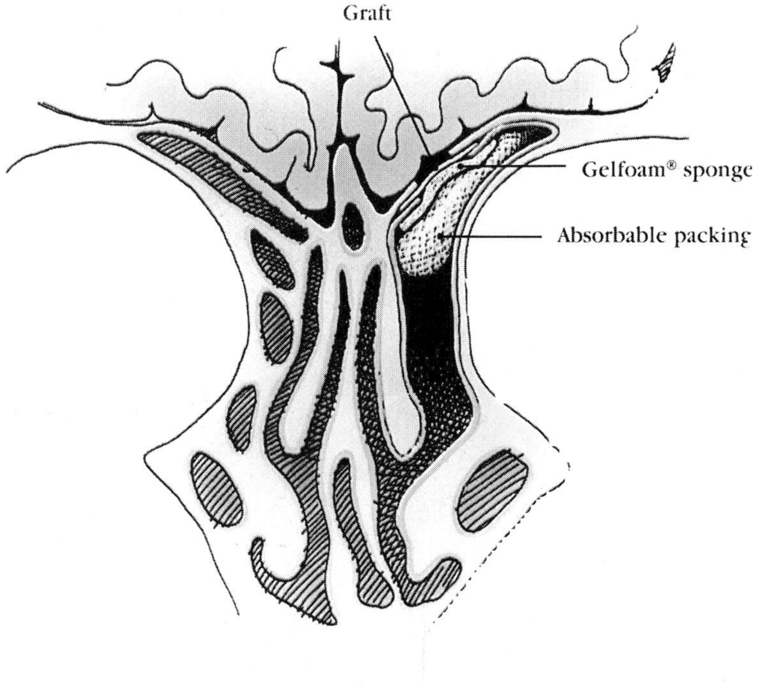

Fig. 6-5. Technique for intranasal repair of CSF rhinorrhea. (From Rice D, Schaefer S: *Endoscopic paranasal sinus surgery*, ed 2, New York, 1992, Raven Press.)

ficient experience with MR cisternography, there is a reluctance to recommend this technology as the primary imaging study.

Once CSF rhinorrhea is confirmed, timing of the repair is important. Iatrogenic fistulas identified at the time of sinus surgery should undergo immediate repair. Repair of both acute and chronic fistulas using a free tissue graft and absorbable packing is recommended, as discussed. Nasal mucosal (septal or turbinate) grafts have been found superior to turbinate or septal flaps because the rotation and size of the flaps has made careful placement difficult.[5] If the acute repair is not watertight, spinal drainage is helpful.[10] As previously discussed, spinal drainage is routinely employed in chronic fistulas. The repair of the chronic fistula is usually made as soon as possible but is not made on an emergent basis. The difficulty of the repair is increased in the presence of active granulation tissue or infection, and surgery may be delayed in such patients pending resolution of these problems. Finally, the routine use of antibiotics in infected patients is problematic, and so these are reserved for intraoperative treatment.[11]

Overall, the intranasal endoscopic repair of patients with acute, chronic, or spontaneous fistulas has resulted in a successful permanent closure rate of 75% to 80%. Intracranial closure is now reserved for patients who have failed the endoscopic approach, have massive defects of the anterior cranial fossa floor, or are anatomically unapproachable from the nose.

REFERENCES

1. Dula DJ, Fales W: The "ring sign": is it a reliable indicator for cerebral spinal fluid?, *Ann Emerg Med* 22:718-720, 1993.
2. Irajala K, Suoupaa J, Laurent B: Identification of CSF leakage by immunofixation, *Arch Otolaryngol Head Neck Surg* 105:447-448, 1979.
3. Skedros DG, Cass SP, Hirsch BE, Kelly HR: Beta-2 transferrin assay in clinical management of cerebral spinal fluid and perilymphatic fluid leaks, *J Otolaryngol* 22:341-344, 1993.
4. Eljamel MS, Pedgeon CN: Localization of inactive cerebrospinal fluid fistulas, *J Neurosurg* 83:795-798, 1995.
5. Dodson EE, Gross CW, Swerdloff JL, Gustafson LM: Transnasal endoscopic repair of cerebrospinal fluid rhinorrhea and skull base defects, *Otolaryngol Head Neck Surg* 111:600-605, 1994.
6. Rice D, Schaefer S: *Endoscopic paranasal sinus surgery*, ed 2, New York, 1992, Raven Press.
7. Eljamel MS: Fractures of the middle third of the face and cerebrospinal fluid rhinorrhoea, *Br J Neurosurg* 8:289–293, 1994.
8. Keros P: Uber die praktische Bedeutung der Niveauunter-scjoede der Lamina cribrosa des Ethmoids, *Laryngol Rhinol Otol (Stuttg)* 41:808-813, 1965.
9. Roth M, Lanza DC, Zinreich J, et al: Advantages and disadvantages of three-dimensional computed tomography intraoperative localization for functional endoscopic sinus surgery, *Laryngoscope* 105:1279-1286, 1995.
10. Shapiro SA, Scully T: Closed continuous drainage of cerebrospinal fluid via a lumbar subarachnoid catheter for treatment or prevention of cranial/spinal cerebrospinal fluid fistula, *Neurosurgery* 30:241-245, 1992.
11. Eljamel MS: Antibiotic prophylaxis in unrepaired CSF fistulae, *Br J Neurosurg* 7:501-505, 1993.

CHAPTER

7

Management of the Obstructing Inferior Turbinate

Richard L. Mabry
Bradley F. Marple

PROBLEM
The patient is a 31-year-old man who presents with unremitting bilateral nasal obstruction that has lasted several years.

The problem of nasal obstruction is a common one. It may be the result of mechanical obstruction from septal deviation and nasal polyps (among other causes) or turbinate enlargement. It is on this problem that this chapter focuses. It is important to establish to the best degree possible an exact cause of nasal obstruction, and to employ appropriate medical management before considering surgical intervention. The primary causes of turbinate hypertrophy are listed in Box 7-1. Turbinate enlargement owing to chronic rhinitis may or may not be reversible with appropriate therapy. However, that which is due to the other causes listed almost always requires surgical correction.

BOX 7-1

Common Causes of Turbinate Hypertrophy

I. Compensatory hypertrophy opposite septal concavity
II. Relative hypertrophy in a narrowed airway
  A. Naturally occurring
  B. After rhinoplasty
  C. After orthognathic surgery
III. Chronic rhinitis medicamentosa
IV. Chronic allergic or vasomotor rhinitis

MEDICAL HISTORY

The patient is an attorney who has a history of bilateral nasal congestion since his late teens. He underwent tonsillectomy and septoplasty at age 21, but his nasal obstruction soon recurred. He was tested for allergy and placed on injections in the past and made no improvement. He likewise did not benefit from antihistamines, decongestants, or nasal corticosteroid sprays. Since his only relief came from nose drops (topical decongestant), he has been using them on a regular basis for about 8 years. His history does not suggest recurrent infections. His symptoms are year-round, worse at night, and otherwise unaffected by season or circumstance. He takes no medications, has no known drug allergies, and is in good general health.

The fact that the patient has been "addicted" to nose drops for years provides an early clue to at least one aspect of the problem. Other considerations include allergic or vasomotor rhinitis, chronic infection, and mechanical nasal obstruction.

The allergic patient typically complains of associated rhinorrhea, sneezing, and having an itchy nose. The symptoms may be associated with certain seasons or circumstances but are perennial in many patients. Vasomotor rhinitis is generally manifested as rhinorrhea and nasal congestion triggered by emotional stress, irritants, cold air, eating, or exercise. Patients with chronic sinus infections describe purulent anterior and/or posterior nasal discharge, with facial pressure, often with a nocturnal cough. In the case of septal deviation, nasal polyps, and other causes of mechanical nasal obstruction, the symptoms may be unilateral or bilateral but do not generally respond to topical nasal vasoconstrictors.

PHYSICAL EXAMINATION

There is no external nasal deformity, nor evidence of valve collapse. On anterior rhinoscopy, the septum is straight. The inferior turbinates are boggy and red and demonstrate poor shrinkage after the topical application of phenylephrine 0.5% with lidocaine 2%. Endoscopic examination confirms diffusely enlarged, obstructing inferior turbinates from anterior to posterior. No polyps or masses are present. The choanae are patent. The nasopharynx and pharynx are clear, and tonsils are absent. The remainder of the examination is unremarkable.

The external nasal structure should be assessed to look for obstruction owing to deformity of the nasal bones or cartilages. Rhinologic examination should begin with anterior rhinoscopy, which will allow assessment of anterior septal deviation, turbinate enlargement, and significant polyps. This should be followed by attempts to shrink the inferior turbinates, with a vasoconstrictor alone or mixed with a topical anesthetic (to facilitate later endoscopic examination). The failure in this patient of the turbinates to decongest indicates irreversible hypertrophy, and although medical management should still be attempted, it is unlikely to succeed. Anterior rhinoscopy should also include palpation of any suspicious areas to differentiate polyps (which are mobile) from polypoid degeneration of the turbinates.

Following repeat rhinoscopy after decongestion, endoscopic evaluation should be carried out. A set routine helps avoid overlooking any area and should include inspection of the inferior turbinates and inferior meatus, middle turbinates and middle meatus, sphenoethmoid recess, choanae and nasopharynx, and nasal septum. Endoscopic evaluation allows examination of the middle meatus and sphenoethmoid recess and may show small polyps that were missed by anterior rhinoscopy, as well as revealing posterior septal deflection or inferior turbinate enlargement that may not otherwise be apparent. Finally, the nasopharynx should be evaluated for masses or other causes of choanal obstruction.

RADIOGRAPHIC EXAMINATION

The patient brings with him a coronal computed tomographic (CT) scan of the paranasal sinuses, which shows no intrinsic sinus abnormalities. The ostiomeatal complex is unobstructed and the middle turbinates are unremarkable. The inferior turbinates are enlarged bilaterally, with very large conchal bones.

Although diagnostic imaging by conventional sinus radiographs or CT scans may be indicated to evaluate coexisting sinus disorders, these studies add little to the information available from direct examination of the nose. To be truly meaningful, the findings of enlarged inferior turbinates on radiographic studies must be correlated with the patient's clinical history and the clinician's findings.

LABORATORY EXAMINATION

A screening radioallergosorbent test (RAST) result for eight seasonal and perennial inhalant antigens was class 0, with a total immunoglobulin E (IgE) of 12 units.

The primary beneficial ancillary study in the work-up and treatment of a patient with obstructing inferior turbinates consists of testing for allergen-specific IgE. Although this patient had previously undergone testing, it was many years earlier, and should be repeated. This may be done by either skin tests or in vitro methods. In either instance, the diagnosis of allergy cannot be made until these test findings are correlated with the patient's history, to establish a pattern compatible with truly significant clinical allergy. The appropriate treatment of inhalant nasal allergy includes environmental control, pharmacotherapy, and immunotherapy where indicated.

The concept of screening with a limited number of inhalant antigens, performing additional testing if positive responses are obtained, has been validated by several authors.[1] In patients in whom the index of suspicion for inhalant allergy is not high, a microscreen, which incorporates six seasonal antigens on one RAST disk and two perennial antigens on another, when combined with measurement of total IgE, is a rapid and cost-efficient method of ruling out inhalant allergy.

Unfortunately, evaluation for food allergy is not so easily performed. Since only a small percentage of food-allergic patients demonstrate IgE-mediated problems, RAST food testing does not provide an adequate answer. If food hypersensitivity is suspected, a diet diary followed by omission and challenge refeeding of the suspected foods remains the diagnostic "gold standard."[2]

TREATMENT

The patient was treated by gentle, submucosal injection of 20 mg triamcinolone acetonide into the anterior tip of each inferior turbinate. This was supplemented by systemic pseudoephedrine, 60 mg three times a day, and saline nasal spray as needed. He was counseled to discontinue the use of topical nasal vasoconstrictors.

He returned 2 weeks later, having discontinued nose drops, continuing to complain of nasal obstruction, especially at night. Examination confirmed continued symptomatic hypertrophy of the inferior turbinates, from anterior to posterior.

Indications

Virtually every patient whose nasal obstruction is primarily the result of turbinate enlargement deserves a trial on medical management. In some instances, such as a hypertrophic turbinate opposite a large septal deviation, it is virtually a foregone conclusion that surgery will be necessary. However, in a surprising number of instances, appropriate therapy for an underlying turbinate dysfunction (such as nasal allergy) affords relief. Even if this is not the case, control of the underlying medical problem often facilitates both the surgery and the patient's recovery and lessens the likelihood of repeat turbinate surgery.

Medical Management

The nonsurgical management of turbinate enlargement consists of nonspecific and specific measures. These are outlined in Box 7-2. General measures include systemic decongestants, the use of nasal steroids (topical or injected) for their anti-inflammatory action, and the avoidance of irritants. These are combined with specific measures for allergic or vasomotor rhinitis and for rhinitis medicamentosa. In this patient, the only appropriate measures were withdrawal of nose drops and the use of nasal steroids (in the form of intraturbinal corticosteroid injection) and decongestants. Unfortunately, the prolonged nature of the patients' nose drops "addiction" had rendered the turbinate hypertrophy irreversible.

Although the increasing use of topical nasal corticosteroids since the mid-1980s has decreased the use of intraturbinal steroid injection (Fig. 7-1), it remains a useful tool.[3] It is especially beneficial in instances of rhinitis medicamentosa, since its action is noted within hours and persists for 4 to 6 weeks, not requiring penetration past congested turbinates nor a period of several days to become effective. Nevertheless, it is a very technique-sensitive procedure, and rare instances of visual loss owing to retinal embolization or vasospasm have occurred when the suggested technique is not closely followed. This involves the application of a topical anesthetic/vasoconstrictor, followed by gentle, submucosal injection into the anterior tip of each inferior turbinate of a repository corticosteroid such as triamcinolone acetonide, using a fine (25-gauge) needle and tuberculin syringe.[4] The reader should consult the appropriate references for further study before attempting the procedure for the first time. However, its safe use for over a third of a century by numerous otolaryngologists attests to its continued utility.

Medical management having failed in our patient, therapeutic options were considered. The patient underwent bilateral partial resection of the inferior turbinates (inferior turbinoplasty) under general anesthesia, without complications. Healing progressed satisfactorily, with an excellent airway from the time of pack removal 1 day postoperatively, and with no bleeding or crusting. He continues free of nasal congestion and has not felt any temptation to resume topical nasal vasoconstrictors.

BOX 7-2

Medical Management of Turbinate Dysfunction

I. General measures
  A. Avoidance of irritants
    1. Cigarette smoke
    2. Chemicals
    3. Dust, fumes
  B. Systemic decongestants
  C. Nasal steroids
    1. Topical
    2. Intraturbinal injection
II. Specific measures (to be combined with above measures)
  A. Allergic rhinitis
    1. Antihistamines (with or without decongestants)
    2. Mast cell stabilizers (e.g., cromolyn)
    3. Avoidance of inciting allergens
    4. Allergen-specific immunotherapy
  B. Vasomotor rhinitis
    1. Topical anticholinergics
  C. Rhinitis medicamentosa
    1. Withdrawal of topical nasal vasoconstrictors
    2. Change from systemic medication causing turbinate congestion (e.g., β-blockers)

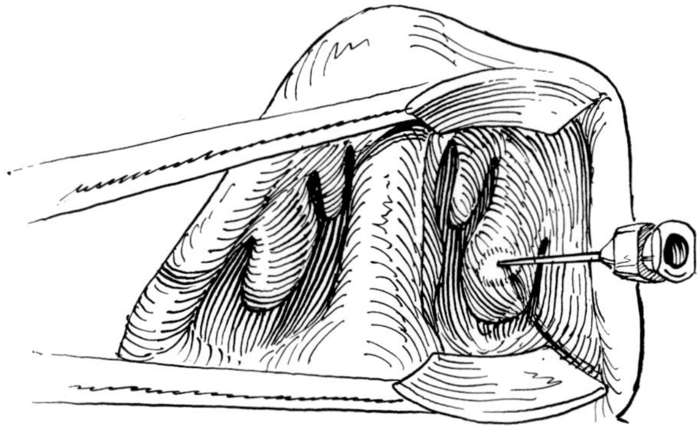

Fig. 7-1. Intraturbinal corticosteroid injection is useful for treating turbinate congestion and assessing whether hypertrophy is reversible. (From *Southern Medical Journal* 71:790, 1978.)

Surgical Management

Surgical reduction of obstructing inferior turbinates can take several forms,[5] which may be classed as mechanical, destructive, or resection (Box 7-3). The choice of procedure depends on a number of factors: whether the patient also requires other nasal and/or sinus surgery, whether the turbinate enlargement involves conchal bone hypertrophy and/or hypertrophy of the stroma, the general condition of the patient (hypertension, other medical problems), and the personal preferences and comfort level of the surgeon with the various procedures.

When only turbinate surgery is necessary, procedures that lend themselves to performance in the clinic rather than the operating room should be considered, such as those listed in Box 7-3 under section II. These procedures tend to produce scarring within the stroma of the turbinate, reducing its size and limiting the degree to which it can become engorged in the future. For rhinologists with ready access to a cryotherapy unit, this may become their procedure of choice. Cauterization (Fig. 7-2), either unipolar or bipolar,[5,6] produces excellent results in patients whose turbinates demonstrate good shrinkage with the application of topical vasoconstrictors (especially when combined with lateral outfracture of the conchal bone). However, care must be given to achieve adequate local anesthesia. The infrared coagulator device (Fig. 7-3) produces local diathermy photocoagulation of the anterior heads of the inferior turbinates and requires only topical anesthesia. Unfortunately, this method is inadequate for hypertrophy involving the entire turbinate.

Various lasers may be used to produce either superficial photocoagulation (with the KTP laser), interstitial photocoagulation (by way of the Nd:YAG laser), or vaporization of a portion of the turbinate (using the CO_2 laser). Specific details of these various methods vary and are generally readily available from the manufacturers and distributors of the equipment involved, as well as from reference sources.[7-9] In a clinic setting, the anterior portions of the inferior turbinates are debulked with a CO_2 laser (Fig. 7-4), using a specially designed waveguide and the superpulse mode, which produces vaporization without charring. In this particular case, the involvement of the entire turbinate made this an inappropriate choice. In addition, the contribution of enlarged conchal bones

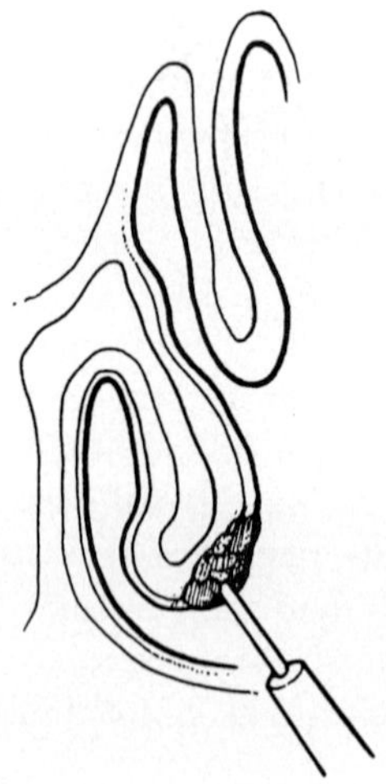

Fig. 7-2. Cauterization of the inferior turbinates is a simple procedure that reduces turbinate bulk by producing fibrosis of the stroma. (Reproduced from *Otolaryngology–Head and Neck Surgery,* 92:572-575, 1984.)

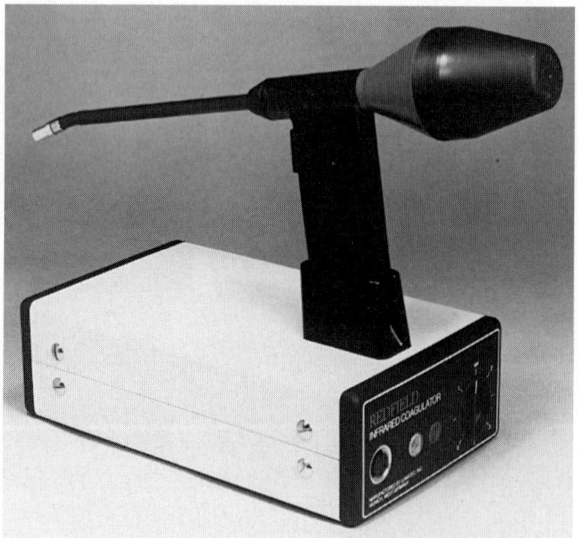

Fig. 7-3. Infrared coagulation produces results similar to electrocautery, through the use of diathermy in a simple, less painful office procedure. It is primarily useful for reducing anterior turbinate bulk. (Courtesy of Redfield Corporation.)

BOX 7-3

Types of Turbinate Reduction Procedures

- I. Mechanical
  - A. Crushing and/or
  - B. Lateral outfracture
- II. Destructive
  - A. Cauterization
    - 1. Extramucosal
      - a. Cautery
      - b. Diathermy (e.g., infrared coagulator)
    - 2. Submucosal
      - a. Unipolar
      - b. Bipolar
  - B. Cryotherapy
  - C. Superficial laser photocoagulation
- III. Resection
  - A. Laser vaporization
  - B. Submucous resection
  - C. Partial resection ("trimming")
  - D. Inferior turbinoplasty

to the size of the inferior turbinates made some type of formal resection a necessity.

The classic operation for diminishing the size of obstructing inferior turbinates by removing the conchal bone is submucous resection of the inferior turbinate (Fig. 7-5). The procedure was originally described in 1924, but the classic modern description is that of House.[10] The technique involves circumferential dissection around the conchal bone to remove as much of it as possible, allowing the soft tissue to fall together. This results in lateralization of the inferior turbinate, plus a reduction in size due to removal of the bone plus internal scarring produced by the surgical procedure. This approach is most beneficial in instances of hypertrophy of the conchal bone, or in patients likely to bleed if more aggressive turbinate resection is carried out.

Many forms of surgical turbinate reduction or "trimming" have been described (Fig. 7-6). The approach used is a matter of choice and personal preference of the surgeon. However, no technique is immune to the potential postoperative complications of crusting and bleeding.[6]

A unique technique of partial inferior turbinate resection is "inferior turbinoplasty" (Fig. 7-7), which was

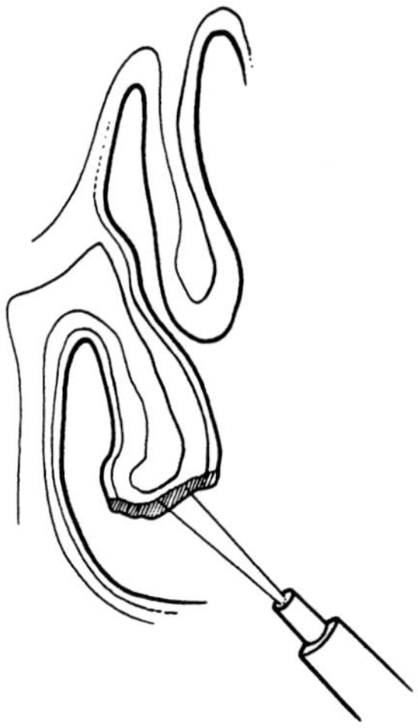

Fig. 7-4. Lasers may be used for either superficial or interstitial photocoagulation, or to vaporize hypertrophic mucosal and submucosal tissue. Different lasers and special delivery systems have increased the usefulness of this modality for treating turbinate disorders. (Reproduced from *Otolaryngology–Head and Neck Surgery,* 92:572-575, 1984.)

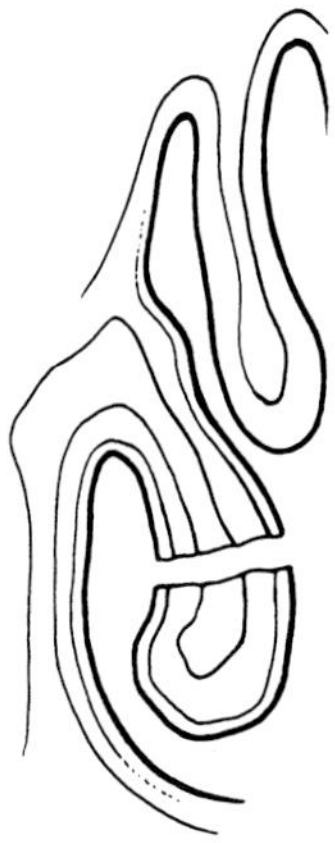

Fig. 7-6. Many methods of partial resection have been espoused, but all carry a significant risk of postoperative bleeding and crusting. Most surgeons clamp across the turbinate before excising tissue inferiorly, and an attempt should be made to leave a cuff of soft tissue to cover exposed bone. (Reproduced from *Otolaryngology–Head and Neck Surgery,* 92:572-575, 1984.)

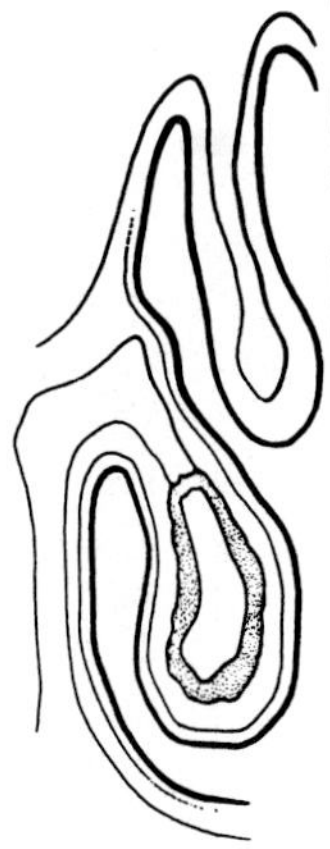

Fig. 7-5. Submucous resection of the inferior turbinate removes the conchal bone, and the stromal scarring produced by the dissection further reduces soft tissue bulk. This technique presents less potential for bleeding and crusting than a "trimming" of the turbinates. (Reproduced from *Otolaryngology–Head and Neck Surgery,* 92:572-575, 1984.)

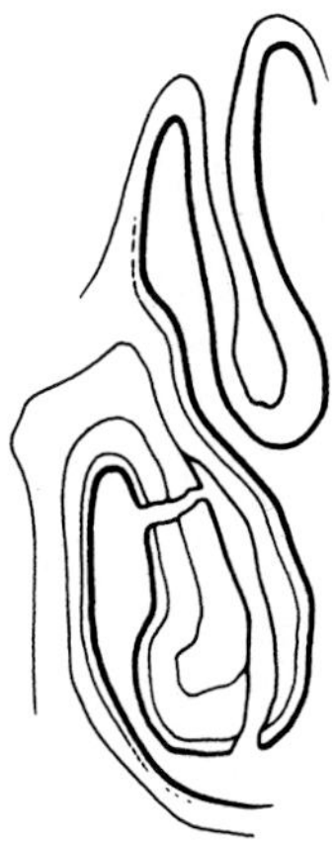

Fig. 7-7. Inferior turbinoplasty removes a wedge containing the conchal bone and soft tissue on its lateral and inferior surface, together with the posterior turbinate tip. Exposed bone should be avoided and suction cautery used for hemostasis. The flap of tissue left forms a functional "neoturbinate." (Reproduced from *Otolaryngology–Head and Neck Surgery,* 92:572-575, 1984.)

adapted by Mabry[11] from earlier techniques described by Freer and others. The procedure involves removal of the conchal bone together with the attached soft tissue lateral and inferior to it (Figs. 7-8 and 7-9). This wedge, including the posterior turbinate tip, is removed with a polyp snare (Fig. 7-10). Suction cautery is then used to achieve hemostasis on the remaining laterally based flap, which ultimately rolls upon itself and heals to form a smaller, but quite functional, neoturbinate (Fig. 7-11). Published follow-up studies indicate no problems with bleeding, prolonged crusting, bothersome postnasal drainage, or other adverse sequelae of inferior turbinoplasty.[12]

When postoperative bleeding is of special concern (e.g., patients with hypertension, anxiety, or a tendency to bleed more freely than usual during septal surgery), it may be preferrable to employ a more conservative turbinate reduction procedure, such as cauterization and outfracture, or submucous resection.

It should also be emphasized that failure to address the underlying cause of turbinate enlargement (e.g., allergy, rhinitis medicamentosa) may result in subsequent hypertrophy and a recurrence of symptoms.

There is a tendency on the part of some surgeons to partially or totally resect middle turbinates in association with endoscopic sinus surgery. The pros and cons of this maneuver are beyond the scope of this chapter, but if such resection is performed, a very conservative inferior turbinate reduction is mandatory to avoid changes in nasal physiology resulting in chronic dryness, thick secretions, and crusting.

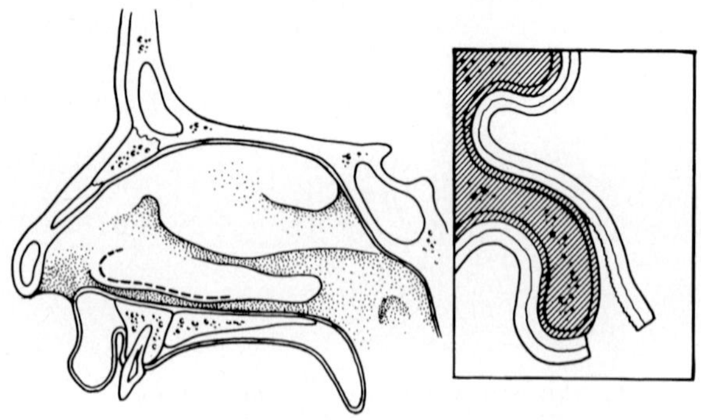

Fig. 7-8. Technique of inferior turbinoplasty: line of incision and flap elevation. (Reproduced from *Operative Techniques in Otolaryngology–Head and Neck Surgery,* 2:183-188, 1991.)

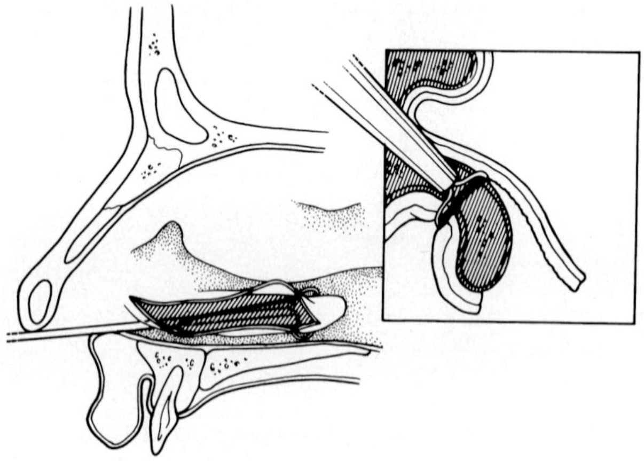

Fig. 7-10. Technique of inferior turbinoplasty: removal of bone and the soft tissue wedge, together with the posterior turbinate tip, with a polyp snare. (Reproduced from *Operative Techniques in Otolaryngology–Head and Neck Surgery,* 2:183-188, 1991.)

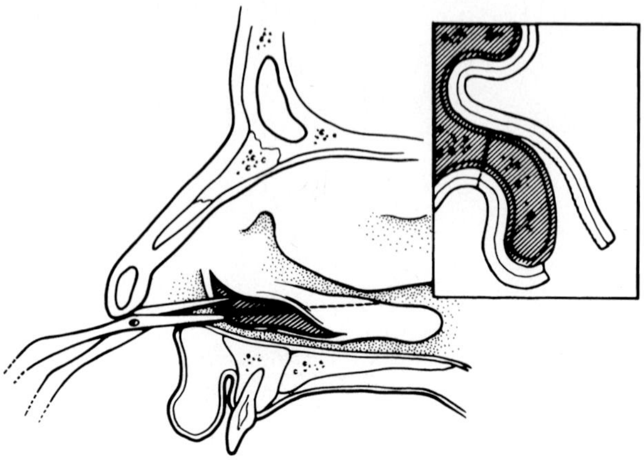

Fig. 7-9. Technique of inferior turbinoplasty: resection of conchal bone and the attached lateral and inferior soft tissue wedge. (Reproduced from *Operative Techniques in Otolaryngology–Head and Neck Surgery,* 2:183-188, 1991.)

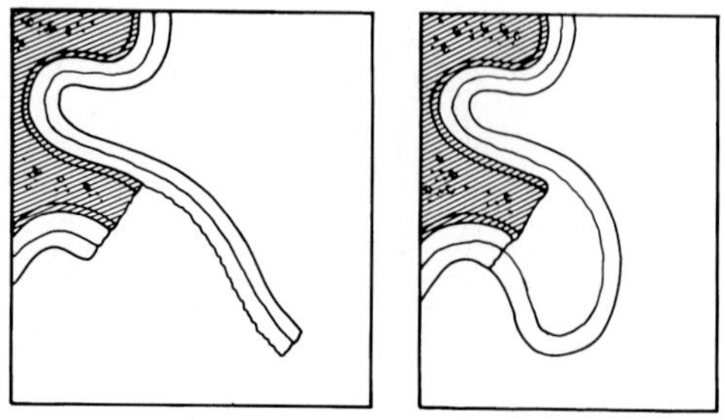

Fig. 7-11. Technique of inferior turbinoplasty: residual inferior turbinate tissue, with mucosa on the medial surface, curls on itself and heals to form a functioning neoturbinate. (Reproduced from *Operative Techniques in Otolaryngology–Head and Neck Surgery,* 2:183-188, 1991.)

DISCUSSION

The case presented as an example was one in which nasal obstruction was due to a single cause. Although chosen for its simplicity and straightforwardness, it is not typical. Most patients who present with nasal obstruction have several causes for their difficulties. Thus, the physician must initially assess for all possible contributing factors, in the form of both mechanical obstruction (e.g., septal deviation, polyps) and turbinate dysfunction (e.g., allergic or vasomotor rhinitis, rebound rhinitis, chronic infection). Rarely does only one therapeutic intervention, whether medical or surgical, offer a "cure" for the patient with nasal obstruction. Rather, it is appropriate to employ appropriate medical management, following this with suitable surgery when necessary. Surgical intervention should be followed by continued management of allergy, avoidance of the chronic use of nasal vasoconstrictors, and prompt treatment of future nasal complaints to avoid the temptation to resort to the regular use of decongestant sprays. In doing so, the rhinologist goes beyond the role of surgical technician and offers patients lasting and complete relief of nasal obstruction.

REFERENCES

1. King WP: Efficacy of a screening radioallergosorbent test, *Arch Otolaryngol* 108:781-786, 1982.
2. King WP: Food hypersensitivity in otolaryngology: manifestations, diagnosis and treatment, *Otolaryngol Clin North Am.* 25:163-179, 1992.
3. Mabry RL: Intranasal steroids in rhinology: the changing role of intraturbinal injection, *Ear Nose Throat* 73:242-246, 1994.
4. Mabry RL: Corticosteroids in otolaryngology: intraturbinal injection, *Otolaryngol Head Neck Surg* 91:717-720, 1983.
5. Goode RL, Pribitkin E II: *Diagnosis and treatment of turbinate dysfunction*, Washington, DC, 1995, American Academy of Otolaryngology–Head and Neck Surgery Foundation, pp 35-58.
6. Mabry RL: *Surgery of the inferior turbinates: when, why, and how?* In Johnson JT, Derkay CS, Mandell-Brown MK, Newman RK, editors: *Instructional Courses, Vol 5,* St Louis, 1992, Mosby–Year Book, pp 137-148.
7. Goldsher M, Joachims HZ, Golz A, et al: Nd:YAG laser turbinate surgery animal experimental study: preliminary report, *Laryngoscope* 105:319-321, 1995.
8. Levine HL: The potassium-titanyl phosphate laser for treatment of turbinate dysfunction, *Otolaryngol Head Neck Surg* 102:247-251, 1991.
9. Krespi YP, Mayer M, Slatkine M: Laser photocoagulation of the inferior turbinates, *Op Tech Otolaryngol Head Neck Surg* 5:287-291, 1994.
10. House HP: Submucous resection of the inferior turbinal bone, *Laryngoscope* 61:637-648, 1951.
11. Mabry RL: Inferior turbinoplasty, *Laryngoscope* 92:459-461, 1982.
12. Mabry RL: Inferior turbinoplasty: patient selection, technique, and long-term consequences, *Otolaryngol Head Neck Surg* 98:60-66, 1988.

CHAPTER

8

Lasers in Nasal and Sinus Surgery

Howard L. Levine

HISTORY

Lasers have been popular tools used for years in laryngology, rhinology, and otology and most recently for oral cavity procedures such as laser-assisted uvular and palatal surgery. The carbon dioxide laser was the first laser used by otolaryngologists, primarily for laryngology. It had limitations for use in the nose and sinuses because of its cumbersome articulating arm and the lack of flexible fibers to reach the recesses and spaces of the nose. The neodymium:yttrium-aluminum-garnet Nd:YAG laser was limited in its intranasal use by its depth of penetration and zone of injury.

When the potassium-titanyl-phosphate (KTP/532) laser was introduced in the early 1980s, it showed promise for use in the nose and sinuses because of its limited depth of penetration; flexible delivery systems; and ability to cut, coagulate, and vaporize tissue.[1]

While there are various methods for managing intranasal and sinus disorders with headlights, nasal speculums, nasal endoscopes, and external nasal procedures, there are roles for the laser in either primary or adjunctive treatment. The laser works well for nasal turbinate dysfunction, nasal vascular disorders, and intranasal scarring. It is also effective in selected nasal polyp and nasal neoplastic problems.

TURBINATE DYSFUNCTION

PROBLEM

A 65-year-old male executive had difficulty breathing through his nose nearly all his life. There had been alternating nasal obstruction and congestion that were worse when sleeping but present even during the day. When the obstruction was present there was pressure over the forehead, medial canthal area, and cheek. This often awakened the patient or created restless sleep to the degree that he was often fatigued in the morning. There was no nasal drainage or itching of the nose or eyes. Cigarette smoke, perfume, beer, and red wine made the symptoms worse.

There had been no significant medical problems. Allergy tests were negative and thyroid function test results were normal. The patient noticed a mild amount of ankle swelling when sitting for long periods.

PHYSICAL EXAMINATION

The otorhinolaryngologic examination was completely within normal limits, except for markedly congested inferior nasal turbinates. These were easily decongested with phenylephrine (Neo-Synephrine), improving the patient's nasal airway. The remainder of the intranasal examination was normal.

TREATMENT

On the basis of the history and physical examination and laboratory testing, vasomotor rhinitis was diagnosed. Because the most distressing symptom was nasal obstruction relieved in the office by a topical decongestant, a systemic decongestant was prescribed. This gave him relief, but he developed intermittent bladder obstruction, making it impossible to continue the medication. A variety of topical steroid sprays were tried, but none provided relief and some even caused nasal bleeding, especially during the winter months. Because of failure of medical management, consideration was given to a laser reduction of the nasal turbinates. This was carried out using the KTP/532 laser with the patient under mild sedation. The laser was used at 8 W and continuous. The laser fiber tip was held just barely in contact with the inferior turbinate tissue. Anterior-to-posterior cuts were made over the anterior two thirds of the inferior turbinate on its medial and inferior surface. These laser cuts were separated by about the same width as the cuts themselves. The inferior turbinate was cross-hatched with vertical cuts in the same manner. Mupirocin ointment was applied over the surface of the turbinate. A saline nasal spray was used three or four times a day for several weeks after surgery.

One week after surgery, typical crusting and eschar was visible over the turbinate. There was slight improvement in the airway. Four weeks after surgery, the crusting and eschar were gone, the turbinates were small, and the airway was excellent. One year later the breathing remained excellent and the patient was pleased with the results.

DISCUSSION

Nasal obstruction caused by turbinate enlargement can be the result of bony hypertrophy of the turbinates or vasoactive turbinates. If the turbinate is enlarged because of bone, the obstruction is generally constant and unrelieved by topical or systemic nasal decongestants. Bony hypertrophy of the turbinates is best treated by submucous resection of the bone.

Vasoactive turbinates cause vasomotor or allergic rhinitis. This is best differentiated by history. The treatment for allergic or vasomotor rhinitis is usually medical with antihistamines, decongestants, and topical nasal steroid sprays. However, some patients do not respond to or cannot tolerate medical management. For nearly all these individuals, laser reduction provides relief.

The laser relieves obstruction by creating a layer of scar tissue in the submucosa. This acts like a "corset" that prevents the turbinate from expanding yet allows it to function, warming and humidifying the inspired air. It may also reduce the number of secreting cells and alter the autonomic innervation minimizing the vasoactive response.[2]

RESULTS

Fukutake and colleagues[3] found 46% of patients operated on with laser with excellent results, 34% with good improvement, and 20% with no change in nasal symptoms. I have used the laser on 425 patients with vasomotor rhinitis (unpublished data) and followed them for 2 to 4 years (mean 3.2 years). Of these patients, 71.1% are asymptomatic and use no medications for the nose; 20.2% are asymptomatic but use moderate amounts of nasal decongestants or topical nasal corticosteroid sprays; 8.7% are no better.

SINUS AND NASAL POLYPS

PROBLEM

A 36-year-old man was referred with a 10-year history of asthma, aspirin sensitivity, and nasal polyps. He had undergone five previous nasal and sinus polypectomies over several years, had been on prednisone frequently because of out-of-control asthma, and used large doses of steroid nasal and pulmonary inhalers. There were large amounts of thick postnasal drainage that the patient believed contributed to the persistent and recurrent asthma symptoms.

PHYSICAL EXAMINATION

The otolaryngologic examination was within normal limits except for the nasal examination, in which massive polyps were seen filling the entire nasal cavity. No anatomic landmarks could be seen because of the size and location of the polyps. The oropharynx and nasopharynx revealed thick postnasal secretions.

Coronal computed tomography revealed opacification of all the sinuses.

TREATMENT

Because the patient had been on steroids and steroid nasal sprays without relief of nasal symptoms and his asthma remained out of control, surgery was performed.

He received 40 mg prednisone once a day for 1 week before surgery to reduce the size of the polyps. An endoscopic sinus procedure was performed, removing polyps and thick, tenacious secretions from all the sinuses. After surgery, he was sent home with a methylprednisolone (Medrol) Dosepak. Once the sinus cavity was healed, a steroid nasal spray was prescribed to minimize the recurrence of the polyps.

Three months after surgery, at a routine office visit, a nasal endoscopy revealed early polypoid change over the roof of the ethmoidal sinus. The use of nasal steroid spray was increased. In spite of this and the use of a Medrol Dosepak, the sense of smell lessened over the next few months, the polypoid change increased, and there were intermittent and more frequent episodes of asthma out of control.

For these reasons, 6 months after the initial sinus surgical procedure, the patient was taken back to surgery and a nasal endoscopic laser photocoagulation of the sinus cavity was performed. The KTP/532 laser was used at 10 to 12 W and an intermittent mode of 0.1 sec on and 0.1 sec off. Once the sinus cavity healed, the patient resumed the nasal steroid spray. He was followed for 4 years with no evidence of any polyps or polypoid change within the sinus cavity.

DISCUSSION

One of the most challenging problems for the rhinologist is the patient with asthma and nasal polyps with or without aspirin sensitivity, because the primary disease process is not being treated as much as the resultant symptoms. It is important to control the nasal and sinus disease in order to prevent the asthma from worsening. However, current medical and surgical management of the nose and sinuses does not "cure" the patient. Traditional sinus surgery and functional endoscopic sinus surgery often control only the symptoms, and polyps frequently recur in spite of the best efforts.

When the laser first became available for nasal and sinus surgery, attempts were made to remove the polyps with the laser in hope of improved results.[1] This was usually tedious and often resulted in increased swelling and delayed healing. The laser could debulk larger pedicled polyps, but it was difficult to completely eradicate all polyps from the nose and sinuses safely with the laser alone. Some of the delay in healing seemed to be due to the accumulation of heat within the tissue transmitted from the laser. Even though these problems occurred in some patients, several individuals had excellent results, and in that some parts of the nose remained free of polyps. For this reason, the idea of completely removing nasal and sinus polyps with the laser was generally abandoned except for a few special circumstances. It was valuable for the patient with a coagulation disorder, because the laser kept the operative site dry.

The laser is also helpful in managing some choanal polyps. It can debulk the choanal polyp at the maxillary sinus ostium and photocoagulate the base of the choanal polyp to prevent recurrences.

Because of the difficulty and generally unpredictable results, attempts were made to remove the nasal polyps with "traditional" endoscopic techniques, treat patients medically with topical nasal steroids, and follow them endoscopically. If there was early discovery of polyps or a polypoid change that was symptomatic, laser photocoagulation of the nose or sinus cavity was performed. The laser was used in an intermittent repeat mode at 0.1 sec on and 0.1 sec off to permit cooling of the tissue between laser pulses. This was to minimize damage to the underlying structures. Most of the patients who have undergone laser photocoagulation of the nose and sinuses have had exuberant rhinitis and sinusitis. For them the laser seemed to be effective by creating a thin layer of scar tissue and reducing the number of mucous-secreting glands. It was almost an attempt to create a small degree of controlled atrophic rhinitis. Even though an attempt was made to achieve this, nearly every patient with nasal polyps, asthma, aspirin sensitivity or nonallergic eosinophilic rhinitis, and polyps continues to have some watery, mucoid discharge. Not a single patient developed true atrophic rhinitis or ozena.

RESULTS

I have followed 46 patients for a minimum of 18 months (unpublished data), all of whom have had nasal polyps with eosinophilia and asthma. All had a traditional endoscopic sinus surgical procedure. All had been managed with nasal corticosteroids and occasional systemic steroids. All had recurrence of the polyps. Laser photocoagulation of the sinus cavity was achieved as described. Some patients did not use any medications after this surgery. In the latter group, seven were asymptomatic and one was improved. Another group required nasal corticosteroid sprays. In this group, 15 were asymptomatic, 17 were improved, 4 were no better, and 2 were worse. Those managed with or without nasal steroid sprays and who were asymptomatic or improved totaled 40 of 46 patients (86.6%). While this number is encouraging for what is a frustrating problem, it will almost certainly decrease as time goes by.

SUMMARY

The laser seems to be an exciting surgical tool, but it is not the answer to every surgical problem. Many patients think that the laser is nonsurgical and will provide relief of frustrating, recurring disorders when other modalities have failed. To the healthcare providers who manage and carefully follow the patient, it is apparent that this is not true.

In the nose and sinus there is excellent improvement for most patients with vasomotor and allergic rhinitis. For the patient with nasal polyps, the excision of polyps is tedious and frequently results in delayed healing and scarring. However, there is some promise in its use as a secondary treatment for the patient who has nasal polyps with eosinophilia and asthma, with or without aspirin sensitivity.

REFERENCES

1. Levine HL: KTP/532 laser for nasal sinus disease, *Ann Otol Rhinol Laryngol* 98:46-51, 1989.
2. Levine HL: KTP/532 laser for treatment of turbinate dysfunction, *Otolaryngol Head Neck Surg* 104:247-251, 1991.
3. Fukutake T, Yamashita T, Tomoda K, Kumazawa T: Laser surgery for allergic rhinitis, *Arch Otolaryngol Head Neck Surg* 112:1280-1282, 1986.

CHAPTER

9

Choanal Atresia

Orval E. Brown

PROBLEM

After term gestation and normal delivery, a newborn girl presented with grunting respiration and sternal retraction followed by crying, which relieved the cyanosis. The patient had a good cry and a good airway but was noticed to have great difficulty with feeding. Slow feeding was noted, accompanied by coughing, choking, and sputtering. There was mucoid discharge from both nares. Further evaluation and diagnostic studies were performed.

Choanal atresia is a relatively rare entity with an incidence of approximately 1 in 7000 to 8000 live births. Choanal atresia is the result of a congenital failure of the posterior nasal cavity to communicate with the nasopharynx. It is approximately twice as common in females as in males, and about 50% to 60% of cases are unilateral. Previous reports have estimated the nature of the obstructing atresia plate in choanal atresia as 90% bony and 10% membranous. New information indicates that the anatomic classification of choanal atresia is about 30% pure bony atresia and 70% mixed bony-membranous; pure membranous atresias without bony abnormalities are very rare, if they exist.[1]

Patients with bilateral choanal atresia usually present early in life with airway obstruction and feeding difficulties, as newborns are obligate nose breathers for a variable period. This nasal airway obstruction can result in marked respiratory distress, which is relieved by crying. Difficulty in feeding is usually seen. Unilateral choanal atresia may escape early detection and present later in life with chronic unilateral nasal discharge and unilateral nasal airway obstruction.

MEDICAL HISTORY

Most patients with bilateral choanal atresia are diagnosed in the neonatal period, presenting with cyclic cyanosis relieved by crying and nasal airway obstruction. Choanal atresia may be associated with other abnormalities, such as the CHARGE associations (coloboma, heart anomaly, choanal atresia, mental retardation, genital and ear anomalies). Patients with unilateral atresia are often diagnosed later in life with a history of unilateral nasal discharge and nasal airway obstruction.

PHYSICAL EXAMINATION

Most newborns are obligate nose breathers. Patients with choanal atresia cannot breathe through the obstructed nasal cavity. They characteristically have marked respiratory distress with sternal retractions that is relieved by crying. The cry (voice and airway) is usually normal. A glass slide may be placed to the nose and the absence of fogging at the nares noted. Further examination entails an attempt to pass a small suction or feeding catheter through the nasal cavity. This fails in patients with choanal atresia. The diagnosis can be confirmed by visualizing the choanae. Topical decongestants are applied to the nose, and the nasal cavity is carefully suctioned to clear secretions. A fiberoptic nasolaryngoscope or rigid telescope can be used to view the nasal cavity and the atretic choanae. Fiberoptic examination through the oral cavity permits visualization of the larynx.

EMBRYOLOGY

The normal choanae begin to develop during the sixth gestational week, when the nasal placodes invaginate to form the nasal pits. These pits deepen and become nasal sacs, which are separated from the oral cavity by the oronasal membrane. The choanae form when the oronasal membranes rupture and the nasal sacs communicate with the oral cavity. As the secondary palate forms, the definitive choanae are located at the junction of the posterior nasal cavity and the nasopharynx.

Neural crest cells migrate from the dorsal neural folds into the region at the developing facial processes, at the time the membranous nasal cavities are developing. These cells differentiate into the cartilaginous framework of the skull base and nasal vaults.[2] Hengerer and Strome[3] proposed that there is abnormal migration of neural crest cells into the region of the developing facial processes. This causes the nasal sacs failure to achieve the proper relationship to the developing nasal cavity, resulting in a lack of perforation and communication with the nasal pharynx. This abnormal mesodermal flow theory explains the local anatomic findings, as well as the existence of anomalies grouped in the CHARGE association. Excess migration of neural crest cells into the developing nasal septum and posterior choanal region may occur at the expense of cells that otherwise form the rest of the ethmoid complex.[2]

ANATOMY

Harner and colleagues[4] described the anatomy of choanal atresia. From tomographic studies, they found that the common abnormalities are a narrowed nasal cavity, lateral bony obstruction, medial bony obstruction from a thickened vomer, and a persistent area of membranous obstruction. This work was done before the availability of computed tomography (CT). In a subsequent study, Brown and associates[5] correlated anatomic and pathologic studies of two patients with choanal atresia and correlated these with CT evaluation. This confirmed the anatomic abnormalities of choanal atresia. Gross examination and light microscopy of axial sections of the posterior atresia plates revealed combined osseous and membranous obstruction of the posterior nasal cavity (Fig. 9-1). The medial pterygoid plates were expanded bilaterally in each case, producing medial deviation of the posterior lateral nasal wall. The posterior vomer was enlarged by endochondral bone formation. These studies confirmed a delicate fibrous membrane invested by respiratory epithelium linking the posterior vomer to the medial pterygoid, causing obstruction of the posterior nasal cavity. No osseous or chondroid islands were identified within the membranous portions of the atresia plates (Fig. 9-2). These anatomic abnormalities were confirmed by CT evaluation, which also provided excellent correlation with the abnormal anatomy.[5] Coniglio and colleagues[6] found in a study of choanal atresia and CHARGE association that these patients have abnormal skull base anatomy with a contracted vertical nasopharynx. They also noted an abnormally prominent bony medial pterygoid lamina and thickened vomer and posterior septum.

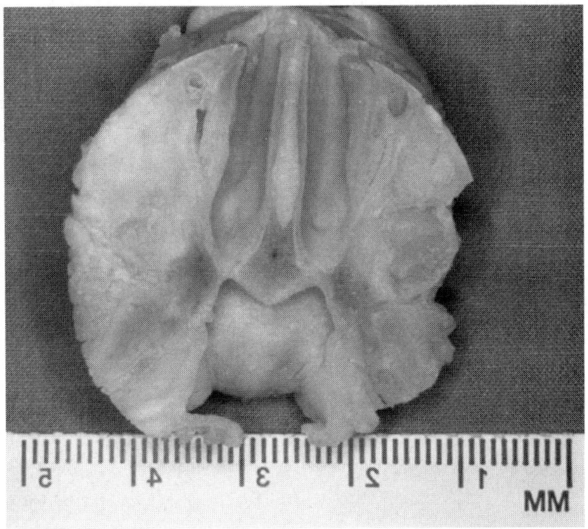

Fig. 9-1. Axial gross section of the nasal cavity and nasopharynx revealing mixed bony-membranous atresia. Medial deviation of the pterygoid plates and a thickened posterior vomer are connected by a thin membrane.

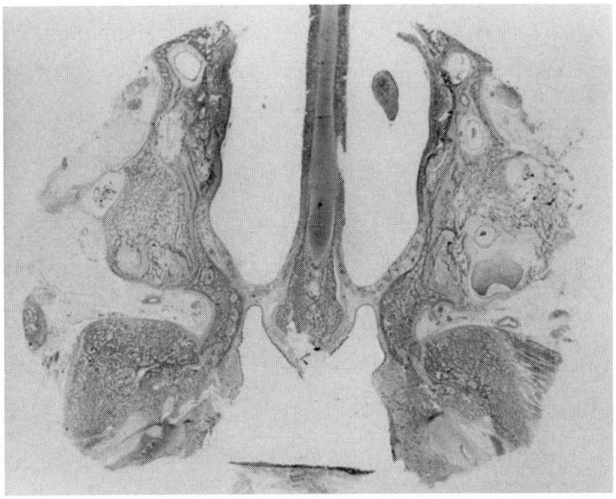

Fig. 9-2. Photomicrograph of the axial section from Fig. 9-1. A fibrous membrane invested by respiratory epithelium links the abnormal vomer and pterygoid plates.

RADIOGRAPHIC EVALUATION

Computed tomography has become the procedure of choice in the evaluation of choanal atresia, as demonstrated by several studies.[7,8] Contrast nasopharyngeal studies have been out of date for several years. The patient's airway is stabilized, usually with an oral airway or McGovern nipple—a feeding nipple with the end cut off. Sedation may be used, and the patients are closely monitored. Before radiographic evaluation the nasal cavity is carefully suctioned and decongestants are applied topically. Scanning is done in the axial plane using 1- to 2-mm slices through the abnormal anatomic areas. Computed tomography shows the narrowing of the pterygoid plates of the choanae, and the thickness and shape of the vomer deformity. It provides accurate delineation of whether the anatomy is bony or membranous, and reveals the thickness of the atresia plate. Sagittal and three-dimensional reconstructions can be done to provide additional information. This anatomic information may influence the choice of surgical repair procedure, depending on the evaluation of the individual patient. The radiation dosage from a CT study is about 1.5 to 2.5 rad and may vary depending on the number of CT sections taken. Computed tomography is an accurate and sensitive imaging technique that provides excellent and accurate delineation of the abnormal anatomy (Figs. 9-3 and 9-4). Magnetic resonance imaging is not a procedure of choice in the evaluation of the bony anatomy of choanal atresia, as the bony abnormalities are poorly revealed.

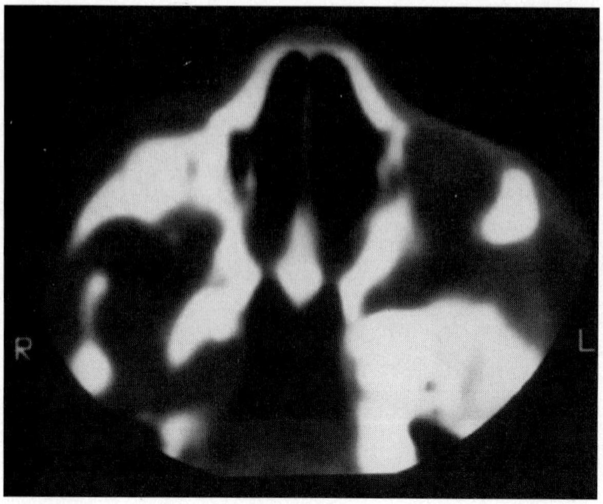

Fig. 9-3. Axial computed tomography (CT) from Figs. 9-1 and 9-2. Delineation of the expanded pterygoid plates and abnormal vomer correlates well with the abnormal gross and microscopic pathology. A mixed bony-membranous atresia plate is demonstrated.

TREATMENT

Medical Treatment

The immediate management of patients with choanal atresia includes stabilization of the airway. A McGovern nipple is inserted into the oral cavity and secured to the face. This provides an oral airway for the child to breathe. Alternatively, an oral airway from the operating room can be inserted into the oral cavity and secured with a surgeon's mask over the occiput (Fig. 9-5). These materials are inexpensive, are easily available within the hospital, and provide an adequate airway for the patient. Feeding can be done by intermittent gavage or placing a small feeding tube through the oral cavity into the stomach.

Most patients stabilize well with an oral airway; however, in the rare patient with multiple anomalies such as CHARGE association, tracheotomy may be indicated. Upon evaluation, some of these patients may not be good candidates for surgical repair for technical reasons, such as abnormalities of the skull base. Underlying medical condition(s) such as associated cardiac or other abnormalities may make them unable to tolerate surgical repair.

A careful work-up for associated anomalies must be undertaken. Patients with CHARGE association present

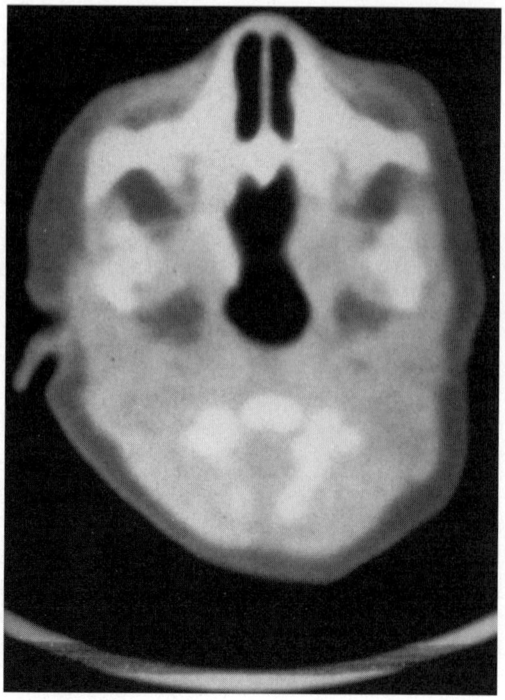

Fig. 9-4. Axial CT of a patient with bilateral bony atresia. Note the absence of membranous atresia plate.

with choanal atresia[9,10] and require a work-up for cardiac problems and other anomalies. Duncan and associates[9] found cardiac anomalies in at least 20% of cases of bilateral atresia. Associated defects are noted in up to 75% of patients with bilateral choanal atresia.[9] These authors also found that cardiac problems and central nervous defects may contribute significantly to infant mortality. A multidisciplinary approach is recommended for the evaluation and management of infants with choanal atresia, including evaluation of the cardiac, nervous, visual, and auditory systems.

Surgical Repair

The choice of surgical technique in the repair of choanal atresia is controversial. In newborns with bilateral choanal atresia, the choice is between a transpalatal or a transnasal approach. Although comparing series with different techniques is difficult, and most results are not directly comparable, Pirsig[11] believes that the success rates of the two procedures are roughly equal. The transpalatal route offers better visualization of the atretic area, and it is a little easier to remove the posterior septum, but there is longer operative time and blood loss plus significant risk of long-term dental cross-bite problems due to the removal of the midpalatal suture.[12] The transnasal route has a shorter operative time, involves low blood loss, and does not interfere with the developing palate growth spurt that occurs within the first 5 years of life.

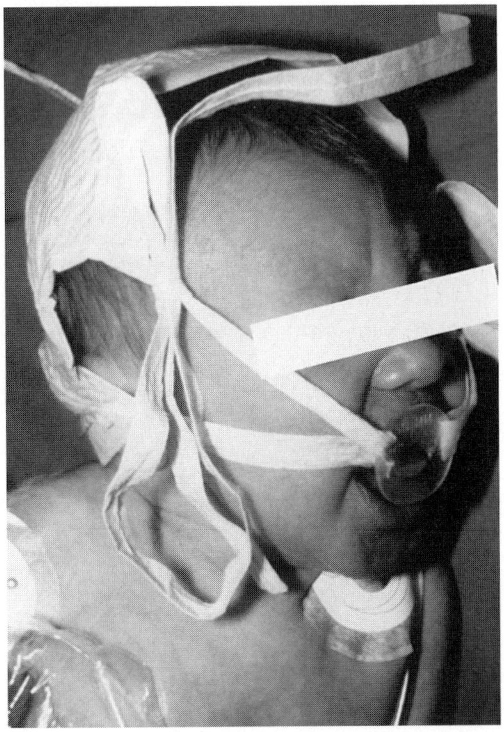

Fig. 9-5. Patient with choanal atresia. The airway is secured with an oral airway and surgeon's mask.

Transnasal perforation techniques have been abandoned; microsurgical techniques with operating microscopes, otologic instruments with burrs, and endoscopic telescopes are employed for the transnasal route.[13] These instruments allow excellent visualization of the atresia plate during repair.

The objective in repair is to provide the best possible chance of a good long-term nasal airway and to correct the anatomic abnormalities. This is accomplished by carefully widening the lateral pterygoid plates and shortening the abnormally thickened posterior vomer to create a common cavity posteriorly. This opens the nasal cavity and provides the best chance to prevent restenosis. Transseptal techniques can be used for revision surgeries or in patients 2 years of age or older. This approach can be used in conjunction with transnasal microsurgical drill-out techniques, and can be particularly useful in patients with CHARGE association and base-of-skull abnormalities. The transseptal technique is done by a careful subperichondrial approach with complete preservation of all the cartilaginous septum. The bony septum can be carefully removed while preserving the mucoperichondrial flaps back to the area of the atresia plate. This provides both transseptal and transnasal access. The risk of significant abnormalities of nasal growth with these techniques should be extremely minimal; they have proved safe in pediatric rhinoplasty.

Patients with bilateral choanal atresia are usually operated on within the first week of life, after careful medical evaluation and work-up. Those with unilateral choanal atresia are often diagnosed later in life and usually operated on after evaluation and work-up at the time of diagnosis. If patients with unilateral choanal atresia are diagnosed very early in life, I usually wait to operate until they are about 1 year of age, as the choanae approximately double in size in the first year of life.

There has been some controversy over the use of flaps in the dissection of choanal atresia. Some consider that mucoperiosteal flaps can be used to cover the raw bony area in the choanal area and reduce the possibility of scar tissue formation and restenosis, but I find it almost impossible to preserve these mucoperichondrial flaps. On a practical basis, it is probably not a useful exercise to try to develop mucoperiosteal flaps.

When the choanae is opened to an adequate size, I use stents for approximately 4 to 6 weeks. This is an arbitrary length of time; no good studies of the optimal timing exist. Easily available Portex endotracheal tubes are cut to length—usually 3.5 or 4.0 in newborns—to pass through the area of the repaired choanae into the nasopharynx, but not past the free edge of the palate. The free edge of the anterior stent is just inside the nasal valve area, and the stents are secured by circumseptal suture (Fig. 9-6). This tech-

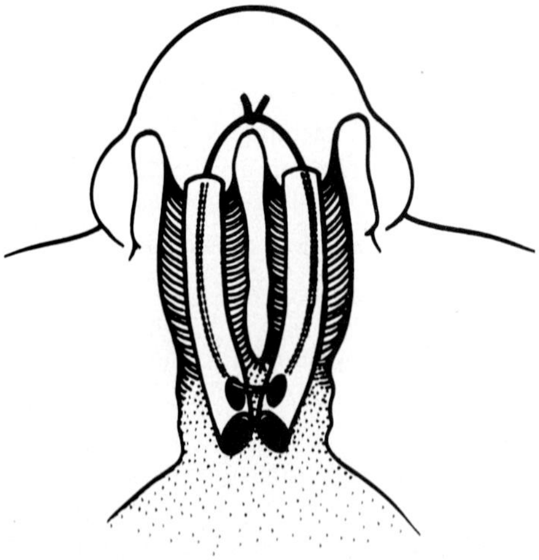

Fig. 9-6. Diagram of nasal stents secured by circumseptal suture.

nique is described by Liston[14]; it has the advantage that there is no suture though the septum. The string can be cut and changed and the stents changed if they become plugged, and the patients do not require anesthesia for removal. The stents also do not protrude through the nose to create a pig-snout type of deformity. While the stents are in place, the patient is usually kept on a regimen of an oral antibiotic, such as cephalexin, to reduce the risk of purulent rhinorrhea. When the stents are removed, nasal steroid sprays, or drops such as beclomethasone, are prescribed in addition to the antibiotics. Beste and colleagues[15] found that gastroesophageal reflux (GER) can complicate the successful repair of choanal atresia; they noted an increased incidence of granulation and stenosis. They believe that recognition and control of GER can reduce operative morbidity. After stent removal, patients are followed-up by periodic fiberoptic nasal examinations. Patients who develop stenosis are treated with nasal dilation under local lidocaine (Xylocaine) anesthesia and oxymetazoline (Afrin) decongestant with female urethral dilators. This can be done weekly in the office until the choanae stabilize.

Patients over 2 years of age with unilateral choanal atresia may be treated with a combined transnasal and transseptal approach. The transantral approach can be utilized in much older patients who have a large, well-ventilated maxillary sinus and completed palatal growth but is rarely indicated.

RESULTS

The author's personal series of 11 patients undergoing transnasal repair has been published.[1] All these patients have functional nasal airways, and 8 of the 11 have required at least one dilation. Two patients needed revision surgery, but one was operated on at an outside institution. In a follow-up of a minimum of 1 year, two patients have unilateral stenosis and nine have bilateral patency. Both patients who required revision surgery have bilateral patency. Of the two patients with unilateral stenosis, both have an acceptable airway function, and revision surgery is not contemplated at this moment.

DISCUSSION

Choanal atresia is a complex nasal anatomic abnormality that requires careful evaluation and considered surgical therapy to obtain a patent nasal airway. After initial stabilization and careful work-up for associated abnormalities, CT is the diagnostic procedure of choice. Axial CT cuts provide excellent delineation of the abnormal anatomy, consisting of narrowed pterygoid plates, an enlarged and thickened vomer, and a connecting or membranous or bony atresia plate.

For surgical repair in newborns, I generally prefer the transnasal approach, because of its safety and reproducibility. There is a high rate of success with this procedure and it does not put the growing palate at risk. The transnasal approach can be repeated if necessary, and patients developing stenosis are treated with outpatient dilation. This is regarded as a continuum of care. With careful selection of surgical procedure and medical management, these patients can be successfully treated.

REFERENCES

1. Brown OE, Pownell P, Manning SC: Choanal atresia: a new anatomic classification and clinical management applications, *Laryngoscope* 106:97-101, 1996.
2. Dunham ME, Miller RP: Bilateral choanal atresia associated with malformation of the anterior skull base: embryogenesis and clinical implications, *Ann Otol Rhinol Laryngol* 101:916-919, 1992.
3. Hengerer AS, Strome M: Choanal atresia: a new embryologic theory and its influence on surgical management, *Laryngoscope* 92:913-921, 1982.
4. Harner SG, McDonald TJ, Reese DF: The anatomy of congenital choanal atresia, *Otolaryngol Head Neck Surg* 89:7-9, 1981.
5. Brown OE, Burns DK, Smith TH, Rutledge JC: Bilateral posterior choanal atresia: a morphologic and histologic study, and computed tomographic correlation, *Int J Pediatr Otorhinolaryngol* 13:125-142, 1987.
6. Coniglio JU, Manzione JV, Hengerer AS: Anatomic findings and management of choanal atresia and the CHARGE association, *Ann Otol Rhinol Laryngol* 97:448-453, 1988.
7. Brown OE, Smith T, Armstrong G., Grundfast K: The evaluation of choanal atresia by computed tomography, *Int J Pediatr Otorhinolaryngol* 12:85-98, 1986.
8. Crockett DM, Healy GB, McGill TJ, Friedman EM: Congenital tomography in the evaluation of choanal atresia in infants and children, *Laryngoscope* 97:174-183, 1987.

9. Duncan NO, Miller RP, Catlin FI: Choanal atresia and associated anomalies: the CHARGE association, *Int J Pediatr Otorhinolaryngol* 15:129-135, 1988.

10. Leclerc JE, Fearon B: Choanal atresia and associated anomalies, *Int J Pediatr Otorhinolaryngol* 13:265-272, 1987.

11. Pirsig W: Surgery of choanal atresia in infants and children: historical notes and updated review, *Int J Pediatr Otorhinolaryngol* 11:153-170, 1986.

12. Freng A: Growth in width of the dental arches after partial extirpation of the mid-palatal suture in man, *Scand J Plast Reconstr Surg* 12:267-272, 1978.

13. Lazar RH, Younis RT: Transnasal repair of choanal atresia using telescopes, *Arch Otolaryngol Head Neck Surg* 121:517-520, 1995.

14. Liston SL: Stenting choanal atresia, *Laryngoscope* 90:1061-1062, 1980.

15. Beste DJ, Conley SF, Brown CW: Gastroesophageal reflux complicating choanal atresia repair, *Int J Pediatr Otorhinolaryngol* 29:51-58, 1994.

SUGGESTED READINGS

Beinfield HH: Bilateral choanal atresia in the newborn, *Arch Otolaryngol* 73:659-671, 1961.

Bergstrom L, Owens O: Posterior choanal atresia: a syndromal disorder, *Laryngoscope* 94:1273-1276, 1984.

Birck HG, Parrish RT: The movable stent in choanal atresia, *Laryngoscope* 96:135-139, 1986.

Caldarelli DD, Friedberg SA: Transnasal microsurgical correction of choanal atresia, *Laryngoscope* 87:2023-2030, 1977.

Carpenter RJ, Neel HB: Correction of congenital choanal atresia in children and adults, *Laryngoscope* 87:1304-1311, 1977.

Cherry J, Bordley J: Surgical correction of choanal atresia, *Ann Otol Rhinol Laryngol* 75:911-920, 1966.

Connelly JP, Montomery WW, Robinson JC: Choanal atresia, *Clin Pediatr* 4:65-76, 1965.

Craig DH, Simpson NM: Posterior choanal atresia, *J Laryngol Otol* 75:603-611, 1979.

Devgan BK, Harkins WB: Congenital choanal atresia, *Int Surg* 62:397-399, 1977.

Dobrowski JM, Grundfast KM, Rosenbaum KN, Zajtchuk JT: Otorhinolaryngic manifestations of CHARGE association, *Otolaryngol Head Neck Surg* 93:798-803, 1985.

Durward A, Lord OC, Polson CJ: Congenital choanal atresia, *J Laryngol Otol* 60:461-500, 1945.

Fearon B, Dickson J: Bilateral choanal atresia in the newborn: plan of action, *Laryngoscope* 78:1487-1499, 1968.

Feuerstein SS, Kresp TP, Sachdev RK: Transnasal correction of choanal atresia, *Head Neck Surg* 3:97-104, 1980.

Flake CG, Ferguson CF: Congenital atresia in infants and children, *Ann Otol Rhinol Laryngol* 73:458-473, 1984.

Frazer JS: Congenital atresia of the choanae, *Br Med J* 2:1698–1701, 1910.

Freng A: Surgical treatment of congenital choanal atresia, *Ann Otol* 87:346-350, 1978.

Hall BD: Choanal atresia and associated multiple anomalies, *J Pediatr* 95:395-398, 1979.

Hall WJ, Watanabe T, Kenan PD, Baylin G: Transseptal repair of unilateral choanal atresia, *Arch Otolaryngol* 108:659-661, 1982.

Hasegawa M, Oku T, Tanaka H, et al: Evaluation of CT in the diagnosis of congenital choanal atresia, *J Laryngol Otol* 97:1013-1015, 1983.

Kleager LE, Nolph MB: Posterior choanal atresia, *Ear Nose Throat J* 58:31-45, 1979.

Lantz HJ, Birck HG: Surgical correction of choanal atresia in the neonate, *Laryngoscope* 10:1629-1634, 1981.

McGill T, Jako GJ, Strong MS, Vaughan CW: Management of choanal atresia with carbon dioxide laser, *Ann Otol* 87:658-662, 1978.

McGovern FH: Bilateral choanal atresia in the newborn—a new method of medical management, *Laryngoscope* 71:480-483, 1961.

McGovern FH: Congenital choanal atresia, *Laryngoscope* 60:815-831, 1950.

McGovern FH, Fitz-Hugh GS: Surgical management of congenital choanal atresia, *Arch Otolaryngol* 73:627-634, 1961.

Osguthorpe JD, Singleton GT, Adkins WT: The surgical approach to bilateral choanal atresia, *Arch Otolaryngol* 108:366-369, 1982.

Owens H: Observations in treating twenty-five cases of choanal atresia by the transpalatine approach, *Laryngoscope* 75:84-104, 1965.

Pagon RA, Graham JM Jr, Zonana J, Yong SL: Coloboma, congenital heart disease, and choanal atresia with multiple anomalies: CHARGE association, *J Pediatr* 99:223-227, 1981.

Peebles EM, Dent JH, Rutledge LJ: Choanal atresia in the newborn infant: report of two cases with detailed anatomic studies, *Laryngoscope* 75:783-792, 1965.

Poch-Vinals R, Calvo RR: Choanal atresia—an embryological, clinical, and therapeutical study, *Arch Otolaryngol* 63:559-575, 1956.

Roopenian A, Stemmer AL: Congenital posterior choanal atresia, *Am J Surg* 96:802-807, 1958.

Ruddy L: A transpalatine operation for congenital atresia of the choanae in the small child or the infant, *Arch Otolaryngol* 41:432-834, 1945.

Schwartz AA, Isaacs HJ: Congenital atresia of the posterior nares, *Arch Otolaryngol* 35:603-612, 1942.

Shirkhoda A, Biggers WP: Choanal atresia: a case report illustrating the use of computed tomography, *Radiology* 142:93-94, 1982.

Singleton GT, Hardcastle B: Reconstructive congenital choanal atresia, *Arch Otolaryngol* 87:74-79, 1968.

Slovis TL, Renfro B, Watts FB, et al: Choanal atresia: precise CT evaluation, *Pediatr Radiol* 155:345-348, 1985.

Smith H, Holmes R: Congenital choanal atresia—a technique for surgical correction, *Trans Am Acad Ophthalmol Otolaryngol* 80:527–535, 1985.

Tadmor R, Ravid M, Millet D, Leventon G: Computed tomographic demonstration of choanal atresia, *AJNR* 5:743-745, 1984.

Weseman CM: Management of choanal atresia in the newborn, *Laryngoscope* 88:1304-1311, 1978.

Williams HJ: Posterior choanal atresia, *Am J Roentgenol* 112:1-11, 1971.

Winther LK: Congenital choanal atresia, *Arch Otolaryngol* 104:72-78, 1978.

Wright WK, Shambaugh GE Jr, Green L: Congenital choanal atresia: a new surgical approach, *Ann Otol Rhinol Laryngol* 56:120-126, 1947.

CHAPTER

10

Surgical Management of Thyroid Eye Disease

James P. Milite
Elizabeth A. Maher
Robert C. Della Rocca

PROBLEM

A 40-year-old woman presents with severe bilateral thyroid orbitopathy and compressive optic neuropathy.

Thyroid orbitopathy, or Graves' disease, is a progressive disorder that may cause significant visual dysfunction and cosmetic deformity in severely affected patients. The presence and type of thyroid disease in these patients is highly variable. This disease is the most common cause of exophthalmos in adults, causing 85% of cases of bilateral and up to 28% of cases of unilateral proptosis.[1,2] In addition to exophthalmos, typical clinical features include upper and lower eyelid retraction and strabismus owing to infiltrative changes of the extraocular muscles. Sequelae of the orbital changes that occur in thyroid orbitopathy include chronic diplopia, corneal exposure, and compressive optic neuropathy.

Medical management of thyroid orbitopathy includes stabilization of the patient's systemic thyroid status, as well as treatment of orbital inflammatory changes with systemic corticosteroids or local radiotherapy. In most patients, surgical correction of proptosis, strabismus, and eyelid position should be delayed until the patient's disease has been stable for at least 6 months. However, this rapidly progressive, vision-threatening disease may necessitate emergent decompression at a relatively acute stage of disease. In this chapter a patient with severe thyroid orbitopathy is presented as a subject for discussion of the role of orbital decompression in the management of this disorder.

MEDICAL HISTORY

The patient was diagnosed with hyperthyroidism 15 months before presentation for ophthalmic disease (Fig. 10-1). She had been treated with radioactive iodine therapy twice, with the last treatment 2 months before presentation. The symptoms included worsening proptosis and periorbital swelling over the previous year, with decreasing vision in the left eye of 2 1/2 weeks' duration. The patient did not complain of diplopia. Three months before presentation she had been told of elevated intraocular pressure by her ophthalmologist, with institution of topical timolol 0.5% twice daily bilaterally. Oral prednisone (20 mg daily) was begun 3 days before evaluation for the worsening orbitopathy. The medical regimen also included oral propranolol and propylthiouracil.

The patient's history provides an example of the typical pattern of presentation seen in acute thyroid orbitopathy. In general, thyroid orbitopathy is a progressive inflammatory process, with a probable, but not clearly defined autoimmune etiology.[3-5] The disease is self-limited and is usually active for 1 to 5 years. The active phase is characterized by an interval of orbital inflammation, vascular congestion, and edema, which is often therapeutically amenable to systemic immune modulation through either corticosteroids or radiation. This is followed by a chronic stage of soft-tissue fibrosis that is resistant to treatment. The severity of the acute inflammation and its responsiveness to medical therapy in a given patient is determinative of the ultimate morbidity related to thyroid orbitopathy. The sexual prevalence of thyroid orbitopathy is defined by a female predominance, and the age of affected patients at onset ranges from the second to the ninth decades. Nunery and colleagues[6] defined a

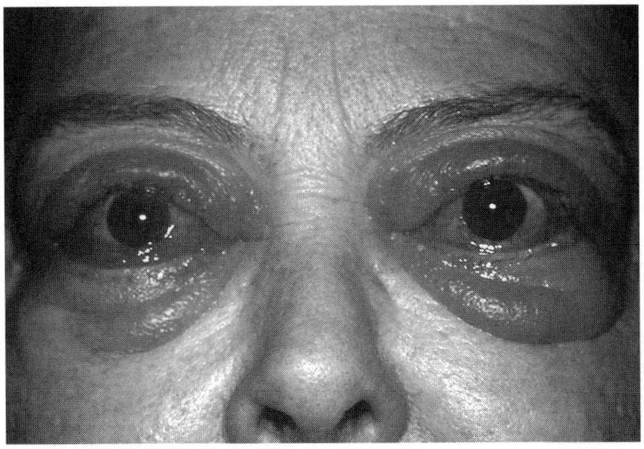

Fig. 10-1. Photograph of the patient presented in the primary position of gaze. Significant proptosis is present, coupled with marked upper and lower eyelid edema and conjunctival chemosis. There is evidence of upper and lower eyelid retraction bilaterally.

classification system of type I disease characterized by proptosis, soft-tissue edema, and full motility; and type II disease with severe restrictive myopathy and a high incidence of exposure keratopathy and optic neuropathy. The severity of disease is influenced by a number of factors, including smoking, stress, and genetic variables.[7-10]

The relationship of orbitopathy to frank dysfunction of the thyroid gland is difficult to define on a patient-to-patient basis. Affected patients are usually hyperthyroid, although hypothyroid and euthyroid cases are not unusual.[11,12] On the basis of observation of the clinical course of these patients and the response of orbital disease to systemic thyroid hormone modulation, it is clear that orbitopathy and thyroid glandular malfunction are related but may progress independently.[13,14] Normalization of thyroid hormone levels often has no effect on orbitopathy; in fact, a worsening of orbitopathy is occasionally noted with normalization of systemic thyroid status. However, to avoid systemic complications of surgery or anesthesia related to a dysthyroid state, as well as to obtain a lasting surgical result, operative intervention in ophthalmic disease should be delayed until a euthyroid state is medically obtained.

The hallmark findings of thyroid orbitopathy at presentation are globe proptosis and eyelid retraction. These two processes interact in a synergistic fashion to cause globe exposure and corneal drying, which, if severe, may be vision threatening. The orbital changes in thyroid orbitopathy are due, at least in part, to tissue deposition of mucopolysaccharides and edema, with subsequent inflammation, tissue ischemia, and late fibrosis.[15] This pathophysiologic mechanism is especially evident in the extraocular muscles, which may become massively enlarged and exhibit altered contractility, resulting in restrictive strabismus.[16] The levator muscle undergoes similar changes that, coupled with sympathetic hyperstimulation of the upper and lower tarsal muscles, cause eyelid retraction. The congestion and enlargement of orbital soft tissues causes forward displacement of the globe, which actually provides a form of anterior decompression of the orbit. However, intraorbital pressure may reach levels significant enough to cause compressive optic neuropathy, usually when there is a "tight" orbital apex with contact of the enlarged rectus muscle bellies upon the optic nerve.[17] Altered optic nerve function and decreased vision occurs in this scenario and will progress unless the compression is relieved. The history of vision loss in the patient presented here is alarming and should make the examiner wary of either corneal decompensation or optic nerve compression.

PHYSICAL EXAMINATION

Best corrected Snellen visual acuity was 20/60 in the right eye, and finger counting at 3 feet in the left eye. Pupils were equal, round, and reactive to light, and there was an afferent pupillary defect in the left eye. Color vision was bilaterally abnormal as tested with Ishihara's plates, and color desaturation of a red object was noted bilaterally, greater in the left eye than in the right. Ocular motility examination revealed a manifest left esotropia of 35 prism diopters. Restriction of ductions in all fields was noted, with marked bilateral limitation of elevation and abduction (Fig. 10-2). Axial proptosis was present with Hertel exophthalmometry measurement of 22 mm bilaterally at a base of 99 mm. Marked resistance to globe retrodisplacement was greater on the left eye than on the right. Significant retraction of the upper (3 mm) and lower (1 mm) eyelids was noted bilaterally, as was lid lag on downgaze. Severe inferior conjunctival chemosis was seen with injection of the insertions of the horizontal rectus muscles. The corneas were clear, with mild punctate epithelial defects inferiorly. Intraocular pressure was 20 mm Hg bilaterally, with elevation of pressure on upgaze to 28 mm Hg in the right eye and 34 mm Hg in the left eye. Fundus examination revealed sharp, pink, optic nerve heads with cup/disc ratios of 0:3. Maculae were flat with normal vessels.

Evaluation of visual function in patients with acute thyroid orbitopathy begins with measurement of Snellen acuity. Acuity may be reduced in these patients for a variety of reasons, including ocular irritation, corneal exposure, and optic neuropathy. Close examination of pupillary reactivity is performed, with attention to the presence of an afferent pupillary defect, indicating impaired optic nerve function on the involved side. However, if bilateral optic neuropathy exists with equal severity, an afferent pupillary defect will not be detected. Color vision testing also allows assessment of optic nerve function.[18]

This is best performed with standardized color testing plates such as the Ishihara or Hardy-Rand-Ritter types. Subjective color desaturation may also indicate optic neuropathy; this is detected by asking the patient to compare the appearance of an illuminated colored test object between the two eyes. Clearly the patient presented here has evidence of significant optic neuropathy with decreased acuity, altered color vision, and an afferent pupillary defect in the left eye.

Evaluation of ocular motility in thyroid orbitopathy typically reveals a restrictive pattern of strabismus, with the inferior and medial rectus muscles most commonly involved. Diplopia may exist in all fields of gaze if the myopathy is severe. Forced duction testing, which involves mechanical manipulation of the globe with a toothed forceps after administration of topical anesthesia, confirms the restrictive nature of the myopathy. Examination of the orbits begins with Hertel exophthalmometry to quantify the degree of proptosis. The amount of orbital congestion can be estimated with gentle manual retrodisplacement of the globes, often correlating with the overall severity of the orbitopathy, although some authors find this test unreliable.[19]

Retraction of the upper and lower eyelids is the hallmark of thyroid eye disease, causing scleral exposure above and below the cornea and a prominent staring appearance of the eyes. Incomplete and delayed excursion of the upper lid on downgaze, or lid lag, is a classic finding in these patients. The eyelid retraction and proptosis may act synergistically in causing incomplete eyelid closure (lagophthalmos) and globe exposure, with poor wetting of the ocular surface. When the orbitopathy is acute, massive edema of the preseptal compartment of the eyelids and subconjunctival space (chemosis) may occur. Hyperemia of the rectus muscle insertions on the sclera may also be noted on examination of the conjunctiva. The status of the cornea must be assessed, with careful attention given to detection of epithelial defects, infectious ulceration, loss of stromal clarity, and neurotrophic changes.

Increased orbital venous pressure and elevation of intraorbital pressure owing to edema and enlargement of native orbital structures may lead to high intraocular

A

B

C

D

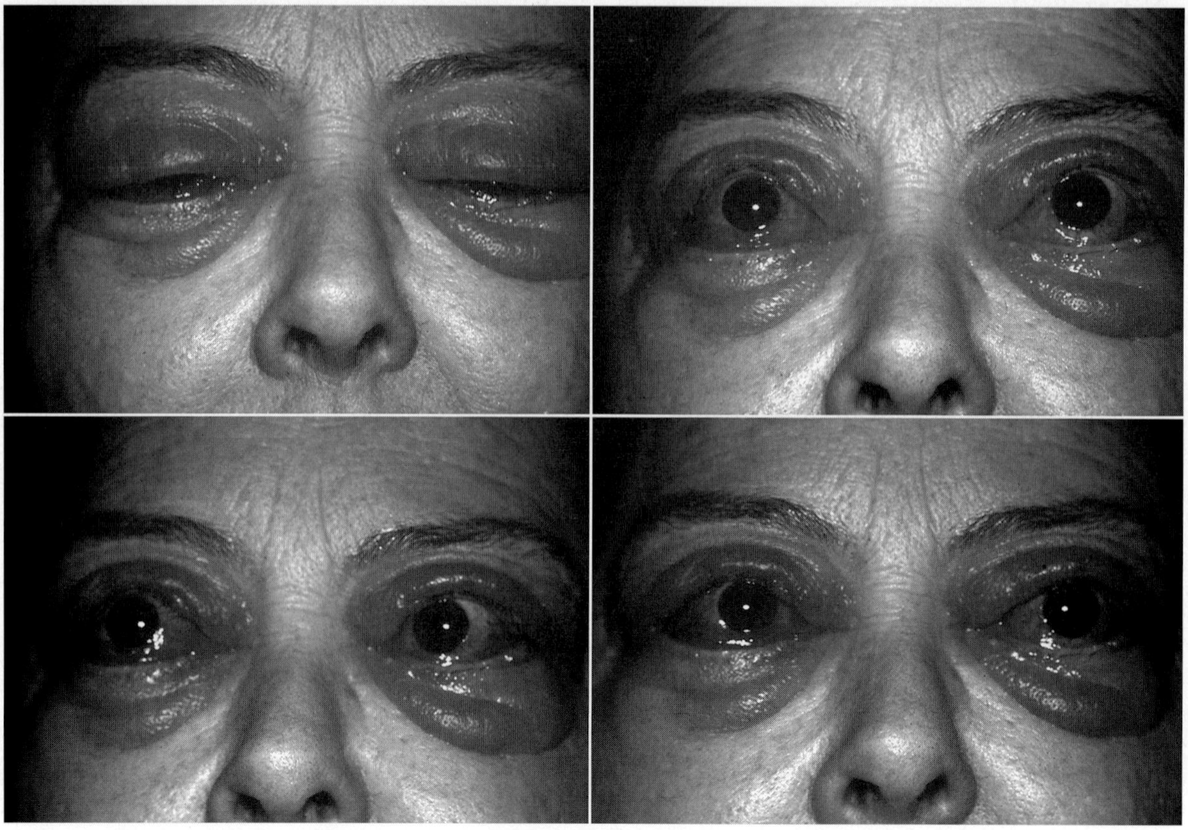

Fig. 10-2. **A**, Lagophthalmos (incomplete eyelid closure) is present bilaterally with inferior corneal exposure. **B**, Marked bilateral upgaze restriction is demonstrated. Upgaze restriction also limits the normal Bell's phenomenon (upward rotation of the globes on eyelid closure), potentiating the development of exposure-related cornea disease. **C** and **D**, In right and left gaze, significant limitation of horizontal motility is seen, especially of abduction of the globes. This is typically due to an enlarged, infiltrated medial rectus muscle.

pressure in thyroid orbitopathy patients. The phenomenon of further elevation of intraocular pressure on upgaze is frequently noted and is probably the result of tethering of the globe by a tight inferior rectus muscle.[20] Dilated fundus examination must be performed to visualize the optic disc, which may manifest cupping owing to chronically high intraocular pressure or may be swollen in cases of compressive optic neuropathy. Chorioretinal folds may also be noted on fundus examination and are due to distortion of the eyewall by the mass effect of the engorged orbital soft tissues.

Adjunctive testing is often helpful in evaluating optic nerve status in thyroid orbitopathy patients. Most important is visual field testing, preferably employing automated techniques that allow detection of small relative central scotomas, and therefore early diagnosis of optic neuropathy.[21] Visual evoked potential testing, a type of focal electroencephalogram obtained from the visual cortex, may also reveal subtle dysfunction of the optic nerve before overt findings are seen on clinical examination.

A

B

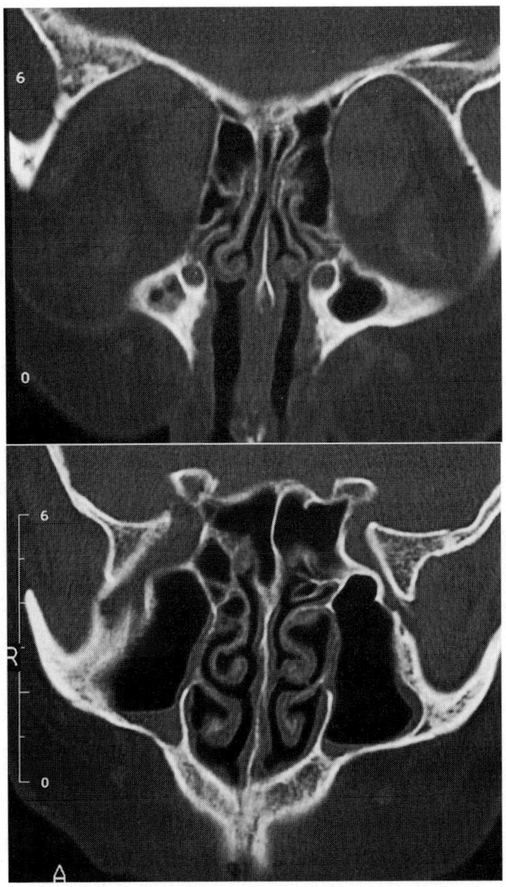

Fig. 10-3. Coronal computed tomography (CT) of the patient's orbits. **A**, Anteriorly, massive enlargement of all four rectus muscles is noted, particularly the medial and inferior recti. **B**, Posteriorly, apical crowding of the orbital contents is evidenced, with the optic nerve vulnerable to compression injury from the enlarged rectus muscle origins.

RADIOGRAPHIC EXAMINATION

Coronal and axial computed tomographic (CT) images of the patient's orbits were obtained (Figs. 10-3 and 10-4). Severe enlargement of all four rectus muscles was noted bilaterally. Additionally, marked crowding of the optic nerve at the orbital apex was seen in both orbits correlating with the clinical diagnosis of compressive optic neuropathy.

Computerized tomography is typically more useful than magnetic resonance imaging (MRI) in cases of thyroid orbitopathy because visualization of the bony orbit is possible. Magnetic resonance imaging has some value in evaluating the orbital apex in cases where optic neuropathy is suspected. The most impressive radiologic finding in these patients is fusiform enlargement of the extraocular muscle bellies with sparing of the muscle tendons.[22] The inferior rectus muscle is most commonly involved, followed by the medical rectus. When all the recti are affected, the optic nerve may be compressed, depending on the degree of muscle enlargement and the bony architecture of the orbital apex.

In addition to extraocular muscle changes, other CT findings are consistently observed in thyroid orbitopathy. Increased vascular markings of the orbital fat compartment may be seen. The lacrimal gland may be noted to be enlarged in an oblong fashion. Anterior bowing of the orbital septum may be present, probably owing to increased orbital pressure and engorgement of the orbital fat compartments. Bone changes may also be noted, especially medial bowing of the medial orbital walls due to extreme enlargement of the medial rectus muscles. In this setting, chronic pressure molds the ethmoid lamina papyracea, providing a form of auto-decompression of the orbit.

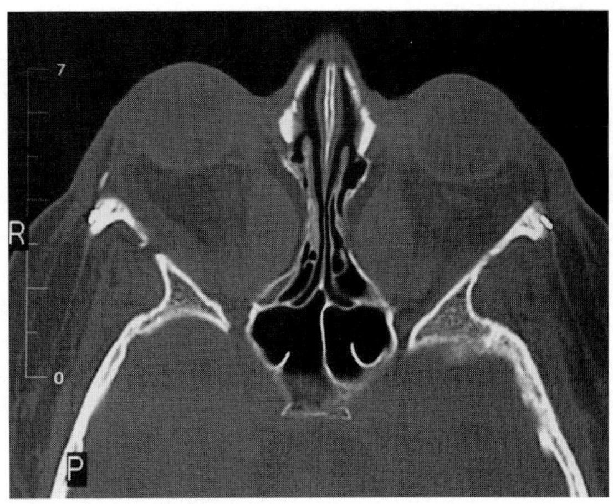

Fig. 10-4. Axial CT reveals massive thyroid myopathy affecting the medial and lateral rectus muscles. Note the inward bowing of the medial wall of the orbit bilaterally, the so-called "coke-bottle" sign.

LABORATORY EXAMINATION

Thyroid function testing is often performed before ophthalmic examination in patients with known thyroid disease. When a systemic diagnosis of thyroid dysfunction is not known, preliminary laboratory testing is indicated at the time of examination as well as prompt endocrinologic consultation. It is important to remember that a significant number of patients with thyroid orbitopathy are euthyroid at the time of presentation with ophthalmic disease. Thyroid function testing in these patients may sometimes reveal a mildly depressed thyroid-stimulating hormone (TSH) level in the face of otherwise normal thyroid values. This low TSH level in euthyroid patients may be the result of suppression in very early subclinical systemic disease, and highly sensitive assays for this hormone have made it the most useful thyroid screening test.[23] Other thyroid function tests of clinical relevance include total T_4 level, T_3 resin uptake, and free T_4 index.

Testing for antithyroid antibodies may be useful in diagnosis of thyroid orbitopathy, especially in euthyroid patients. Antimicrosomal antibodies have been reported in both hyper- and hypothyroidism. Most important is the so-called *thyroid-stimulating immunoglobulin,* an antibody to the TSH receptor that exercises a stimulatory effect on the thyroid gland. Numerous theories exist regarding the role these antibodies play in orbital disease, ranging from reaction to antigens shared by orbital tissue and the thyroid gland to reaction against thyroid hormonal fragments entrapped in orbital tissues. The true nature of this immune mechanism is still a matter of debate.

MEDICAL TREATMENT

Treatment of thyroid orbitopathy begins with local therapy oriented toward protecting the eyes and minimizing globe exposure. Corneal drying may be helped by topical lubricant drops and ointments, nocturnal lid taping, moist chambers, and surgical tarsorrhaphy if necessary. Adnexal edema can be reduced with head elevation and judicious use of diuretics. Topical α-adrenergic blockers have been used to treat eyelid retraction.

The mainstay of medical treatment for thyroid orbitopathy is corticosteroids, which act by reducing edema and inflammation. In the acute setting, high doses are often required, with the occasional need for megadose intravenous methylprednisolone in very severe cases.

In using steroids, it must be kept in mind that rebound inflammation may occur with cessation of therapy. This is especially true of optic neuropathy, which often recurs when steroids are tapered below some threshold dose. It appears that in such cases, radiotherapy or surgical decompression offers more stable results. In addition, the complications and contraindications of prolonged corticosteroid use must be weighed, especially in patients who have multiple medical problems. Immunosuppressive agents have been used as an alternative to steroids. Of these alternatives, the most frequently used agent is cyclosporine, which is generally less effective than steroids and may cause sterility, hypertension, and toxicity to the kidneys and marrow.

Patients who are not surgical candidates or cannot tolerate steroids may benefit from local radiotherapy to the orbits. The mechanism of radiotherapy involves lymphocyte inhibition and fibroblast suppression. This modality is most effective against early inflammatory changes and optic neuropathy, which is stabilized or improved in 65% to 85% of cases.[24] Virtually no change is seen, however, in proptosis or strabismus. The effects of radiotherapy are usually seen in 1 to 8 weeks, but a transient worsening of the orbitopathy may be noted early in the treatment. This often necessitates a temporary increase in the steroid dosage until the radiation effect occurs. Complications of radiotherapy include dry eye, cataracts, and retinopathy.

Surgical intervention in thyroid orbitopathy is guided by four main indications: optic neuropathy, strabismic diplopia, globe exposure and corneal drying, and cosmesis. Surgical treatment of optic neuropathy requires orbital decompression. Correction of strabismus involves extraocular muscle surgery. Globe exposure may be treated with tarsorrhaphy, eyelid-lengthening procedures, or orbital decompression if severe. Cosmetic appearance may be improved with lid lengthening, blepharoplasty, or orbital decompression. The recommended sequence of surgical management of thyroid orbitopathy is to perform orbital decompression first if it is indicated, then strabismus repair, and finally any eyelid surgery. In general, it is prudent to delay any surgical intervention until the thyroid function and orbital inflammation are stable for 6 months, unless the indications are emergent and vision threatening.

ORBITAL DECOMPRESSION

The principle of central-to-orbital decompression is expansion of orbital volume through removal of all or part of the individual orbital walls. Surgery may be performed by removing one wall or several walls in a variety of combinations and employing a number of anatomic approaches.[25-30] The net result of all these approaches is enlargement of orbital volume, allowing orbital soft tissues to expand into the anatomic cavities adjacent to the orbit. This allows posterior displacement of the globe into a more normal anatomic position and also substantially reduces intraorbital pressure. In general, these procedures require bone removal from the selected orbital walls and lysis of the periorbita to allow prolapse of soft tissue out of the orbit. The number and pattern of walls operated on depends on the indications for surgery and the aesthetic desires of the patient. Some authors have championed fat removal without bony decompression for patients with mild-to-moderate cosmetically deforming proptosis, however, this technique offers minimal benefit for severe proptosis or apical optic nerve compression.[31,32]

Indications for orbital decompression include compressive optic neuropathy, intractable corneal exposure, repeated prolapse of the globe anterior to the eyelids, and severe acute inflammatory exophthalmos. To achieve adequate decompression in cases of optic neuropathy, attention must be given to the posterior orbital apex in order to sufficiently relieve pressure on the optic nerve and restore vision. Decompression for other indications does not need to be as aggressive posteriorly but enough bone removal must be performed to allow the globe to move posteriorly into the desired position. As with all thyroid-related eye surgery, it is always preferable to wait until the orbit has stabilized for at least 6 months before decompression. This allows for more predictable surgical results and results in less systemic and local surgical complications. However, patients who have been chronically stable may have significant orbital fibrosis and relatively noncompliant soft tissues, limiting the ultimate results of decompression. Emergent decompression is often required for severe optic neuropathy or when corneal integrity is threatened by globe exposure. In these cases the patient is temporized with high-dose corticosteroids and surgery is performed as promptly as possible.

In selecting an operative approach, consideration is given to the degree of proptosis and to the effect desired from the decompression as outlined previously. A preoperative CT scan is vital not only for diagnostic purposes, but also for evaluation of orbital and periorbital structures. The configuration of the orbital bones should be noted, as well as any orbital apex crowding. The degree of decompression can be estimated by comparing the size of the extraocular muscles with the volume of the orbital cavity. The paranasal sinuses must also be carefully evaluated for size and condition, as the sinuses provide an important role for most decompression techniques.

With the exception of transpalpebral fat decompression, all anatomic approaches to orbital decompression depend on the fact that all orbital walls are shared with other cavities. The medial wall of the orbit is shared with the ethmoidal air cells, and the lateral wall is shared with the temporal region. The orbital roof is also the floor of the anterior cranial fossa, and the floor of the orbit is the superior wall of the maxillary sinus. Therefore, removal of a given wall allows prolapse of soft tissue into an adjacent space. Of the available adjacent anatomic spaces, the anterior cranial fossa provides the least decompression of orbital contents. This is because inferior sagging of the intracranial contents may limit the decompressive effect of removal of the orbital roof.

A variety of surgical approaches have been developed to achieve orbital decompression. The currently preferred method is to combine transnasal endoscopic ethmoidectomy and medial wall decompression with a transconjunctival subperiosteal approach to orbital floor decompression. In selected patients with severe proptosis, the lateral wall may be decompressed in combination with the medial wall and floor. In some patients, decompression of the medial and lateral walls may be performed, and the floor is spared to prevent excessive inferior displacement of the globes and to avoid aggravating any strabismic component of the orbitopathy. Other techniques to approach the medial wall and floor include external ethmoidectomy and a transantral approach to the medial and inferior walls through a Caldwell-Luc operation. Regardless of the approach used, adequate medial decompression must be performed if optic neuropathy is present. The methods used to effect orbital decompression by way of both the two- and three-walled techniques are described later.

Preoperatively, the number of walls to be decompressed is determined. Three-walled decompression is reserved for patients with severe proptosis and congestive orbitopathy in whom two-walled techniques would be unlikely to give adequate decompression. Surgery may be performed bilaterally if the orbitopathy is symmetric, or unilaterally if one orbit is primarily affected. We generally prefer to decompress the medial wall through an endoscopic approach and the orbital floor through a transconjunctival approach similar to that employed in blowout fracture repair. On occasion, medial wall decompression is combined with lateral decompression, leaving the floor intact. This is appropriate for cases with significant strabismic features, which may be worsened by floor decompression. However, less decompression is obtained with the medial/lateral wall approach, and this must be borne in mind in patients with severe orbital congestion.

At the initiation of surgery, forced ductions and posterior ballotment of each globe are performed to allow for intraoperative comparison of these parameters with their preoperative status. A local anesthetic with epinephrine is injected subcutaneously into the lower eyelids and into each lateral canthus. Injection of the nasal mucosa is performed bilaterally, and the nasal cavity is packed with Codman sponges soaked with a vasoconstrictor (typically 0.25% neosynephrine). This is performed before the sterile preparation of the patient to allow time for vasoconstriction to occur.

The rectus muscles correspondent to the walls to be decompressed are then tagged by placing 6-0 silk sutures transconjunctivally about the insertion of each muscle. Decompression of the medial wall of each orbit is first performed using a transnasal approach with a rigid endoscope. Bilateral ethmoidectomy is performed endoscopically to provide exposure of the nasal aspect of the medial wall of each orbit. When the medial walls are clearly identified, the bone of the lamina papyracea is carefully removed with forceps, leaving the periorbita uninjured. The posterior extent of the decompression depends on the presence and degree of optic neuropathy. If optic neuropathy is severe, bone removal may be carried out posteriorly into the sphenoid sinus. This allows medial unroofing of the optic canal, to maximally decompress the optic nerve. Bone removal should not extend superior to the level of the ethmoidal foramina; otherwise, the anterior cranial fossa may be entered and a cerebrospinal fluid leak created.

When the periorbita of each medial wall is completely exposed, a sickle knife is used to open the periorbita. These openings are made as linear anteroposterior incisions of sufficient depth to penetrate the periosteum without injuring the adjacent orbital soft tissues. Orbital fat can be seen to prolapse readily through the incisions created in the periorbita, and the fat may be teased through these vents to further the effect of the decompression. During this part of the procedure, it is helpful to have an assistant actively pull and release the tagged medial rectus muscle so that it may be identified and avoided during the endoscopic decompression. After the periorbita is opened, the globe may be gently retroplaced manually to potentiate the decompressive effect created by the endoscopic procedure. A dramatic difference from the preoperative degree of retroplacement is often noted at this stage. If decompression of the orbital floor is to be performed, endoscopic maxillary antrostomies are created to avoid maxillary sinus outflow problems caused by the obstructive effect of orbital soft tissue prolapsing into the sinus. Each nasal cavity is then packed with Codman sponges, and decompression of the orbital floors and/or lateral walls may then progress.

The approach to the orbital floor begins with an incision extending from the lateral commissure laterally and slightly inferiorly for a distance of approximately 8 to 10 mm, using a No. 15 blade. A curved hemostat is then placed over the exposed lateral canthal tissues directed toward the lateral orbital rim, and a lateral canthotomy is created with Stevens scissors. The inferior crus of the lateral canthal tendon is then exposed and lysed (Fig. 10-5). Double-armed 4-0 silk sutures may be placed through the upper and lower eyelid margins to facilitate exposure. Inferior traction is then placed on the lower eyelid margin over a Desmarres lid retractor, and the conjunctiva of the inferior fornix is marked for incision. This incision should be 6 mm inferior to the lower tarsal border centrally and 3 mm inferior to the tarsus medially and laterally. After subconjunctival injection of local anesthetic with epinephrine, this incision is made with a Westcott scissor or No. 57 Beaver blade. The superior edge of the conjunctival incision is then placed on a 4-0 silk double-armed traction suture, and a plane is created anterior to the orbital septum with blunt dissection. The lateralmost aspect of the incision should be joined to the lateral canthotomy to provide for maximal exposure.

A 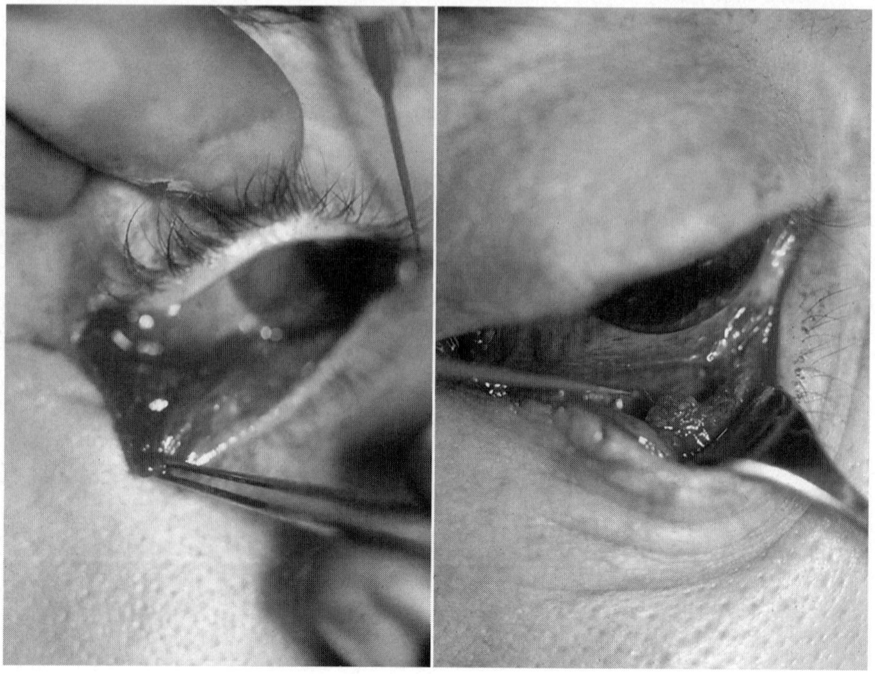 B

Fig. 10-5. Transconjunctival approach to the orbital floor. **A**, Lateral canthotomy and inferior cantholysis are performed to improve access to the inferior orbit. **B**, The conjunctival incision is made in the inferior fornix. Through this incision, the orbital rim periosteum is exposed and may be elevated, revealing the orbital floor, which may then be osteotomized.

If possible, it is helpful to avoid perforation of the orbital septum as this dissection is carried inferior toward the inferior orbital rim. This will keep the orbital fat from prolapsing anteriorly into the surgical field and limiting exposure. However, the orbital fat is often significantly herniated anteriorly through a rarefied septum in most thyroid patients, and debulking of this fat is necessary at this stage before entry into the orbit. When the orbital rim is clearly identified for the full horizontal extent of the incision, cutting cautery may be used to lyse the overlying soft tissues down to the periosteum. The periosteum is then incised and mobilized superiorly, and then posteriorly along the orbital floor with periosteal elevators to expose the orbital plate of the maxilla and the zygoma.

At this stage, identification of the infraorbital neurovascular bundle in the infraorbital groove and canal is necessary to avoid traumatization of the nerve. In addition, the opening in the medial wall created endoscopically should be found. Retraction of the globe and orbital tissue is provided by malleable ribbon retractors. During the procedure, retraction should be periodically released and the pupil checked to ensure adequate circulation to the globe and optic nerve. This is especially important in patients in whom optic nerve function may be already compromised by orbitopathy. The thin bone making up the medial half of the orbital floor, medial to the infraorbital nerve, may then be osteotomized using a fine osteotome and mallet. During creation of the osteotomy, a strut of bone should be left intact at the junction of the medial wall and floor to provide support for the globe and orbital tissues and prevent the so-called *sunset syndrome.*

Enlargement of the osteotomy is achieved with Kerrison and straight rongeurs, with bone removal performed in a careful, piecemeal fashion. Attention must be paid to the infraorbital neurovascular bundle to ensure that it is not injured during creation of the osteotomy. When the area of bone removal is approximately 20 mm^2, incision of the periorbita may commence. A toothed forceps is used to tent the periorbita, and sharp Westcott scissors or a No. 57 Beaver blade may be employed to incise the periosteum. These incisions should be made in a linear anteroposterior direction and should be of sufficient depth to open the periorbita without injuring the soft tissues contained within. Orbital fat should readily prolapse through the periorbital openings. Gentle posterior manual pressure placed on the globe will cause further herniation of fat through the periosteal openings. Some authors recommend debulking of orbital fat at this point, but we do not do this as part of our routine decompressions.

At the conclusion of the procedure, the periosteum is left unsutured. The conjunctival incision is closed with a running 6-0 plain or chromic gut suture from medially to laterally. The edges of the conjunctiva should be carefully opposed during this closure, to avoid foreshortening the inferior fornix. The lateral aspect of the tarsus is resuspended from the lateral orbital rim with a horizontal mattress 4-0 Polydek or Prolene suture. The lateral commissure is reformed with 6-0 chromic gut sutures placed across the mucocutaneous junctions of the upper and lower eyelids. The remaining lateral skin incision is closed with 6-0 silk interrupted sutures. When lateral wall decompression is desired, the lateral canthal skin incision described above is extended laterally about 20 mm toward the ear. Lateral canthotomy and inferior cantholysis are performed as is dissection of the lateral canthal subcutaneous tissues to expose the superficial temporalis fascia and the lateral orbital rim. The periosteum is exposed and incised 2 to 3 mm external to the rim with a No. 15 blade. With periosteal elevators, the periosteum is mobilized from the internal and external surfaces of the zygoma. Externally, the temporalis muscle must be partially disinserted from its attachment to the zygoma.

Osteotomies are then made with an oscillating saw in the lateral orbital rim. The superior cut is made just above the frontozygomatic suture; the inferior cut is made at the junction of the lateral and inferior orbital rims. A malleable ribbon retractor is placed between the lateral orbital wall and the periorbita to protect the globe and orbital contents during this maneuver. An osteotome and mallet may be used to vertically fracture the bone at the zygomaticosphenoidal suture, and the large, mobilized portion of the lateral rim may be removed and placed in saline for later refixation. Rongeurs are used to remove the remaining lateral orbital bone. Care is exercised as the process extends posteriorly, to avoid entry through the dura of the middle cranial fossa. The more posterior portions of the greater sphenoid wing may be contoured if necessary by means of a powered drill with a cutting burr.

Periosteal incisions are again made to allow prolapse of orbital fat after bone removal is complete. Cutting cautery may be used at this point to debulk the adjacent temporalis muscle, to further the decompressive effect afforded by this approach. The bone fragment removed initially from the rim may then be refixated with microplates.[33] The internal surface of this fragment may be hollowed out and recontoured with the cutting drill bit. When the fragment is plated into position, it may be placed so as to anteriorize the forward projection of the lateral rim and mask any residual proptosis. If significant bony stepoffs are created by this placement, the cutting drill burr may be used to round off these deformities.

Closure is similar to that described for the approach to the orbital floor. However, resuspension of the lateral aspect of the tarsus may prove problematic, especially if the rim has been anteriorly repositioned or if insufficient periosteum is present to allow placement of sutures. Occasionally, drill holes must be made in the bone at the desired level of tarsal fixation. In addition, the degree of tension placed on the lower lid margin with this placement must be carefully adjusted; failure to do so may result in "slinging" of the lower eyelid below the globe.

The patient presented here was placed on high-dose intravenous corticosteroids immediately, and after becoming sufficiently medically stabilized she underwent bilateral decompression of the orbital floors and medial walls 4 days later. Three weeks postoperatively, her vision had improved to 20/70 OD and 20/50 OS, with complete improvement of color vision in both eyes. Oral prednisone was gradually tapered to a maintenance dose of 5 mg per day 1 month postoperatively. Six months after decompression, vision improved to 20/30 OU, but the patient experienced continued intractable diplopia (Fig. 10-6). Seven months postoperatively, bilateral inferior rectus recession and left medial rectus recession was performed, and single vision in primary and reading positions was obtained after surgery. Two years after decompression, repair of upper eyelid retraction and blepharoplasty were performed, with satisfactory eyelid levels obtained postoperatively.

COMPLICATIONS OF DECOMPRESSION

A number of possible complications of orbital decompression exist. As with any orbital surgery, hemorrhage is a possible complication, especially if the anterior ethmoidal, posterior ethmoidal, or infraorbital arteries are injured. Most commonly, hypoesthesia in the dermatome of the infraorbital nerve is noted and may last up to 6 months postoperatively, even if the nerve is carefully spared during surgery. In addition, worsening of strabismus is common resulting from potentiation of muscle imbalance caused by alteration of globe position and orbital wall removal.[34] All patients should be made aware of the likelihood of worsened diplopia after orbital decompression. For this reason, extraocular muscle surgery is typically triaged behind orbital decompression in the care of thyroid orbitopathy patients; however, in a select group of patients with high intraocular pressure, recession of the inferior rectus muscles is performed simultaneously.

Ptosis of the globes, or the sunset syndrome, may be present if excessive bone removal from the orbital floor is performed.[35] This effect is lessened by preserving an inferomedial strut of bone to better support the orbital contents.[36] Excessive inferomedial bone removal may also cause trauma to the nasolacrimal duct with secondary obstruction. In addition, excessive bone removal from the medial wall in a superior direction may result in cerebrospinal fluid leak.

Other complications include traumatization of intraorbital structures, specifically the globe, extraocular muscles, and optic nerve. The optic nerve may most easily be injured during posterior medial wall decompression, where it is most closely opposed to the adjacent bone.

A

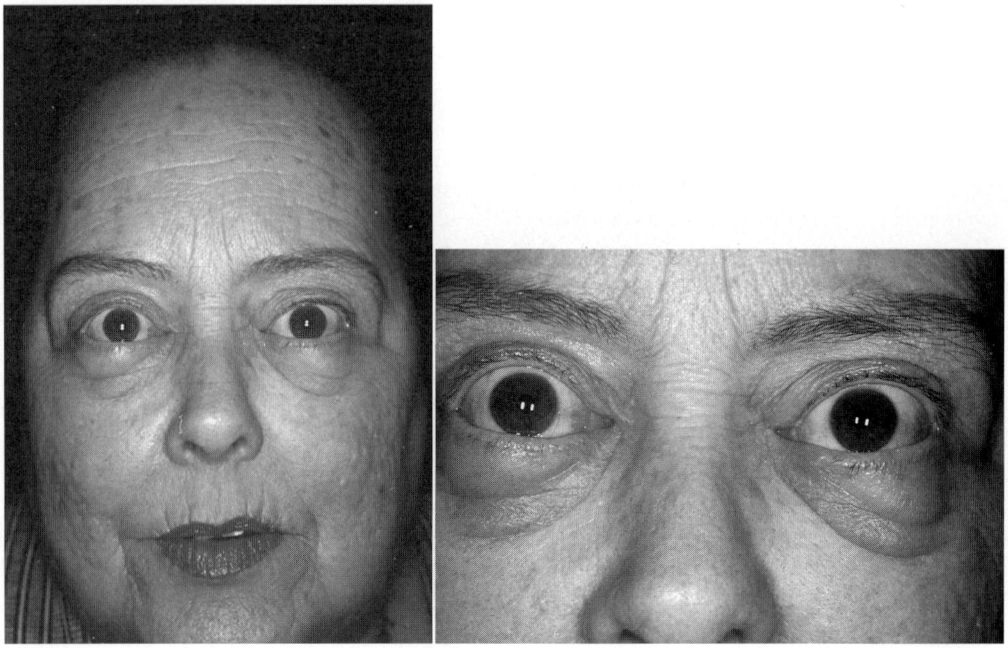

B

Fig.10-6. Full face **(A)** and close-up **(B)** photographs of the patient presented here approximately 1 year after initial presentation. After three-wall orbital decompression bilaterally, she underwent orbital external beam radiotherapy and hard palate mucosal grafts to both lower eyelids. Vision at this point is 20/20 OU with markedly improved cosmesis, but the patient has residual horizontal and vertical diplopia currently corrected by prisms.

Tagging of the rectus muscles is helpful for identification during decompression, as these muscles may be easily incised because of their considerable girth and proximity to the orbital walls.

Poor drainage of the sinuses, especially the maxillary sinus, may follow orbital decompression. Obstruction of sinus outflow by prolapsed orbital contents should be expected and may be obviated by adequate maxillary antrostomy. This procedure should be performed at the time of the initial decompression.

REFERENCES

1. Grove AS: Evaluation of exophthalmos, *N Engl J Med* 292:1005, 1975.
2. Lawton NF: Exclusion of dysthyroid eye disease as a cause of unilateral proptosis, *Trans Ophthalmol Soc UK* 99:226, 1979.
3. Adams DD, Purvis HD: Abnormal response in assay of thyrotrophin, *Proc Univ Otaga Med Sch* 34:11, 1956.
4. Strakosch CR, Wenzel BE, Row VV, et al: Immunology of autoimmune thyroid diseases, *N Engl J Med* 307:1499, 1982.
5. Rose NR, Kong YM, Okayasu I, et al: T-cell regulation in autoimmune thyroiditis, *Immunol Rev* 55:299, 1981.
6. Nunery WR, Martin RT, Heinz GW, Gavin TJ: The association of cigarette smoking with subtypes of ophthalmic Graves' disease, *Ophthalmic Plast Reconstr Surg* 9:77, 1993.
7. Theofilopoulos AN, Dixon FJ: Autoimmune diseases: immunopathology and etiopathogenesis, *Am J Pathol* 108:321, 1982.
8. Adams DD, Adams YJ, Knight JG, et al: On the nature of the genes influencing the prevalence of Graves' disease, *Life Sci* 32:3, 1983.
9. Weiss M, Ingbar SH, Winblad S, et al: Demonstration of a saturable binding site for thyrotropin in *Yersinia enterocolitica, Science* 219:1331, 1983.
10. Hagg E, Asplund K: Is endocrine ophthalmopathy related to smoking? *Br Med J* 295:634, 1987.
11. Solomon DH, Chopra IJ, Chopra U, et al: Identification of subgroups of euthyroid Graves' ophthalmopathy, *N Engl J Med* 296:181, 1977.
12. Kendal-Taylor P: The pathogenesis of Graves' ophthalmopathy, *Clin Endocrinol Metab* 14:331, 1985.
13. Peter SA: Euthyroid Graves' disease: report of a case observed over a 12 year period, *Am J Med* 80:1197, 1986.
14. Stridama V, DeGroot LJ: Treatment of Graves' disease and the course of ophthalmopathy, *Am J Med* 87:70, 1989.
15. Riley FC: Orbital pathology in Graves' disease, *Mayo Clin Proc* 47:975, 1972.
16. Hufnagel TJ, Hickey WF, Cobbs WH, et al: Immunohistochemical and ultrastructural studies on the exenterated orbit of a patient with Graves' disease, *Ophthalmology* 91:1411, 1984.
17. Kennerdell JS, Rosenbaum AE, El-Hoshy MH: Apical optic nerve compression of dysthyroid optic neuropathy on computed tomography, *Arch Ophthalmol* 99:807, 1981.
18. Niegel JM, Rootman J, Belkin RI, et al: Dysthyroid optic neuropathy. The crowded orbital apex syndrome, *Ophthalmology* 95:1515, 1988.
19. Frueh BR, Musch DC, Grill R, et al: Orbital compliance in Graves' eye disease, *Ophthalmology* 92:657, 1985.
20. Pohjanpelto P: The thyroid gland and intraocular pressure: tonographic study of 187 patients with thyroid disease, *Acta Ophthalmol (Suppl)* 97:1, 1968.
21. Gasser P, Flammer J: Optic neuropathy of Graves' disease. A report of perimetric follow-up, *Ophthalmologica* 192:22, 1986.
22. Trokel SL, Hilal SK: Recognition and differential diagnosis of enlarged extraocular muscles in computed tomography, *Am J Ophthalmol* 87:503, 1979.
23. Toft AD: Use of sensitive immunoradiometric assay for thyrotropin in clinical practice, *Mayo Clin Proc* 63:1035, 1988.
24. Dallow RL, Netland PA: *Management of thyroid ophthalmopathy (Graves' disease).* In Albert DM, Jakobiec JA, editors: *Principles and practice of ophthalmology*, Philadelphia, 1994, WB Saunders, p 1909.
25. McCord CD Jr: Current trends in orbital decompression, *Ophthalmology* 92:21, 1985.
26. Ogura JH, Lucente FE: Surgical results of orbital decompression for malignant exophthalmos, *Laryngoscope* 84:637, 1974.
27. Stranc M, West M: A four-wall orbital decompression for dysthyroid orbitopathy, *J Neurosurg* 68:671, 1988.
28. Naffzinger HC: Surgical treatment of progressive exophthalmos following thyroidectomy, *JAMA* 99:638, 1932.
29. Kennerdell JS, Maroon JC: An orbital decompression for severe dysthyroid exophthalmos, *Ophthalmology* 89:467, 1972.
30. Wolfe SA: Modified three-wall orbital expansion to correct persistent exophthalmos or exorbitism, *J Plast Reconstr Surg* 64:448, 1979.
31. Olivari N: Transpalpebral decompression of endocrine ophthalmopathy (Graves' disease) by removal of intraorbital fat: experience with 147 operations over 5 years, *Plast Reconstr Surg* 87:627, 1991.
32. Hecht SD, Guibor P, Wolfley D, Wiggs EO: Orbital dissection defatting technique for Graves' disease, *Ann Ophthalmol* 16:314, 1984.
33. Shore JW, Carvajal J, Westfall CT: Miniplate reconstruction of the lateral orbital rim after orbital decompression for Graves' disease, *Ophthalmology* 99:1433, 1992.
34. Shorr N, Neuhaus RW, Baylis HI: Ocular motility problems after orbital decompression for dysthyroid ophthalmopathy, *Ophthalmic Plast Reconstr Surg* 89:323, 1982.
35. Long JA, Baylis HI: Hypoglobus following orbital decompression for dysthyroid ophthalmopathy, *Ophthalmic Plast Reconstr Surg* 6:185, 1990.
36. Goldberg RA, Shorr N, Cohen MS: The medial orbital strut in the prevention of post-decompression dystopia in dysthyroid ophthalmopathy, *Ophthalmic Plast Reconstr Surg* 8:32, 1992.

CHAPTER

11

Dacryocystorhinostomy

Dale H. Rice

PROBLEM

A 38-year-old woman presents with a history of right-sided epiphora that began approximately 5 to 6 days after endoscopic sinus surgery 1 year previously.

Epiphora as a symptom will result from any malfunction in the drainage system. In broad generalizations, the causes are (1) malposition of the drainage system or (2) obstruction of the drainage system. Malposition is commonly seen with facial nerve paralysis in which lower lid laxity allows the inferior punctum, in particular, to pull away from the globe. However, anything that causes ectropion will lead to the same result. Obstruction of the drainage system is most commonly owing to stenosis of the nasolacrimal duct from trauma, a calculus, or chronic infection.

For problems of malposition, the treatment should be directed at the primary cause. In this situation, dacryocystorhinostomy would be inappropriate and would not solve the basic problem. On the other hand, dacryocystorhinostomy is the treatment of choice for chronic obstruction of the nasolacrimal duct. It does not, however, address canalicular obstruction, which is not helped by dacryocystorhinostomy.

MEDICAL HISTORY

The medical history of a patient with epiphora should be directed toward which of the two above-mentioned causes is pertinent and to what caused the problem itself. Thus, one would want to know if the patient had a history of anything that would lead to malfunction of the facial nerve, such as parotid surgery, penetrating trauma, or Bell's palsy. In addition, a history should be elicited of any eyelid surgery or eyelid trauma that might lead to ectropion of the lower lid.

Causes of ductal obstruction

The cause of nasolacrimal duct obstruction may be obvious, such as a long history of chronic dacryocystitis or penetrating trauma in the area of the duct. On occasion, the cause may be more subtle, such as a neoplastic process within the nasal cavity or paranasal sinuses invading or obstructing the duct. Physical examination of a patient with epiphora should be centered around the eyelids themselves and the nasal cavity and the sinuses. The function and position of the eyelids for proper drainage should be determined. If these are normal and nasolacrimal duct obstruction is suspected, a Jones test may be performed, but not before a thorough endoscopic intranasal examination. The Jones test involves injecting saline into either the superior or inferior canaliculus, observing where the saline exits. If the nasolacrimal duct is obstructed, the saline will emerge from the other canaliculus; if it is open, it will run into the nose.

RADIOGRAPHIC EXAMINATION

The best first study after the endoscopic examination and the Jones test is axial and coronal computed tomography of the sinuses without contrast. The thin-section scans are taken in the area of the nasolacrimal system and the anterior ethmoidal sinuses. Much can be learned about the status of the sac and duct.

TREATMENT

Indications

If the cause of the epiphora is found to be obstruction of the nasolacrimal duct, the treatment is dacryocystorhinostomy. This can be done by either an external or internal approach. The first comprehensive report of lacrimal sac surgery was apparently made around 1770 by Wolfgang Van Goethe, who witnessed an operation performed by an ophthalmologist in Straussburg who connected the lacrimal duct with the nasal cavity and inserted a horse hair to keep the sac open.[1] An external approach was not again described until 1904 by Toti,[2] and then by Dupuy-Dutemp and Borquet in 1921.[3] The first intranasal approach was described by Caldwell in 1893[4] and modified by West[5] and then Mosher.[6]

Endoscopic intranasal dacryocystorhinostomy was originally described by Rice in 1988,[7] by McDonogh and Meiring in 1989,[8] and again by Rice in 1990.[9] For the purposes of this chapter, the discussion of technique will be limited to endoscopic intranasal dacryocystorhinostomy.

Technique

The technique of this operation is relatively straightforward to someone with reasonable experience in endoscopic sinus surgery and in dacryocystorhinostomy. It is generally performed with the patient under general anesthesia, and after its induction the nasal cavity on the side in question is vasoconstricted with a topical application of the vasoconstrictor of choice. Next, the lateral nasal wall just anterior to the anterior superior insertion of the middle turbinate and the middle turbinate itself is infiltrated with 1% lidocaine (Xylocaine) and 1:100,000 epinephrine. This injection should also include the septum, if the space is narrow. Occasionally the anterior end of the middle turbinate will need to be resected, but this is more an exception than a rule. After the attainment of good local vasoconstriction, an approximately 1-cm circular incision is made through the mucosa on the lateral nasal wall immediately anterior to the middle turbinate (Fig. 11-1). This mucosa is dissected off the bone and discarded. The bone is next removed by any of a variety of techniques, although it is usually best done with a cutting burr. Once the bone has been satisfactorily removed, a lacrimal probe is placed through the inferior canaliculus into the lacrimal sac. At this time one should be able to see the sac being prolapsed into the nasal cavity by the probe intranasally. An incision is then made over the lacrimal probe to expose it, and some portion of the medial wall of the lacrimal sac is removed (Fig. 11-2). A polyethylene stent is then placed through both the superior and inferior canaliculi (Fig. 11-3), brought intranasally, tied together and left in place for 4 to 6 weeks for final healing.

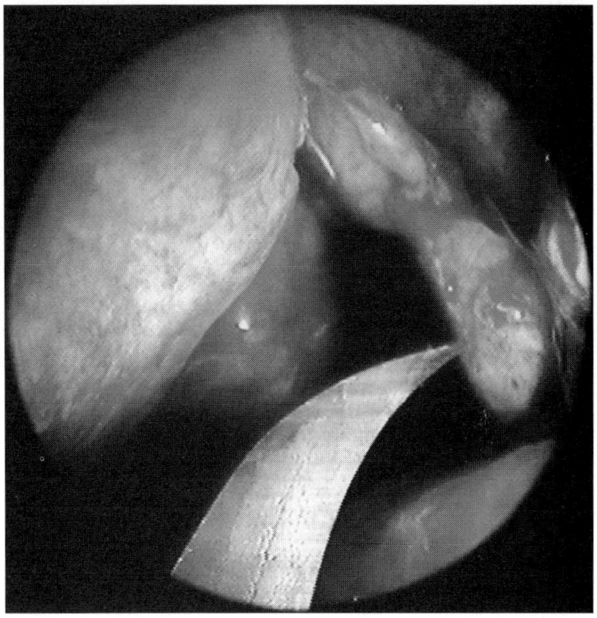

Fig. 11-1. Sickle knife making an incision in the lateral nasal wall.

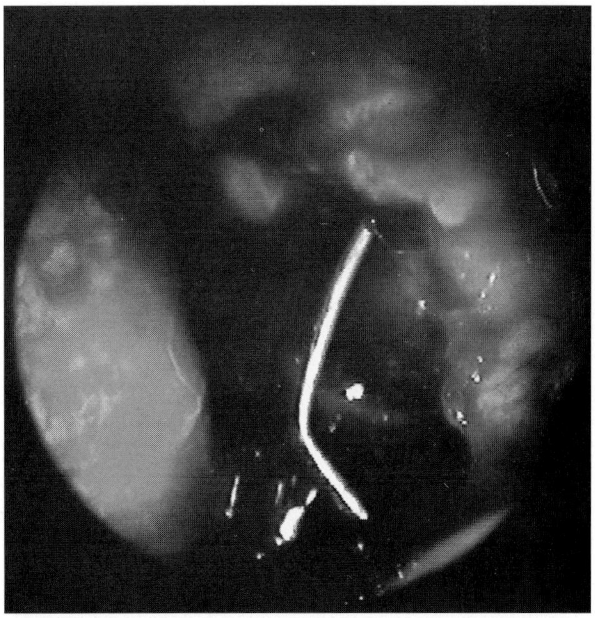

Fig. 11-2. Lacrimal probe passing through the lacrimal sac into the nasal cavity.

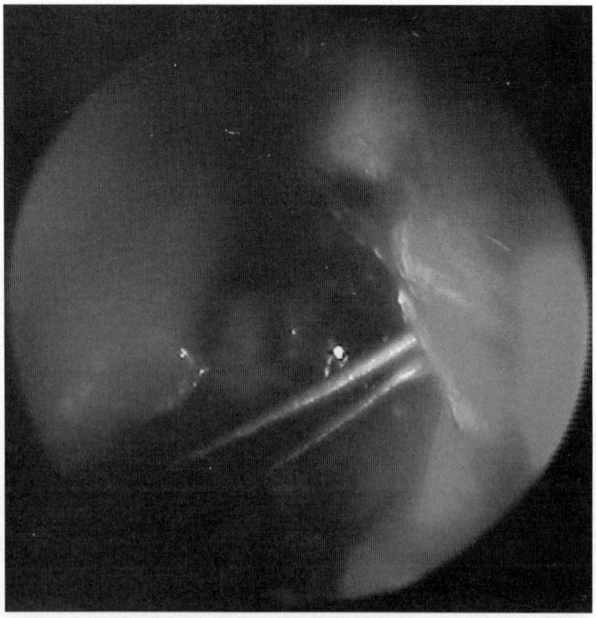

Fig. 11-3. Polyethylene tubing being placed through the superior and inferior canaliculi into the nasal cavity.

RESULTS

The author has experience with this procedure, not only for chronic dacryocystitis or calculi, but also in cases of stenosis secondary to craniofacial surgery and radiation therapy, as well as sinus surgery. In every case to date the procedure has been successful, although some patients have been lost to follow-up in less than 1 year. The long-term patency rate with other authors has varied from 75%[10] to 95%.[11]

DISCUSSION

The symptom of epiphora can be caused by many different entities, but it falls into two broad categories: those that malposition the canaliculi to inhibit drainage and those that obstruct the drainage system. In the latter situation, the most common cause is obstruction of the nasolacrimal duct, and this is best managed, if chronic, by dacryocystorhinostomy.

The dacryocystorhinostomy can be done by an external approach through an incision placed between the medial canthus and the dorsum of the nose. The lacrimal sac is then dissected out after removal of the overlying bone, and connected to the mucosa intranasally.

A more contemporary procedure involves the endoscopic intranasal technique previously described. In most series, the results obtained with the endoscopic intranasal approach are at least as good as those obtained by the external approach. In addition, the intranasal approach is ideal for revision surgery after failure by either technique, as the bone is already removed, and identification of the sac intranasally with an endoscope is easy in experienced hands.

REFERENCES

1. Cited by Weidenbecker M, Hoseman W, Buhr W: Endoscopic endonasal dacryocystorhinostomy: results in 56 patients, *Ann Otol Rhinol Laryngol* 103:363, 1994.
2. Toti A: Nuevo metodo conservatore di cura radicale delle suppurazoni croniche del sacco lacrimale (dacrio cistorhinostomia), *Clin Moderna (Firenze)* 10:385, 1904.
3. Dupuy-Dutemp L, Borquet M: Procede plastique de dacryocystorhonostomie et results, *Ann Ocul* 158:241, 1921.
4. Caldwell GW: Two new operations for obstruction of the nasal duct with preservation of the canaliculi and an incidental description of a new lachrymal probe, *NY Med J* 57:581, 1893.
5. West J: A window resection of the nasal duct in cases of stenosis, *Trans Am Ophthalmol Soc* 12:659, 1910.
6. Mosher HP: Re-establishing intranasal drainage of the lachrymal sac, *Laryngoscope* 31:492, 1921.
7. Rice DH: Endoscopic intranasal dacryocystorhinostomy: a cadaver study, *Am J Rhinol* 2:127, 1988.
8. McDonogh M, Meiring JH: Endoscopic transnasal dacryocystorhinostomy, *J Laryngol Otol* 103:585, 1989.
9. Rice DH: Endoscopic intranasal dacryocystorhinostomy: results in four patients, *Arch Otolaryngol Head Neck Surg* 116:1061, 1990.
10. Metson R: Endoscopic surgery for lacrimal obstruction, *Otolaryngol Head Neck Surg* 104:473, 1991.
11. Weidenbecker M, Hoseman W, Buhr W: Endoscopic endonasal dacryocystorhinostomy: results in 56 patients, *Ann Otol Rhinol Laryngol* 103:363, 1994.

S E C T I O N

THREE

SINUS DISEASE

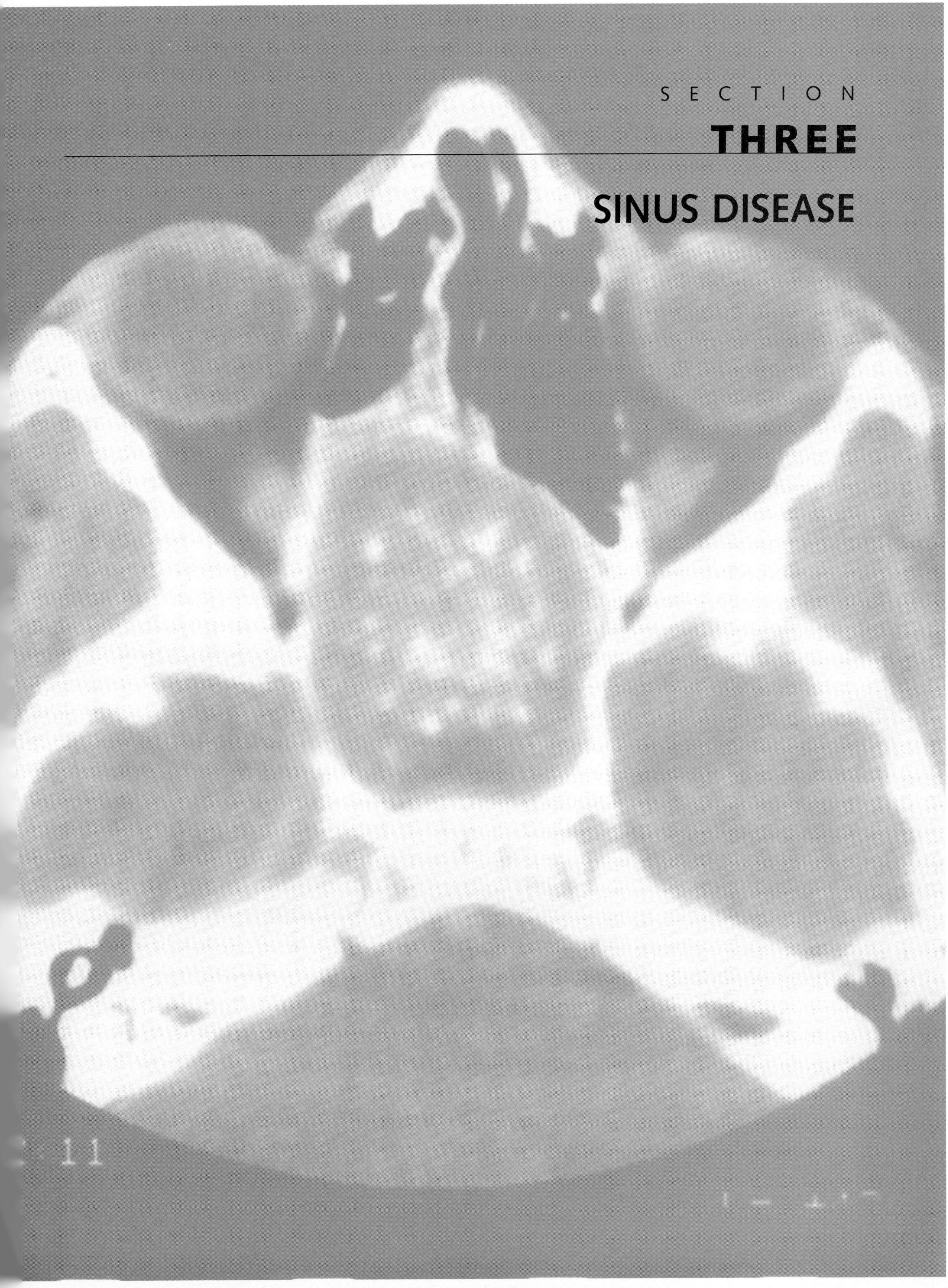

CHAPTER

12

Fungal Sinusitis

Scott C. Manning

PROBLEM
A 20-year-old man presents with a 6-month history of progressive left proptosis, nasal congestion, and headache.

Fungal sinusitis can be divided clinically and histologically into four distinct categories (Table 12-1). Mycetoma or fungus ball is most commonly reported from desert areas in the Sudan. It is characterized histologically by a tangled mass of fungal hyphae within the involved sinus, with minimal surrounding mucosal inflammation and no tissue invasion. *Aspergillus* species are the fungal organisms most commonly cultured, and the disease is considered to be a saprophytic process rather than an infection. Treatment consists of surgical drainage and ventilation of involved sinuses.

Indolent invasive fungal sinusitis occurs rarely in seemingly immunocompetent patients. The slow process of tissue invasion can progress over years, and again *Aspergillus* is the most common fungus recovered on culture. Histologically, the disease is characterized by granulomas with rare vascular invasion. Multiple biopsies may be required before the disease can be confirmed histologically or by cultures. Treatment consists of surgical excision of involved tissue, along with administration of systemic antifungal agents such as amphotericin B. Patients may experience a waxing and waning course, with multiple recurrences over many years.

Fulminant invasive fungal sinusitis occurs only in immunocompromised patients. Diabetics in ketoacidosis are at risk for invasive disease primarily from fungi within the Zygomycetes class (*Mucor, Rhizopus, Absidia*), which prefer high-acidity, high-glucose environments. Patients receiving steroids as part of their immunosuppressive regimen in the first year after organ transplantation are also at significantly increased risk for invasive fungal disease, including sinusitis. Similarly, patients with acquired immunodeficiency syndrome (AIDS) are at risk for invasive fungal disease.

At autopsy, approximately 25% of patients dying from leukemia are found to show evidence of invasive fungal infection.[1] Overall, the most frequent offending organisms are *Aspergillus* and *Candida* species, with Zygomycetes (*Mucor*) found less frequently. The lungs are the most commonly involved organ (usually with *Aspergillus*), and invasive fungal sinusitis relatively rarely reported. The true incidence of invasive fungal sinusitis is probably underestimated, since it often presents concurrently with terminal lung infection. The highest incidence is seen in neutropenic patients undergoing treatment for acute myelogenous leukemia (AML). This observation is probably related to the more severe and more prolonged granulocytopenia produced by chemotherapy regimens for AML. Acute lymphocytic leukemia (ALL) is diagnosed with much greater frequency than AML, but the incidence of fungal sinusitis is less in these patients. The net effect is that the overall prevalence of invasive fungal sinusitis is about the same among AML and ALL patient groups. *Aspergillus* organisms are the most commonly cultured fungi in patients with nondiabetic immunodeficiency and invasive fungal sinusitis.

Allergic fungal sinusitis (AFS) was first characterized in the early 1980s by Lamb and colleagues[2] in Great Britain and Katzenstein and colleagues[3] in the United States. These authors noted histologic similarity between allergic mucin from certain sinusitis patients and that from patients with allergic bronchopulmonary aspergillosis. Since the mid-1980s, studies have demonstrated that AFS is most commonly caused by fungi in

Table 12-1. Spectrum of fungal sinusitis

FUNGAL SINUS DISEASE	MOST COMMON ORGANISM	HISTOLOGIC FINDINGS	HOST CHARACTERISTICS	TREATMENT	OUTCOME
Mycetoma	*Aspergillus* species	Mass of hyphae, little tissue reaction, no invasion	Immunocompetent	Surgical drainage	Good
Allergic fungal sinusitis	Dematiaceous class (*Bipolaris, Curvularia*)	Pronounced tissue reaction with allergic mucin, scattered fungal forms, no invasion	Young, atopic, immunocompetent	Surgical drainage, topical and systemic steroids	Good
Indolent invasive	*Aspergillus* species	Noncaseating granulomas, minimal or no vascular invasion	Immunocompetent	Excision of involved tissue, systemic antifungals	? Fair
Fulminant invasive—diabetic	Zygomycetes (*Mucor, Rhizopus, Absidia*)	Tissue necrosis, vascular invasion, broad non-septated fungal forms	Poorly controlled glucose, ketoacidosis	Correct metabolic abnormalities, amphotericin B, excision of involved tissues	30%-80% survival
Fulminant invasive—other immuno-suppressed	*Aspergillus* species	Necrosis, vascular invasion, septated fungal forms with acute angle branching	Profound granulocytopenia, steroids by causing system immunodeficiency, intravenous antibiotics by altering the balance of normal flora, then by potentiating growth of pathogenic fungi	Try to reverse underlying immuno-deficiency, amphotericin B, excision of involved tissues	Poor

From Gates GA: *Current therapy in otolaryngology–head and neck surgery*, ed 5, St. Louis, 1994, Mosby–Year Book, p 407.

the Dematiaceous class such as *Bipolaris, Curvularia, Alternaria,* and *Exserohilum,* rather than by *Aspergillus* organisms. Studies provide evidence that AFS is an immunologically mediated response involving specific antifungal IgE and IgG antibodies and a late-phase type of eosinophilic inflammation, rather than an infection or a point along a spectrum leading to infection.[4]

MEDICAL HISTORY

Patients with mycetoma have no history of immunodeficiency or allergy. Likewise, patients with indolent invasive fungal sinusitis usually do not have a history of a definite immunodeficiency. By contrast, diabetics are at greatest risk for invasive disease during periods of ketoacidosis, and post-transplant patients are at greatest risk during periods of treatment with steroids or other immunosuppressive agents. Those undergoing treatment for lymphoreticular malignancies are at greatest risk for invasive fungal sinusitis during periods of profound neutropenia (white blood cell counts below $100/mm^3$) while receiving broad-spectrum antibiotics for other infections.

Initial symptoms of indolent or fulminant invasive fungal sinusitis may be subtle, including mild pains or paresthesias of the nose, face, palate or eye, along with congestion and thin, clear rhinorrhea. Spiking fevers without an obvious source in a neutropenic patient should always prompt the suspicion of fungal sinusitis.

Allergic fungal sinusitis patients are immunocompetent, generally young, and atopic as in the case presented here. Most have a history of inhalant allergies, and up to 40% have a history of asthma. The most common presenting symptom is progressive nasal obstruction, with headache and anosmia reported less frequently.

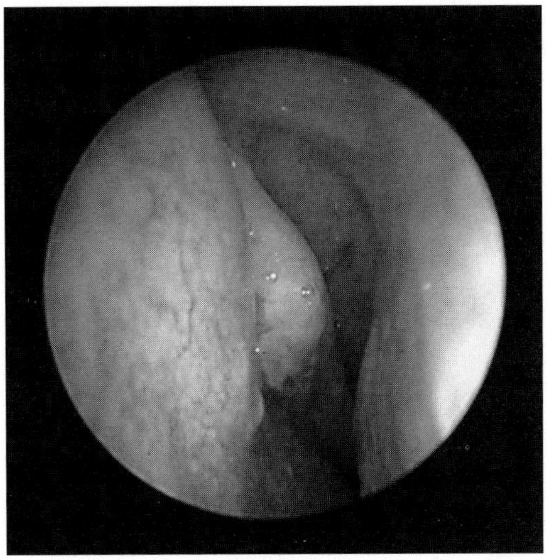

Fig. 12-1. Endoscopic view of the left nasal cavity in an 8-year-old boy with spiking fevers. The patient was neutropenic and taking steroids after a kidney transplant. The middle turbinate head appears yellow, with adjacent areas of mucosal excoriation. Subsequent biopsy and culture yielded a diagnosis of invasive *Aspergillus* sinusitis.

PHYSICAL EXAMINATION

With invasive fungal sinusitis, presenting physical findings are usually subtle and may include thin clear rhinorrhea with redness or edema around the nostril or lower eyelid. Rhinoscopy can be easily performed in the clinic or at the bedside with a sinus endoscope or an otoscope. The earliest findings with invasive disease may be pale yellow mucosa of the middle turbinate head that is relatively insensate when touched (Fig. 12-1). Excoriated, bleeding adjacent mucosa of the septum or lateral nasal wall may indicate more advanced disease. Ischemic necrosis with black eschar indicates advanced vascular invasion and tissue necrosis. The oral cavity should be inspected for evidence of extension through the nasal floor creating palatal ulceration or defect.

With allergic fungal sinusitis, up to 20% of patients demonstrate proptosis or other facial bony deformity such as widening of the canthal area or expansion and flattening of the malar eminence. Rhinoscopy always reveals polyposis, which is usually unilateral. At times, the polypoid expansion within one nasal cavity is enough to push the septum to the contralateral nasal wall.

In this case rhinoscopy revealed left-sided polyposis that appeared to arise from the sphenoethmoidal recess. The patient had mild left proptosis without other facial deformity.

RADIOGRAPHIC EXAMINATION

Plain sinus radiographs are generally not very helpful in establishing the diagnosis of fungal sinusitis. They may show sinus expansion with areas of high attenuation in cases of mycetoma or AFS. Computed tomography (CT) is recommended whenever the diagnosis of fungal sinusitis is considered. Unfortunately, with both indolent and fulminant invasive disease, initial CT findings consist only of nonspecific mucosal inflammation. Bone destruction with evidence of inflammation of surrounding structures is an ominous late finding with invasive disease. Magnetic resonance imaging (MRI) may be more sensitive than CT in detecting evidence of invasive fungal sinusitis by demonstrating optic nerve or orbital inflammation or early intracerebral abscess formation.

In both mycetoma and AFS, CT demonstrates central areas of speckled or linear high attenuation. In AFS, CT also shows significant inflammation of surrounding mucosa within involved sinuses. Often in AFS, the sinuses are expanded and areas of bone erosion are common. Presumably the mechanism for bone resorption involves pressure necrosis and/or elaboration of cytotoxic proteins such as major basic protein from allergic mucin. Extension of disease intraorbitally or intracranially is not unusual, and postobstructive mucoceles upstream to the areas of allergic mucin are common. At surgery, disease is always found to be extraperiorbital or extradural even in cases of massive bone erosion.

Magnetic resonance imaging is very helpful in confirming the diagnosis of AFS. The thick central allergic mucin has a very high protein content and results in low signal on T1 imaging and signal loss on T2 imaging. The surrounding sinus mucosal inflammation yields bright signal on T1 image. The combination of irregular areas of high attenuation on CT with low signal on T1 and T2 MRI is virtually pathognomonic for AFS. Magnetic resonance imaging is also useful in precisely delineating areas of allergic mucin with hypertrophic polypoid sinus mucosa in order to allow for total surgical removal.

In the case presented here, CT demonstrated speckled areas of high attenuation within a greatly expanded sphenoid sinus (Fig. 12-2). Coronal views (not shown) demonstrated extension through the roof of the sphenoid into the middle cranial fossa. T1 MRI demonstrated peripheral mucosal high signal with central signal void corresponding to the areas of high attenuation on CT (Fig. 12-3).

LABORATORY EXAMINATION

In cases of suspected fungal sinusitis, nasal swabs used for fungal staining or culture may increase suspicion of the diagnosis if positive, but they are not in themselves diagnostic. When invasive fungal sinusitis is considered, biopsy of suspicious mucosa is necessary to confirm the diagnosis and initiate proper treatment. Fungi present within tissue or evidence of granuloma formation or vascular invasion in an immunocompromised patient should

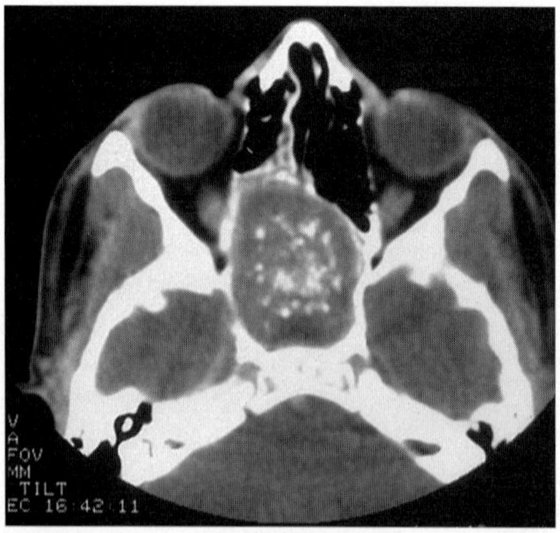

Fig. 12-2. Expanded sphenoid with central areas of high attenuation on computed tomography.

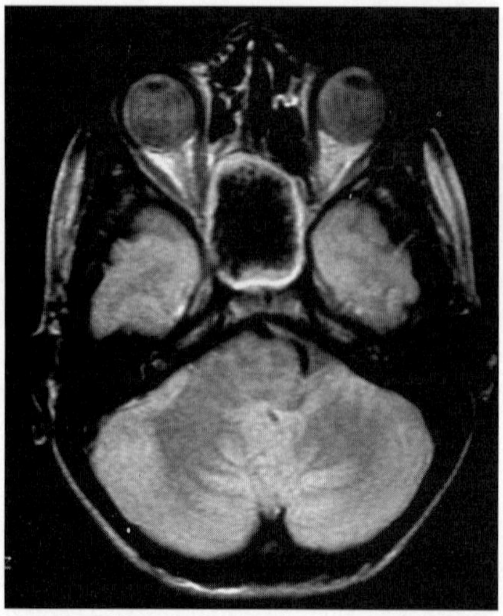

Fig. 12-3. T1-weighted magnetic resonance imaging shows a central signal void with a peripheral high signal from inflamed mucosa, typical of allergic fungal sinusitis.

prompt therapy with systemic amphotericin B even before final culture results are available.

In AFS cases, mucosal biopsies show nonspecific inflammation without evidence of fungal invasion. Serologic and skin testing can be helpful, however, in establishing the diagnosis. Studies suggest that virtually 100% of patients with AFS demonstrate positive skin test or radioallergosorbent test (RAST) results for at least one commercially available fungal antigen in the Dematiaceous or *Aspergillus* family compared with a 5% to 20% rate of positive response in normal populations. *Bipolaris* is the most common isolated fungus in reported cases of AFS, and no commercial *Bipolaris* antigen is available. However, *Bipolaris* patients usually show positive responses to other fungal antigens in the Dematiaceous class such as *Helminthosporium* or *Curvularia.*

In the patient presented above, a RAST demonstrated class 4 responses to *Helminthosporium* and *Curvularia.* Multiple other inhalant allergies were also demonstrated.

TREATMENT

Patients with invasive fungal disease are gravely ill and represent extremely complex management problems. Their treatment requires a team approach involving hematologist-oncologists, infectious disease specialists, and surgeons. When invasive fungal sinusitis is demonstrated by biopsy or strongly suspected while biopsy results are awaited, amphotericin B should be given immediately. A test dose is given initially by slow infusion while patients are monitored for signs of hypersensitivity. Treatment dosing is then begun at 0.25 mg/kg over 2 to 6 hours. On subsequent days, dosing is usually increased in increments of 0.25 mg/kg until maintenance dosing is achieved at 0.25 to 1.0 mg/kg per day as limited by side effects or toxicity. The therapeutic plan is usually to give a total of 2 to 4 g over 6 to 8 weeks. Amphotericin B is toxic to kidneys, causing some degree of renal tubular acidosis that is usually reversible. Patients are monitored for development of hypomagnesemia, hypokalemia, and azotemia. They are generally given pain medication, antinausea medication, and acetaminophen to minimize common side effects including rigors, fever, and nausea. Liposomal amphotericin B preparations may result in both higher transfer of drug through fungal cell walls and lower overall host toxicity. Studies of the efficacy of liposomal amphotericin B in the treatment of fungal sinusitis are limited at present. Other antifungal agents have limited usefulness in the treatment of invasive *Aspergillus* or Zygomycetes disease. 5-Flucytosine possibly augments the effectiveness of amphotericin B in the treatment of *Aspergillus* infection, but it also potentially increases renal toxicity.

Hyperbaric oxygen may be helpful in the treatment of invasive fungal sinusitis. High oxygen partial pressures are fungicidal or fungistatic in vitro, and a few anecdotal reports have suggested a benefit from hyperbaric oxygen treatment for invasive fungal sinusitis. Ferguson and associates[5] reported a series of 12 patients with rhinocerebral zygomycosis treated with amphotericin B and surgical debridement. Four of six patients receiving hyperbaric oxygen survived compared with two of six in the group not treated with hyperbaric oxygen.

The role of surgery in the treatment of invasive fungal sinusitis is principally that of establishing the diagnosis through biopsy and of debriding devitalized tissue. At my institution, endoscopic techniques have taken on a greater role, replacing more radical open approaches such as maxillectomy. Serial endoscopic debridements of devitalized tissue, in conjunction with systemic administration of amphotericin B, is a relatively practical, low-morbidity way to manage these patients. Maxillectomy with orbital exenteration may be considered for advanced rhinoorbitocerebral zygomycosis. However, it is probably not possible to achieve a surgical margin in these cases, as fungal invasion has usually crossed the anterior or middle cranial fossa floor along vascular channels. The prognosis for rhino-orbitocerebral invasive disease is extremely poor unless the underlying immunodeficiency can somehow be reversed.

Patients with sinus mycetoma are adequately treated with surgical drainage and ventilation of the involved sinus. Likewise, complete surgical removal of all sinus allergic mucin is often adequate therapy for AFS. I give all AFS patients oral steroids at a dose of 1 to 2 mg/kg prednisone, beginning at least 1 week before surgery and continuing at least 1 week afterward. The goal of steroid therapy is to reduce mucosal inflammation in order to improve visualization at surgery and decrease surgical bleeding, in addition to blunting postsurgical edema. After surgery, patients are started on topical nasal steroids and saline lavage, and immunotherapy is strongly recommended for other inhalant allergies. Specific antifungal immunotherapy is controversial because of theoretical concerns that it may amplify the immune response and aggravate the disease process. However, reports of decreased disease recurrence in AFS patients given specific fungal immunotherapy are now appearing (R. Mabry, personal communication).

In my practice, patients with AFS are managed with endoscopic surgical techniques even if imaging studies reveal extensive bone destruction with disease adjacent to periorbita or dura. Microdebrider instruments are extremely helpful for atraumatic removal of inflamed polypoid mucosa, and large straight and curved suctions are usually the best instruments for removing allergic mucin. Allergic fungal sinusitis tends to expand the outflow tracts of involved sinuses, including the frontal sinuses, allowing better endoscopic access. Frequent irrigation with saline can help mobilize and flush out allergic mucin. This technique is especially useful with the frontal sinuses. If all the allergic mucin is not removed, the fungal antigen–triggered immune response continues and recurrence of clinical disease is rapid.

The patient presented here was managed with endoscopic removal of hypertrophic mucosa and allergic mucin. Mucin was noted to extend to dura in one area of the lateral sphenoid, but it was removed without difficulty. Postoperatively, the patient was given immunotherapy for multiple inhalant allergies plus topical nasal steroids.

RESULTS

Results of treatment of invasive fungal sinusitis are poor unless the underlying immunodeficiency can be reversed. Published series of diabetic patients report a 30% to 80% overall survival rate for invasive fungal sinusitis, but my own experience with rhinoorbitocerebral disease in these patients has been less encouraging. Neutropenic patients undergoing treatment for lymphoreticular malignancies have a very poor prognosis when diagnosed with invasive fungal sinusitis. They often have concurrent fungal pneumonia and profound bone marrow suppression.

Mycetoma is usually cured with surgery alone. Allergic fungal sinusitis has a relatively low rate of recurrence if (1) all allergic mucin is removed at surgery and (2) patients comply with a postoperative regimen of topical nasal steroids and immunotherapy for other inhalant allergies. Careful follow-up is required, and bursts of systemic steroids may be necessary during periods of seasonal flare-up of inhalant allergy. Rapid clinical recurrence after initial surgery implies missed allergic mucin and are an indication for MRI.

DISCUSSION

Many authors have a tendency to lump all forms of fungal sinusitis together in discussions of diagnosis and treatment. However, the four types of fungal sinusitis represent different, nonoverlapping conditions with different issues in diagnosis and treatment (Fig. 12-4). They do not constitute points along a continuous spectrum. With rare exceptions (usually involving deep tissue injury), invasive fungal disease occurs only in immunocompromised patients. This group includes patients with AIDS, patients taking steroids and/or other immunosuppressive agents after organ transplant, and diabetics (usually with ketoacidosis). Patients with profound marrow suppression, such as leukemics receiving chemotherapy, are at greatest risk for developing fulminant invasive fungal sinusitis. The diagnosis should be considered early in any neutropenic patient with recurrent fever even if nasal symptoms are minimal. The greatest potential contribution for the otolaryngologist in these situations is early diagnosis by way of rhinoscopy and biopsy. Unfortunately, the prognosis for these patients remains poor. Sometimes the only hope for successful outcome is through bone marrow transplantation, which most transplant centers will not consider in the face of invasive fungal disease.

The biggest problem with AFS lies in the diagnosis. The often dramatic initial CT findings sometimes lead to an erroneous clinical diagnosis of possible malignancy, resulting in overradical surgical approaches. A fungal cul-

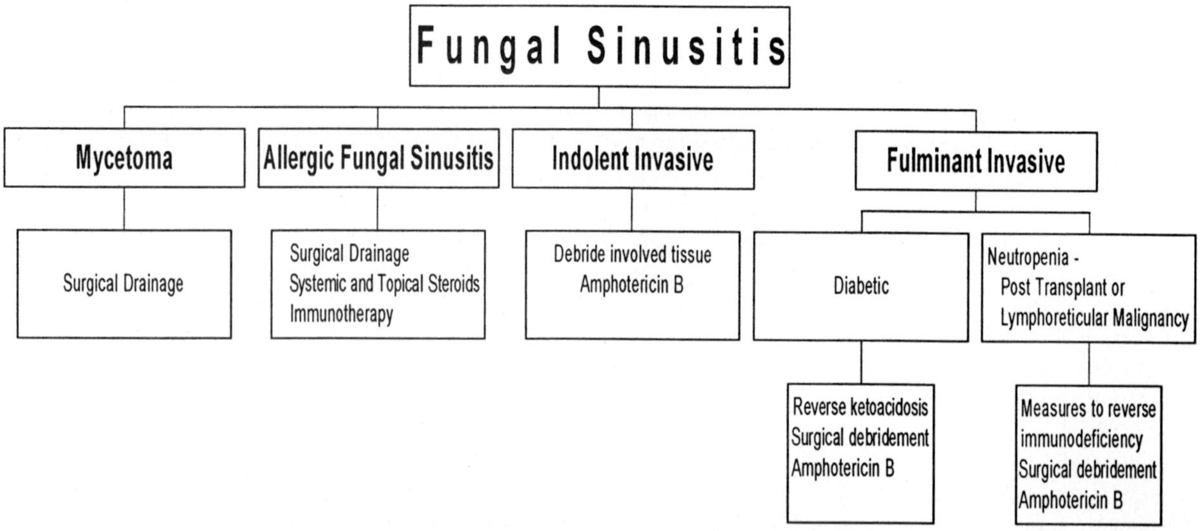

Fig. 12-4. Fungal sinusitis algorithm.

ture often leads to an institutional reflex to treat the patient with potentially toxic antifungal medication even in the absence of histologic evidence of invasive disease. Allergic fungal sinusitis is an allergy, and treatment consists of complete drainage of involved sinuses along with appropriate management of other inhalant allergies. The patient presented here was initially treated in such a manner and remains disease free.

REFERENCES

1. Drakos P, Nagler A, Or R, et al: Invasive fungal sinusitis in patients undergoing bone marrow transplantation, *Bone Marrow Transplant* 12:203-208, 1993.
2. Lamb D, Millar J, Johnston A: Allergic aspergillosis of the paranasal sinuses, *J Pathol* 137:56, 1982.
3. Katzenstein A, Greenberger P, Sale S: Allergic *Aspergillus* sinusitis: a newly recognized form of sinusitis, *J Allergy Clin Immunol* 72:89–93, 1983.
4. Manning S, Mabry R, Schaefer S, et al: Evidence of IgE-mediated hypersensitivity in allergic fungal sinusitis, *Laryngoscope* 103:717-721, 1993.
5. Ferguson B, Mitchell T, Moon R, et al: Adjunctive hyperbaric oxygen for treatment of rhinocerebral mucormycosis, *Rev Infect Dis* 10:551-559, 1988.

CHAPTER

13

Management of Sinusitis in Infants and Young Children

Peter A.R. Clement

PROBLEM

An 8-year-old girl is referred by her pediatrician for recurrent purulent rhinorrhea despite several years receiving intermittent oral antibiotic therapy. The pediatrician relates that he is unable to visualize the nose well, but he suspects that the patient has polyps. Computed tomography (CT) shows bilateral opacification of the ethmoidal and maxillary sinuses. Sweat chloride test results are interpretated as normal.

Management of sinusitis, especially in young children, has been and still is one of the most controversial issues in the medical community and especially among ear, nose, and throat (ENT) specialists.[1] One extreme was the complete denial of the very existence of sinusitis based on early radiologic evidence that sinuses had not yet developed in young children (especially the maxillary sinuses, because these were the only sinuses well visualized by standard x-ray examination), and the belief that the runny nose of a child was mainly due to rhinitis or adenoid hypertrophy. Since the introduction of CT scanning, it has been demonstrated that chronic nasal complaints in children are often accompanied by extensive inflammation of the sinus mucosa, especially in the younger child, yet rhinorrhea and nasal obstruction are by far the most common complaints in children. In fact, infection of the upper respiratory tract is the single most common organic disease presenting to the primary care physician.[2]

EPIDEMIOLOGY AND PATHOPHYSIOLOGY

From a survey of 635,874 ear, nose, and throat (ENT) visits at 45 Dutch hospitals in 1993, it was obvious that more than 30% of these visits involved children under the age of 14 years. An age breakdown of ENT visits in this pediatric outpatient clinic showed that 80% concerned children under the age of 8 years.[3] These figures clearly showed the importance of the pediatric ENT population in an average ENT practice. Most of these children had chronic nasal complaints, although our knowledge of the existence and prevalence of sinusitis in this group is still far from complete. Zuckerkandl[4] described in detail in 1892 the anatomy of the sinuses in adults, in embryos, and in newborns. Later, many authors[5-7] measured the height, width, and depth of the different sinuses in a pediatric population, from the newborn to the adult subject. (In our clinic, children under the age of 14 years are seen in the pediatric department and over the age of 14 are seen in the adult department.) As early as 1895,[8] it was shown that sinusitis is fairly common in children, and in 1940 with standard x-ray examination[9] this finding was reconfirmed. In that same period, it was already demonstrated not only that certain children with complaints showed a high frequency of sinus changes on x-ray examination, but also that this was observed in children not immediately suspected of suffering from sinusitis and examined for other conditions, e.g., adenoid and tonsillar problems.

Unfortunately, most studies in the pediatric ENT literature deal with patient populations (children with nasal complaints) and few involve normal populations, so that not much is known about the *epidemiology* of sinusitis in young children. A first prospective epidemiologic study on sinusitis was performed by Maresh and Washburn.[9] It was started in 1925 and they followed on a regular basis 100 healthy children from birth to maturity, looking at the history and performing a physical examination and a routine posteroanterior radiograph of the paranasal sinuses four times a year (a total of 3501 roentgenograms); the oldest children underwent over 50 radiographs of the sinuses. It was noted that there existed a relatively constant percentage (30%) of "pathologic" antrums in the films taken between 1 year and 6 years of age, the range being 23% to 35%. From 6 to 12 years, this percentage dropped steadily to approximately 15%. Interestingly, the authors noted that variations in size of the sinuses occur frequently, without any demonstrable relation to the amount or frequency of infections as seen in the radiographs and without following any definitive pattern. When there was a recent upper respiratory tract infection (in the previous 2 weeks), less than 50% showed clear sinuses. Tonsillectomy had no demonstrable effect on the radiographic appearance of the sinuses. Another very extensive epidemiologic study was performed by Bagatsch and colleagues,[10] who followed the total pediatric population (24,000) representing 30% of a newly developed residential area in the neighborhood of Rostock consisting of 80,000 people who were followed for 1 year in the only available medical center of that area. Eighty-four percent of the children aged between 0 and 2 years, 47% of those between 4 and 6 years, and 18% of those over 7 years had one or more episodes of respiratory tract infection in that period. In a closer look at the 0- to 3-year-old group, 72% of these children staying in day care centers and 27% of those staying at home had one or more episodes of upper respiratory tract infection. Of the 84% of children aged 0 to 3 years (n=4103), 32% suffered from rhinosinopharyngitis. The peak of this disease occurred in the months of November to February. Lind[11] and Bjuggren and colleagues[8] also found a much higher prevalence of up to 100% of maxillary sinusitis in children staying in day care centers compared with the same age group staying at home or older children in schools. Sometimes, children in day care centers also induce recurrent sinusitis in the adults watching over them ("young child to young adult sick sinus syndrome").[1] Desterbeck and associates[12] studied eustachian tube function and nasal patency in 154 schoolchildren (age range 5 to 12 years) for a period of 24 weeks (summer time was not included because of the school holidays). After routine ENT examination, eustachian tube function and nasal patency were followed in an objective way twice weekly, using tympanometry and passive anterior rhinomanometry, respectively. Distribution of nasal patency was significantly ($p \leq .05$) more favorable in older children (10 to 12 years better than 7 to 9 years, the latter better than 5 to 6 years) and better during the spring and summer periods ($p \leq .001$). Another finding was that satisfactory nasal patency was mostly associated with a good middle ear function. The influence of swimming was studied in all children in a cross-over pattern, revealing an overall favorable effect especially in the 3 days after swimming ($p \leq .001$).

The relationship between poor nasal patency and rhinosinusitis was confirmed by van Cauwenberge,[13] who showed a significant relationship between the results of passive anterior rhinomanometry and pronounced edema of the nasal mucosa (p .09 for the right side, .03 for the left side) and the presence of purulent rhinitis (p .006 for the right side and $<.05$ for the left side).

Therefore, it seems from these studies that in younger children with chronic sinusitis there exists a spontaneous tendency toward recovery after the age of 6 to 8 years. This finding of decrease in prevalence of sinusitis in older children was also confirmed by other authors in patient populations.[14-16]

Breast feeding seems to have a beneficial influence on lower respiratory disease, but such an influence on sinusitis in infants and young children has not yet been demonstrated. Passive smoking is a putative risk factor, especially in allergic children.[17-22] There is a clearly increased risk for recurrent coryza (odds ratio 3.00) and sinus problem (odds ratio 4.73) in children with smoking mothers compared with children from nonsmoking families.[23] Breast feeding has little or no effect on the incidence of infantile respiratory disease in children in developed countries.

These epidemiologic studies already yield important information on the pathophysiology of rhinosinusitis in children:

1. There is a clear-cut decrease in the prevalence of rhinosinusitis after 6 to 8 years of age. This is the natural history of the disease and is probably related to an immature immune system in the younger child.
2. In temperate climates, there is a definite increase in the occurrence of chronic rhinosinusitis in children during the fall and winter time, so that the season seems to be another important factor.
3. Younger children staying in day care centers show a dramatic increase in the prevalence of chronic or recurrent rhinosinusitis compared with children staying at home.

Exposure to infection is therefore a determinant factor for the prevalence. The influence of the season and the exposure to viral infections are linked parameters, and this has been demonstrated very well in adults by Jones and colleagues,[24] who studied more than 1.5 million patients. These showed a monthly point prevalence pattern with a very high correlation between upper respiratory tract infection and chronic sinusitis during wintertime. Most interestingly, 71% of the upper respiratory infections (common cold) in the 0- to 9-year-old age group occurred within the 90 days preceding a first episode of chronic sinusitis. Gwaltney and associates[25] showed that of healthy adults with common colds of 48 to 96 hours' duration and no active allergic rhinitis or history of sinus disease or nasal polyposis, 77% had occluded infundibula, 87% had abnormalities in one or both maxillary cavities, 65% had ethmoid sinus abnormalities, 32% had frontal sinus disease, and 39% had sphenoid sinus abnormalities on CT examination. Although such a study has not been performed yet in children, there is no reason to think that the results would be different. Saito and colleagues[26] demonstrated the relationship between viral infections and sinusitis. Viral infections in children are very common. Together with the clinical signs, the age of the child, and the month of the year, the viral agent can already be determined with a high degree of accuracy.[27] The same authors state that colds occur more frequently in younger children, with an average of five colds a year, whereas older children and their adult family members average two to three colds a year. Rhinovirus infections are the most frequent viral infections (30% to 40% of upper respiratory tract infections according to Wald[2]), but they seldom induce high fever and never require hospitalization. Destruction of the nasal epithelium during symptomatic rhinovirus infections has not been detected in any of several studies.[28] In the temperate climate zone, common colds occur mainly at the start of the school year and in March or April. From two consecutive serum samples in 138 children who were hospitalized with signs of upper respiratory tract infections and high fever, Clement and associates[29] were able to determine the virus involved. *Mycoplasma pneumoniae* infection occurred more frequently after the age of 6; parainfluenza virus, enterovirus, and respiratory syncytial disease are more common before the age of 5 years. The distribution during the year correlated with the literature: influenza A, respiratory syncytial virus, parainfluenza virus, and *M. pneumoniae* mainly in wintertime; enterovirus in summertime. The ratio of the number of cases in wintertime (October to March) compared with summertime (April to September) in children under age 6 years was 2.9:1 and even higher in children aged 6 to 12 years (4.3:1). Viruses have been recovered twice (rhinovirus) by Evans and colleagues[30] from 65 needle punctures in adults. Hamory and associates[31] found viruses in 81 aspirates from 11 sinuses. These isolates included rhinovirus (n=6), influenza A (n=3), and two types of parainfluenza. Piskunov and Piskunov[32], however, using an immunofluorescent technique, frequently demonstrated viral antigens (67%, n=46) in the nasal and paranasal mucosa of adult patients suffering from chronic maxillary sinusitis. They mainly found paraadenovirus, adenovirus, parainfluenza, influenza B, and respiratory syncytial virus and showed evidence of a virus-carrying state and latent virus infection of the upper respiratory mucosa.

However, viruses are recovered infrequently from sinus aspirates in children: adenovirus was found in one patient; parainfluenza in combination with a bacterial isolate was recovered from a second.[33]

Most authors[24,25] agree that viral infections are the trigger for acute and recurrent rhinosinusitis, but after a few days only the bacteriologic infection remains.[34] According to the consensus meeting on rhinosinusitis,[34] the acute viral infection—the common cold—is often the precipitating factor, while the most common microorganisms found in sinus washings are bacteria secondary to obstruction of the ostiomeatal complex. Although bacterial infection is not the original cause of rhinosinusitis, it contributes considerably to the ongoing inflammation. Since the 1950s, after the introduction of antibiotics, bacterial culture of maxillary sinus lavage fluid in children was performed regularly.[2,8,29,35-40] Although many different antibiotics have been used in the last 40 years, it is obvious from Table 13-1 that the pathologic microflora found in antral washings in children has not shown a tremendous shift. Also, the introduction of the antibiotic spectrum of the microflora did not change at all the microflora involved. Because of frequent antibiotic use, the microorganisms became resistant (pneumococci) or produced β-lactamase (*Haemophilus influenzae*). Few systematic investigations of the bacterial etiology of sinusitis in children have been performed.[41]

Material recovered from sinuses shows positive culture in the proportion of 72%[38] to 89%.[39] From Table 13-1, it follows that *Haemophilus influenzae* and *Streptococcus pneumoniae* are still scoring very high in sinusitis in children (60%),[38] especially acute and recurrent sinusitis. Since the 1970s, *Branhamella catarrhalis* has been cultured more frequently. Before the organism was first called *Neisseria catarrhalis* and was considered to be an inoffensive commensal. Branham discovered in the 1950s that it was structurally and biochemically different from *Neisseria*. In 1970, a new genus was introduced called *Branhamella*, but in 1991 it was officially accommodated in the *Moraxella* family as *Moraxella catarrhalis*. Interestingly, *B. catarrhalis* is not cultured during the summer months and is not protected against the secretory IgA dimers, as it is not producing any IgA protease. *M. catarrhalis* is β-lactamase positive in 85% of cases and frequently found in combination with *H. influenzae* and *S. pneumoniae.* In this combination it renders the other microorganisms penicillin resistant,[42] forming the well-known "infernal trio".[43] Poole[44] states that these three microorganisms are common findings in 60% of 2-year-olds with chronic rhinosinusitis. Multiple isolates in one specimen are fairly common. Bjuggren and colleagues[8] found it in 21%, Wald and colleagues[36] found it in 26%, and Brook[35] stated that 38% of the anaerobes were mixed with aerobes.

Some authors also demonstrated the importance of gram-negative enteric bacteria[40] and anaerobes,[35,45] which seem to be more common in chronic sinusitis. The

Table 13-1. Number and percentage of pathologic aerobic bacteria found in sinuses of children (antral washings or sinus surgery) from 1982 until 1991

YEAR AUTHOR	1952 BJUGGREN ET AL	1981 BROOK	1981 WALD ET AL	1988 OTTEN ET AL	1989 CLEMENT ET AL
Number of children	**40**	**37**	**30**	**59**	**25**
Number of sinuses	**60**	**NM**	**47**	**NM**	**45**
Age in years	**3-7**	**6-16**	**1-6**	**3-10**	**2-9**
Streptococcus pneumoniae	24 (60) 30 (50)		17 (36)	14 (26)	15 (33)
Haemophilus influenzae	14 (35) 16 (26)	2 (5)	11 (23)	26 (48)	10 (22)
Staphylococcus aureus	8 (20) 9 (15)	7 (19)		3 (6)	1 (2)
β-hemolytic streptococci	0 0	4 (11)	1 (2)		1 (2)
α-hemolytic streptococci		7 (19)	2 (4)		
Moraxella catarrhalis			9 (19)	4 (7)	
Remarks		Many anaerobes (mainly chronic sinusitis)	Acute sinusitis		Chronic rhino-sinusitis

NM, Not mentioned.

most common gram-negative enteric bacteria were *Pseudomonas aeruginosa* and *Proteus mirabilis*[40]; the most common anaerobes were *Peptostreptococcus* and *Bacteroides.*[35] The child population studied by Brook, however, was quite heterogeneous (allergy, cystic fibrosis).

One should remember, however, that a high bacterial colony count ensures that the culture results reflect actual sinus infection rather than contamination. Counts greater than 10^4 colony-forming units per millimeter give a high degree of assurance of in situ infection.[2] Thus, quantification of bacterial growth from maxillary aspirates can also help distinguish contamination from real sinus infection,[46] and isolates should be considered positive only when any type of bacteria is present in a quantity of at least 10,000 colonies per milliliter.

Since antral punctures are not frequently performed anymore, it is interesting to know from the study of Orobello and associates[39] that in children there exists a good correlation between the maxillary sinus and the middle meatus specimen (83%) and a poor correlation between those of the nasopharynx and of the maxillary sinus (45%). The positive culture of antral washings has been the "gold standard" in the diagnosis of sinusitis, but Wald[37] and van Buchem and their respective colleagues[15] failed to find a significant difference between positive and negative cultures in relation to the clinical picture and to the nature of the washings (turbid or clear).

DEFINITIONS

The American Rhinologic Society and the International Rhinologic Society have published a guide to first-line management in sinusitis[34] describing the following consensus on the definition of acute and chronic sinusitis in children. The definition of acute sinusitis is the same for adults and children, but that for chronic sinusitis is different, especially with respect to duration and recurrence rate.

Acute sinusitis is defined as a symptomatic sinus infection in which symptoms persist no longer than 6 to 8 weeks or in which there are fewer than four episodes per year of acute symptoms of 10 days' duration. Sinusitis is acute when episodes of infection resolve with medical therapy, leaving no significant mucosal damage.

Chronic sinusitis is a persistent disease that cannot be alleviated by medical therapy alone and involves radiographic evidence of mucosal hyperplasia. In children, it is defined as 12 weeks of persistent symptoms and signs (in adults, 8 weeks), or six episodes per year of recurrent acute sinusitis (in adults, four episodes), each lasting at least 10 days, in association with persistent changes on CT, 4 weeks after medical therapy without intervening acute infection.

Recurrent sinusitis is defined as repeated acute episodes that resolve with medical therapy, leaving no significant mucosal damage.

From these definitions, it is clear that for the diagnosis of acute sinusitis, history taking and observation of symptoms are sufficient, whereas for the diagnosis of recurrent and chronic sinusitis a CT scan together with history and symptomatology is mandatory. According to the latest consensus meeting in Brussels (1996; see addendum) a CT scan is not required for the diagnosis of chronic sinusitis in children.

COMPLAINTS, SYMPTOMS, AND SIGNS

Wald[2] states that commonly recognized symptoms of sinusitis in adults and adolescents are facial pain, headache, and fever. However, children with acute sinusitis fre-

Table 13-1. Number and percentage of pathologic aerobic bacteria found in sinuses of children (antral washings or sinus surgery) from 1982 until 1991—cont'd

YEAR AUTHOR	1989 WALD ET AL (IN LUSK 1992)	1991 OROBELLO ET AL
Number of children	**40**	**39**
Number of sinuses	**52**	**NM**
Age in years	**NM**	**1 to 19**
Streptococcus pneumoniae	12 (23)	3 (8)
Haemophilus influenzae	11 (21)	3 (8)
Staphylococcus aureus		9 (23)
β-Hemolytic streptococcus	2 (4)	1 (2)
α-Hemolytic streptococcus	1 (2)	14 (35)
Moraxella catarrhalis	8 (15)	
Remarks	Chronic sinusitis	Chronic sinusitis (few anaerobes and other gram$^-$ bacteria)

NM, Not mentioned.

quently have complaints that are less specific. Wald further stresses that two common clinical developments should alert the clinician:

1. Signs and symptoms of a cold are persisting beyond 10 days (any nasal discharge; daytime cough, worse at night time).
2. A cold that seems more severe then usual (high fever, copious purulent nasal discharge, periorbital swelling and pain).

Some authors studied the presenting symptoms of rhinosinusitis in children.[15,29,36,47,48] From Table 13-2, it is clear that rhinorrhea is the most frequent presenting symptom in all forms of sinusitis (71% to 80%). Cough seems to be a frequent symptom (50% to 83%). In acute sinusitis, however, nasal obstruction does not appear to be the most prominent symptom, probably because it is masked by more severe symptoms such as fever (50% to 63%) and pain (29% to 33%). On the other hand, in chronic sinusitis, nasal obstruction and mouth breathing are very frequent (70% to 100%) and it is often accompanied by ear complaints (recurrent purulent otitis media or chronic otitis media with effusion: 40% to 68%). This relationship between sinusitis and otitis is not unusual, as the middle ear can be considered a kind of specialized paranasal space. The correlation between upper respiratory tract infection and middle ear pressure has been documented by Bonding and Tos.[49] A special condition that needs to be differentiated from acute sinusitis is acute osteomyelitis of the maxilla in the infant (from a few days to 2 years of age), which is now a rare condition. Osteomyelitis is a staphylococcal infection of an unerupted deciduous tooth and the surrounding bone. The swelling in that condition is usually considerably more extensive than in sinusitis and involves the cheek and hard palate as well as the eyelids.[50] Orbital cellulutis as a complication of ethmoiditis is the most common complication of sinusitis in young children. Untreated, this can lead to cavernous sinus inflammation with or without thrombosis.[51-54] Intracranial abcess formation is mostly due to an extension of frontal sinusitis that does not occur in children under the age of 7 years.[55,56]

In children with cystic fibrosis, sinusitis appears to be common. Brihaye and associates[57] found the following complaints in 84 patients (mainly children): cough (62%), nasal blockade (60%), rhinorrhea (53%), recurrent spells of rhinosinusitis (51%), headache (32%), and anosmia (12%). Another symptom was the poor quality of sleep, with agitation and snoring during the night (37%). Thus, nasal blockade is the main problem in these children, as in children who have chronic sinusitis without cystic fibrosis.

PHYSICAL EXAMINATION

Physical examination of a child's nose is often extremely difficult, and only limited rhinoscopy is tolerated by these young patients.[58] The examination may be accomplished in a simple way by tilting the tip of the nose upward (young children have wide noses with round nostrils, allowing easy examination of the condition of the inferior turbinate). Another convenient method is to use an otoscope.[59,60] Because of the difficulty of performing anterior rhinoscopy in a young child, most studies provide only limited information about the condition of the nasal cavity in sinusitis. Mostly the nasal (boggy turbinates) and pharyngeal mucosa appear erythematous. Yellow to greenish purulent rhinorrhea of varying viscosity can be seen. Lymphoid hyperplasia may be seen in the oropharynx. There may be tonsillar and adenoidal hypertrophy; the cervical lymph nodes may be moderately enlarged and slightly tender.[2,58,60]

Table 13-2A. Presenting symptoms and complaints of sinusitis in young children according to the literature (%): Acute sinusitis (needing hospitalization or with complications)

AUTHOR	CHERRY ET AL	WALD	RIDING ET AL
Year of publication	**1981**	**1981**	**1987**
Age of children	**NM**	**1-16**	**<6**
Number	**NM**	**30**	**26**
Presenting symptoms			
Rhinorrhea	80	76	71
Nasal obstruction and mouth breathing		NM	33
Cough	50	83	
Fever	50	63	52
Pain/headache	30	33	29
Sore throat	20	23	
Fetor ex ore (halitosis)		50	
Ear complaints	40		
Irritability			
Snoring			

NM, Not mentioned.

Table 13-2B. Presenting symptoms and complaints of sinusitis in young children according to the literature (%): Chronic sinusitis

AUTHOR	KOYAT ET AL	CHERRY ET AL	CLEMENT ET AL	LUSK ET AL	MUNTZ ET AL	VAN BUCHEM ET AL	PARSON ET AL	WOLF ET AL
Year of publication	**1973**	**1981**	**1989**	**1990**	**1992**	**1992**	**1993**	**1994**
Age of children	**7 mo-14 yr**	**NM**	**2-9 yr**	**6.6 yr**	**NM**	**2-12 yr**	**7.4 yr**	**3-16 yr**
Number	**100**	**NM**	**80**	**31**	**58**	**79**	**200**	**145**
Presenting symptoms								
Rhinorrhea	77	80	83	100	90	67	90	54
Nasal obstruction and mouth breathing			83		31	70	100	44
Cough	48	75	67	48	40	50	71	12
Fever	21	20	13	55	38	13		
Pain/headache	13	30	8	45	36		90	30
Sore throat		20			12	9		
Fetor ex ore (halitosis)			13				67	
Ear complaints	68	60	50			40		11
Irritability			40					
Snoring						52		

NM, Not mentioned.

The only data on rhinoscopy in young children in the literature are given by Clement and associates,[29] showing a postnasal drip in 60% and pus in the middle meatus in 50%, and by Riding and Irvine,[47] showing turbinate mucosal swelling in 29%.

Although examination of the nasal cavity and of the nasopharynx with a 3.6-diameter fiberoptic rhinolaryngoscope was possible under local anesthesia alone in 93% of children under 1 year of age and in 89% of children aged 4 to 6 years, it was possible in only 33% without

Table 13-3. Nasal rigid endoscopic findings (%) of 40 children scheduled for minor ENT surgery (Cools GHE, Clement PAR: The use of a rigid nasal endoscope in children with special interest in the middle meatus, *Acta Otolaryngol Belg* **45:399-404, 1991).**

Age group (yr)	**1-4**	**5-8**
Number	**17**	**15**
Nasal secretions in middle meatus	68	60
Prominent uncinate process	18	37
Polypous or congestive bulla	6	20
Septal deviation	41	60

ENT, Ear, nose, and throat.

premedication in the 3-year-old age group.[61] In another study,[62] it was shown that 14 children with confirmed sinusitis (by CT scan, or by pus in the middle meatus on fibroscopy) had continuous (43%) and periodic (57%) nasal obstruction. As already stated by Lusk and colleagues[60] and confirmed by Wang and colleagues,[61] flexible endoscopy allows good visualization of the nasopharynx and nasal cavity but does not give sufficient information about the middle meatus, which is the key area in rhinosinusitis, being the site of the ostiomeatal complex.

Cools and Clement[63] performed nasal endoscopy, mainly with a 2.7-mm rigid endoscope, after nasal decongestion and medialization of the middle turbinate in 40 children scheduled for minor surgery (adenotomy, tonsillectomy, placement of ventilation tubes). In 60% to 68% of cases, they found secretions in the middle meatus. With age, the uncinate process became more prominent (medial displacement) and the bulla became more congestive or polypous. Also, the occurrence of septal deviations increased (Table 13-3).

DIAGNOSIS

The value of transillumination and ultrasonography is certainly limited, and these procedures are not recommended for diagnosis of adult sinusitis.[34] The increased thickness of both the soft tissue and the bony vault of the palate in children under 10 years of age limits the clinical usefulness of transillumination in the younger age group even more.[2] Wald and colleagues[36] stated that a study, correlating ultrasound and sinus aspiration, showed indeterminate patterns in children under 4 years of age; using the A-mode ultrasound and radiographs in a population of allergic children and adults, they found sharp discrepancies even when ultrasound tracing and radiographs could be interpreted unambiguously.[64] van Buchem and associates[15] also found no correlation between the radiographic and ultrasound images in children.

To confirm a suspected diagnosis of chronic sinusitis in adults, a radiographic evaluation needs to be performed. The value of plain sinus films in assessing the extent of the disease, especially in young children, is questionable. As might be expected, Riding and Irvine[47] found on plain x-rays that those under 6 years old have only maxillary and ethmoid sinus involvement. Typical air-fluid levels most diagnostic for bacterial sinusitis are an uncommon radiographic finding in children under 5 years of age.[2] Lazar and colleagues,[65] however, found CT signs of sinus disease in 40% of patients with normal sinus x-ray results. The interpretation of sinus plain films in infants and young children may be difficult and the significance of sinus clouding uncertain.[66] Maresh and Washburn[9] found sinus opacification in 60% of subjects under 1 year of age, and in 30% of those under 5 years in a study of normal children without complaints or signs of clinical sinusitis. Maes and Clement[67] in a group of 50 children 2 to 9 years of age with sinusitis, found a 71% correlation between the antroscopy findings and the standard x-ray film performed the day before surgery. A similar figure (70%) was found by Arruda and colleagues.[46] Interestingly, however, these last authors found bacterial growth of the nonpathogenic flora in the maxillary sinus washings (*Streptococcus viridans* being the most common) of six children with normal x-ray findings, while these bacteria were not recovered from the nasal cavity, making contamination highly improbable.

Lusk and associates[60] studied 70 children who had symptoms compatible with chronic sinusitis, and compared plain films with coronal CT scans within a few hours of one another. When all the sinuses were evaluated or considered, they found a lack of correlation between both methods in 74% of the patients. Forty-five percent of the normal plain radiographs showed abnormalities on CT, and 34% of the abnormal plain radiographs were actually normal on CT. These authors found that plain films both over- and underestimated the amount of sinus disease. Thus, for the evaluation of pediatric sinusitis, CT remains the imaging modality of choice, because of its ability to resolve both bone and soft tissue.[59] Furthermore, visualization of the ostiomeatal complex, which is the cornerstone in the diagnosis of sinusitis,[34] is not possible with a standard x-ray investigation.

The significance of radiographic sinus abnormalities in infants and children remains a controversial and confusing topic.[68] On the other hand, Kogutt and Swischuk[69] stated that although sinusitis can often be suspected clinically, its unequivocal documentation can be accomplished only with radiography. In fact, during the consensus meeting, everybody agreed that CT is the modality of choice to identify and evaluate each frontal sinus, frontal recess, uncinate process, infundibulum, maxillary sinus, ostium, ethmoidal bulla, sinus lateralis, sphenoid sinus, and sphenoethmoidal recess.[34]

According to the Princeton[34] consensus meeting, the indications for CT scanning, for adults and children, in the diagnosis of sinusitis were:

1. When nasal endoscopy is unrevealing and severe symptoms persist, CT is indicated to search for disease predominantly in the anterior ethmoid sinuses.
2. When the patient is a candidate for surgery, a full CT examination is necessary to define sinal anatomy.
3. To obtain optimal information, the mucosa should be as free as possible from inflammation, so that an appropriate course of medical therapy should precede CT examination.
4. When CT is performed after medical therapy, it can reveal the extent of mucosal disease deep in the ostiomeatal complex and, once secondary inflammation changes have resolved, serve as a guide to the precise surgical anatomy before an invasive procedure is undertaken.

For the indications of CT scanning in children according to the most recent consensus meeting in Brussels, see addendum.

Before a definition of which CT scan findings are abnormal in children, it is interesting to discuss the incidental paranasal sinus abnormalities on CT scans of children and their clinical correlation. Glasier and associates[68] performed a prospective study on a group of infants and children (n=101) undergoing cranial CT for indications unrelated to upper respiratory inflammation. They found sinus abnormalities in 62% of asymptomatic children (n=13) under the age 1 and in 17% of the 1- to 6-year-old age group (n=30). The same authors compared these percentages with those children in this group who had a history of recent upper respiratory tract infection and found a clear-cut increase in CT scan abnormalities (in 100% and 35% of the sinuses, respectively, for the corresponding age groups).

Diament and colleagues[70] studied 137 pediatric patients referred for skull CT scans and were unable to find any relative higher rate of opacification of the maxillary (33%) and the ethmoid (30%) in children under 1 year of age (n=31) compared with the group (n=30) 1 to 2 years of age (55% and 52%) and the group (n=17) 3 to 5 years of age (9% and 41%). They did not, however, differentiate between patients with or without a recent history of upper respiratory tract infection. Glasier and associates[71] studied 100 infants under 1 year of age, of whom 16% had maxillary hypoplasia (81% under the age of 2 months) and 70% had opacification on CT. These authors concluded that radiographic opacification in this group is of uncertain significance and is not diagnostic for upper respiratory infection, much less for sinusitis.

Looking at the percentage of CT signs of sinus disease in a symptomatic pediatric population, the prevalence of CT sinus abnormalities increases from 64% to 81%.[66,72,73] Thus most authors are in agreement that a symptomatic child with an incidental paranasal sinus finding on CT needs no further work-up unless clinical symptoms and signs are elicited.[74] van der Veken and colleagues[72,75,76] studied 196 children with chronic nasal complaints and concluded that in the younger child (under age 6) there is more bilateral and more severe involvement of the sinuses and less anatomic anomalies than in the older children and adults, pleading for the major role of an immature immune system in the pathogenesis of sinusitis at this age. An examination of the different sinuses (Table 13-4) shows that the percentage of sinusitis as a whole (average 64%) and of maxillary sinusitis (average 50%) stays somewhat constant for all age groups. For all other sinuses, there is a constant decline in the prevalence percentage with increasing age. In this study,[72-75] it was also obvious that there existed a close correlation between the occurrence of maxillary sinusitis and infundibulum ethmoidale pathology (p =.00, X^2=149, n=354), but that in all age groups maxillary sinus disease exceeded ethmoidal and infundibulum pathology. This means that maxillary sinusitis is mostly an extension of ethmoidal infundibulum pathology, but not always. The occurrence of maxillary sinusitis remains constant in all age groups and tends to be more unilateral in older children. Isolated maxillary sinusitis was found in 5% of the youngest age group, rising to 31% in the oldest age group.

Table 13-5 clearly shows that anatomic anomalies such as septal deviations, concha bullosa, and Haller's cell are seldom found in the younger child, and that these show a clear-cut increase in prevalence with increasing age. The authors therefore assume that the higher prevalence of maxillary sinusitis in the older child is probably due to anatomic variations, while the more severe bilateral maxillary sinusitis in combination with inflammation of the other sinuses in the younger child is more often due to an immature immune response.

Table 13-5 shows also a clear-cut decrease in the total number of children with chronic nasal complaints and sinusitis after the age of 8 years, which again reconfirms the hypothesis of an immature immune system in the younger child, responsible for the higher prevalence of sinusitis, and showing the natural history of the disease, which tends to heal spontaneously after the age of 8 years. This natural history must be considered in the evaluation of any kind of therapy.

Stammberger and Kopp[77] described the important anatomic variants in adults that can be responsible for chronic or recurrent sinusitis, such as the relation of the uncinate process to the ethmoidal infundibulum and the frontal recess, the size of the bulla, the presence of a concha bullosa, Haller's cell, paradoxically bent middle turbinate, and a medially bent uncinate process. van der Veken and colleagues[72] (Table 13-5) had already demonstrated the presence of some of these variants in children and also showed that their prevalence increases with age.

If the prevalence of these anatomic variants (Table 13-6) in the older children is compared, similar percentages can be seen for some of these variants in the van der Veken study (concha bullosa, Haller's cells). Only the prevalence of septal deviations is much higher in the van

Table 13-4. Prevalence of sinusitis as a whole (abnormal) compared with disease of the separated sinuses for different age groups (%)

AGE (YR)	NUMBER	ABN	MAXILLARY	ETHMOIDAL	SPHENOID
3-4	38	72	63	58	29
5-6	46	50	39	35	13
7-8	42	70	52	40	26
9-10	21	62	33	23	19
11-12	20	65	45	20	10
13-14	29	66	65	10	0
Total	196				

ABN, abnormality of sinus mucosa in all sinuses.

Table 13-5. Prevalence of anatomic variants (%) for different age groups

AGE (YR)	NUMBER	SEPTAL DEVIATION	CONCHA MEDIA BULLOSA	HALLER CELL
3-4	38	16	0	0
5-6	46	37	8	3
7-8	42	55	4	2
9-10	21	48	2	2
10-12	20	65	15	10
13-14	29	72	20	3

Table 13-6. Anatomic variants in children with chronic sinusitis (%)

AUTHOR	APRIL ET AL	MILCZUK ET AL
Year	**1993**	**1993**
Number of children	**74**	**114**
Age (median) (yr)	**8.8**	**6**
Anatomic variants		
Concha bullosa	19	10
Haller cell	18	5
Septal deformity	13	
Paradoxical middle turbinate	7	4
Atelectatic maxillary sinus	3	17
Prominent ethmoidal bulla	2	

der Veken study, but this depends on the definition of septal deviation (slight bending or well-developed septal spur). Milczuk and associates[78] found a high prevalence of hypoplastic maxillary sinuses (17%) and also noted that these hypoplastic sinuses had diseased mucosa. For these authors, a hypoplastic maxillary sinus was an absolute indication for surgery (middle antrostomy, anterior ethmoidectomy, nasal antral window, sphenoidectomy, antral lavage and sphenoidectomy). The median age of these children at surgery was 6 years, and lateral deviation of the uncinate process was found in 57%. As the maxillary sinus is the only sinus that can be visualized very well on standard x-ray films in children, it is interesting to compare the Milczuk and colleagues[78] results of hypoplastic maxillary sinuses with the only available longitudinal study in children over 10 years by Maresh and Washburn.[9] The latter emphasized that variations in size of the maxillary sinus occur frequently, without any demonstrable relation with the amount or frequency of infection and without following any definite pattern. They observed children who had one antrum that appeared to be definitively infected in every film for several years, but for whom later films showed normally clear antrums over a period of years. They also showed an appreciable increase in the number of clear sinuses after 6 years of age. April and colleagues[79] found a clear-cut positive correlation between size and age (p .007) and no significant relation between the maxillary sinus size and average severity of the disease (p .6). All these findings suggest that the growth of the maxillary sinus is not impaired by extensive or chronic disease of the maxillary sinus, unlike the temporal bone, which becomes sclerotic with chronic middle ear disease. In looking at the evidence from the Maresh[9] and April[79] studies, it seems that the presence of a hypoplastic maxillary sinus per se is not a real indication for surgery.

Riding and Irvine[47] found preexisting disease in 50% of children with chronic sinusitis (mainly allergy in 12% and immune deficiency in 13%). In the literature, many authors attribute a great importance to allergy (asthma, allergic rhinitis) in the etiology of rhinosinusitis.* Some authors even stated that in children allergy is regarded as the most important condition that predisposes to sinus infection.[84,86-88] van der Veken and colleagues[76] found no difference in the involvement of the different sinuses of atopic children and of children with chronic nasal complaints without atopy. In their study, the prevalence of rhinosinusitis clearly decreased after the age of 8 years, while the prevalence of atopy increased with age. Therefore, it seems that atopy itself is not a major cause of chronic rhinosinusitis in young children. However, the prevalence of rhinosinusitis is higher in atopic children than in normal children; when rhinosinusitis exists, the involvement of the different sinuses is the same as in children with infectious chronic rhinosinusitis. This was confirmed by Iwens and Clement,[89] who found CT signs of sinus mucosa inflammation in 61% of atopic children (n=59) and 58% of atopic adults (n=62) compared with 64% of children (n=169) and 57% of adults (n=350) with chronic nasal complaints, mainly of infectious origin (Table 13-7).

When the atopic adults and children (Table 13-8) are compared, different sinuses are involved in a similar percentage. In children under the age of 8 years, the number of cases is lower (allergic rhinitis in children tends to occur after the age of 6), but the percentage of severe sinusitis is higher (probably because of concomitant infection that is more frequent in this age group). Also, Yaniv and associates[14] demonstrated that chronic rhinitis (rhinosinusitis?) in preschoolers is more frequently caused by bacterial infection (58% good results with antibiotic treatment), while in schoolchildren allergy is more frequently the reason (49% good response on antihistamine therapy). It is therefore obvious that the diagnosis of atopy needs to be confirmed by skin testing and eventually total and specific IgE levels, when there is any suspicion of allergy in the history.

All young children have a physiologic primary immune deficiency.[59,80] Umetsu and associates[90] studied 20 children with recurrent sinopulmonary infections and found serum IgG levels within the normal range. They showed, however, selective IgG-subclass deficiency (60% were deficient for IgG_2, 25% for IgG_3, 15% for IgG_2 and IgG_3, and 15% for IgA). Defense against polysaccharide-encapsulated bacteria via immunoglobulin G subclasses 2 and 4 may not reach adult levels until the age of 10 years.[91] IgG subclass deficiency can lead to protracted or chronic sinusitis.[78,82,87,90,92] According to Polmar,[82] recurrent and chronic sinusitis is the most common clinical presentation of common variable immunodeficiencies (CVID). CVID is a disorder in which patients have significantly reduced levels of two or more immunoglobulin classes (usually IgG and IgA) in the serum. Also, IgA production increases slowly and is dependent on the number of plasma cells in the mucosa, reaching the adult level at the age of 10 years.[58,80] Although not all patients who lack secretory IgA antibodies have an increased number of more severe respiratory infections, the subject who has IgA deficiency and chronic sinusitis is a difficult management problem, and substitution therapy cannot be provided.[87,92] Other less common immunodeficiencies are C_4 deficiency, X-linked agammaglobulinemia, ataxia-telangiectasia, and hyper IgM immunodeficiency.[82] Patients with primary or acquired immunodeficiencies (e.g., treatment for malignancies, organ transplants, maternally transmitted AIDS or blood-transmitted AIDS in hemophiliacs, drug-induced conditions) are at increased risk for developing a difficult-to-treat sinusi-

* References 14, 46, 47, 58, 59, 79-85, 170.

Table 13-7. Computed tomography of sinus mucosal inflammation in atopic children and adults (%)

	CHILDREN (N=59) UNDER 14 YR	ADULTS (N=62)
Without sinus disease	39	42
With sinus disease	61	58
Maxillary sinus	83	89
Anterior ethmoid	55	44
Posterior ethmoid	30	28
Sphenoid	39	11
Frontal sinus	14	5

Table 13-8. Prevalence of sinusitis in allergic children (according to age) and adults (%)

	N	NO SINUSITIS	MILD SINUSITIS	SEVERE SINUSITIS
Children				
Age (yr)				
3-6	8	50	0	50
6-9	19	37	31	31
10-12	14	36	50	14
13-15	18	39	44	17
Adults				
15-55	62	42	45	12

tis with resistant microorganisms and fungi.[58] Also, the initial signs and symptoms may be nonspecific, with thin rhinorrhea, mild congestion, and chronic cough.[59]

Sethi and Legsold[93] recommend a number of investigations in patients with (1) a persistence of sinus infection, despite sinus surgery that restored normal microbiology transport and corrected ventilation problems; (2) an inadequate response to appropriate antimicrobial therapy; (3) a culture of unusual pathogens from the sinuses; and (4) a history of infections at other sites. After careful history taking and physical examination, the following investigations are indicated: serum immunoglobulin levels, IgG subclasses, and assessment of response to immunization with protein antigens (i.e. diphtheria and tetanus toxoid) and polysaccharide antigens (pneumococcal vaccine).

Not much is known about the influence of cellular immunology and cytokines in rhinosinusitis.[94] It has been shown that interleukin II-8 transcript was detected in only 45% of adults with chronic sinusitis.[94] Interleukin II-8 is a macrophage-derived cytokine displaying potent activating properties toward neutrophils, and in this way its decrease may contribute to the pathogenesis of chronic sinusitis. Down syndrome,[81,87] cyanotic heart disease,[42,95] and hypothyroidism[42] can also predispose to sinusitis. In children with cystic fibrosis, sinusitis seems to be a common problem. The relationship among cystic fibrosis, polyposis and chronic sinusitis was first described by Shwachman and colleagues.[96] Brihaye and colleagues[57] found the following complaints in 84 patients (mainly children) with cystic fibrosis: cough (62%), nasal blockade (60%), rhinorrhea (53%), recurrent spells of rhinosinusitis (51%), poor quality of sleep (agitation and snoring during the night, 37%), headache (32%), and anosmia (12%). Thus, in children with cystic fibrosis, nasal blockade is certainly the main nasal problem, as it is in children with chronic rhinosinusitis without cystic fibrosis. Jones and associates[24] also found nasal obstruction to be the main symptom in children with cystic fibrosis (n=16) (65%), followed by cough (56%), purulent discharge (51%), and halitosis (42%).

Although the prevalence of nasal polyposis in children with cystic fibrosis was previously estimated to be between 6% and 20%,[97-99] Lieberman and colleagues[100] estimated it to be 40%, and Brihaye and colleagues[57] reported that performing rigid endoscopy in 84 patients with cystic fibrosis revealed inflammatory polyps in 45% (mean age 15 years) and medial bulging of the lateral nasal wall in 12% (mean age 5 years). In patients with cystic fibrosis and chronic rhinosinusitis, CT almost always (99%,[99] 100%[57]) showed opacification of the anterior complex (anterior ethmoid, maxillary, and, if developed, frontal sinus, Fig. 13-1), and 57% showed clouding in the posterior complex (posterior ethmoid and sphenoid). In all children with a medial displacement of the lateral wall, there was a soft tissue mass in the maxillary antrum (large quantity of secretions, surrounded by a polypous mucosa, representing mucopyosinusitis). In 80% of these children the displacement was so extreme that the lateral nasal wall touched the septum, resulting in a total nasal blockade. In the study by Brihaye and colleagues,[57] massive nasal polyposis was never found before the age of 5 years. Mucopyosinusitis of the maxillary sinus can occur at a younger age (3 months to 8 years), and the maxillary sinus seems to be the first sinus affected by the disease. The youngest child ever reported

A

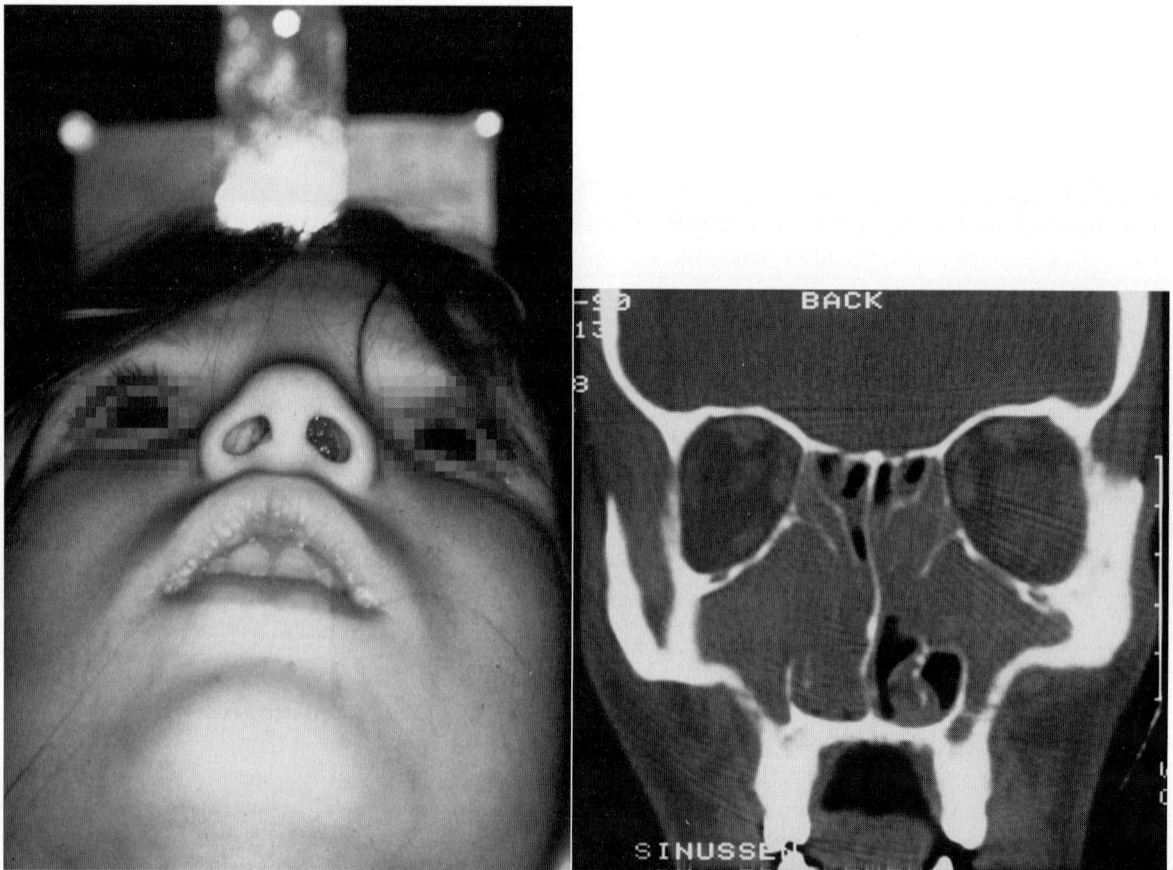

B

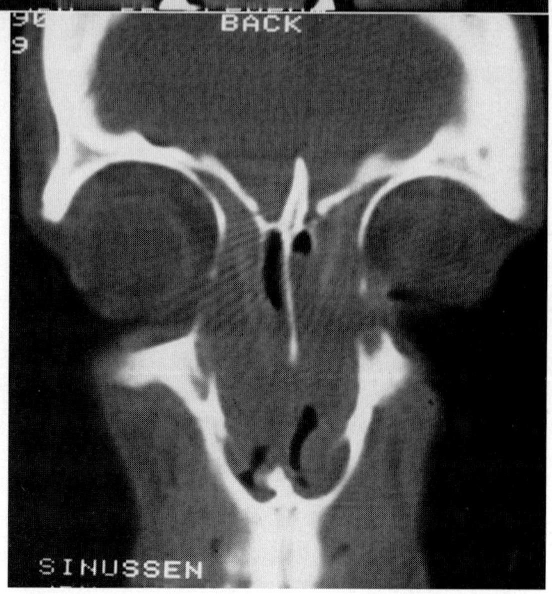

C

Fig. 13-1. **A**, A 7-year-old girl with cystic fibrosis and massive polyposis; note the typical polyps in the nasal vestibulum and hypertrophy of the gingiva because of continuous mouth breathing. **B**, Coronal computed tomographic (CT) scan showing total opacification of the middle ethmoid, maxillary sinus, and nasal cavity. **C**, Coronal CT scan showing total opacification of the anterior ethmoid and frontal recess.

with this disease (mucopyosinusitis with medial displacement of the nasal lateral wall, resulting in nasal blockade) was a 3-month-old infant presenting symptoms similar to those of children with bilateral choanal atresia (nasal blockade, stridor, and feeding problems), except that the symptoms occurred only gradually following a symptom-free period after birth, requiring acute surgical treatment (Fig. 13-2). A similar case was described by Tunkel and associates,[101] but in an older child (13 months of age), resulting in nasal obstruction, but without stridor. An interesting observation was also made by April and colleagues,[79] who found no anatomic abnormalities (concha bullosa, Haller's cell, septal deformity, paradoxal middle turbinate, atelectatic maxillary sinus, prominent ethmoidal bulla) whatsoever in these children, but found bilateral uncinate process erosion in 100% and increased attenuation in maxillary sinus in 75% (n=12). Brihaye and colleagues[57] found one case of extreme septal deviation (a vertical fracture of the septum, probably due to trauma) in their series of cystic fibrosis children with polyposis. Although the CT signs of cystic fibrosis are typical, the diagnosis is of course made on the basis of a positive sweat test.

By definition, patients with Kartagener's syndrome (the classic syndrome described by Kartagener in 1933[102] for the first time consisted of a hereditary disease involving the classic triad of sinusitis, bronchiectasis, and situs inversus) have chronic rhinosinusitis, but not from the start. The neonatal group with Kartagener's syndrome do not have sinusitis or bronchiectasis, and therefore the term *immotile or dysmotile cilia syndrome* was introduced in the seventies to describe these infants[103-105] in whom an ultrastructural

A

B

C

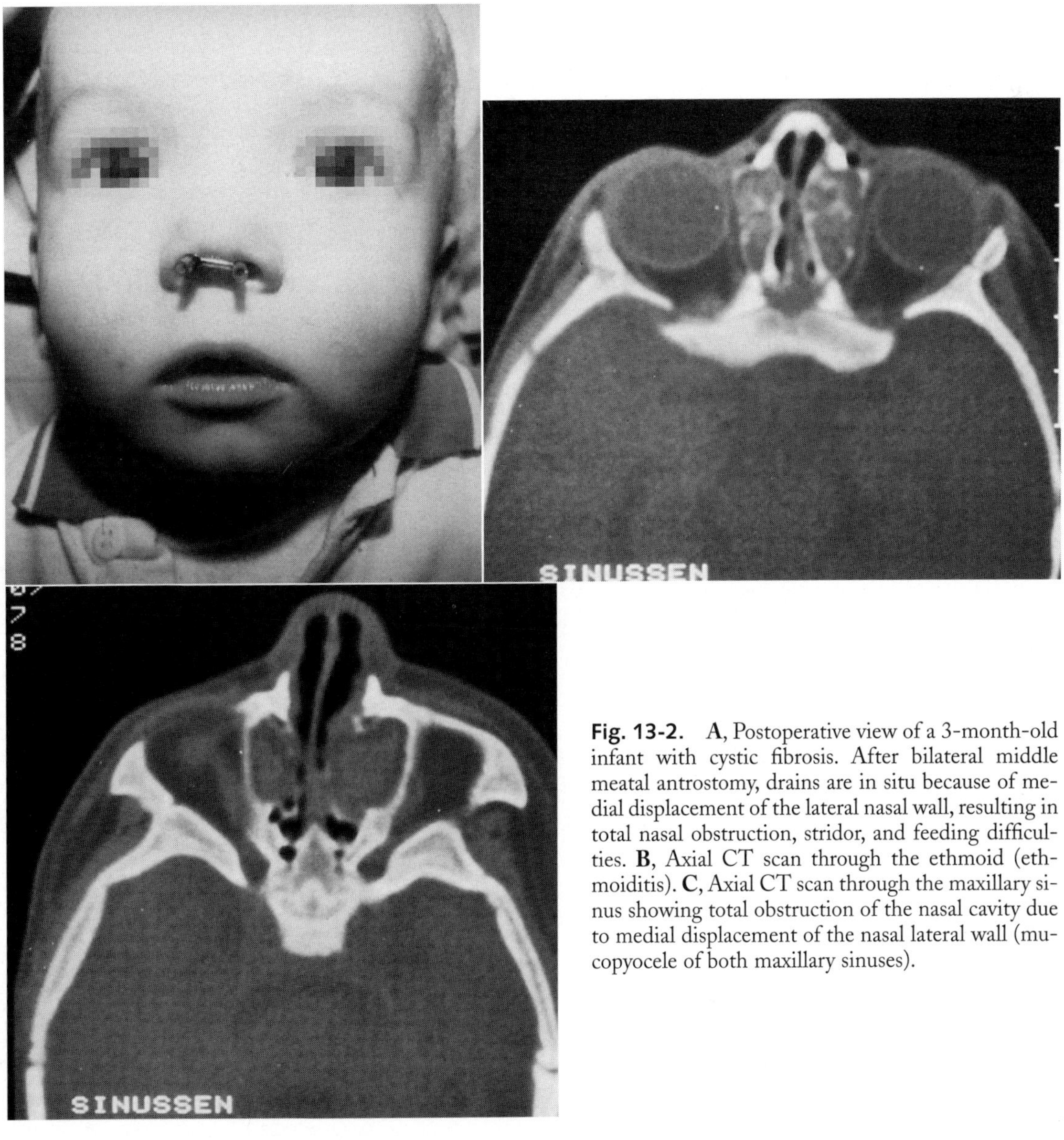

Fig. 13-2. **A**, Postoperative view of a 3-month-old infant with cystic fibrosis. After bilateral middle meatal antrostomy, drains are in situ because of medial displacement of the lateral nasal wall, resulting in total nasal obstruction, stridor, and feeding difficulties. **B**, Axial CT scan through the ethmoid (ethmoiditis). **C**, Axial CT scan through the maxillary sinus showing total obstruction of the nasal cavity due to medial displacement of the nasal lateral wall (mucopyocele of both maxillary sinuses).

anomaly was found: lack of dynein arms on the peripheral doublets of the cilia. As ultrastructural changes of the cilia were also found after chronic infections or polyposis, and situs inversus did not seem to be essential, the name of this autosomal recessive disease was changed to *primary ciliary dyskinesia*.[106] de Boeck and Jorissen[107] described 15 cases (only four with situs inversus) in which the diagnosis was made at a median age of 5 years and 9 months. Fourteen of these patients showed chronic sinus disease, and none had massive nasal polyposis.

Therefore, when situs inversus is present, the diagnosis of Karagener's syndrome is not difficult. In the absence of situs inversus (50% according to Ramet and associates[108]), however, the diagnosis can be difficult in a neonate, as sinusitis and bronchiectasis develop only later. Therefore, one should always consider the diagnosis in any neonate with respiratory or ENT problems of unknown origin, and the diagnosis should be confirmed by nasal biopsy for transmission electromicroscopic examination showing the typical ultrastructural ciliary lesions: absence of dynein arms from the outer doublets, abnormal orientation of the cilia, and variations of the normal nine plus two microtubular arrangements (an extra central pair and missing peripheral microtubules). These typical anomalies were first shown to be present already in nasal biopsies at birth[108,110,111] and were proved not to be acquired.[109] Table 13-9[29] describes the different ultrastructural anomalies for different nasal diseases.

According to the literature, the diagnosis of primary cilia dyskinesia is made at an average age of 5 years. It appears that bronchiectasis may be delayed or can even be prevented if early diagnosis is made followed by adequate symptomatic therapy.[110,111] All patients with primary ciliary dyskinesia show an important decrease of the mucociliary transport rate[112] and abnormal ciliary beating patterns.[113] In vitro tests are also being developed to assist the diagnosis.[114]

Jaffe and Deblanc[115] described a high prevalence of purulent rhinorrhea (71%) and signs of maxillary sinusitis (72%) in 21 Navajo children. Ishikawa and Amitani[116] found on x-ray examination a high prevalence (47%) of sinusitis in children (n=60) with congenital velopharyngeal insufficiency without overt or submucosal cleft palate, and in 44% of children (n=333) with cleft palate. In the first group, there was a low prevalence of septal deviation (27%), and the mucociliary clearance was normal. Although in children with cleft palate chronic rhinosinusitis can be the result of anatomic variants (septal deviation, abnormal configuration of the ostiomeatal complex), these cannot be the cause in the children of the first group with only velopharyngeal insufficiency. Other possible factors, such as regurgitation of saliva and food, may induce chronic irritation of the mucosa leading to chronic rhinosinusitis.

Although inflammation and anatomic variants can cause mechanical obstruction of the ostiomeatal complex, obstruction caused by abnormal masses may also be contributory. Mechanical obstruction of the nasal cavity, congenital as well as acquired (e.g., antral choanal polyp, adenoid hyperplasia, nasogastric tube, foreign body, tumors, nasal trauma), can also cause chronic rhinosinusitis in infants and children.[47,117]

The most common type of mass occurring in the nasal cavity in children is the benign nasal polyp. According to the literature, the most common polyp in children is the antral choanal polyp.[99] In 100 children[117] with polyps the antrochoanal polyp was found in 36%, and cystic fibrosis was responsible for another 22% of cases; 42% were just inflammatory polyps (21% unilateral and 21% bilateral). The antral choanal polyp is extremely rare in children under the age of 10.[118] Hardy[119] described one case involving a 9-year-old girl, and Sirola[120] found five cases of choanal polyps in children under the age of 10, the youngest being a boy of 6. The youngest child seen was a 4-year-old boy with bilateral chronic pansinusitis and also adenoid hypertrophy (Fig. 13-3).

Among benign tumors, hemangiomas and tumors of neural derivation (gliomas) are the next common. Gliomas present at a very early age (2 to 6 weeks) with symptoms of acquired choanal atresia, with a reddish or bluish mass in the nasal cavity that does not change color with cry-

Table 13-9. Transmission electronmicroscopic findings of the cilia in 17 children with chronic respiratory infections

ABNORMAL MORPHOLOGY	KARTAGENER'S SYNDROME (N=3)	CHRONIC SINOBRONCHIAL SYNDROME (N=11)	NASAL POLYPS (N=3)
Absence of dynein arms	3 (100%)	8 (72%)	1 (33%)
Random orientation of central pair of microtubules	3 (100%)	8 (72%)	1 (33%)
Compound cilia	3 (100%)	4 (36%)	3 (100%)
Absence of radial spokes	0 (0%)	0 (0%)	1 (33%)
Variation of the 9 + 2 configuration	2 (66%)	4 (36%)	1 (33%)

ing.[117] The differential diagnosis from mycopyosinusitis caused by cystic fibrosis is easy and can be made on a clinical and radiologic basis (Table 13-10). Sarcomas (mainly rhabdomyosarcomas) are predominant nasal malignancies.

The most common benign tumor of the sinuses in children is fibrous dysplasia; the corresponding most common malignant tumor is carcinoma (transitional and squamous cell) and again sarcoma (rhabdomyosarcoma).[117]

In conclusion, one can state that the diagnosis of acute maxillary sinusitis with empyema is straightforward, as these children have acute signs and symptoms, such as ill patient, local swelling, marked pain and fever, opacification of the sinuses on CT, and positive cultures.[15,86] As van Buchem and colleagues[15] mentioned, the number of children suffering from acute sinusitis is small. The diagnosis of chronic sinusitis is more difficult.[121] Neither a positive CT scan[1] nor culture alone can be considered the "gold standard" in the diagnosis. The "gold standard" should be a combination of findings such as long-standing complaints of rhinorrhea and/or nasal obstruction, cough, positive culture from an antral washing or from the middle meatus, and signs of sinus inflammation on CT. The real "gold standard," however, for diagnosing inflammation is histology. Goldwyn and associates[122] found from specimens taken in an adult population during surgery a significant difference in the histologic findings between patients with sinusitis and those with no sinus disease. Furthermore, any attempt at evaluating the histology of sinusitis on a quantitative basis should use detailed cell counts (400x magnification) rather than a low-power estimate of severity (40x magnification). Finally, these authors found no significant correlation between infiltrate (as measured by lymphocytes, eosinophils or total cell count) and the extent of the disease as demonstrated by CT.

Thus, a patient with limited infundibular disease may have intensive inflammation in the particular area and otherwise normal sinuses on CT, while a patient with pansinus polyposis of all sinuses may have markedly little inflammatory infiltrate. The problem with histology, however, is that the representative specimens can be obtained only during surgery, so that this "gold standard" is of no use as an indication for surgery.

THERAPY

The most controversial part in the pediatric sinusitis debate is probably the therapy aspect, ranging from therapeutic nihilism, conservative medical therapy, to the most aggressive surgery such as complete sphenoethmoidectomy. According to Rachelefsky and colleagues,[87] treatment of chronic sinus disease in children should be aimed at promoting drainage, controlling infection, and providing symptomatic relief. Most important, however, in the evaluation of any kind of therapy, if it is not compared with a placebo-controlled group, is the need to correlate the results with the natural history of the disease, keeping in mind that in most cases chronic sinusitis in the younger child is a self-limiting disease, resolving spontaneously after the age of 6 to 7 years. As discussed, this natural history has been documented by many authors[1,9-11,14-16,39,123] and in fact is comparable with the natural history of otitis media with effusion.[124-126] Mann and Jonas,[127] in a 5-year follow-up study in children aged 7 to 13 years, showed that even then there was a high self-cure rate of up to 94%.

In the preantibiotic era, treatment of sinusitis consisted of topical decongestants, local heat or cold application, and analgesics[128-130]; in more severe cases, antral lavage or limited surgery was performed, such as turbinate fracture, partial turbinectomy, and removal of polyps.[129-131] Furstenberg[128] reflects very well the general opinion of the preantibiotic era, noting that there was a surgical axiom of long standing in the ENT department of Michigan University to avoid bone work in the pres-

Table 13-10. Differential diagnosis in infants with stridor (improving during crying) and feeding difficulties from nasal origin

	BILATERAL CHOANAL ATRESIA	GLIOMA	CYSTIC FIBROSIS
Symptoms	Occur from birth	Occur after a latency of 2-6 wk	Occur after a latency of 4 wk or more
Rhinoscopy	Impossible to pass catheter or dye via nose into naso- and oropharynx Purulent secretions present	Reddish to bluish mass in nasal cavity, mostly attached to septum Not changing with crying	Medial displacement of lateral nasal wall Purulent secretions (no polyps in nasal cavity)
Computed tomography	Bilateral atretic plate Sinusitis	Tumor mass Eventual sinusitis	Mucopyocele of maxillary sinus

A B C D

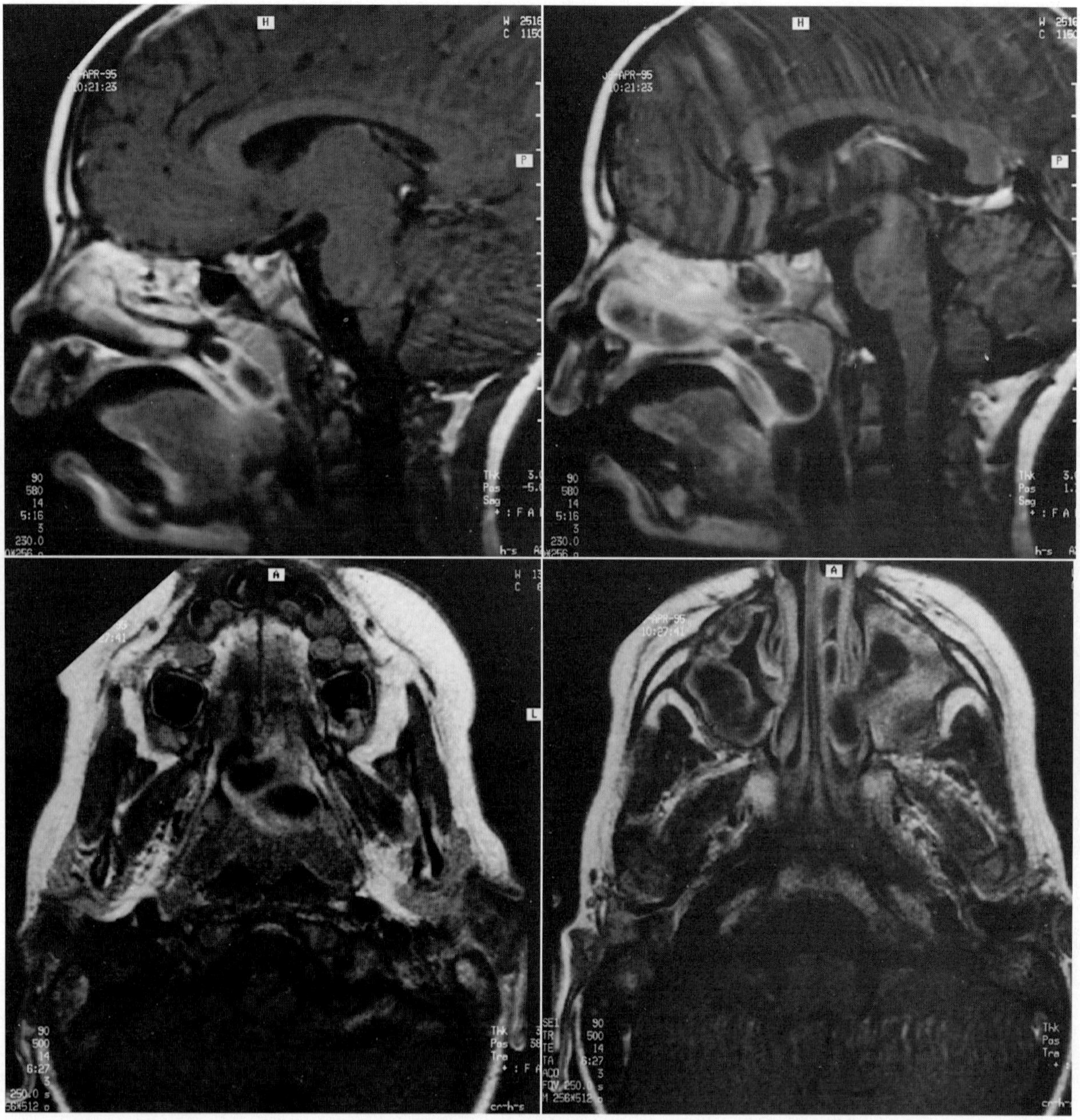

Fig. 13-3. **A** and **B**, T1-weighted sequence (magnetic resonance imaging or MRI) with gadolinium, parasagittal scans showing ethmoiditis and a huge antral choanal polyp extending in the nasopharynx in this 4-year-old boy (with gadolinium the stroma of the polyp does not enhance with gadolinium). **C** and **D**, T1-weighted MRI with gadolinium, axial scans showing an antral choanal polyp in the left maxillary sinus, left nasal cavity, and nasopharynx. *Continued*

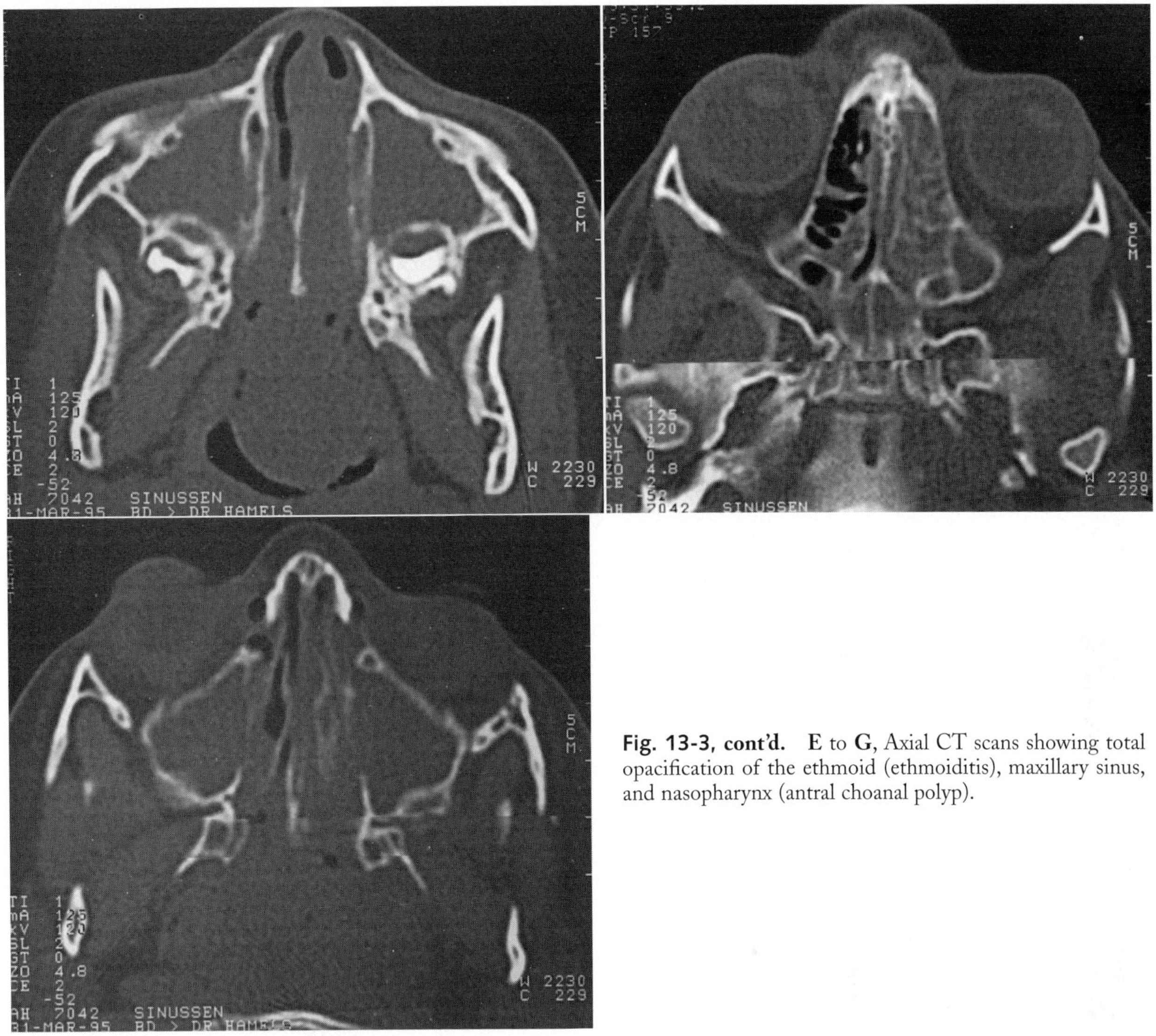

Fig. 13-3, cont'd. E to G, Axial CT scans showing total opacification of the ethmoid (ethmoiditis), maxillary sinus, and nasopharynx (antral choanal polyp).

ence of an acute infection in the sinuses, and that this immutable law was enforced even to the extent of discouraging the practice of antral lavage. Of course, at that time the rate of serious postoperative infections was very high, and so the statement made sense.

Preventive methods are mentioned by many authors,[10,132] such as reducing air pollution, informing parents about the connection between smoking and airway disease, awareness of pediatric allergy, and avoiding day care centers; all are valuable, but they are not always easy to achieve.

Medical treatment

In 1994, Poole[1] stated that chronic rhinosinusitis in the young child does not necessarily have to be treated, as spontaneous resolution is the norm. With regard to the natural history of the disease and the growing resistance and β-lactamase production of many microorganisms, one should refrain from overtreating a runny nose in a young child. One should not treat every common cold with antibiotics or smash any minor superinfection of a common cold self-limited in time with the sledgehammer of broad-spectrum antibiotics.

Some physicians prescribe antibiotics for minor upper respiratory infections, in the hope of preventing serious complications. van Buchem and colleagues[15] followed 169 children with a runny nose for 6 months, treating them only with decongestants or saline nose drops. They did not find a single child who developed a clinically serious disease with general symptoms such as marked pain, pressure on sinuses, local swelling, or empyema, which proved that rhinosinusitis complications in a child are not very frequent.

The question remains, which child should be treated and which not? Poole[133] noted that while there are wide variations in defining rhinosinusitis, discussions about the necessity and thresholds for initiating therapy are even more complicated. In view of all the foregoing, a conservative approach to the treatment of rhinosinusitis in the young child appears appropriate and should include at a minimum one or more of the following (modified according to Poole[1,44]):

1. A marked acute exacerbation of the runny nose: more copious secretions, pressure and pain over the sinuses, local swelling.
2. A systematically ill patient: fever, general malaise.
3. Associated worsening of lower respiratory symptoms: e.g., cough, wheezing.
4. An association with otitis media (acute or chronic with effusion).

The initial treatment of sinusitis (acute as well as recurrent or chronic) consists of eradicating microorganisms with appropriate antibiotics and additional treatment promoting drainage and ventilation, such as decongestants, analgesics, anti-inflammatory drugs, and antipyretics.[123] With regard to the medical treatment of sinusitis in children, only a few double-blind placebo-controlled studies have been performed. In a short-term follow-up study, Furukawa and Rachelefsky[86] showed a superior result from erythromycin-sulfisoxazole plus topical decongestants compared with placebo plus topical decongestant, and Rachelefsky and associates,[87] studying 84 children, demonstrated on the basis of radiographic and clinical response a better result in the group treated with amoxicillin, although trimethoprim-sulfamethoxazole was an adequate alternative, while erythromycin was not any better than an antihistamine-decongestant combination. These studies prove a well-known fact, that an adequate antibiotic will promptly result in cessation of clinical symptoms.[1]

The only long-term follow-up in the treatment of children with chronic maxillary sinusitis (n=141),[38] comparing oral amoxicillin combined with decongestive nose drops, drainage of the maxillary sinus (antral lavage), a combination of the previous two regimens, and placebo, showed that the therapeutic effects of these four forms of treatment did not differ significantly or have a significant curative effect. The conclusion was that none of these forms of therapy can be recommended as an active treatment policy. With this in mind, antibiotics are seen to be still the cornerstone of medical treatment for sinusitis, as they resolve the symptoms of acute or recurrent sinusitis (within 24 to 48 hours, Wald and colleagues[36]) and decrease the symptoms of chronic sinusitis in the short term. Sometimes this short-term result can be just enough to help the child recover and reach the summer period in relative good condition, or sometimes keeping the child out of the day care center will avoid reinfection.

The usual duration of antimicrobial therapy is 10 to 14 days. This recommendation is based on experience in adults. Hamory and colleagues[31] showed negative cultures in adults (n=81) with symptoms of acute sinusitis after a 10-day treatment with an antibiotic to which the organism was susceptible in 42 out of 44 (95%) repeated sinus aspirates. When the patient's condition has improved but without complete recovery, or when chronic sinusitis exists, this treatment can be extended for another 10 to 14 days.[1,2]

The only exception to the normal 10- to 14-day treatment regimen is with the antibiotic azithromycin. The recommended duration for the treatment of acute sinusitis[134,135] and otitis[136] with this drug is 3 to 5 days. This agent is selectively transported to the site of infection by the phagocytes, resulting in high tissue concentrations.[137] The choice of antibiotic depends on the microorganisms involved. From the literature, the most common organisms are the well-known infernal trio: *Haemophilus influenzae*, *Streptococcus pneumoniae*, and *Moraxella catarrhalis*. According to Poole[1,44] there is a 50% resistance of pneumococci to oral antibiotics in the United States, and *H. influenzae* strains are becoming less sensitive to β-lactams and show a frank resistance to sulfa drugs. Poole therefore encourages nonantibiotic measures as often as possible. If it is decided to use antibiotics, the guide to first-line management[34] recommends the following oral agents for treatment of acute and recurrent sinusitis in an empiric way:

1. Trimethoprim (6 mg/kg/day)–sulfamethoxazole (30 mg/kg/day) bid
2. Loracarbef bid
3. Amoxicillin and clavulanate potassium, 30 mg/kg/day tid
4. Cefuroxime axetil 20 mg/kg/day for a child bid (exists more in syrup form).

In some countries the choice of a first-line antibiotic can be different depending on the percentage of the local resistance and β-lactamase–producing microorganisms.

The first case of ampicillin-resistant *H. influenzae* infection was described by Gunn and colleagues.[138] Since 1981 the percentage of β-lactamase–producing strains of *H. influenzae* have been monitored in the Department of Microbiology (Chairman S. Lauwers) of the University Hospital of the Free University of Brussels (AZ-VUB), which studies every year an average of 300 to 600 strains. Table 13-11 shows since 1981 a steady increase of β-lactamase–producing strains from 6% to about 20% in the late 1980s and early 1990s, with a peak of 25% in 1992. In Belgium the rate of resistance of *S. pneumoniae* strains highly resistant to penicillin is negligible. The rate of resistance to clarithromycin is approximately 20% and to doxycycline approximately 30%.[139] So, in this country amoxicillin can still be used as a good first-line antibiotic. When recovery is insufficient after 10 days of therapy or when there is no improvement of clinical symptoms within 24 to 48 hours, one can take a culture or switch to an appropriate β-lactam–resistant antibiotic such as amoxicillin-clavulanate or cefuroxime for at least 10 days.

In this country the combination of trimethoprim and sulfamethoxazole (bid), although it is 10 times less expensive than the combination amoxicillin-clavulanate and cefuroxime for a full course of treatment, and shows a good activity against *H. influenzae* (up to 90%), is not considered a good first-line antibiotic because of the serious and sometimes lethal side-effects. Since 1976, the Belgian Center for the Surveillance of Drugs[140] received reports of 70 skin reactions to co-trimoxazole (three with Lyell's syndrome—one lethal and nine with Stevens-Johnson syndrome), two cases of bone marrow aplasia (one lethal), two cases of agranulocytosis and one of trombopenia, five cases of serious anaphylactic reactions (five with shocks, two with Quincke's edema). Since the introduction of co-trimoxazole in the United Kingdom in 1969, there are 113 documented deaths due to the drug (Committee on Safety of Medicines). Finally, the drug is not very active against β-hemolytic streptococci.

Other antibiotics such as chloramphenicol[50] and clindamycin[141] have been advocated but cannot be considered first-line treatments because of some serious side effects.

Additional therapy

This mainly consists of topical or oral decongestants. Most authors prefer topical α_2 agonists (xylo- and oxymetazoline) in an appropriate concentration. Careful dosage, however, is important when treating infants and young children, to prevent toxic manifestations.[142] The ratio of the area of nasal mucosa to body weight is an important factor in infants. It is three times as high in neonate, as in adults, and twice as high in children aged 2 to 3 years (Table 13-12).

Care should be taken not to use these decongestants for longer than 1 week, because they also decrease local blood flow,[59] have a ciliotoxic influence,[65,143] and involve a potential rebound.[60] On the other hand, they give rapid symptom relief,[53] especially of nasal blockade. Oral decongestants in young children are less appropriate because of their influence on cardiac rhythm and because they are often combined with the older generation of antihistamines, which have an anticholinergic effect resulting in the thickening of secretions. Besides their immediate effect on nasal congestion, their further role is unclear.[86]

Other treatments with some decongestant effect include the use of a humidifier[58,59,141,144] or the inhaling of moist heat.[144] Inhalation of hot air saturated with water will result in a temporary decongestion of the nasal mucosa.

Oral or topical mucolytics (guaifenesin, acetylcysteine) in sinusitis have never proved very effective in sinus clearance. Analgetics and antipyretics[47] effect a symptomatic treatment of the pain and of elevated temperature if any. Antihistamines are inappropriate in the treatment of common cold or sinusitis[34] unless allergy is

Table 13-11. Survey of β-lactamase–producing Haemophilus influenzae strains from 1981 to 1994 on average of 300 to 600 strains per year (%) Data from Chairman S. Lauwers, Department of Microbiology of the University Hospital of the Free University, Brussels.

YEAR	1981	1982	1983	1984	1985	1986	1987	1988	1989	1990	1991	1992	1993	1994
	6	5	8	5	12	14	NP	18	22	21	20	25	18	17

NP, Not performed.

Table 13-12. Use of a 0.1 nasal solution of xylometazoline (Brewinger H: Konservative Behandlung der Nase Ihren Nebenhohlen, Hals-Nasen-Ohern-Helkunda. In Berendes J, Link R, Zöllner F, editors: Praxis) und Klinick, Stuttgart, 1977, Georg Thieme Verlad, Bond Obere und Untere Luftweg, pp 1-28.)

	TOTAL DAILY DOSAGE (MA)	DOSE/KG/BODY WEIGHT/DAY (MG)
Adult (70 kg)	4 × 3 drops = 1.2	0.015
Infant (3.4 kg)	4 × 2 drops = 0.8	0.24
	4 × 1 drop = 0.4	0.12
6-month-old child	4 × 2 drops = 0.8	0.11
	4 × 1 drop = 0.4	0.055
1-year-old child	4 × 2 drops = 0.8	0.08
	4 × 1 drop = 0.4	0.04
3-year-old child	4 × 2 drops = 0.8	0.056

involved. In allergic rhinitis, preference should be given to the newer antihistamines such as loratadine and cetirizine, which are histamine antagonists without any known cardiotoxicity so far.

Topical steroids are indicated when allergy is involved or in chronic rhinosinusitis, especially for their anti-inflammatory effect (decrease of the influx of inflammatory cells and release of mediators, thereby reducing mucosal edema). They are also often used in nasal polyposis, especially during the postoperative phase, to decrease the volume of the polyps or to reduce the recurrence rate.[58-60,145,147]

In young children, even topical steroids administered for a long period can decrease bone turnover rate.[146]

Saline nose drops or nasal douches are popular with pediatricians.[58,59,141,144] As long as the saline is isotonic and is at body temperature, it can help eliminate nasal secretions.

The Proetz procedure[2,148] is difficult to perform in children younger than 8 years[47] and it can even spread the infection to other sinuses.[53] Its efficacy has never been proved. It has been shown that with this method mainly the posterior ethmoid and sphenoid sinuses are irrigated, while the irrigation of the anterior ethmoid is more difficult and the maxillary sinus is irrigated in only 20% to 25%.[149]

In allergic children, different other antiallergic drugs can be used, such as cromolyn sodium,[59,65] immunotherapy,[59,145] and antihistamines.[14,144,148] Topical steroids have already been discussed. Oral steroids[59,145] should be given with extreme caution in young children[48] and only in close collaboration with the pediatrician.

Intravenous gamma globulin is useful only when a gamma globulin deficiency has been demonstrated. The result of vaccination against pneumococci is not yet very successful in young children, but in the future it could prove to be a better alternative than repetitive antibiotic therapy.

Surgical treatment

Adenoidectomy. Adenoidectomy has been recommended by many authors for different indications.* These include recurrent sinusitis combined with adenoiditis as a source of recurrent infection,[87,144] in a case of adenoid hypertrophy with an almost total nasal obstruction by an adenoid pad resulting in stasis,[60,144] or in a case of serous otitis media with effusion.[58,151] Clement[168-169] did not find any significant correlation between the size of the adenoid and the presence of purulent secretions in the middle meatus on fiberscopic examination in 420 children between the ages of 1 and 7 years, while there is a very significant correlation between the size of the adenoid and the complaint of mouth breathing ($p < .001$) and snoring ($p < .001$). Thus, it is important to differentiate between the symptoms typical for chronic rhinosinusitis and those for adenoid hypertrophy. Hilbert[152] showed that nasal obstruction, snoring, and speech defects occur more frequently in children with adenoid hypertrophy, while symptoms of rhinorrhea, cough, headache, signs of mouth breathing, and abnormality on anterior rhinoscopy occur as frequently in children with chronic sinusitis as in children with adenoid hypertrophy.

Some authors, however, are not certain of the benefit of adenoidectomy[144,153] and note that the effect of adenoidectomy on sinusitis is not well documented[60] or has not been proved statistically.[147] Although the beneficial effect of adenoidectomy on otitis media with effusion has been demonstrated by different authors,[154,155] only one study[151] performed in 78 children showed a significant improvement ($p < .01$) of the sinusitis signs on x-ray examination 6 months after surgery, compared with a control group. Accordingly, in cases in which chronic sinusitis is accompanied by clear-cut signs of adenoid hypertrophy resulting in nasal obstruction, snoring, and speech difficulty, adenoidectomy should be performed before more extensive surgery is considered.

With the introduction of antroscopy at the end of the 1970s, antral lavage in children became more popular. As the trocar of the endoscope had a 4-mm diameter, it was easy to leave a ventilation tube in position, making frequent irrigation of the maxillary sinus possible in children without any need for repetitive anesthesia. The main indications were chronically opacified maxillary sinuses* in children who were clinically and radiologically unresponsive to appropriate therapy for 5 to 6 weeks, and acute sinusitis (with or without complications) when the patient failed to show significant improvement within 48 hours[50] of initiating antibiotic therapy, or when the patient experienced pain.[2,144] It was shown, however, that in children with chronic rhinosinusitis, irrigation of the maxillary sinus does not lead to a better cure after 3 weeks, compared with a control group,[67,92] or is not statistically significantly more successful.[60] It is the author's opinion that since antral lavage requires general anesthesia in children, it is justified only when pain is present, or when maxillary sinusitis is accompanied by complications not responsive to intravenous antibiotic therapy within 48 hours and when CT shows complete opacification of the maxillary sinus.

It having been demonstrated that the results of antral lavage in children were not long-lasting, the logical consequence, in children who required continuous antral lavage,[144] was to resort to permanent antrostomy in the inferior meatus or to a nasal antral window. A further advantage of this window is that it allows frequent fiberscopic examination.[53] The technique of antral lavage and nasal antral window has been very well described by Ritter and Fritsch.[145] Some authors claim good results with this technique.[156] Lund,[157] however, demonstrated that, especially in children under the age of 16 years, there oc-

* References 58, 60, 86, 144, 146, 150, 151.

* References 38, 53, 58, 67, 81, 92, 144.

curs a high rate of closure of this nasal antral window. She concluded that the inferior meatus in children is smaller than in adults, making it impossible to create an adequately sized antrostomy. As a consequence, Lusk and colleagues[60] and Muntz and Lusk[158] were able to show that in a 6-month follow-up the success rate of the nasal antral window procedures dropped to 27%. All patients remained symptomatic, and 28% needed further functional endoscopic sinus surgery.

As demonstrated by Stammberger and Kopp,[77] even in patients with a patent nasal antral window in the inferior meatus, the mucosal transport is still deviated toward the natural ostium. The current indication for this technique is therefore mainly limited to primary ciliary dyskinesia,[145] where one hopes to achieve a kind of gravitational drainage.[2]

Caldwell-Luc operation

The Caldwell-Luc operation is contraindicated in children[2,59,144] as it can cause damage to the unerupted teeth.

As mentioned, most of the controversies seem to dwell on the indication for functional endoscopic sinus surgery (FESS) in children. The "functional" in FESS means that the function of the ostiomeatal complex is restored.[159] This can be done by a minimal procedure such as infundibulotomy, nasal antral window in the middle meatus, total or partial middle turbinectomy, ethmoid air cell exenteration, and proceeding finally to extensive sphenoethmoidectomy.* The frontal recess and frontal sinus do not represent a problem in children under the age of 7 because they are not developed at that age. The indications for surgery are chronic sinusitis† lasting for at least 6 months,[141] with symptoms and CT signs severe enough to warrant surgery after failed prolonged medical therapy.[54,55,60,160] The CT scan should be obtained after a 4- to 6-week course of an antibiotic that will cover β-lactamase–producing bacteria to evaluate residual disease. Some authors also include acute sinusitis with orbital or intracranial complications.[53,150,156] The goal of the surgery is to reestablish normal mucociliary clearance of the sinuses by opening the ostiomeatal complex, removing ethmoidal disease, and opening when indicated the natural ostia of the other sinuses.[65] The dispute over paranasal sinus surgery in young children appears to involve more an emotional argument than a real controversy among the different authors. Poole,[1] who is very much against surgery, sees only five to 20 cases each year (excluding cystic fibrosis, polyps, and suppurative complications) from referral centers serving well over 1 million patients with practically no cases of pre-school age sinusitis. Wolf and Greistorfer,[162] in a series of 105 children, operated on only seven children under 6 years of age, and three under 5 years of age (including children with choanal polyp, immunodeficiency, cystic fibrosis, and primary ciliary dyskinesia). Gross and colleagues[150] operated on 57 children, of whom only seven were under the age of 6 (also including those with cystic fibrosis and complications of acute sinusitis). Surgeons who operate on larger numbers of young children are Lazar and colleagues[65]: 26 children between the age of 0 and 5 years; Lusk and Muntz[160]: about 15 under the age of 6.6 years; and Parsons and Philips,[153] with approximately 100 children under the age of 7.4 years.[65,153,160] Their main indication is recalcitrant severe chronic sinusitis often combined with allergy and asthma. The age group in the Stankiewicz study[161] is not well determined. Triglia and associates[164] and Jones and associates[24] operate mainly on children with cystic fibrosis or polyposis, each on respectively 24 and 17 children with a mean age of 12 and 10 years.

Clement operated mainly on 11 children under the age of 6 (the youngest patient being 3 months of age), all cystic fibrosis cases; on one child of 4 years with antral choanal polyp; and on six neonates with bilateral choanal atresia. In the child with antral choanal polyp, a wide middle meatal antrostomy was performed to remove the choanal polyp on one side and the polypous degeneration of the maxillary sinus mucosa that was starting on the other side (Fig. 13-3). In the choanal atresia cases (Fig. 13-4), only the atretic bony plate was drilled away under nasopharyngeal endoscopic control.[165] In the children with cystic fibrosis, two showed a medial displacement of the nasal lateral wall, one causing total nasal obstruction with stridor and feeding problems in a 3-month-old child. In both cases, both maxillary antra were cleared of polyps, leaving a wide middle meatus antrostomy. In all the other cases of cystic fibrosis, a total sphenoethmoidectomy was performed. These children with cystic fibrosis are, however, the most difficult to operate on, since not one single landmark can be seen at the start of the operation because of the massive polyposis. When the children are 4 years or over, the 4-mm diameter, 25-degree wide-angle (Panoview) endoscope and the small-size adult instruments can be used. In the younger child, the 2.7-mm diameter, 25-degree endoscope and ear instruments (small ear Blakesley and aspiration canulas) must be used. Most of the children with cystic fibrosis are already under long-term antibiotics. Surgery is performed with the child under general anesthesia with hypotension (systolic pressure between 80 and 90 mm Hg). To decongest the nasal mucosa, I use cottonoids soaked in xylometazoline 0.05%. Lusk and colleagues[54] showed that an α_2 agonist scored best for perioperative bleeding and visualization, compared with phenylephrine 0.25% and cocaine 4% ($p < .02$). When satisfactory hypotension is reached, infiltration of the mucosa with lidocain-epinephrine is not necessary.

In massive polyposis, one has first to remove delicately the polyps, starting from the floor of the nose and staying

* References 50, 53, 54, 58-60, 65, 141, 145, 150, 153, 160-162.

† References 54, 65, 73, 113, 141, 150, 159, 161-163.

A B C D

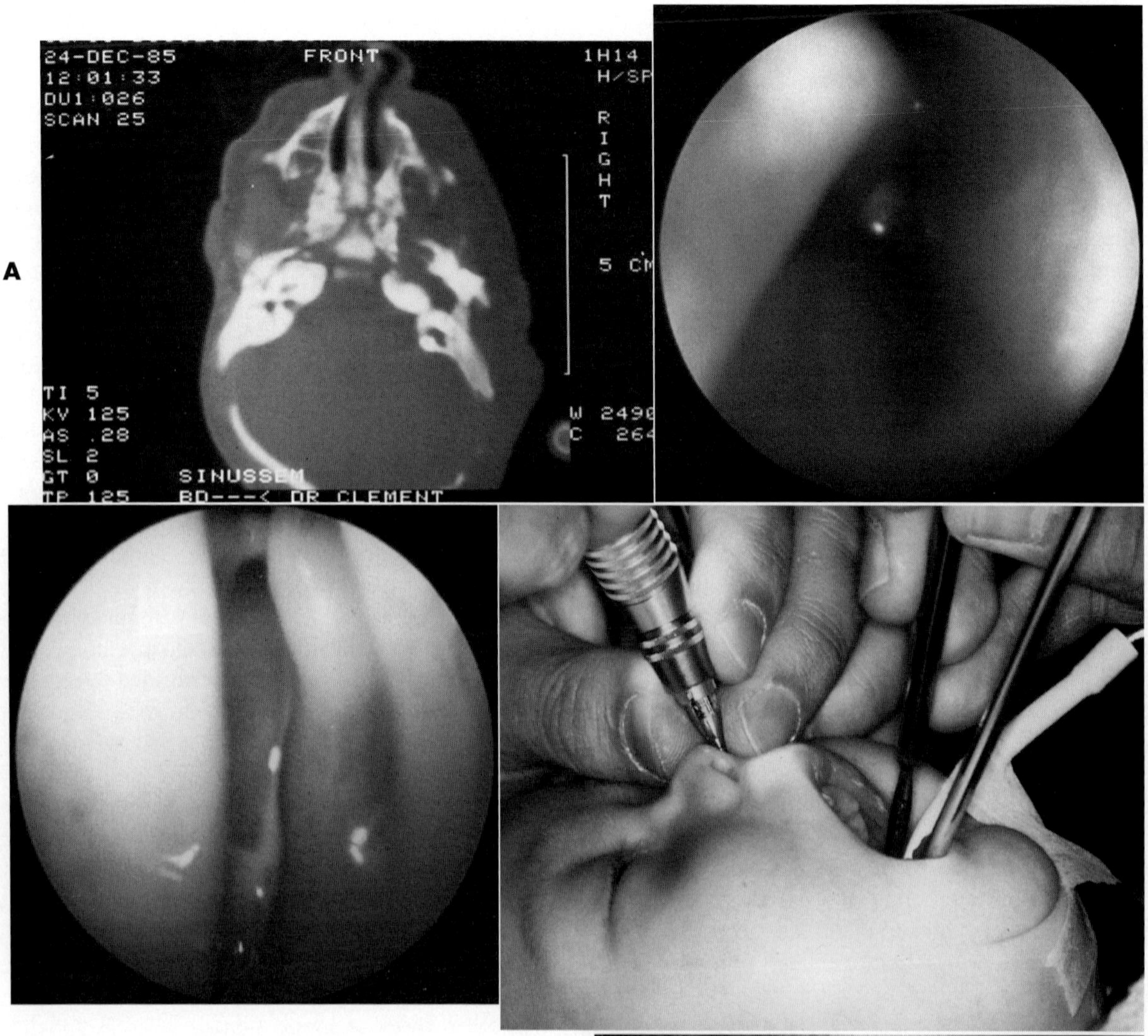

E

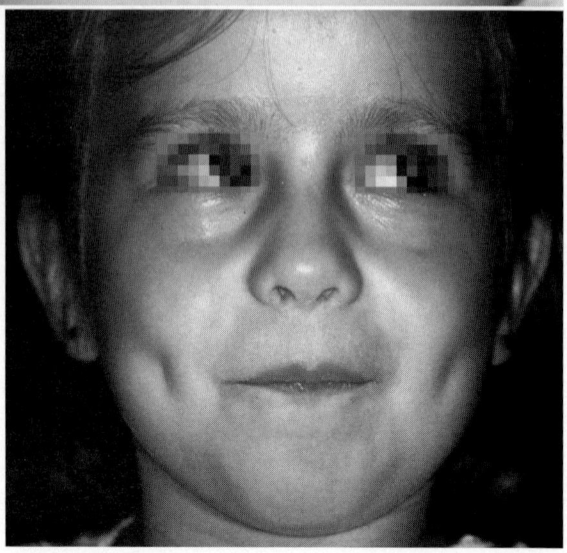

Fig. 13-4. **A**, Coronal CT scan of bilateral choanal atresia and maxillary sinusitis in a neonate with multiple mandibulofacial anomalies. **B**, endoscopy of the right nasal cavity in a 3-month-old girl with bilateral choanal atresia, stridor, and feeding difficulties. Note the curvature of the inferior turbinate and pus at the level of the atretric choanal bony plate (0-degree endoscope). **C**, endoscopy of the right nasal cavity (same patient as in **B**; 70-degree endoscope). Note the inferior turbinate, edema of the middle meatus, and the presence of pus. **D**, Opening of the atretic plate under endoscopic control. **E**, Postoperative view at age 4 years.

medially until the inferior turbinate is identified. One can also use the microdebrider (Hummer or Shaver) to debulk the nasal cavity. Then the rest of the polyps are removed, taking care not to remove bony parts, until the middle turbinate can be identified, which in most cases (over 90%) does not show any major polypous degeneration. Only in three cases was a partial middle turbinectomy necessary. Once the middle turbinate is completely visualized, the middle meatus is cleared in a lateral inferior way, entering the maxillary sinus just over the edge of the inferior turbinate. When the maxillary sinus is cleared of polyps, the posterior wall of the sinus indicates the level of the anterior wall of the sphenoid more superiorly and medially. Finally the roof of the ethmoid is reached, the superior turbinate removed, and the anterior wall of the sphenoid palpated with a suction cannula medially from the attachment of the superior turbinate until the ostium is identified. Once the ostium of the sphenoid is palpated, it can be widened to make one cavity with the ethmoid. A dressing containing no petrolatum or Vaseline (to avoid myospherulosis)[166] is left in the cavity and removed after 1 day, again with the patient under general anesthesia, allowing cleaning of the cavity (of blood clots and some remaining polyps). As postoperative control in these young children is nearly impossible, one or two more procedures with anesthesia are needed after 1 week and 3 weeks to remove possible granulation tissue and synechiae. The author does not use any pre- or postoperative topical steroids in these young children. Corticosteroids do not improve the healing process and are not recommended in young children, as they can interfere with bone growth and bone metabolism. Postoperative nasal lavage with saline (and an appropriate antibiotic) is helpful in cleaning the nose.[167] Most of these children stay 5 days postoperatively in the hospital, not because of the surgery but to optimize their pulmonary condition. They also remain under systemic broad-spectrum antibiotics. The average blood loss in these children with massive polyposis was 130 ml. No complications occurred during surgery. After surgery, two children had a fever that disappeared after removal of the packing, and one child showed benign heart arrhythmias during the first postoperative day. One child had a hemorrhage after removal of the packing; this was easily stopped with local decongestants.

If one looks at the total population of cystic fibrosis patients operated on (n=19, age range <1 year to 27 years, mean age at surgery 8.5 years), the average follow-up time was 6 years (endoscopic and CT scan control). Of the 19 patients operated on, 11 had no recurrence, five had a single recurrence, and two had a second and one a third recurrence, requiring surgery. The average number of surgical procedures per child was 1.6, with a recurrence rate of 42% (Table 13-13). In these 19 children the average age of the group without recurrence at first surgery was 12 years (n=11); in those with one recurrence the average age at first surgery was 4 years (n=5); in those with a second recurrence it was 5 years (n=2); and in the one child with three recurrences it was 6 years at first surgery. From these figures, it is obvious that most recurrences are seen in younger children (under the age of 6 years), probably because the postoperative care is so difficult and a thorough cleansing of the operative cavity always necessitates gen-

Table 13-13. Cystic fibrosis

	NUMBER OF SURGICAL PROCEDURES	
	AVERAGE	RANGE
Jaffe 1977	3.6	1-10 (nasal polypectomy)
	1.5	1-3 (ethmoidectomy)
Schramm 1979	2.5	NM
Reilly et al 1985	2.2	1-12 (nasal polypectomy and ethmoidectomy)
Clement 1991	1.6	1-4 (ethmoidectomy)
	RECURRENCE RATE (%)	TYPE OF PROCEDURE
Jaffe 1977	87	Nasal polypectomy
	45	Ethmoidectomy
Reilly et al 1985	53	Nasal polypectomy and ethmoidectomy
Schramm 1979	52	NM
Clement 1991	42	Ethmoidectomy

NM, not mentioned.

eral anesthesia. With regard to the recurrence rate and follow-up in years, the average follow-up of the children without a recurrence was 2 years, of those with one recurrence 4 years, of those with two recurrences 6 years, and of the one child with three recurrences 8 years, which means that the longer the duration of the follow-up period, the more recurrences there will be. It is also interesting to know how long it takes for a recurrence to be seen. The first recurrence was after an average period of 2 years (sometimes as soon as 6 months); the second and third recurrence were 4 years after the second and third surgeries. The important conclusions are that in children under the age of 6 years with cystic fibrosis and massive nasal polyposis, the first massive recurrence will be within 2 years, and later recurrences can be expected after another 4 years.

The percentages of the recurrence rate in cystic fibrosis are difficult to compare. In the Clement group the mean follow-up was 6 years, and the control was done by CT and endoscopy. In comparison with other authors, the mean follow-up time in the Triglia and colleagues[164] group is 3 years and only seven out of 23 have cystic fibrosis, while in the Jones and colleagues[24] group the average follow-up time (done by telephone) is 29 months. As I did not perform surgery in children for chronic sinusitis under the age of 7 year without systemic disease, one needs to consult the literature for some information about results. Most results are judged on symptom relief and not on endoscopic examination or CT scan. Willner and colleagues[58] reported that there is no standardized method for assessing the efficacy of FESS. The comparison of the success rate in chronic sinusitis is even more difficult for several reasons: heterogeneity of material (isolated chronic sinusitis), chronic sinusitis with systemic disease, different age groups, variable follow-up times, and variable ways of assessing success rate (phone call or questionnaire, endoscopy, CT scan). Comparison of the success rate between surgical techniques and medical therapy is even more difficult, as most of the children receive a broad-spectrum antibiotic therapy postoperatively.

In conclusion, the management of chronic sinusitis in infants and young children needs thorough history taking and examination, carefully noting all complaints, signs, and symptoms. If chronic sinusitis is suspected, the necessary preventive measures must be taken (as far as possible) and systemic diseases sought. If any systemic disease is present, an optimal therapy must be instituted. If all these measures fail and the chronic or recurrent sinusitis is long-lasting with symptoms and complaints justifying antibiotic therapy, this should be started on the basis of at least a middle meatus specimen culture for an adequate time. Only when all these measures have failed should surgery be considered, keeping in mind that it is very rarely indicated in infants and children.

Addendum to the Management of Sinusitis in Children

Consensus Meeting Brussels, 1996

Moderator: Clement P. (Brussels, Belgium)

Participants: Bluestone C.D. (Pittsburgh, USA), Gordts F. (Brussels, Belgium), Lusk R. (St. Louis, USA), Otten F. (Leiden, The Netherlands), Goossens H. (Antwerp, Belgium), Scadding G.K. (London, UK), Takahashi H. (Kyoto, Japan), Van Buchem F.L. (Tilburg, The Netherlands), Van Cauwenberge P. (Ghent, Belgium), Wald E.R. (Pittsburgh, USA).

The members of the Consensus Meeting consisted of an international panel of experts with long-standing experience in the management of chronic sinusitis in children and a well-established scientific reputation.

The authors prefer to speak of rhinosinusitis, because in children it is difficult to differentiate between rhinitis and sinusitis. Guided by the agreement reached during the Princeton Conference on Sinus Disease (1993) (8), the author suggested the following definitions:

Acute rhinosinusitis in children is a sinus infection in which complete resolution of symptoms (judged on a clinical basis only) without intermittent upper respiratory tract infection may take up to 12 weeks. Acute rhinosinutis is subdivided into a severe and a nonsevere form (Box 13-1).

Chronic rhinosinusitis in children is defined as a sinus infection with low-grade symptoms and signs that persist longer than 12 weeks.

BOX 13-1

Symptoms and Signs of Pediatric Rhinosinusitis

Nonsevere acute rhinosinusitis	Severe acute rhinosinusitis
Rhinorrhea (of any quality)	Purulent (thick, colored, opaque) rhinorrhea
Nasal congestion	Nasal congestion
Cough	Facial pain or headache
Headache, facial pain, and irritability (variable)	Periorbital edema (variable)
Low-grade or no fever	High fever (>39°C)

Recurrent rhinosinusitis in children consists of multiple acute episodes in which symptoms and signs resolve completely between episodes.

Frequently, however, patients suffer of chronic sinusitis with acute exacerbations, in which symptoms and signs do not resolve completely between episodes.

The diagnosis of rhinosinusitis in children is usually made on clinical grounds alone. Imaging is not necessary to confirm the diagnosis. CT scans are indicated in a severely ill or toxic child, in an acutely ill child who does not improve on medical therapy in 48 to 72 hours, in an immunocompromised host, and in the presence of suppurative (intraorbital or intracranial) complications (orbital cellulitis excepted).

Additional investigations are needed in the presence of recalcitrant rhinosinusitis such as allergy (Box 13-2), immune deficiency (Box 13-3), cystic fibrosis, ciliary dyskinesia, and gastroesophageal reflux.

Antimicrobial therapy is mainly indicated in the severely ill or toxic child with suspected or proven suppurative complications (parenteral antibiotics are preferred), in severe acute rhinosinusitis, and in nonsevere acute rhinosinusitis in children with protracted symptoms or accompanying disease such as asthma, chronic bronchitis, and acute otitis media.

The duration of the antimicrobial therapy should be at least 10 to 14 days, and can be prolonged to 1 month if the symptoms have clearly improved but are not resolved completely. However, if symptoms are unchanged at 72 hours or worsen at any time, the clinician should either change antibiotics or obtain a specimen of sinus secretions for culture and make a thorough reevaluation of the child's condition.

In chronic rhinosinusitis, especially when there are frequent exacerbations, an initial course of 2 weeks of oral antimicrobial treatment is advised. If there is no response within 5 to 7 days, the antibiotic should be changed. If there is again no response within 5 to 7 days, a specimen of sinus secretion should be obtained for culture or a noninfectious condition should be considered. If, however, the patient responds rather slowly, a second 2-week course can be prescribed. In rare cases when there is a clear-cut improvement but still persisting symptoms, a third course can be given before any surgery is considered. Parenteral antimicrobial therapy may be administered before surgery is considered.

Adenoidectomy can be effective in some patients but definite conclusions are not available yet.

Extensive sphenoethmoidectomy (Boxes 13-4 and 13-5) is usually not necessary in children.

BOX 13-2

History and/or Examination Suggestive of Allergy

History

Nasal symptoms:
- Itching of nose, ears, eyes
- Paroxysms of sneezing (exacerbated by factors such as dust, animal exposure)

Personal history
- Infantile eczema
- Asthma
- Food allergy in infancy
- Previous good response to antihistamine or to intranasal anti-inflammatory drugs

Family history
- Atopy in a first-degree relative

Examination
- Allergic nasal crease, allergic salute
- Pale, swollen, purple inferior turbinates
- Other evidence of atopy such as eczema, urticaria, or asthma

BOX 13-3

Immunologic Evaluation

Complete blood count
Quantitative immunoglobulins
Measurement of IgG-subclass levels in serum
Antipneumococcal antibody titers

BOX 13-4

Indications for Sinus Surgery

Complete nasal obstruction in cystic fibrosis due to massive polyposis or closure of nose by medialization of lateral nasal wall
Antrochoanal polyp
Intracranial complications
Mucoceles and mucopyoceles
Orbital abscess
Traumatic injury in optic canal (decompression)
Dacryocystorhinitis due to sinusitis and resistant to appropriate medical treatment
Fungal sinusitis
Some meningoencephaloceles
Some neoplasms

BOX 13-5

Possible Indications for Sinus Surgery

In chronic rhinosinusitis that persists despite optimal medical management and after exclusion of any systemic disease, endoscopic sinus surgery is a reasonable alternative to continuous medical treatment
Optimal medical management includes 2-6 wk of adequate antibiotics (IV or oral) and treatment of concomitant diseases

Partial anterior ethmoidectomy (removal of the uncinate process) with or without a maxillary antrostomy (opening of the bulla) is often sufficient. In other cases, extensive sphenoethmoidectomy may be necessary (cystic fibrosis).

REFERENCES

1. Poole MD. Pediatric endoscopic sinus surgery: the conservative view, *Ear Nose Throat J* 73:221-227, 1994.
2. Wald ER. *Rhinitis and acute and chronic sinusitis.* In Bluestone CD, Stool SE, Scheetsz MD, editors: *Pediatric otolaryngology,* Philadelphia, 1990, WB Saunders, pp 729-744.
3. De Groot RRM, Van Zanten ME: Oto-rhino-laryngology in outline 1984-1993, SIG Health Care Information, Utrecht, 1-24, 1993.
4. Zuckerkandl E: *Normale und pathologische Anatomie der Nasenhöhle und ihrer Pneumatischen Anhänge,* Vienna, 1892, W Braumüller.
5. Killian G: *Zur Anatomie der Nase menschlicher Embryonen,* Vol II, 1895, pp 2-47.
6. Peter K: *Vergleichende Anatomie und Entwicklungsgeschichte der Nase.* In *Denker's Handbuch der Hals-Nasen-Ohren-Heilkunde,* 1925, Springer, Berlin, pp 96-136.
7. Anderhuber W, Kuhn F. Development of the paranasal sinuses in children: implications for paranasal sinus surgery, *Am Otol Rhinol Laryngol* 102:705-711, 1993.
8. Bjuggren G, Kraepelien S, Lind J, Tunevall G: Occult sinusitis in children, *Acta Otolaryngol (Stockh)* 42:4-5, 287-310, 1952.
9. Maresh MM, Washburn AH: Paranasal sinuses from birth to late adolescence. Clinical and roentgenographic evidence of infection, *Am J Dis Child* 60:841-861, 1940.
10. Bagatsch K, Dietzel K, Pathenheimer F, Ritter B: Morbiditätsanalyse der unspezifisch-infektbedingten akuten Erkrankungen der Respirationstraktes und der Mittelohrräume des Kindesalters in einem Ballungsgebiet mit modernen Wohnbe-dingungen, *HNO Praxis* 5:1-8, 1980.
11. Lind J: Über das Vorkommen von Nebenhöhlenaffektionen bei Kindern, *Arch Kinderheilk* 131:143-155, 1944.
12. Desterbeck R-AES, Clement PAR, Kaufman L, Derde MPR: *The influence of swimming on the nasal patency and tube function in children.* In Sade J, editor: *The eustachian tube,* Kugler Publications Amsterdam, Berkeley, 1987, pp 129-135.
13. van Cauwenberge P: Secretoire otitis media. Een epidemiologische, klinische en experimentele sudie. Thesis, 1988.
14. Yaniv E, Oppenheim D, Fuchs C: Chronic rhinitis in children, *Int J Pediatr Otorhinolaryngol* 23:51-57, 1992.
15. van Buchem FL, Peeters MF, Knotterus JA: Maxillary sinusitis in children *Clin Otolaryngol* 17:49-53, 1992.
16. Clement P, van der Veken P, Iwens P, Buisseret TH: *X-ray, T-scan, MR-imaging.* In Mygind N, Nacleirio RM, editors: *Allergic and nonallergic rhinitis. Clinical aspects,* 1993, Munksgaard, Copenhager, pp 58-65.
17. Myers MG, Fomon SJ, Koontz FP, et al: Respiratory and gastrointestinal illness in breast- and formula-fed infants, *Am J Dis Child* 138:629-632, 1984.
18. Agre F: The relationship of mode of infant feeding and location of care to frequency of infection, *Am J Dis Child* 139:809-811, 1985.
19. Chen Y, Li W, Yu S: Influence of passive smoking on admissions for respiratory illness in early childhood, *Br Med J* 293:303-306, 1986.
20. O'Connor GT, Weiss S, Tager I, Speizer FE: The effect of passive smoking on pulmonary function and nonspecific bronchial responsiveness in a population-based sample of children and young adults, *Am Rev Respir Dis* 135:800-804, 1987.
21. Cogswell JJ, Mitchell EB, Alexander J: Parental smoking, breast feeding, and respiratory infection in development of allergic diseases, *Arch Dis Child* 62:338-344, 1987.
22. Geller-Bernstein G, Kenett R, Weisglass L, et al: Atopic babies with wheezy bronchitis, *Allergy* 42:85-91, 1987.
23. Barr MB, Weiss ST, Segal MR, et al: The relationship of nasal disorders to lower respiratory tract symptoms and illness in a random sample of children, *Pediatr Pulmonol* 14:91-94, 1992.
24. Jones JW, Parsons DS, Cuyler JP: The results of functional endoscopic sinus surgery (FESS) on the symptoms of patients with cystic fibrosis, *J Pediatr Otorhinolaryngol* 28:25-32, 1993.
25. Gwaltney JM, Philips CD, Miller RD, Riker DK: Computed tomographic study of the common cold, *N Engl J Med* 330:25-30, 1994.
26. Saito H, Taneka H, Hoshino A, Mizokoshi O: Antiviral defence mechanism of the nasal mucosa, *Rhinology* suppl 1:19-27, 1981.
27. Glezen WP: *Respiratory viruses and* Mycoplasma pneumoniae. In Drew L, editor: *Viral infections: a clinical approach,* Philadelphia, 1976, FA Davis, pp 69-99.
28. Winther B, Gwaltney JM, Mygind N, et al: Sites of rhinovirus recovery after point inoculation of the upper airway, *JAMA,* 256:1763-1767, 1986.
29. Clement PAR, Byloos J, Kaufman L, et al: Incidence and etiology of rhinosinusitis in children, *Acta Otorhinolaryngol Belg* 43:523-543, 1989.

30. Evans FO, Sydnor JB, Moore WEC, et al: Sinusitis of the maxillary antrum, *N Engl J Med* 293:735-739, 1975.

31. Hamory BH, Sande MA, Sydnor A Jr, et al: Etiology and antimicrobial therapy of acute maxillary sinusitis, *J Infect Dis* 139:197-202, 1979.

32. Piskunov GZ, Piskunov SZ: Role of virus infection in the chronic disease of nose and paranasal sinuses, *Am J Rhinol* 8:294, 1994.

33. Wald ER: *Microbiology of acute and chronic sinusitis.* In Lusk RP, editor: *Pediatric sinusitis*, New York, 1992, Raven Press, pp 43-47.

34. Kennedy DW, editor: *Sinus disease. Guide to first-line management*, Philadelphia, 1994, Health Communications, Darien, Connecticut, pp 1-44.

35. Brook I: Bacteriologic features of chronic sinusitis in children, *JAMA* 246:967-969, 1981.

36. Wald ER, Milmoe GJ, Bowen A, et al: Acute maxillary sinusitis in children, *N Engl J Med* 304:749-754, 1981.

37. Wald ER, Reilly JS, Casselbrant M, et al: Treatment of acute maxillary sinusitis in childhood: a comparative study of amoxicillin and cefaclor, *J Pediatr* 104:297-302, 1984.

38. Otten FWA, Grote JJ: Treatment of chronic maxillary sinusitis in children, *J Pediatr Otorhinolaryngol* 15:269-287, 1988.

39. Orobello PW, Park RI, Belcher LJ, et al: Microbiology of chronic sinusitis in children, *Arch Otolaryngol Head Neck Surg* 117:980-983, 1991.

40. Bolger WE: Gram negative sinusitis: an emerging clinical entity, *Am J Rhinol* 8:279-283, 1994.

40a. Falser N: Kinozilienanomalien beim Kartagner-Syndrom, *Laryng Rhinol Otol (Stuttg)* 62:129-133, 1983.

41. Shurin PA: *Inflammatory diseases of the nose and paranasal sinuses.* In Bluestone C, Stool S, editors: *Pediatric otolaryngology*, Philadelphia, 1983, WB Saunders, pp 781-790.

42. McLeod DT: *Moraxella catarrhalis*: it's importance as a respiratory pathologic agent, *Spectrum* 38:1-4, 1995.

43. Nord CE: Efficacy of penicillin treatment in purulent maxillary sinusitis. A European multicenter trial, *Infection* 16:209-214, 1988.

44. Poole MD: The young child to young adult sick sinus syndrome, *Ear Nose Throat J* 73:342, 1994.

45. Brook I, Thompson DH, Frazier EH: Microbiology and management of chronic maxillary sinusitis, *Arch Otolaryngol Head Neck Surg* 120:1317-1319, 1994.

46. Arruda LK, Mimica IM, Solé D, et al: Abnormal maxillary sinus radiographs in children: do they represent bacterial infection? *Pediatrics* 85:553-558, 1990.

47. Riding KH, Irvine R: Sinusitis in children, *J Otolaryngol* 16:239-243, 1987.

48. Muntz HR, Lusk RP: *Signs and symptoms of chronic sinusitis.* In Lusk R, editor: *Pediatric sinusitis*, New York, 1992, Raven Press, pp 1-5.

49. Bonding P, Tos M: Middle ear pressure during brief pathological conditions of the nose and throat, *Acta Otolaryngol (Stockh)* 92:63-69, 1981.

50. Jazbi B: *Sinusitis in infants and children.* In Jazbi B, editor: *Pediatric otorhinolaryngology. A review of ear, nose and throat problems in children,* New York, 1980, Appleton-Century-Crofts, pp 143-157.

51. Fearon B, Edmonds B, Bird R: Orbital facial complications of sinusitis in children, *Laryngoscope* 89:947-953, 1979.

52. Fearon B, McMillin BD: *Sinusitis in infants and children.* In Blitzer A, Lawson W, Friedman W, editors: *Surgery of the paranasal sinuses*, Philadelphia, 1985, WB Saunders, pp 287-298.

53. Fearon B, McMillin BD: *Sinusitis in infants and children.* In Blitzer AB, Lawson W, Friedman W, editors: *Paranasal sinuses*, ed 2, Philadelphia, 1991, WB Saunders, pp 421-432.

54. Lusk RP: *Surgical management of chronic sinusitis.* In Lusk RP, editor: *Pediatric sinusitis*, New York, 1992, Raven Press, pp 77-125.

55. Lusk RP, Tychsen L, Park TS: *Complications of sinusitis.* In Lusk RP, editor: *Pediatric sinusitis*, New York, 1992, Raven Press, pp 127-146.

56. Lerner DN, Choi SS: Intracranial complications of sinusitis in childhood, *Am Otol Rhinol Laryngol* 104:288-293, 1995.

57. Brihaye P, Clement PAR, Dab I, Desprechin B: Pathological changes of the lateral nasal wall in patients with cystic fibrosis (mucoviscidosis), *Pediatr Otorhinolaryngol* 28:141-147, 1994.

58. Willner A, Lazar RH, Younis RT, Belkford NS: Sinusitis in children: current management, *Ear Nose Throat J* 73:485-490, 1994.

59. Manning SC: Pediatric sinusitis, *Otolaryngol Clin North Am* 26:623-638, 1993.

60. Lusk RP, Lazar R, Muntz HR: The diagnosis and treatment of recurrent and chronic sinusitis in children, *Pediatr Clin* 36:1411-1421, 1989.

61. Wang D, Clement PAR, Kaufman L, Derde MP: Fiberoptic examination of the nasal cavity and nasopharynx in children, *J Pediatr Otorhinolaryngol* 24:35-44, 1992.

62. Wang D, Clement PAR: Fiberoptic imaging of the pediatric nasopharynx, *Diagn Ther Endosc* 1:153-157, 1995.

63. Cools GHE, Clement PAR: The use of a rigid nasal endoscope in children—with special interest in the middle meatus, *Acta Otolaryngol Belg* 45:399-404, 1991.

64. Shapiro GG, Furukawa CT, Pierson WE, et al: Blinded comparison of maxillary sinus radiography and ultrasound for diagnosis of sinusitis, *J Allergy Clin Immunol* 77:59-64, 1986.

65. Lazar RH, Younis RT, Gross CW: Pediatric functional endonasal sinus surgery: review of 210 cases, *Head Neck* 14:82-97, 1992.

66. McAllister WH, Herman TE, Wippold FJ: *Imaging of sinusitis in infants and children.* In Lusk RP, editor: *Pediatric sinusitis,* New York, 1992, Raven Press, pp 15-42.

67. Maes JJ, Clement PAR: The efficacy of antral lavage in children with maxillary sinusitis, *Acta Otorhinolaryngol Belg* 40:570-581, 1986.

68. Glasier CM, Ascher DP, Williams KD: Incidental paranasal sinus abnormalities on CT of children: clinical correlation, *Am J Neur Radiol* 7:861-864, 1986.

69. Kogutt MS, Swischuk LE: Diagnosis of sinusitis in infants and children, *Pediatrics* 52:152-155, 1973.

70. Diament MJ, Senac MO, Gilsanz V, et al: Prevalence of incidental paranasal sinuses opacification in pediatric patients: a CT study, *J Comput Assist Tomogr* 11:426-431, 1987.

71. Glasier CM, Mallory GB, Steele RW: Significance of opacification of the maxillary and ethmoid sinuses in infants, *J Pediatr* 114:45-50, 1989.

72. van der Veken PJV, Clement PAR, Buisseret Th, et al: CAT scan study of the incidence of sinus involvement and nasal anatomic variations in 196 children, *Rhinology* 28:177-184, 1990.

73. Lazar RH, Younis RT, Gurucharri MJ: *Endoscopic sinus surgery in children.* In Levine HL, May M, editors: *Endoscopic sinus surgery*, New York, 1992, Thieme Medical, pp 244-256.

74. Lesserson JA, Kieserman SP, Finn DG: The radiographic incidence of chronic sinus disease in the pediatric population, *Laryngoscope* 104:159-166, 1994.

75. van der Veken PJV, Clement PAR, Buisseret Th, et al: CT scan study on the prevalence of sinus disease and anatomical variations in 196 children, *Acta Otorhinolaryngol Belg* 43:51-58, 1989.

76. van der Veken PJ, Clement PAR, Buisseret Th, et al: Age-related CT-scan study of the incidence of sinusitis in children, *Am J Rhinol* 6:45-48, 1992.

77. Stammberger J, Kopp W: *Functional endoscopic sinus surgery.* In Stammberger H, editor: *The Messerklinger technique,* Philadelphia, 1991, BC Decker.

78. Milczuk HA, Dalley RW, Wessbacher FW, Richardson MA: Nasal and paranasal sinus anomalies in children with chronic sinusitis, *Laryngoscope* 103:247-252, 1993.

79. April MM, Zinreich J, Baroody FM, Nacleirio RM: Coronal CT scan abnormalities in children with chronic sinusitis, *Laryngoscope* 103:985-990, 1993.

80. Albegger K: Zur Rhinosinusitis des Kindes aus HNO ärztlichen Sicht, *HNO* 28:321-328, 1980.

81. Benjamin B: Sinusitis in children—general considerations, *J Pediatr Otorhinolaryngol* 5:281-284, 1983.

82. Polmar SH: *Sinusitis and immune deficiency.* In Lusk RP, editor: *Pediatric sinusitis,* New York, 1992, Raven Press, pp 53-58.

83. Shapiro GG: *Sinusitis and allergy.* In Lusk RP, editor: *Pediatric sinusitis,* New York, 1992, Raven Press, pp 49-52.

84. Slavin RG: *Sinusitis and asthma.* In Lusk RP, editor: *Pediatric sinusitis,* New York, 1992, Raven Press, pp 59-64.

84. Sharpe M, Furukawa CT, Bierman CW, et al: Allergic patients have more frequent sinus infections than nonallergic patients, *J Allergy Clin Immunol* (abstr) 751:332, 1992.

85. Sircar M, Karol R, Bhatia P: Radiological abnormalities of paranasal sinuses in asthmatics with rhinitis, *Am J Rhinol* 9:99-101, 1995.

86. Furukawa CT, Rachelefsky GS: Children with sinusitis, *Pediatrics* 71:133-134, 1983.

87. Rachelefsky GS, Katz RM, Siegel SC: Chronic sinusitis in the allergic child, *Pediatr Clin North Am* 35:1091-1101, 1988.

88. Savolainen S: Allergy in patients with acute maxillary sinusitis, *Allergy* 44:116-122, 1989.

89. Iwens P, Clement PAR: Sinusitis in allergic patients, *Rhinology* 32:65-67, 1994.

90. Umetsu DT, Ambrosino DM, Quinti I, et al: Recurrent sinopulmonary infection and impaired antibody response to bacterial capsular polysaccharide antigen in children with selective IgG-subclass deficiency, *N Engl J Med* 313:1247-1251, 1985.

91. Oxelius VA: IgG subclass levels in infancy and childhood, *Acta Paediatr Scand* 68:23-27, 1979.

92. Berdal P, Henriksen SD, Skrede S: Immunodeficiency syndromes with otorhinolaryngological manifestations, *Acta Otolaryngol (Stockh)* 82:185-192, 1976.

92. Maes JJ, Clement PAR: The usefulness of irrigation of the maxillary sinus in children with maxillary sinusitis on the basis of the Waters x-ray, *Rhinology* 25:259-264, 1987.

93. Sethi DS, Leopold DA: Diagnosis and management of chronic recurrent sinusitis and immunoglobulin deficiency, *Curr Opin Otolaryngol Head Neck Surg* 3:21-25, 1995.

94. Takeuchi K, Yuta A, Sakakura Y: Interleukin-8 gene expression in chronic sinusitis, *Am J Otolaryngol* 16:98-102, 1995.

95. Rosenthal A, Fellow KE: Acute infectious sinusitis in cyanotic congenital heart disease, *Pediatrics* 52:692-696, 1973.

95. Marcy SM: Prevention of respiratory infections, *Pediatr Infect Dis J* 4:442-446, 1985.

96. Shwachman H, Kulczycki LL, Mueller HL, Flake CG: Nasal polyposis in patients with cystic fibrosis, *Pediatrics* 30:389-401, 1962.

97. Neely JG, Harrison GM, Jerger JF, et al: The otolaryngologic aspects of cystic fibrosis, *Trans Am Acad Ophthalmol Otol* 76:313-324, 1972.

98. Cepero R, Smith RJH, Catlin FI, et al: Cystic fibrosis—an otolaryngologic perspective, *Otolaryngol Head Neck Surg* 97:356-360, 1987.

99. Batsakis JG, Sciubba JJ: *Pathology.* In Blitzer A, Lawson W, Friedman WH, editors: *Surgery of the paranasal sinuses,* ed 2, Philadelphia, 1991, WB Saunders, p 121.

100. Lieberman A, Cole Ph, Corey M, et al: Otolaryngological und rhinomanometric findings in cystic fibrosis, *Am J Rhinol* 5:61-65, 1991.

101. Tunkel DE, Nacleirio RM, Barody FM, Rosenstein BJ: Bilateral maxillary sinus mucoceles in an infant with cystic fibrosis, *Otolaryngol Head Neck Surg* 111:116-120, 1994.

102. Kartagener M: Zur Pathognese der Bronchieectasien, *Beitr Klin Tuberkulose* 33:489-501, 1933.

103. Afzelius BA: The immotile-cilia syndrome and other ciliary diseases, *Int Rev Exp Pathol* 19:1-43, 1979.

104. Friday GA, Yunis EJ, Agostine RM: Immotile cilia syndrome, *Pediatr Clin North Am* 28:807-812, 1981.

105. Rott HD: Genetics of Kartagener's syndrome, *Eur J Respir Dis* 64, suppl 127:1-4, 1980.

106. Sleigh MA: Primary ciliary dyskinesia, *Lancet* 11:476, 1981.

107. De Boeck K, Jorissen M: Primary ciliary dyskinesia. Paper on Pediatric Otolhinolaryngology Symposium, Ghent, 1995.

108. Ramet J, Byloos J, Delree M, et al: *Neonatal diagnosis of the immotile cilia syndrome.* In Oski Stockman, editor: Yearbook of Pediatric, Chicago, 1988, Mosby-Year Book, pp 287-288.

109. Carson JL, Collier AM, Hu SS: Acquired ciliary defects in nasal epithelium of children with acute viral upper respiratory infections, *N Engl J Med* 321:463-468, 1985.

110. Ramet J, Byloos J: To the editor, *Chest* 91:292, 1987.

111. Ramet J, Byloos J, Delree M, et al: Neonatal diagnosis of the immotile cilia syndrome, *Chest* 89:138-140, 1986.

112. Kärjä J, Muutinen J: Immotile cilia syndrome in children, *J Pediatr Otorhinolaryngol* 5:275-279, 1983.

113. Rossman CM, Forrest JB, Lee RMKW, Newhouse MT: The dyskinetic cilia syndrome. Ciliary motility in immotile cilia syndrome, *Chest* 78:580-582, 1980.

113. Parsons DS: *Sinusitis and cystic fibrosis.* In Lusk RP, editor: *Pediatric sinusitis,* New York, 1992, Raven Press, pp. 14-40, 65-70.

114. Jorissen M, Cassiman JJ: Relevance of the ciliary ultrastructure in primary and secondary ciliary dyskinesia: a review, *Am J Rhinol* 5:91-101, 1991.

115. Jaffe BF, Deblanc CB: Sinusitis in children with cleft lip and palate, *Arch Otolaryngol* 93:479-482, 1971.

116. Ishikawa Y, Amitani R: Nasal and paranasal sinus disease in patients with congenital velopharyngeal insufficiency, *Arch Otolaryngol Head Neck Surg* 120:861-865, 1994.

117. Schramm VL: Inflammatory and neoplastic masses of the nose and paranasal sinus in children, *Laryngoscope* 89:1887-1897, 1979.

118. Batsakis JG: The pathology of head and neck tumors: nasal cavity and paranasal sinuses, part 5, *Head Neck Surg* 2:410-419, 1980.

119. Hardy G: The choanal polyp, *Am Otol Rhinol Laryngol* 66:306-326, 1957.

120. Sirola R: Choanal polyps, *Acta Otolaryngol (Stockh)* 61:42-48, 1966.

121. Kovatch AL, Wald ER, Ledesma-Medina J, et al: Maxillary sinus radiographs in children with nonrespiratory complaints, *Pediatrics* 73:306-308, 1984.

122. Goldwyn BG, Sakr W, Marks SC: Histopathologic analysis of chronic sinusitis, *Am J Rhinol* 9:27-30, 1995.

123. Clement PAR: Conservative sinusitis treatment in children, *Rhinology*, suppl 1:77-92, 1981.

124. Portmann M: *The natural history of serous otitis media (SOM) and mucous otitis media (MOM).* In Sade J, editor: *Acute and secretory otitis media*, part I, Amsterdam, 1986, Kugler Publications, pp 91-93.

125. Tos M, Stangerup S-E, Hvid G, et al: *Epidemiology and natural history of secretory otitis media.* In Sade J, editor: *Acute and secretory otitis media,* part I, Amsterdam, 1986, Kugler Publications, pp 95-106.

126. Bluestone CD, Klein JO: *Epidemiology.* In Otitis media in infants and children, Philadelphia, Tokyo, 1988, WB Saunders, pp 31-43.

127. Mann W, Jonas I: Untersuchungen zur Spontanheilung der Sinusitis maxillaris, *HNO* 29:92-94, 1981.

128. Furstenberg AC: The treatment of acute nasal accessory sinus disease, *Am Otol Rhinol Laryngol* 47:902-909, 1937.

129. Ballenger WL, Ballenger HC: Ethmoiditis, sphenoiditis, sinusitis in children. Aero-sinusitis. In *Diseases of the nose, throat and ear. Medical and surgical,* London, 1942, H Kimpton, pp 158-167.

130. Jents EJ: *Entzündliche Prozesse der Nebenhöhlen. Rhinologie in Oto-Rhino-Laryngologie in Kindesalter. Einschliesslich der Endoscopie,* Vienna, 1949, Verlag W Maudrich, pp 134-143.

131. Veeneklaas GMH: Clinical lesson. Chronic maxillary sinusitis, a frequent cause of general complaints in children, *Ned Tijdschr Geneesk* 92:2886-2890, 1948.

132. Westrin KM: Prevention of rhino-sinusitis in children, *Am J Rhinol* 8:292-293, 1994.

133. Poole MD: Medical therapy of pediatric sinusitis, *Otolaryngol Head Neck Surg*, 226, 1993.

134. Casiano RR: Azithromycin and amoxicillin in the treatment of acute maxillary sinusitis, *Am J Med* suppl 3A, 91:27S-30S, 1991.

135. Feldstead SJ, Daniel R, European Azithromycin Group: Short course treatment of sinusitis and other respiratory tract infections with azithromycin: a comparison with erythromycin and amoxicillin, *J Int Med Res* 19:363-372, 1991.

136. Mosh E, Rodriguez-Solares E, Rivas E, el Hosby Z: A comparative study of azithromycin and amoxycillin in pediatric patients with acute otitis media, *J Antimicrob Chemother* suppl E:73-79, 1993.

137. Carlier M, Zenebergh A, Tulkins P: Cellular uptake and subcellular distribution of roxithromycin and erythromycin in phagocytic cells, *J Antimicrob Chemother* 20 suppl B:47-56, 1987.

138. Gunn BA, Woodall JB, Jones JF: Ampicillin-resistant *Haemophilus influenzae, Lancet,* 845:5, 1974.

139. Verbist L: In vitro susceptibility of recently isolated respiratory tract pathogens to microcycline and comparable antibiotics. A multicentre study, *Acta Clin Bel,* 49:268-273, 1994.

140. Bogaert M: Ernstige ongewenste effecten van co-trimoxazole, *Folia Pharmacother* 21:9, 71, 1994.

141. Lusk RP, Mair EA, Poole MD: *Chronic sinusitis in a child.* In Smith JH, editor: *Controversies, Head Neck* 252-257, 1995.

142. Breuninger H: *Konservative Behandlung der Nase and ihren Nebenhöhlen, Hals-Nasen-Ohren-Heilkunde.* In Berendes J, Link R, Zöllner F, editors: *Praxis und Klinick,* Stuttgart, 1977, Georg Thieme Verlag, Band Obere und Untere Luftweg, pp 1-28.

143. Ingels KJAJ, Meeuwsen F, Graamans K, Huizing EH: Influence of sympathetic and parasympathetic substances in clinical concentrations on human nasal ciliary beat, *Rhinology* 30:149-160, 1992.

144. Rachelefsky GS, Katz RM, Siegel SC: Chronic sinusitis in children with respiratory allergy: the role of antimicrobials, *J Allergy Clin Immunol* 69:382-387, 1982.

145. Ritter FN, Fritsch MH: *Atlas of paranasal sinus surgery,* New York, 1991, Igaku-Shoin.

146. Juntunen-Backman K, Sorva R, Tähtelä R, et al: Bone turnover during inhaled budesonide in childhood asthma, *Allergy Clin Immunol News,* suppl 2, abstr 76:21, 1994.

147. Westrin KM: Pathogenesis of pediatric sinusitis, *Am J Rhinol* 8:291-292, 1994.

148. Ingels K., Hertveldt K, van Cauwenberge P: Conservative management of rhinosinusitis in children, *Am J Rhinol* 8:293, 1994.

149. Naumann HH: *Konservative Behandlung der Nase und ihrer Nebenhöhlen.* In Berendes J, Link R, Zöllner F, editors: *Handbuch der Hals-Nasen-Ohrenheilkunde,* Stuttgart, 1964, Thieme Verlag.

150. Gross CW, Gurucharri MJ, Lazar RH, Long TE: Functional endonasal sinus surgery (FESS) in the pediatric age group, *Laryngoscope* 99:272-275, 1989.

151. Takahashi H, Fujita A, Honjo I: Effect of adenoidectomy on otitis media with effusion, tubal function, and sinusitis, *Am J Otolaryngol* 10:208-213, 1989.

152. Hilbert J: The occurrence of adenoidal signs and symptoms in normal children, *Clin Otolaryngol* 6:97-100, 1981.

153. Parsons DS, Philips SE: Functional endoscopic sinus surgery in children: a retrospective analysis and results, *Laryngoscope* 103: 899-903, 1993.

154. Paradise JL, Bluestone CD, Rogers KD, et al: Efficacy of adenoidectomy for recurrent otitis media: results from parallel random and nonrandom trials, *Pediatr Res* 21:674, 1987.

155. Maw AR, Herod F: *The effect of adenoidectomy, tonsillectomy, and grommets on otoscopic, impedence and audiometric findings in glue ears.* In Sadé J, editor: *Acute and secretory otitis media,* Amsterdam, 1986, Kugler Publications, pp 539-543.

156. Hellmich S: Die operatieve Behandlung von Nasennebenhöhlenerkrankungen im Kindesalter, *HNO* 32:91-98, 1984.

157. Lund VJ: Inferior meatal antrostomy. Fundamental considerations of design and function, *J Laryngol Otol,* (suppl 10):1-18, 1988.

158. Muntz HR, Lusk RP: Nasal antral windows in children: a retrospective study, *Laryngoscope* 100:643-646, 1990.

159. Flottes LP, Clerc R, Riu R, Devilla F: *La physologie des sinus* Paris, 1960, Librairie Arnette.

160. Lusk RP, Muntz HR: Endoscopic sinus surgery in children with chronic sinusitis: a pilot study, *Laryngoscope* 100:654-658, 1990.

161. Stankiewicz JA: Pediatric endoscopic sinus surgery: results in 83 children (abstr) *Otolaryngol Head Neck Surg* 109:281, 1993.

162. Wolf G, Greistorfer K: Unsere Erfahrungen mit der endoskopisch-endonasalen Operationstechnik bei der Therapie der Sinusitis in Kindesalter, *Laryngol Rhinol Otol (Stuttg)* 73:258-263, 1994.

163. Wald ER: *Medical management of sinusitis in pediatric patients.* In Lusk RP, editor: *Pediatric sinusitis*, New York, 1992, Raven Press, pp 71-75.

164. Lazar RH, Younis RT, Long TE: Functional endonasal sinus surgery in adults and children, *Laryngoscope* 103:1-5, 1993.

165. Triglia JM, Dessi P, Cannoni M, Pech A: Intranasal ethmoidectomy in nasal polyposis in children. Indications and results, *J Pediatr Otorhinolaryngol* 23:125-131, 1992.

166. Dehaen F, Clement PAR: Endonasal surgical treatment of bilateral choanal atresia under optic control in the infant, *J Otolaryngol* 14:95-98, 1985.

167. Paugh DR, Sullivan MJ: Myospherulosis of the paranasal sinuses, *Otolaryngol Head Neck Surg* 1:117-119, 1990.

168. Davidson TM, Murphy C, Mitchell M, et al: Management of chronic sinusitis in cystic fibrosis, *Laryngoscope* 105:354-358, 1995.

169. Wang D, Clement PAR, Kaufman L, Derde MP: *Fiberoptic examination of the nasal cavity and nasopharynx in children.* In Papanella MM, Holt GR, editors: *The yearbook of otolaryngology-head neck surgery*, St. Louis, 1993, Mosby-Year Book, pp 320-322.

170. Wang D, Clement PAR, Kaufman L, Derde MP: Fiberoptic evaluation of the nasal cavity and nasopharyngeal anatomy in children with snoring, *J Otolaryngol* 23:57-60, 1994.

171. Sharpe M, Furukawa CT, Berman CN, et al: Allergic patients have more frequent sinus infections than non-allergic patients, *J Allergy Clin Immunol* (abstr) 751:332, 1992.

172. Falser N: Kinozilienanomalien bein Kartagner-Syndrom, *Laryng Rhinol Otol (Stuttg)* 62:129-133, 1983.

173. Koay B, Cox GJ: The emerging role of multi-drug resistant *streptococcus pneumoniae*—a cause for concern *Clin Otolaryngol* 21:289-291, 1996.

CHAPTER

14

Management of Sinusitis in Adolescent Children

Jay N. Dolitsky

PROBLEM

An 11-year-old boy presents with an 8-month history of purulent rhinorrhea, nasal obstruction, cough, halitosis, and occasional frontal headaches. These symptoms have improved temporarily on 10-day courses of antibiotics. He does not routinely snore nor breathe through the mouth. His medical history is significant for asthma, for which he is treated with oral and inhalant bronchodilators, inhaled steroids, and occasional short courses of oral steroids. He has been previously evaluated by an allergist, with prick and intradermal testing, all of which were negative for atopy.

Physical examination reveals mucopurulent discharge in both nasal cavities. After topical nasal decongestion and suctioning, examination of the nasal cavities with an endoscope reveals scant mucopurulent discharge in both middle meatus. There is mild erythema and hypertrophy of the adenoids, with mild obstruction of the choanae. There is no sinus tenderness, but there is mucopurulent postnasal discharge. The lungs are clear to auscultation. A fine-cut coronal computed tomographic (CT) scan of the paranasal sinuses is undertaken, as well as other diagnostic studies.

MEDICAL HISTORY

The symptoms of sinusitis generally include nasal obstruction, purulent rhinorrhea, headache, facial pain or pressure, halitosis, cough, fever, stomach upset, and exacerbations of lower airway disease.

Sinusitis can be categorized into acute, subacute, chronic, and recurrent forms. Wald defines acute sinusitis as clinical presentation of sinusitis lasting no more than 3 weeks. Symptoms and signs of sinusitis lasting 3 weeks to 3 months are considered subacute; those lasting longer than 3 months are chronic. Most patients with sinusitis present with only a selection of the above complaints. It is therefore incumbent upon the physician to suspect sinusitis as a cause of one or more of these symptoms, particularly when there is little or no response to seemingly appropriate treatment. Three episodes of sinusitis occurring over 6 months or four episodes occurring within 1 year, with completely lucid intervals, would be considered recurrent sinusitis.

The signs and symptoms of sinusitis are consistent with those of a viral upper respiratory infection, or the "common cold." Differentiation between a cold and acute sinusitis is usually based on duration. If the clinical presentation clears within 10 days, it is likely to have been a routine viral upper respiratory infection. If it persists beyond 10 days, this is probably acute sinusitis. Aside from duration, the presentation of acute sinusitis is frequently different from that of subacute or chronic sinusitis in that facial pain, headache, and fever are more likely to be present; purulent rhinorrhea and cough are more likely to be present in the subacute or chronic variety.

Our sample patient exhibits several of the symptoms discussed above, and as the symptoms have been persistent for 8 months, a working diagnosis should include chronic sinusitis. It is not unusual for a patient with such a presentation to be given multiple forms of medical therapy for asthma before being referred for an evaluation by an otolaryngologist. It is also common for such a patient to have undergone an allergy work-up, as a possible aggravating factor for the asthma. In our sample patient, it may appear evident that sinusitis is present, but many patients may manifest only one symptom such as chronic cough, headache, or intractable asthma, making the diagnosis of sinusitis less obvious. In such cases the diagnosis of sinusitis is frequently delayed. In addition, the primary care physician may have already treated the patient for suspected sinusitis, but the treatment may have been inadequate or the sinusitis may be refractory to medical treatment (Figs. 14-1 and 14-2).

PHYSICAL EXAMINATION

One of the most challenging aspects of diagnosing sinusitis is that there is no direct way to examine the paranasal sinuses. At best, in a cooperative patient, one can examine the middle and possibly superior meatus. Although this does not afford a direct view into the sinuses, examination of the nose and middle meatus with both 0- and 30-degree telescopes is the best way to obtain meaningful clinical information regarding the sinuses. Also, examination of the nasopharynx with either a rigid telescope or flexible endoscope is very useful to determine both the size and appearance of the adenoids. This can frequently be accomplished in children 6 years of age and older if the nose is prepared before endoscopic examination in the following way. A cotton pledget impregnated with a topical decongestant such as 0.25% phenylephrine or 0.05% oxymetazoline and a topical anesthetic such as 4% lidocaine (Xylocaine) should be placed for 10 to 15 minutes in each nasal cavity. This not only decongests and anesthetizes the nasal cavity, but also acquaints the child with intranasal manipulation. After removal of the pledgets, the nasal cavities should be suctioned with either a Frazier tip suction or a flexible suction catheter.

Examination of the nose should begin with anterior rhinoscopy. This is best performed initially with an otoscope by passing the speculum just beyond the nasal hairs. This allows assessment of the nasal septum, the turbinates, the presence or absence of secretions and crusts and of lesions such as polyps, and the overall patency of the nasal airway. If the child is cooperative, additional evaluation can be undertaken using a nasal speculum and head mirror or headlight.

Examination of the middle meatus and superior meatus should then be performed using a zero- and if possible a 30-degree endoscope. Particular attention should be

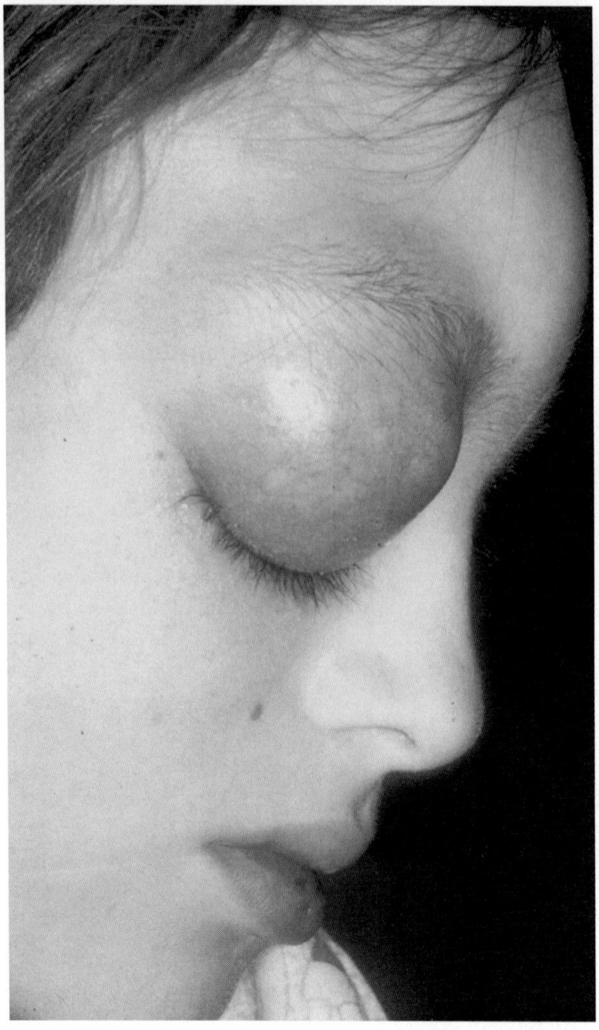

Fig. 14-1. Child with right preseptal cellulitis and abscess.

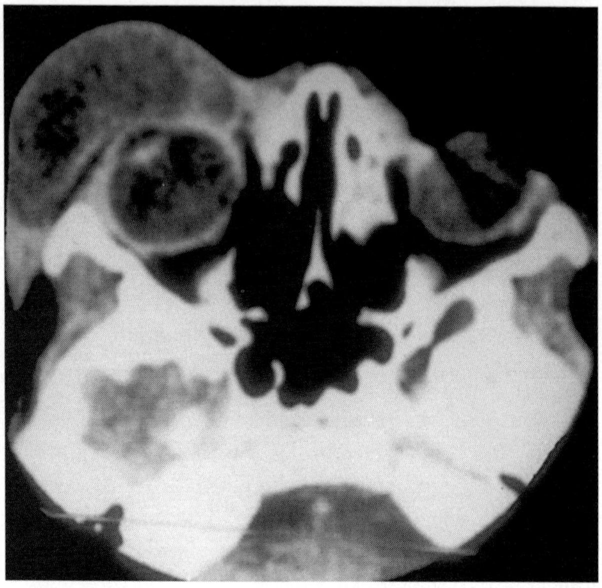

Fig. 14-2. Axial computed tomography (CT) scan of the child in Fig. 14-1.

directed toward the presence or absence of secretions and/or tissue in the meatus. Examination of the choanae and nasopharynx should focus on the size of the adenoidal pad and its impact on the choanal airway, as well as the presence of erythema or debris. The absence of secretions in the middle meatus does not rule out sinusitis, as the sinuses may be completely obstructed, thereby preventing drainage of the secretions into the nasal cavities. After endoscopic evaluation, the frontal and maxillary areas should be palpated for sinus tenderness, which is more likely to be present in acute sinusitis.

Examination of the oropharynx is important to determine the presence of posterior nasal discharge. Also, the posterior pharyngeal wall can be assessed for lymphoid hypertrophy when the palate elevates. This is particularly useful in a patient who is not cooperative for nasopharyngoscopy.

In our patient, the physical findings were not overwhelming. Specifically, aside from a small amount of mucopurulent material in the middle meatus, the nasal and sinus examinations were unremarkable. It is this inability for direct visualization that makes the definitive diagnosis of sinusitis based on physical examination so difficult.

RADIOGRAPHIC EXAMINATION

Of the various modalities of radiographic imaging of the paranasal sinuses, a fine-cut CT scan without intravenous contrast, in the coronal plane, is the most useful. It allows visualization of the sinus cavities, the bony structure surrounding the sinus cavities, and the outflow tracts of the sinuses, specifically the middle meatus and infundibulum. Computed tomography also complements the examination of the nasal cavity and nasopharynx in uncooperative patients.

The advantages of a fine-cut coronal CT scan are many. The presence and degree of disease within the sinuses can be assessed. These findings may be extensive, such as complete opacification of one or more of the sinuses. There may be indications of acute disease, such as air-fluid levels within the maxillary, frontal, or sphenoid sinuses. The findings may also be subtle, limited to mucosal thickening within the sinuses.

A computed tomographic scan is also useful in evaluating the bony architecture of the sinuses and surrounding areas (Fig. 14-3). Abnormalities identified may include a hypoplastic sinus, paradoxical curvature of the middle turbinate, concha bullosa of the middle turbinate (Fig. 14-4), deviated nasal septum with obstruction of the middle meatus, or a Haller cell (Fig. 14-5). Computed tomography also provides detailed information regarding orbital or intracranial extension of sinus disease. When there is evidence of intracranial disease, magnetic resonance imaging (MRI) is the radiographic study of choice.

Computed tomography also has its limitations. Several studies have shown that it may display abnormalities of the sinuses in the absence of clinical disease. At The New York Eye and Ear Infirmary, 42% of children who underwent a CT evaluation of the orbit, with no clinical evidence of rhinitis or sinusitis, were found to have some form of radiographic evidence of sinus disease. Therefore, one cannot rely solely on CT for evidence of clinical sinusitis. I have frequently been asked for a consultation on patients found to have minimal mucosal thickening

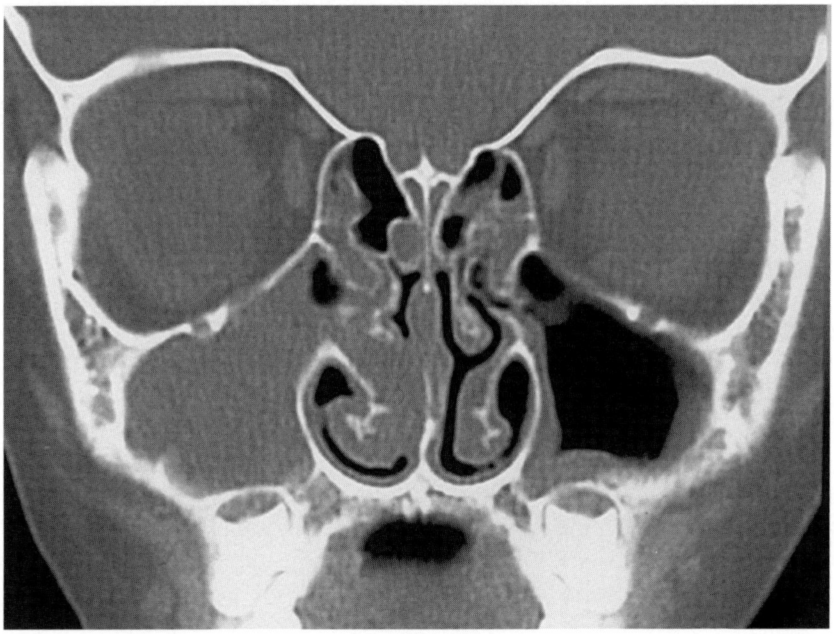

Fig. 14-3. Coronal CT of the paranasal sinuses. Note the bilateral opacification, greater on the right.

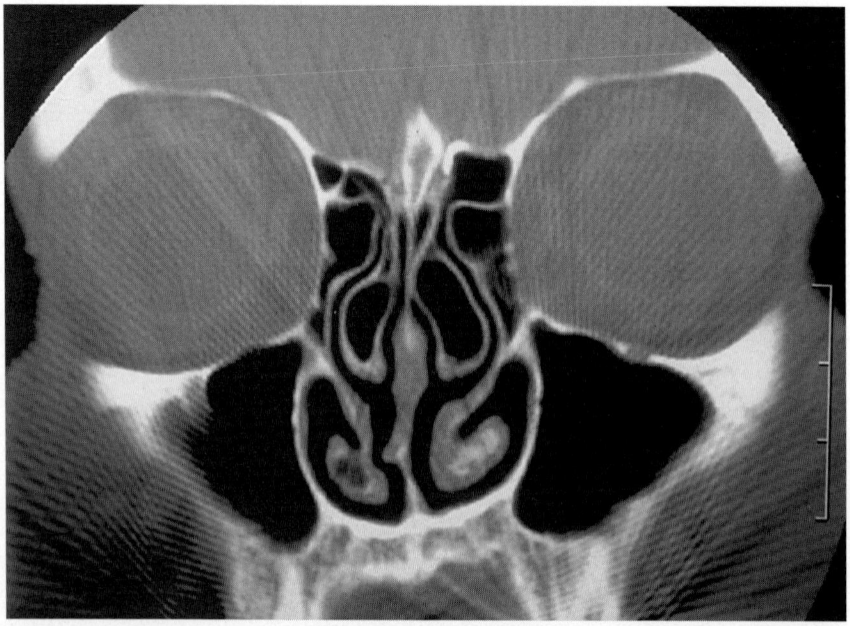

Fig. 14-4. Coronal CT of the nose and paranasal sinuses depicting bilateral concha bullosa of both middle turbinates.

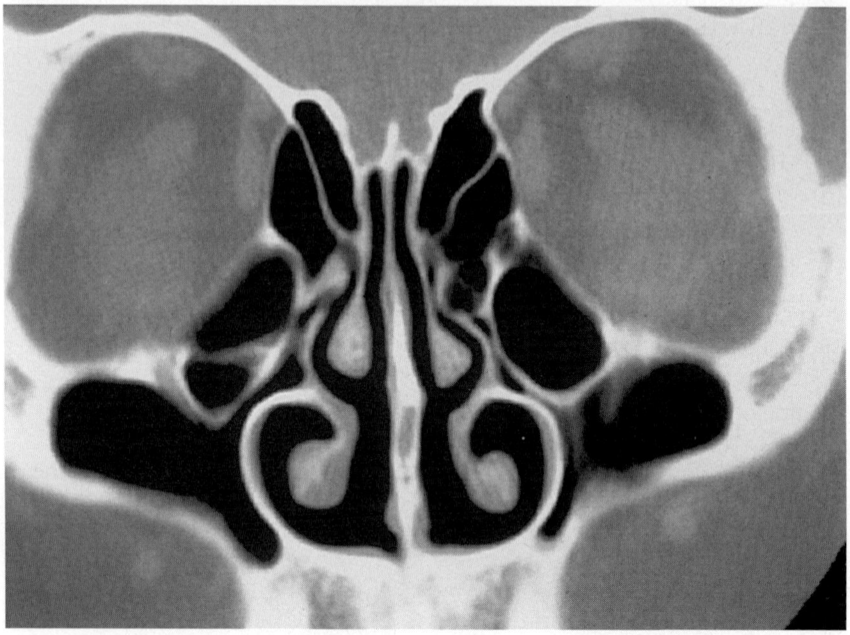

Fig. 14-5. Coronal CT of the nose and paranasal sinuses depicting bilateral Haller cells, larger on the left.

within a sinus or a mucuos retention cyst, as an incidental finding on a CT scan of the brain or orbit (Fig. 14-6). I have also been asked to perform antral puncture and lavage on patients undergoing a fever work-up in whom there was only the subtlest indication of sinus abnormality on CT. Another consideration regarding CT is the stillness required on the part of the patient in order to obtain a high-resolution study. With the newer generation scanners, this is taking less and less time, but occasionally even an adolescent has difficulty with this task.

Magnetic resonance imaging of the paranasal sinuses is helpful in determining the presence and extent of soft-tissue disease within the sinuses. It is limited, however, in its ability to provide detailed information about the bony aspects of the sinuses. Magnetic resonance imaging also takes considerably longer to perform, is very noisy, and is more likely to induce claustrophobia in an adolescent. It is the imaging modality of choice when there is suspicion of an intracranial complication of sinusitis (Fig. 14-7).

Routine x-ray films have limited usefulness in evaluating sinusitis. The advantage of plain radiographs is that the technology is more readily available than CT or MRI and is much quicker. There has also been more literature correlating the presence of routine x-ray findings and

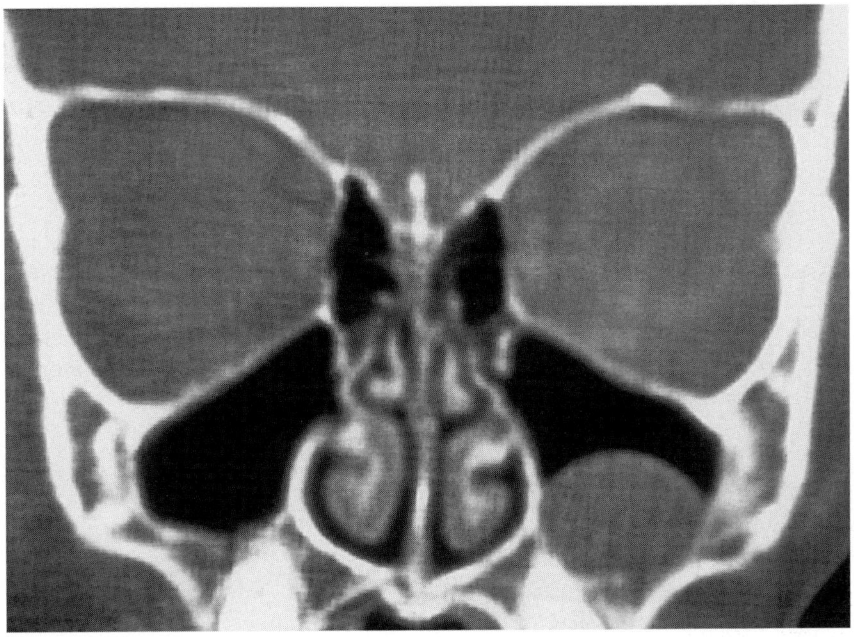

Fig. 14-6. Coronal CT of the maxillary sinuses depicting a left mucous retention cyst. Note the absence of disease elsewhere in the sinus.

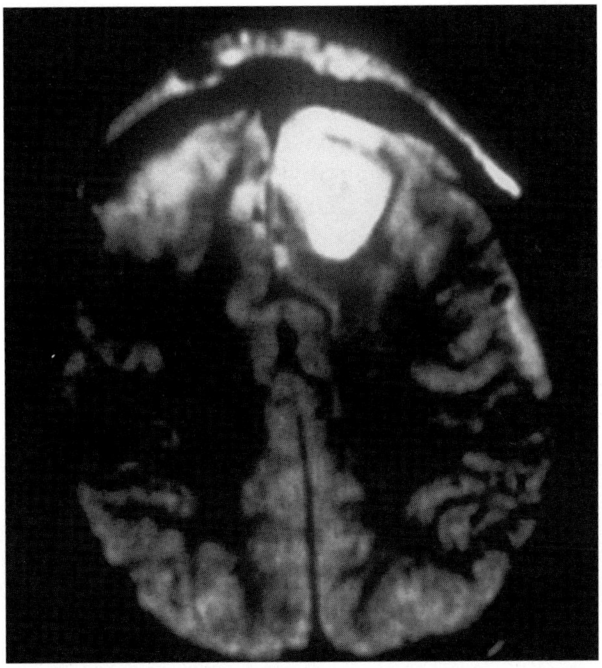

Fig. 14-7. T2-weighted magnetic resonance image of the brain showing a left frontal lobe abscess.

bacteriologic sinusitis. Radiography is therefore useful as a screening tool in evaluating a patient with acute sinusitis, particularly when an air-fluid level is observed. It is least useful in evaluating the ethmoidal sinuses. There is also no significant advantage in the amount of radiation exposure to the patient when four views are obtained (Caldwell, Waters, lateral, and base views) over a CT scan. In evaluating chronic sinusitis, it has almost no role when CT is available. The lateral radiograph is also helpful in determining the size of children's adenoids if they are uncooperative with nasopharyngoscopy. Unfortunately, the size of adenoidal tissue alone does not necessarily correlate with chronic inflammation. Radiographic examination therefore does not replace nasopharyngoscopy for adenoidal evaluation.

Ultrasonography has a very limited or no role in evaluating sinusitis in children, particularly when other radiographic tools are available.

Scintiscanning and barium swallowing with fluoroscopy are useful in evaluating gastroesophageal reflux (GER) as an underlying cause of chronic or recurrent sinusitis. Of the two, scintiscanning is more sensitive and exposes the patient to less radiation, but it usually requires several hours to complete the study. A barium swallow is more helpful when a structural abnormality in the esophagus leading to reflux is suspected. The diagnostic study of choice for GER is the dual-channel, 24-hour pH probe monitor. When this is unavailable or when the child refuses to cooperate, the above tests are useful.

A CT examination was performed in our patient to confirm the diagnosis of sinusitis and to look for possible structural causes. Evaluation to rule out GER also seems appropriate at this time. If the patient is uncooperative for a pH probe study, a scintiscan may be considered.

LABORATORY EXAMINATION

Routine laboratory testing of the blood and urine has limited or no usefulness in the diagnosis of sinusitis. In a child with acute sinusitis or a complication of sinusitis, following the white blood cell count along with fever and other clinical findings may be helpful in gauging response to treatment. In a child who has recurrent or chronic sinusitis, laboratory testing can help assess underline diatheses. Serum IgE test, as well as a radioallergosorbent test (RAST) is helpful in screening for allergy. In a child strongly suspected of having allergies, skin testing may also be necessary. To rule out an immunologic deficiency, quantitative serum immunoglobulin levels (IgG, IgA, IgM) and response to *H. influenzae* type B and pneumoccal vaccines should also be determined. Sweat testing to rule out cystic fibrosis, and electron microscopic evaluation of nasal or carinal mucosa to rule out ciliary dyskinesia, may also be necessary.

In the sample patient, an allergy evaluation had already been performed and the child was found to be nonallergic. A child with such a refractory history should be evaluated for cystic fibrosis, immunologic deficiencies, and possibly ciliary motility disorder. The above studies are therefore helpful at this point in the evaluation.

TREATMENT

Medical treatment

The treatment of sinusitis must include appropriately targeted antimicrobial agents, as well as improved ventilation and drainage of the sinuses.

Acute sinusitus. The bacterial organisms most commonly responsible for acute sinusitis are *Streptococcus pneumoniae, Haemophilus influenzae*, and *Moraxella catarrhalis*. The appropriate first-line antibiotic is therefore amoxicillin or (in the penicillin-allergic patient) sulfamethoxazole/trimethoprim. When there is no evidence of clinical response within 48 to 72 hours, one must consider the possibility of a β-lactamase–producing organism and should therefore employ an agent stable to that enzyme. An exhaustive review of antimicrobial selection is not possible in this chapter, but examples of β-lactamase–stable antibiotics include amoxicillin/clavulanate, cefuroxime axetil, cefprozil, loracarbef, clarithromycin, and azithromycin. Antimicrobial therapy should continue for 10 to 14 days. In addition to an appropriate antibiotic, a topical decongestant such as oxymetazoline or phenylephrine should be applied for 2 to 5 days. The use of a saline nasal spray for 2 weeks to improve mucociliary clearance is also strongly recommended.

Recurrent and/or chronic sinusitus. The medical treatment for these conditions begins with a prolonged course of a β-lactamase–stable antibiotic. The exact duration of antimicrobial use remains unclear in the literature, but 3 to 6 weeks of treatment is generally recommended, depending on the severity and duration of illness. Recurrent or chronic sinusitis may result from acute sinusitis in which the bacterial load has been decreased but not eradicated owing to an inadequate course of antibiotic. Nasal decongestion with an intranasal steroid should be used to improve ventilation and drainage of the paranasal sinuses. Use of a topical decongestant for more than 5 days is not recommended, and therefore intranasal steroids, which are safe for prolonged use, are recommended in these situations. Humidification of the nasal airways is very important to improve mucociliary function, and can best be accomplished with intranasal normal saline or hypertonic saline spray. Also, a cold air, ultrasonic humidifier can be used in the patient's room at night. In patients with recurrent sinusitis, the use of antimicrobial prophylaxis during the seasons when they are most prone to sinusitis, as is frequently done in recurrent acute otitis media, may be considered. One must take into account the potential for growth of resistant organisms when using antibiotics for a prolonged period.

If an underlying medical condition has been diagnosed that may have a causal relationship to a patient's sinusitis, it should be treated at this time as well. When possible, known allergens should be avoided. Antihistamines have not been shown to have a directly beneficial effect on sinusitis, but they may be used in atopic individuals for symptomatic relief. Allergy desensitization may be worthwhile in selected patients, but their secondary effects for alleviating chronic or recurrent sinusitis may take considerable time. Gamma globulin is rarely necessary in individuals with minor immune deficiencies; administration should be under the direction of an immunologist. Gastroesophageal reflux may initially be treated with antacids and reflux precautions (avoidance of oral ingestion 2 hours before bedtime and avoidance of lying flat). If this is not successful, one can use a histamine blocker to reduce gastric acidity coupled with a prokinetic agent to hasten gastric emptying. The medical treatment of cystic fibrosis is not pertinent to this chapter.

The sample patient had been treated with multiple short courses of antibiotics and had been evaluated by an allergist. However, he had not undergone an evaluation for an immune deficiency, GER, or cystic fibrosis, and had not been given a longer duration of antibiotics. In this case because there is evidence of temporary improvement on antibiotics, and there remains the possibility that the asthma is inadequately controlled owing to sinusitis, I would first place the patient on a 6-week course of a β-lactamase–stable antibiotic, hypertonic nasal lavage, and intranasal steroids. I would also refer him for an immune work-up as previously described, a sweat test, and an evaluation for GER.

Surgical Treatment

Indications. In the patient presenting with sinusitis who has not responded to maximal medical therapy, or who has a complication of sinusitis in which there is impending threat to vision or to intracranial extension, surgical intervention must be considered. The type and extent of surgery will be dictated by the individual situation.

Acute sinusitis. When an adolescent has unrelenting facial pain or headache that has been refractory to 72 hours of appropriate antimicrobial therapy coupled with humidification and topical nasal decongestion, one should confirm the diagnosis of acute sinusitis with a plain radiograph. If there is an air-fluid level or complete opacification in the maxillary sinus, an inferior meatal antrotomy can be performed in a cooperative patient. This can be done in the outpatient setting by decongesting and anesthetizing the inferior meatus, as described earlier. With a straight or curved trocar, the inferior meatus can be punctured into the maxillary sinus with relatively little discomfort. The puncture should be placed at least 1 cm posterior to the nasal sill to avoid injury to the nasolacrimal duct. Alternatively, this procedure can be performed through the canine fossa. Once the maxillary sinus is entered, the fluid can be aspirated and the sinus gently irrigated with sterile saline. This will provide a specimen for culture to direct the selection of antibiotics and immediate relief to the patient.

When the radiograph confirms opacification or an air-fluid level in the frontal sinus, a frontal trephination can be performed with the patient under general anesthesia. Alternatively, the frontal sinus can be drained through endoscopic techniques. The decision to approach the frontal sinus externally or endoscopically should depend on the surgeon's personal level of comfort and experience in draining a frontal sinus endoscopically. If there is doubt whether the sinus can be drained adequately using endoscopic techniques, external trephination is recommended. When performed properly, the resultant scar is very acceptable. When the ethmoidal sinuses are involved, one must choose between an external or intranasal approach. Again, this decision should be based on the extent of disease and on the surgeon's level of confidence in performing the procedure endoscopically.

When there is evidence of preseptal orbital extension, a complete ophthalmologic evaluation is imperative. If after 48 to 72 hours of aggressive medical therapy, there is no significant improvement, or if there is evidence of worsening, a CT scan should be obtained and the appropriate sinuses drained. If there is evidence of postseptal disease, particularly when there is any loss of vision or continuing decrease in extraocular motility, surgical intervention is indicated after high-resolution CT. Surgery should be directed to draining the affected sinuses and the orbit. The intranasal versus external approach is again dependent on the confidence and experience of the surgeon. In my experience, the external approach provides better exposure. One must consider that, in an acute process, there is usually a greater amount of granulation tissue and bleeding, which makes endoscopic eradication of disease more difficult and time consuming. Also, when the incision is planned properly and the periosteum and skin are reapproximated carefully, the scar is minimal. If there is intracranial extension such as with an epidural empyema, the neurosurgeon should be consulted immediately.

Chronic sinusitis. When a maximal medical effort, as guided by an appropriate medical work-up, fails to provide symptomatic relief to a patient with CT evidence of chronic sinusitis, surgery is indicated. In children in whom there is still evidence of adenoiditis, either endoscopically or radiographically, the initial surgical approach to chronic sinusitis may be limited to adenoidectomy. This is a low-risk, low-morbidity procedure that can be combined with inferior meatal antrostomy if there is maxillary sinus disease.

When there is evidence of nasal polyposis, a bony obstruction of the sinus ostium, or extensive sinus disease unlikely to be improved by adenoidectomy alone, or when adenoidectomy has not been successful in resolving the sinusitis, surgical treatment directed at the sinuses is indicated. The goal of surgery in the treatment of sinus disease is the same as that of medical therapy: to remove disease and provide the sinuses with adequate ventilation and drainage. In many cases, this can be accomplished successfully with endoscopic techniques. Although endoscopic sinus surgery in children is relatively safe, one must consider the potential risks involved and address these issues with the parents. These include the potential for adverse effect on the growth of the midface; injury to the eye; and penetration through the dura causing cerebrospinal fluid rhinorrhea, meningitis, and intracranial abscess. The potential for recurrence must be acknowledged, and it should be stressed that the success of sinus surgery depends not only on the surgical procedure but also on the postoperative care.

The precise surgical procedure to be performed is determined by the location and extent of sinus disease as evidenced on the CT scan. The most commonly involved sinuses are the maxillary sinuses and the anterior ethmoids. In these situations I follow the techniques described by Lusk, in which endoscopic techniques are used to perform a complete uncinectomy followed by a middle meatal antrostomy. This is accomplished by enlarging the natural maxillary sinus ostium posteriorly, inferiorly, and to a lesser degree anteriorly. After the antrostomy, an anterior ethmoidectomy is performed by entering the ethmoidal bulla and opening the anterior ethmoidal cells from anterior to posterior until the basal lamella is reached. With a 30-degree telescope as described by Schaefer, the superior ethmoidal cells are further opened from posterior to anterior. Lusk then recommends placing a rolled piece of Gelfilm into the ethmoid to prevent synechiae formation. The Gelfilm is removed 2 to 3 weeks later using general anesthesia as a second-look procedure, at which time crusts and granulation tissue can be removed. In cooperative children, this can be performed in the office using topical anesthesia.

When the posterior ethmoids, sphenoid sinuses, and frontal sinuses are involved, it may be necessary to open the sinuses also. The necessary techniques have been described elsewhere and will not be reviewed in this chapter.

The postoperative care in children after endoscopic sinus surgery is critical to the success of the procedure. In addition to the second look performed by the surgeon at 2 to 3 weeks, the patient must irrigate the nose with saline solution, two or three times daily. This is best performed using a Waterpik with a Grossan nasal adaptor. The patient should also use intranasal steroids to help prevent granulation tissue. Continued close follow-up for additional removal of crusts, secretion, and granulation tissue is critical. It is also necessary for the patient to continue the medical treatment of any underlying medical illness that may have contributed to the sinusitis. A follow-up CT scan is necessary only when there has been no significant symptomatic improvement, and this should not be performed before 3 months after surgery.

In my experience, aggressive medical treatment of contributing diseases and state-of-the-art imaging of the paranasal sinuses permits an appropriate selection of patients in whom sinus surgery is necessary. Continued treatment of these diseases, appropriate surgical intervention, and careful thorough postoperative care will increase the rate of success of the surgical procedure and satisfaction of the patient and family.

CHAPTER

15

Management of Asthma and Sinusitis in Adults

Gillian M. Shepherd

PROBLEM

A 68-year-old woman presented with a 6-year history of steroid-dependent asthma.

Management of asthma and sinusitis in adults is often a complex task. Recent years have seen major advances in our understanding of the pathophysiology of asthma.[1] It is predominantly an inflammatory disease: the airway walls are infiltrated, particularly with neutrophils and eosinophils. The airways become obstructed, partly because the lumen becomes smaller from the inflammation and swelling and partly because of increased smooth muscle constriction.

The primary problem is heightened sensitivity of the airways to a variety of factors such as allergens, viral infections, cold temperature, irritant odors, and particulate matter. One of these factors may be chronic sinusitis. Depending on the stimulant, different pathways are triggered, allergic or neural, with the common result of inflammation and airway obstruction. Asthma is a vicious cycle: the greater the airway inflammation, the greater is the hyperresponsiveness.

Chronic sinusitis generally results from obstruction of the outflow tracts from the sinuses to the nasal cavity. This may be caused by nasal congestion with a swollen mucosal lining, enlarged nasal turbinates, and/or nasal polyps. Adequate sinus drainage has to be established for antibiotic treatment to be effective.

The challenge in the patient presented here was to manage her difficult steroid-dependent asthma, both by therapy and by identifying all possible aggravating factors, including chronic sinusitis.

MEDICAL HISTORY

This patient initially presented for a second opinion regarding the management of her asthma. She has a history of one brief episode of asthma at age 4 years and of sinusitis in her twenties, finally treated with bilateral puncture of the maxillary antrum. She was then asymptomatic until 6 years earlier at the age of 62, when she abruptly redeveloped asthma without any obvious precipitating factors. In retrospect, however, she had a persistent mild cough in the winter for the preceding 2 years. At the time she presented, she had experienced a flare of her asthma for several days.

Her symptoms were perennial with no obvious change associated with exposure or locations, except for environments with markedly increased particulate matter and changing temperature and humidity, especially cold air. The asthma was often flared by upper respiratory infections and when she was under unusual stress. At the time of presentation, she was taking the following medications: Azmacort (triamcinolone), four puffs tid; prednisone, 5 mg bid; Ventolin (albuterol) metered dose inhaler prn—for the preceding week she had averaged one puff each hour at night; and Ventolin, via a nebulizer prn.

The patient had never been hospitalized for her asthma, but over the preceding 6 years she had six flares sufficient to require an increased dose of prednisone. For the past year she had been on 5 mg bid. Previously she had been on theophylline, but she felt she was intolerant to it. She had a peak flow meter and the average value was 250 L/sec; during the preceding days this had fallen to 150 L/sec. Her lowest recorded level was 100 L/min. She had no current symptoms of an associated viral syndrome. Some of this flare she attributed to recent severe weather changes. She was normally able to play nine holes of golf, but over the last week she had experienced increasing shortness of breath climbing the stairs in her house.

She had associated symptoms of perennial nasal congestion with some clear postnasal drip but no rhinorrhea or sneezing. There was no history of nasal polyps. The patient denied pain or tenderness in the area of the sinuses or head fullness, and had no known episodes of sinusitis since her twenties. For years she complained about frequent headaches and was told these were "probably migraine headaches." A hiatus hernia was diagnosed some years before, but there were no symptoms suggestive of reflux. She was able to tolerate aspirin and eat dried apricots (high concentration of sulfite preservative). There was a history of two episodes of pneumonia. There was no history of known allergies to inhalants, foods, or drugs and no family history of asthma.

The review of the patient's environment was unremarkable. She had no pets and did not smoke or live with smokers. The remainder of her medical history, including a review of systems, was otherwise unremarkable except for surgery for a ruptured appendix as a child. She was only taking the medications for asthma as noted above.

PHYSICAL EXAMINATION

On initial physical examination the patient was in no respiratory distress with no appreciable use of accessory muscles of respiration. Blood pressure was 130/85 with no detectable pulsus paradoxus (>12 mm Hg fall in systolic blood pressure during inspiration often noted with moderate to severe asthma). The heart rate was 84 beats/min and respiratory rate 16 breaths/min. The examination was otherwise remarkable for moderate congestion of the nasal turbinates with clear mucus and no tenderness over the maxillary sinuses. The oral cavity was clear. Examination of the chest was notable for diffuse end-expiratory and end-inspiratory wheezing with scattered rhonchi. There were no abnormal cardiac sounds.

EVALUATION

The patient brought a chest x-ray film taken several months previously, which was reviewed and found to be normal except for hyperinflation of the lungs. Pulmonary function testing was done and the results are noted in Table 15-1.

The FEV_1/FVC ratio is 73% because, in addition to the low FEV (forced expiratory volume 1 second), the FVC (forced vital capacity) is also low. The average normal ratio is 75%; a higher ratio suggests restrictive disease and a lower indicates obstruction. When the small airway flow ratio (FEF25-75) is severely reduced, as in this case, the vital capacity is often low also. There may be associated restrictive disease, but with a chest radiograph showing hyperinflation, this is most likely due to air trapping from the severe obstruction. The FEF 25%-75% is more effort independent than the FEV_1 and is indicative of obstruction in small airways. This improved 50% after use of a bronchodilator, suggesting that significant airway constriction existed beforehand. Neither the FEV_1 nor the FEF 25%-75% reversed completely because of underlying airway inflammation.

TREATMENT

This patient had steroid-dependent asthma with an acute flare that was not adequately controlled on her present regimen. The first priority was to stabilize the disease with an adequate therapeutic regimen; the second was to evaluate factors that might precipitate or aggravate the asthma. The actual severity of asthma is very difficult to judge clinically; objective spirometry is essential. Several studies have shown that physicians' and patients' judgments regarding severity are often flawed, usually in terms of under-assessing the degree of asthma. Full spirometry is desirable. Lacking that, a measure of the peak expiratory flow rate is acceptable. This is very effort

Table 15-1. Results of pulmonary function testing)

	BEFORE BRONCHODILATOR		AFTER BRONCHODILATOR (2 PUFFS ALBUTEROL)		% CHANGE
	PREDICTED	MEASURED	PREDICTED	MEASURED	
FVC	2.72	1.64 (60%)	2.72	1.80 (66%)	9%
FEV_1	1.93	1.64 (62%)	1.93	1.26 (65%)	4%
FEF 25%-75%	2.23	.58 (26%)	2.23	.89 (39%)	50%

For abbreviations, see text.

dependent, so patients must be instructed carefully in correct technique. This patient's spirometric measurements showed significant obstruction.

The most important treatment for any asthma patient with moderate to severe symptoms consists of corticosteroids, since the primary pathology is inflammation.[2] This patient presented with an acute flare of the chronic asthma, most likely exacerbated by recent severe weather changes. Although she was not in acute respiratory distress according to the physical examination, the peak flow and small airway flow rates were very low, especially considering that she was on prednisone, 5 mg bid. Although the long-term management goal was to decrease or eliminate this patient's steroid dependence, at present she required an increased dose to treat this flare. I recommended that she increase the prednisone to 20 mg bid for 4 days and then taper by 10-mg increments, pending determination of the peak flow values. It is hard to prescribe automatic steroid tapers for patients with asthma flares because of the difficulty in predicting the course of recovery. I recommend strongly that they follow their peak flow rate as well as their symptoms. I suggest that they maintain the initial prednisone dose until their peak flow rate starts to improve. The average patient may then be able to decrease by 10 mg every 4 to 7 days as long as the peak flow rate continues to improve. I usually see the patient again in 3 to 7 days. I also speak with them once or twice a week to check symptoms, flow rates, and prednisone dosing. I generally prescribe prednisone rather than methylprednisolone (Medrol) because the former is cheaper; it is converted to methylprednisolone in the liver. A commercial steroid taper pack (Medrol Dosepak) provides 24 mg Medrol (equals 30 mg prednisone) decreasing over 6 days. This is convenient and simple to use, but it is more expensive than prednisone and provides no flexibility in dosing. After a flare, the expiratory flow rate may take a considerable time to return to the best pre-flare baseline. The main concern is not to taper steroids too fast, if the patient's airways are not responding.

This patient was on inhaled Azmacort, 4 puffs tid, plus prednisone, 5 mg bid. The goal is always to maximize inhaled steroids so as to minimize oral dosing. A change from Azmacort (triamcinolone, 100 μg/puff) to AeroBid (flunisolide, 250 μgs/puff) was recommended because the latter is stronger and fewer puffs are needed. Although triamcinolone and flunisolide are not directly comparable, 12 puffs per day of Azmacort is 1200 μg/day, which approximates five puffs per day of AeroBid. Because the patient needed further control, the dose was increased to five puffs bid (2500 μg/day). The additional benefit of tid vs. bid dosing, factoring in decreased compliance, is minimal, so most patients can manage with bid regimens.

The patient was urged to decrease her use of Ventolin to an absolute maximum of eight puffs per day. Some studies have linked use of more than eight puffs per day or one canister per month with an increased death rate from asthma (a canister has 200 puffs = average 6.6 puffs a day). Other studies have shown that regular use of a β-agonist spray (two puffs qid for 1 month) results in increased airway reactivity.[3] Assuming this is cause and effect, the reasons are not clear. One possible theory is that β-blockers may block the glucocorticoid receptor, therefore downregulating the ability of endogenous steroids to modify airway reactivity.

The patient was also urged to use the peak flow meter before and after using the bronchodilator spray. Many patients reach for their bronchodilator β-agonist sprays when they have the mildest chest symptoms. Some of these sprays may not be necessary. I urge patients to check their peak flow when they feel the need for a bronchodilator and, if it is not significantly decreased from their normal baseline, to hold off using it. This sometimes has to be done for several months until patients can determine when they truly need the spray and until the baseline asthma improves following the other treatments.

Because this patient was having primarily nocturnal symptoms, Serevent was recommended on a temporary basis. This is salmeterol, a 12-hour bronchodilator and very close relative of albuterol. Potentially it may have the same negative effects as short-acting β-agonist sprays. She was instructed to use this before bedtime to minimize the nocturnal symptoms. She was warned that this occasionally causes insomnia and told that if this occurred, she should use the spray earlier in the evening.

Proper use of metered dose inhalers is essential. Improper use has been found to be widespread.[2] In most patients, use of a spacer should be recommended, particularly with steroid inhalers. These are a variety of essentially empty tubes. The metered dose inhaler is sprayed into the spacer; the patient breathes in from the opposite end, usually through a valve. By doing this, the patient will breathe in the medication mixed with air, which significantly enhances the deposition of the medication in the small airways. Without a spacer, much of the medication will deposit on the posterior pharyngeal wall. This patient was previously taking Azmacort, which is often used, as it has a spacer built into the metered dose inhaler device. AeroBid does not have this, so a spacer was prescribed with it, in this case an Aerochamber spacer.

Use of a spacer with the bronchodilator metered dose inhalers is less critical but certainly helps. If a spacer is not used, correct technique is essential. Although there has been much debate, most physicians believe the inhaler should be held approximately 1 inch from the mouth. The patient should exhale maximally and then start to inhale coincident with pressing for spray release. This represents an attempt to increase the distance between the spray and the pharynx in order to minimize medication deposition there, and an attempt to mix the medication with inhaled air. To facilitate this, it is essential that the inhaled breath be slow and that the breath (each puff) be held for a least 5 seconds so that the medication has a chance to encounter its receptor and bind.

COURSE

The patient was instructed to return in 1 week. At this time she was somewhat improved on prednisone, 30 mg/day. Her Ventolin use had decreased to one or two puffs bid and she was sleeping through most nights with Serevent. Her peak flow had increased to 200 L/mm. The physical examination was otherwise unchanged.

At this visit, further testing was done to determine any factors that might precipitate or aggravate the asthma, with the goal of avoiding or treating these factors to minimize disease. A list of common precipitating or aggravating factors is shown in Box 15-1.

Allergy skin testing was done using the common allergens noted in Box 15-2. This was completely negative except for the positive histamine control.

Because of her history of sinusitis in her twenties and symptoms consistent with chronic nonallergic rhinitis, the patient was referred to an ENT specialist for fiberoptic nasopharyngolaryngoscopy. This was clear except for a white postnasal discharge. No nasal polyps were seen. There were no symptoms of gastroesophageal reflux. She tolerated aspirin and sulfite exposure in the past without incident.

Because of the past sinusitis and two recent episodes of pneumonia, quantitative immunoglobulins were obtained to rule out an IgG or IgA deficiency. A total gamma globulin count was normal on a recent biochemistry profile, so a specific deficiency was unlikely. A specific IgA deficiency could exist, however, with a normal total level. In this patient's case, all levels were normal.

She was instructed to continue AeroBid, five puffs bid through the Aerochamber; Serevent, two puffs at bedtime; and Ventolin prn. The prednisone dose was decreased to 20 mg/day for 4 days followed by a baseline dose of 10 mg/day (5 mg bid) if the peak flow did not decrease during this taper.

At this time other treatments were considered:

1. Intal (cromolyn). This basically coats airways and blocks allergic reactions through an unknown mechanism. The spray should ideally be used every 6 hours, so this presents a compliance problem. This patient did not have a demonstrable allergic component contributing to the asthma, so the addition of cromolyn was unlikely to be beneficial. *Tilade* (nedocromil) inhaler is similar to cromolyn.
2. Atrovent (ipatropium bromide). This is an atropine derivative that helps dry up watery secretions. In general it is not very helpful for asthma unless ac-

BOX 15-1

1. Allergies: 90% of children and 50% of adults have significant allergies that can flare asthma
2. Upper respiratory infections
3. Changing temperature, especially cold air, humidity, and barometric pressure
4. Exposure to particulate matter and irritant odors, e.g., ammonia, insecticides, and pollution, including ozone and sulfur dioxide
5. Aggravated stress or other emotional upset, or laughing
6. Sinusitis
7. Gastroesophageal reflux
8. Sulfite sensitivity
9. Aspirin sensitivity

BOX 15-2

Trees
Mix of 15 different trees that produce pollen in the spring

Grasses
Mix of five different grasses (fewer than the number of trees because many grasses are similar antigenically and cross-react)

Ragweed
Major fall allergen

Other weeds
Mix of 12 different weeds that pollinate, mainly in the summer through the fall

Molds
Mix of seven different molds including the main outdoor ones that produce spores throughout most of the year, except mid-winter in snow-covered areas.

Cats and dogs
Even though patients may not have animals, they may have frequent exposure

Cockroaches
A major city antigen; even though patients may claim they have no direct exposure, airborne exposure in buildings with central ventilation systems is common

Dust mites
The most common allergen worldwide; it is ubiquitous except in very dry climates (including high altitudes).

Pigeons
Another city antigen; pigeons may sit above air intake equipment of large buildings, and external droppings are everywhere.

companied by copious mucus secretions, which this patient did not have.

3. *Theophylline.* This is an older oral medication for asthma, relative to the metered dose inhalers. Surprisingly the mechanism responsible for its efficacy is still not fully elucidated. It is used less frequently now since (1) very effective topical steroid sprays are available that treat the underlying inflammation, (2) the therapeutic to toxic range is narrow, and (3) interactions with multiple drugs are a problem. This patient was previously treated with theophylline but experienced unacceptable side effects of feeling shaky.

FURTHER COURSE

After improving initially with increased inhaled steroids and prednisone, 10 mg/day, the patient did not improve further, and the peak flow rates continue to average 200 L/min. One month after her initial visit, she went to Florida for Thanksgiving. During this time she had a moderate flare of asthma, again requiring an increased dose of prednisone. Coincidentally for the first time she had symptoms of fullness in the area of the maxillary sinuses and was given Bactrim DS (trimethoprim and sulfamethoxasole), 10 days bid, for presumptive sinusitis. She returned 2 months later improved, with a peak flow averaging 250 L/min now on AeroBid-M, five puffs bid; prednisone, 5 mg bid; and Ventolin prn. She had discontinued Serevent and was sleeping through the night.

At this time a sinus computed tomographic (CT) scan was ordered despite lack of specific sinus symptoms. This was done because of her history of sinusitis in her twenties, the postnasal drip, and the recent symptoms of maxillary fullness in Florida that had responded to a 10 day course of Bactrim. The surprising results are shown in Fig. 15-1. This was read as the following: "Extensive opacification of the paranasal sinuses sparing only a portion of each frontal sinus. The sphenoid sinus is only partially pneumatized. The nasal septum is deviated with a convexity to the right in its midportion and displacement inferiorly to the left. There is nodular and polypoid soft tissue filling the superior half of the nasal fossa, particularly posteriorly. There is total occlusion of the ethmoidal recesses and the ostiomeatal complexes bilaterally. There is lateral deviation of the uncinate processes bilaterally and erosion with thinning of the left uncinate process. The osseous structures of the sinuses are otherwise remarkable for marked attenuation of the ethmoid septa."

The remarkable aspect of this case is the degree of chronic sinusitis seen on CT and the comparative lack of associated clinical symptoms. In retrospect, some of the "migraine headaches" may have been sinusitis symptoms. The patient was placed on a 3-week course of Ceftin (cefuroxime), 500 mg bid; Neo-Synephrine (phenylophrine) 1%, bid for 3 days; and Flonase (fluticasone), two sprays in each nostril bid. It is difficult to achieve adequate antibiotic levels in the paranasal sinuses, so a course of at least 3 weeks is necessary for chronic symptoms.

A number of studies link chronic sinusitis and asthma, particularly steroid-dependent asthma. These show that in many cases, if the sinusitis is treated aggressively, the asthma improves, often eliminating the need for oral steroids.[4,5] It is difficult to obtain pure microbacteriologic cultures in an individual patient. Antibiotic coverage is selected on the basis of the most common organisms known to be responsible for sinusitis: *Streptococcus pneumoniae*,

A

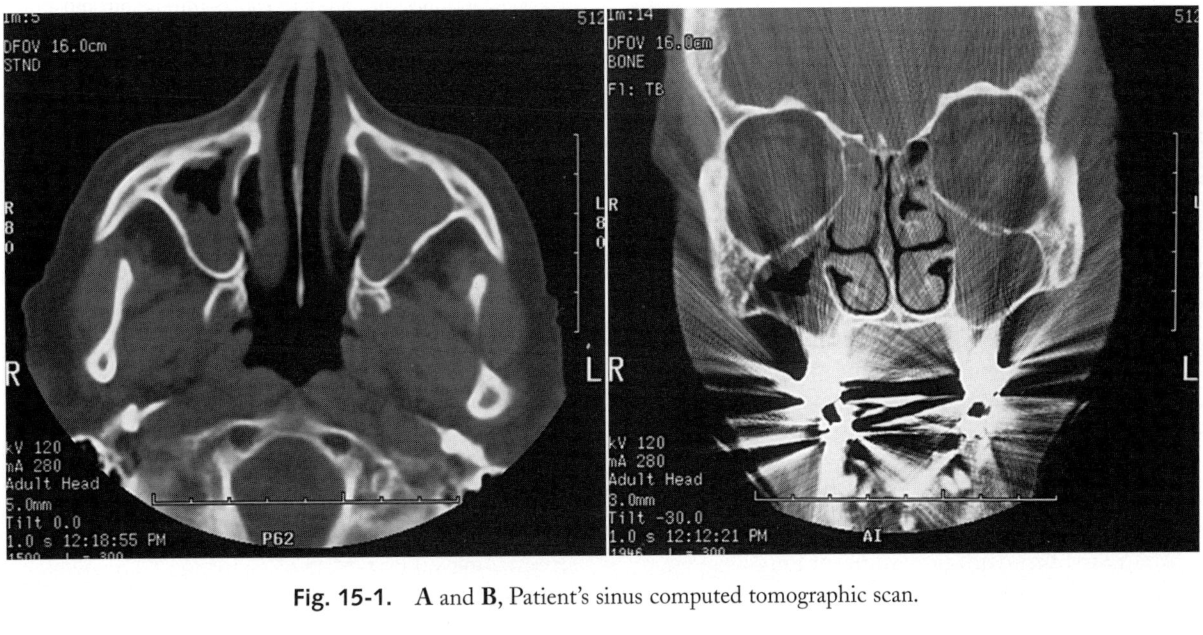

B

Fig. 15-1. A and B, Patient's sinus computed tomographic scan.

Haemophilus influenzae, *Moxarella catarrhalis*, and *Streptococcus pyogenes*. Data regarding local susceptibility of bacteria to various antibiotics also need to be considered. Most physicians elect to treat adults initially with amoxicillin, 500 mg tid; Augmentin, 250 mg tid; or a third-generation cephalosporin such as Ceftin (cefuroxime) or Lorabid (loracarbef). Bactrim and Biaxin (clarithromycin) are also very effective.

Besides antibiotics, the other critical aspect of aggressive treatment consists of establishing open drainage to the nasal cavity. This can be done momentarily with decongestant nasal sprays (e.g., Afrin [pseudoephedrine] or Neo-Synephrine) as prescribed for this patient. Rebound congestion is a common side effect that limits such a treatment to approximately 3 days. Corticosteroid nose sprays should also be used. In this case, Flonase was chosen because it is stronger than other steroid nose sprays and can be used once daily as maintenance. This patient was initially placed on bid dosing because of the significant nasal soft-tissue swelling. If this shrank sufficiently to open up the ostiomeatal complex area, the plan was to decrease the Flonase dose to once a day.

If there is an anatomic blockage and the problem is chronic, surgery may be indicated. This is especially true if significant nasal polyps are present or if there is blockage of the ostiomeatal complex area between the maxillary sinuses and nasal passage. This patient had occlusion of the ostiomeatal complexes bilaterally. If this was not cleared adequately with antibiotics and steroid nose spray, surgery was a definite consideration.

The patient had not had symptoms consistent with chronic rhinosinusitis at the time of treatment, and therefore there was no obvious change in symptoms after treatment. She thought her headaches might have decreased. The asthma symptoms, however, improved significantly. Within 2 months, she was able to discontinue prednisone and decrease the inhaled AeroBid dose to four puffs bid along with albuterol prn. The peak flow increased from an average of 250 to 300L/min, and exercise tolerance was excellent.

This improvement was sustained for approximately 4 months. At this time, the patient had another flare of asthma with no obvious cause. Clinically, she had no symptoms suggestive of repeat sinusitis. Steady use of Flonase nose spray had been recommended, but she had not done this. Empirically, she was placed on another 3-week course of Ceftin, along with Flonase, an increase in AeroBid to six puffs bid, and a return to prednisone, 10 mg/day for 2 weeks. Again, she had an excellent response with clinical improvement of the asthma and peak flow test results.

One month after the second course of Ceftin, a repeat sinus CT scan was obtained. The results were almost identical to the first, with no significant improvement.

Clinically the patient again did well for another 3 months. In the past, flares of her asthma had to be treated with higher doses of oral steroids, and improvements in status lasted for shorter periods. The prolonged improvements in the asthma noted after these antibiotic treatments was therefore presumed to be due in part to improvement in the chronic sinusitis. The mechanism responsible for this association of increased asthma in the setting of sinusitis is not clear. It is not completely accepted that there even is an association, although most physicians today believe sinusitis to be an aggravating factor. This is supported by data from the 1980s; no recent trials have been reported.[14]

Three months after the second course of Ceftin, the patient had a third flare of asthma despite steady use of Flonase. This time she was treated, again empirically, with Augmentin, 250 mg tid for 3 weeks. A 500-mg dose was considered, but she had a sensitive gastrointestinal tract that might have been aggravated by a higher dose. Coincidentally, she was placed back on prednisone, 10 mg per day, with increased AeroBid spray.

The possibility of sinus surgery had been repeatedly discussed with the patient. After the second antibiotic course and CT scan, she was again referred to an ENT specialist, who recommended an ethmoidectomy and surgery to open the maxillary sinuses. The patient was very hesitant. At this time, I urged her strongly to consider surgery because I believed that (1) the sinusitis was contributing to the asthma; (2) the asthma was moderately severe and required constant steroid treatment, both inhaled and frequent oral; and (3) she was at risk of osteoporosis from this as well as other side effects, so that every effort should be made to minimize her steroid requirement.

The patient finally refused surgery for the present because (1) she never had any symptoms of sinusitis, except questionably her flares of asthma; (2) she was very concerned that surgery would result in some symptoms when she didn't have any to begin with; (3) despite long discussions and explanations, she still felt her asthma was not a significant problem, as she was usually functional, and when her asthma flared, her symptoms were adequately treated with prednisone; and (4) she believed she had no side effects from prednisone.

Many years previously, she had refused a recommended regimen of estrogen and progesterone. At this juncture, I referred her to an endocrinologist for bone densitometry analysis. Not surprisingly, this showed mild to moderate osteoporosis. She was started on Fosamax but could not tolerate it because of gastrointestinal side effects. She was also started on Accolate (a lenkotruine inhibitor that may help asthma) but felt no improvement, therefore, she discontinued the use of this. Most recently the patient has been taking varying doses of AeroBid and Serevent.

SUMMARY

This patient has moderate steroid-dependent asthma aggravated by viral infections, changing weather, stress, and probably sinusitis. The asthma has required constant steroids to treat and she has osteoporosis; therefore, all measures should be taken to improve the asthma in order to minimize the steroids needed. In the long term, osteoporosis is probably the greatest risk to her health.

Although the CT scans show massive opacification of the sinuses, the patient remarkably has no associated clinical symptoms. Treatment of the sinusitis with three courses of antibiotics was associated with marked improvement in the asthma. She coincidentally took increased steroids, but the improvement in the asthma lasted much longer than usual after the steroid courses were taken. This suggests that improvement in the sinusitis was contributory. In conjunction with the ENT specialist, I urged her to consider sinus surgery, but she was reluctant in case it resulted in symptoms where none existed before. A possible compromise might be two-step surgery with a lesser procedure first.

Moderate-to-severe asthma is a complex disease to manage and requires consideration of all the aspects mentioned in this case. These include identifying all factors that may flare the disease, including sinusitis, and fine-tuning medical and other therapy accordingly. Success depends in large part on patient education, which requires a considerable commitment from the physician or other medical personnel.

REFERENCES

1. Guidelines for the diagnosis and management of asthma. Bethesda, Md, DHHS Publication No 91-3042, 1991 and 1997 update in publication, U.S. Department of Health and Human Services.

   The national multidisciplinary expert panel report, which is considered the current best guide to asthma and establishes the practice parameters that all physicians should meet. International guidelines also exist with essentially the same recommendations.

2. Hartert TV, Windom HH, Stokes Peebles R Jr, et al: Inadequate outpatient medical therapy for patients with asthma admitted to two urban hospitals, *Am J Med* 100:386-394, 1996.

   In this population of patients (Baltimore), antiinflammatory treatment was underutilized, β-agonist treatment was overutilized, and patients did not use their metered dose inhalers correctly.

3. Executive Committee of the American Academy of Allergy, Asthma, and Immunology: Position statement: Inhaled β_2-adrenergic agonists in asthma, *J Allergy Clin Immunol* 91:1234-1237, 1993.

   Summarizes data on the use of β-agonists in asthma: "Although there is no proof that regular use of inhaled β_2-agonists increases morbidity and mortality rates in patients with asthma, such a possibility exists."

4. Slavin RG: *Nasal polyps and sinusitis.* In Middleton E, Reed CE, Ellis EF, et al, editors: *Allergy: principles and practice*, ed 3, St. Louis, 1988, Mosby–Year Book, pp. 1291-1304.

   Reviews the association between asthma and sinusitis. Slavin aggressively treated 33 adults with asthma and sinusitis with medical and/or surgical therapy. A total of 28 of 33 patients were symptomatically better and 15 were able to significantly decrease their previous steroid dose.

5. Senior BA, Kennedy DW: Management of sinusitis in the asthmatic patient, *Ann Allergy Asthma Immunol* 77:6-19, 1996.

   Good discussion of clinical management.

CHAPTER

16

Management of Asthma and Sinusitis in Children

David S. Mazza

PROBLEM

A 9-year-old girl presents with a 1-year history of nocturnal cough. For the past 2 years she has had nasal congestion with intermittent rhinorrhea. The nasal discharge is green tinged in the early morning and then becomes clear as the day progresses. She also complains of shortness of breath with chest tightness. This is accompanied by cough with laughing and exertion. In the past, the child has had wheezing with viral infections. She has received three separate courses of amoxicillin during the past year. Each course is 10 days in duration and symptoms do abate, but they return each time in 2 to 4 weeks.

The child presents with nocturnal cough, which is seen in up to 40% of children with sinusitis. The additional observation of purulent nasal discharge points to an underlying sinus infections as a possible cause. The child also has a history of airway hyperactivity with viral infections and is now manifesting increased signs of respiratory involvement, as evidenced by cough with exertion and laughing.

Figure 16-1 is a schematic diagram of the above information.

A number of other conditions should be considered, particularly in the younger child (Table 16-1). Appropriate studies should be performed based on the history and clinical findings to rule out the possible etiologies. The clinical presentation of sinusitis is presented in Table 16-2. Predisposing factors are listed in Table 16-3.

The interrelationship between sinusitis and asthma was proposed by Gottleib in 1925.[1] Although clinical improvement in sinusitis often results in a similar change in airway symptoms, studies in this regard have been mixed.

MEDICAL HISTORY

In any upper or lower respiratory complaint in children, the birth and neonatal history is of primary importance. In our case, the girl was a product of a 9-month gestation with normal, spontaneous vaginal delivery. There were no complications in the neonatal period and the child was breast fed for the first 5 months of life. Foods were introduced one at a time and no dermatologic or gastrointestinal symptoms occurred. She had three episodes of otitis media between 1 and 3 years of age. At age 7, she developed symptoms of wheezing with an upper respiratory viral infection and required a 2-week course of albuterol syrup. Since that time, she has needed albuterol in the winter season with viral infections. In the past 2 years, the mother has noted cough with exertion and has been instructed by the pediatrician to give albuterol inhaler 15 minutes before exercise.

The child often coughed and sneezed when the mother cleaned the house and complained of palatal itching during the months of May and June. The present symptoms developed 2 years before their evaluation. At that time, the child had developed a viral respiratory infection. Initially she was absent from school for 3 days with cough and fever. The mother called the school and learned that several children were absent because of respiratory symptoms. The child subsequently felt well but had persistent rhinorrhea and nocturnal cough that continued for the next year, as noted above. That spring, the symptoms of rhinitis in-

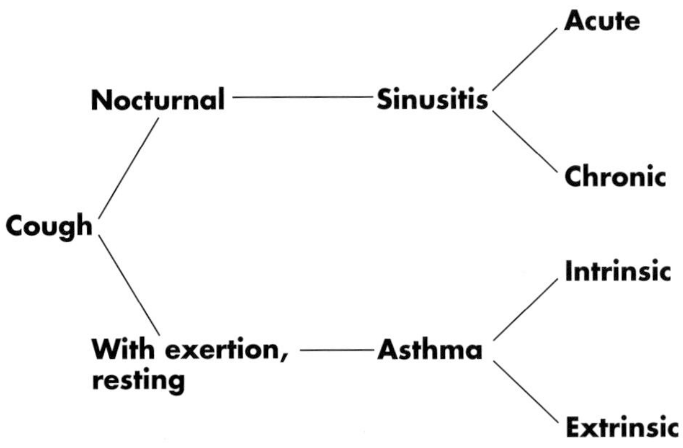

Fig. 16-1. Algorithm for case study.

creased and were accompanied by palatal itching. As mentioned, the child was treated three times (in January, April and November of that year) with a 10-day course of amoxicillin and had minimal improvement each time. During that same year, she required the use of an albuterol inhaler four or five times a week, exclusive of albuterol prophylaterally prior to exercise. The child's growth and development are normal.

Environmental history is significant for a cat present in the house for 5 years, as well as many stuffed animals in the bedroom and wall-to-wall carpeting throughout the house. The family lives on the sixteenth floor of a 25-story building. No environmental problems are present. There is no smoking in the house nor at the baby sitter's apartment.

There is no history of snoring, nor is there any food, insect, or medication allergy or atopic dermatitis. The family history is positive for allergic disease on both the paternal and maternal sides of the family. The patient's 15-year-old brother has seasonal allergic rhinitis but no symptoms of asthma.

The above history illustrates several key points in the approach to a child with cough, nasal symptoms, and wheezing. Given the normal neonatal and early childhood history, congenital abnormalities are unlikely. The fact that the present complaints began after a respiratory infection is highly suggestive of chronic sinusitis. In the course of a viral infection, mucosal edema may cause blockage of the sinus ostia, with a subsequent inflammatory response. Figure 16-2 depicts the anatomic landmarks of the paranasal sinuses. The ethmoidal and maxillary sinuses are present at birth. The ethmoids may not be visible radiographically until 6 months to 1 year of age. The postnatal growth of the frontal sinuses is slow and in most children can be demonstrated radiographically after 6 years of age. Significant increase occurs in size until the late teens. The sphenoid sinus is the last to develop; by the age of 7 it is visible, but it also continues to grow until the late teens. The ostia of the maxillary, frontal, and anterior ethmoidal sinuses drain into the middle meatus. The sphenoidal and posterior ethmoidal sinuses drain into the superior meatus. Only the nasal lacrimal duct empties into the inferior meatus. In the pathophysiology of sinus disease the patency of the sinus ostia, the function of the ciliary apparatus and the nature of the nasal secretions are critical factors. The ostiomeatal complex is the point between the middle and inferior turbinates that represents the common drainage tract for the frontal, ethmoidal, and maxillary sinuses. This narrow passage is prone to blockage by thickened nasal secretions

Table 16-1. Differential diagnosis of cough and/or wheezing during childhood

Upper respiratory tract
- Foreign body
- Mucus in the nose creating "wheeze"
- Sinusitis (acute/chronic)

Middle respiratory tract
- Epiglottitis
- Foreign body
- Laryngomalacia/tracheomalacia
- Laryngotracheobronchitis
- Laryngeal webs
- Pertussis
- Toxic inhalation (dust, gas, talc)
- Tracheoesophageal fistula
- Tracheostenosis/bronchiostenosis

Lower respiratory tract
- α_1-antitrypsin deficiency
- Asthma
- Bronchiectasis
- Bronchiolitis
- Bronchopulmonary dysplasia
- Congenital anomalies
- Cystic fibrosis
- Foreign body
- Gastroestophageal reflux
- Hypersensitivity lung disease (e.g., molds, fibers)
- Pulmonary eosinophilia (Loeffler's syndrome)
- Pulmonary hemosiderosis
- Pulmonary interstitial emphysema
- Toxic inhalation (dust, gas, fumes)
- Tumor

Cardiovascular system
- Mitral valve prolapse
- Vascular rings (around airways)

Nervous system
- Hyperventilation
- Swallowing mechanism dysfunction (aspiration)

Adapted from Virant FS, Shapiro GG: *Evaluation of the child with chronic cough/wheezing.* In Tinkelman DG, Naspitz CK, editors: *Childhood asthma, pathophysiology and treatment,* New York, 1987, Marcel Dekker.

Table 16-2. Clinical presentation of sinusitis

ACUTE	CHRONIC
Symptoms	**Symptoms**
Persistent upper respiratory infection	Persistent nasal obstruction
Mucopurulent nasal drainage	Purulent postpharyngeal drainage
Cough	Fetor oris
	Sore throat
	Hyposmia
	Malaise
Signs	**Signs**
Nasal mucosal edema/erythema	Nasal mucosal edema/erythema
Purulent rhinorrhea	Mucopus (nasal and pharyngeal)
Postpharyngeal drainage	Nasal polyps

From Slavin RG, Toffel PH: Sinusitis—a medical and surgical approach. Current Views in Allergy, 1991, Medical College of Georgia.

Table 16-3. Factors resulting in predisposition to sinus ostial obstruction[4]

MUCOSAL SWELLING	MECHANICAL OBSTRUCTION
Systemic disorder	Choanal atresia
Recurrent viral upper respiratory infection	Deviated septum
Allergic inflammation	Nasal polyps
Cystic fibrosis	Haller cells
Immune disorders	Agger nasi cells
Dysmotile cilia syndrome	Concha bullosa
Local insult	Uncinate process bullosa
Facial trauma	Paradoxically curved turbinate
Swimming, diving	Foreign body
Rhinitis medicamentosa	Tumor

From Wald ER: Chronic sinusitis in children, *J Pediatr* 127:339, 1995.

and mucosal edema. Thus, inflammation in this area also causes secondary inflammation and/or infection in the maxillary, ethmoidal, and frontal sinuses. The patency of this area is of paramount importance in maintaining normally functioning sinuses.

In our patient, the history is highly suggestive of allergic disease. Given the seasonal symptoms in the spring, together with coughing and sneezing during house cleaning as well as a positive family history of allergic disease, an allergy evaluation is indicated.

PHYSICAL EXAMINATION

The child appeared well developed and in the 75th percentile for height and weight. Blood pressure was 100/60, respiratory rate 20, and heart rate 76. "Allergic shiners" (a darkening of the skin below the eyes) with Dennies lines and a transverse nasal crease were present. Adenoidal facies were noted. The ear examination was unremarkable. Nasal examination revealed edematous nasal mucosa that was erythematous in color. The septum was midline and thick, green-tinged secretions were visible. After this, the nasal mucosa was constricted with topical phenylephrine. Twenty minutes after this procedure, the nose was reexamined with a nasal speculum and headlight. No nasal polyps were visualized. Pharyngeal examination revealed marked posterior pharyngeal hypertrophy with thick, green-tinged mucus in the posterior pharynx. The tonsils were normal in size with no evidence of abcess. Tenderness upon percussion over the maxillary sinuses was appreciated. Chest examination revealed a normal anteroposterior diameter with occasional end-expiratory wheezing upon deep expiration. No tachypnea or retrac-

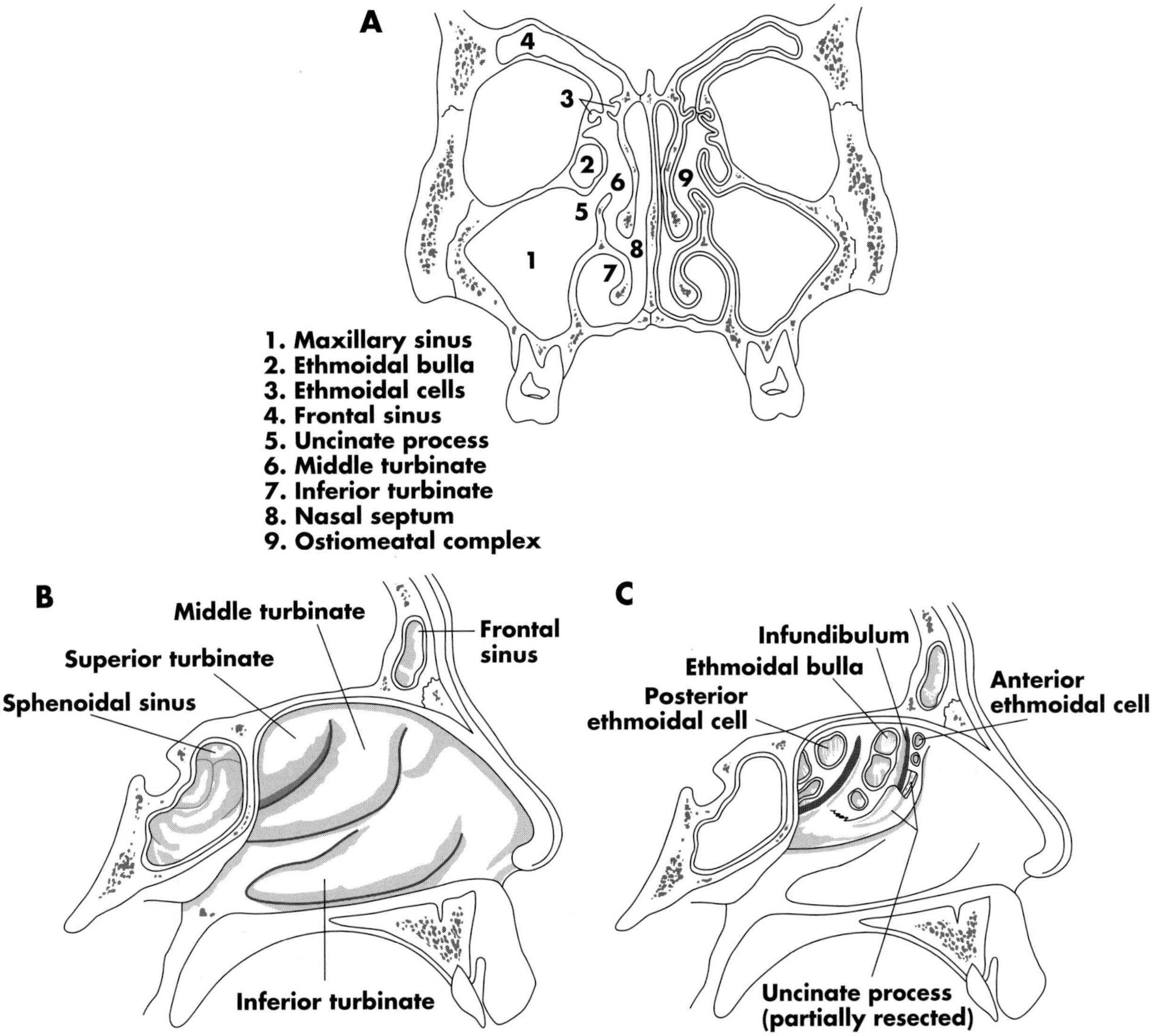

Fig. 16-2. Coronal **(A)** and sagittal **(B** and **C)** sections of the nose and paranasal sinuses. The shaded area in **A** represents the ostiomeatal complex. **C,** View through the middle and superior turbinates, displaying the ethmoidal cells. (From Wald ER: *N Engl J Med* 326:319-323, 1992. Sinusitis in children. Reprinted by permission of *The New England Journal of Medicine.* Copyright 1992. Massachusetts Medical Society. All rights reserved.)

tions were present. The skin examination was unremarkable. No clubbing or cyanosis was present. The remainder of the physical examination was noncontributory.

Normal growth and development are important parameters to assess, since children with chronic diseases or recurrent infections often exhibit a failure to grow normally and may appear malnourished.

The presence of "allergic shiners," may be secondary not only to allergy but also to sinus disease. This finding results from blockage of the venous return below the eyes with exudation of fluid and resultant edema. Abnormal ear examination results are often seen in children with respiratory symptoms. In children with chronic otitis media there may be an abnormal appearance of the tympanic membranes. Eustachian tube dysfunction may be suggested by middle ear fluid or retracted and/or immobile drums. The nasal examination was consistent with mucosal inflammation and infection. Constriction of the mucosa is important with enlarged nasal turbinates to appreciate any visible tumors, polyps, or foreign bodies that would be obscured by the edematous tissue. The consistency and color of nasal secretions is variable, and green-tinged secretions can be seen in chronic sinusitis.

Marked posterior pharyngeal hypertrophy is indicative of chronic postnasal drip, most commonly caused by rhinitis and/or sinusitis. Rhinitis can in turn be caused by allergy, but vasomotor as well as nonallergic rhinitis–eosinophilia syndrome (NARES) must also be considered. Careful assessment of the soft palate should also be performed, as some children with chronic infections may have a potential cleft that has been overlooked. Tonsillar size should also be assessed. Normally, tonsillar tissue increases with age through puberty and then shrinks in size. Halitosis may also be noted and may be an indication of sinusitis.

The chest examination should be assessed with respect to shape and excursions. In our patient, no signs of chronic airway disease such as increased airway diameter or digital clubbing were appreciated. Digital clubbing is unusual in uncomplicated asthma but if present, heart disease or cystic fibrosis should be considered. The occasional end-expiratory wheezing implicates involvement of the lower respiratory tract, but clear lungs may be found in so-called *cough-variant asthma*.

The dermatologic examination in our patient was normal. However, one should look carefully for signs of chronic skin disease such as atopic dermatitis that suggest a possible allergic factor as well as chronic dermatitis that may be seen with acquired or congenital immunodeficiency.

RADIOGRAPHIC EXAMINATION

Plain films of the sinuses were obtained (Fig. 16-3) showing bilateral mucosal thickening of the maxillary sinuses. The anteroposterior and Waters views best demonstrate the frontal and maxillary sinuses. However, plain films do not adequately visualize the ethmoidal sinuses because of structural superimposition. Two weeks after a 4-week treatment with amoxicillin-potassium clavulanate, a corona computed tomographic (CT) scan was obtained and was normal. With regard to imaging of the sinuses, the primary goals are to accurately depict the regional anatomy and document the extent of disease. Accordingly, plain films are of limited value since they do not adequately assess the ethmoidal sinuses and ostiomeatal complex, which are the most common locations of sinus disease. Ideally, CT is performed in children refractory to adequate treatment or whose history reveals significant recurrent infections. This is best obtained 2 weeks after an adequate course of antimicrobial treatment and in children in whom surgery is being contemplated. Such studies offer excellent delineation of the ostiomeatal complex, and since they are obtained after treatment, obstructing lesions of the ostiomeatal complex can be distinguished from adjacent mucosal edema and fluid. In children whose initial presentation is complicated by such findings as proptosis or periorbital edema, an axial as well as a coronal CT scan should be obtained immediately. Magnetic resonance imaging (MRI) is performed if possible intracranial involvement is seen on CT. MRI is best for soft tissue examination.

A chest radiograph was also obtained and was normal. This should be taken in all patients presenting with symptoms referable to the lower respiratory tract if film has not been previously obtained. Underlying congenital abnormalities, infection, and masses may be detected and may all present with the symptom of wheezing.

LABORATORY EXAMINATION

A nasal smear revealed cellular contents consisting of neutrophils. Nasal cytology can be particularly helpful when viewed in conjunction with the clinical history. A predominance of neutrophils with or without intracellular bacteria, is seen in sinusitis, although this finding can also be noted with an acute upper respiratory infection. If the percentage of eosinophils is greater than 5%, atopy must be considered. The entity of NARES is most uncommon in children. In cases of sinusitis, it is possible that neutrophils will predominate to such an extent that eosinophils are not seen, even if a patient is allergic. Nasal cytology is not definitive, but it may indicate that further studies such as skin testing or radiologic evaluations are advisable.

In any case of suspected sinusitis and lower airway symptoms, an allergy evaluation should be obtained. If a patient is allergic to environmental allergens, symptoms may not resolve or may recur despite adequate antimicrobial therapy until environmental controls are instituted

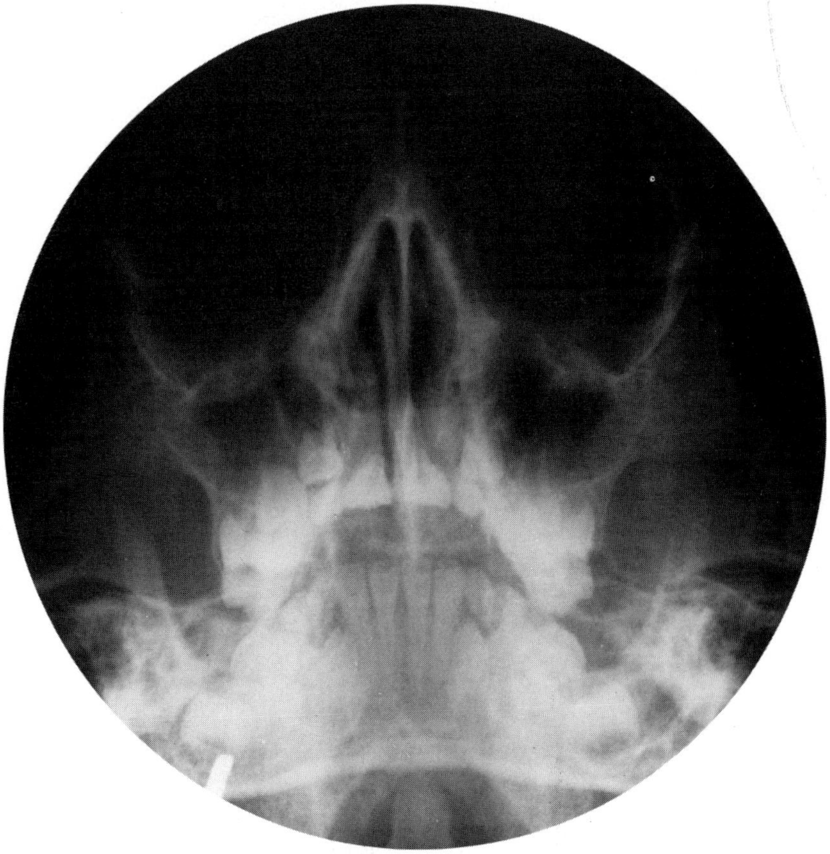

Fig. 16-3. Radiograph revealing bilateral mucosal thickening in the maxillary sinuses.

also. In this case, skin testing was performed to a representative panel of common indoor allergens as well as to outdoor allergens appropriate for the geographic location. Positive skin tests to dust mite, grass, and trees were noted. Subsequent intradermal testing to those allergens negative on prick testing were negative, including ragweed, mold, cockroaches, and feathers. Skin tests should be interpreted in light of the patient's history, particularly with regard to environment. A careful environmental history with particular emphasis on the bedroom should be obtained. Possible exposures to such perennial allergens as dust mite, cockroaches, animals, and mold should be obtained. Any exposure to cigarettes in the home, at relatives' residences, or at a baby sitter's house should be elicited. Several studies have documented exposure to cigarette smoke as causing an increased incidence of infection in both the upper and lower respiratory tract as well as exacerbating allergic rhinitis. Skin testing should be directed by the clinical history; in very young children it is usual to perform a prick test only to those allergens for which environmental controls would make a difference. In older children, prick testing to seasonal allergens is also performed and followed by the more sensitive intradermal testing to those allergens that are negative by prick testing. Food is very seldom an allergic factor in upper and/or lower respiratory symptoms of this nature.

Fiberoptic rhinoscopy is not usually performed in younger children, because cooperation is necessary and the procedure may provoke anxiety and fear in this age group.

Spirometry in our patient revealed a borderline obstructive pattern that showed a significant improvement to normal values after an aerosol albuterol treatment. It should be emphasized that in cough-variant asthma the spirometric result may be normal, and a trial of antiinflammatory therapy may be utilized to make the diagnosis. Alternatively, a methacholine challenge can be performed, but this is rarely indicated in clinical practice and is usually done only if the therapeutic trial is unsuccessful. If a recent purified protein derivative (PPD) test has not been performed, this should be done. In our case, the child had a PPD test 4 months before the initial visit and this was negative. An immunologic work-up was not performed in our patient, with the exception of serum immunoglobulins, which were normal. Usually the type of immunodeficiency associated with recurrent sinusitis is a defect of antibody production. If such an evaluation is undertaken, quantitative measurements of IgG, IgA, IgM, IgE, and IgG subclasses and complement screening with C3, C4, and CH50 should be obtained. A functional assessment of the IgG subclass system should be evaluated for both protein and polysaccharide antigens by measuring response before and after vaccination with diphtheria and tetanus toxoid (IgG 1 and 3) and 23-valent pneumococcal vaccine (IgG 2 and 4). Consideration may also be given to testing for the human immunodeficiency virus, a biopsy for the dysmotile cilia syndrome, and a sweat test for cystic fibrosis. In our patient, because of normal growth and development and positive findings of allergic disease, the preponderance of evidence points to allergy as the underlying cause.

TREATMENT

At this point the diagnosis in our patient is chronic sinusitis, allergic rhinitis, and asthma. For the allergic rhinitis, the child was begun on intranasal beclomethasone, 1 spray in each nostril bid. Saline nasal washes were advised to remove crusted mucus and improve mucociliary clearance. Dust mite precautions were recommended. For the chronic sinusitis the child was treated for 4 weeks with amoxicillin-potassium clavulanate. A subsequent CT scan was normal. For the asthma, in addition to the above environmental controls, the child was begun on sodium cromolyn, two puffs tid through InspirEase, and an albuterol inhaler, one or two puffs every 4 hours as needed. Peak flow monitoring three times a day was also begun.

Medical management of chronic sinusitis involves antimicrobial therapy in conjunction with treatment of underlying allergic diseases and maintenance of nasal hygiene; surgery is rarely indicated. The three organisms most often implicated are *Streptococcus pneumoniae*, *Moraxella catarrhalis*, and *Haemophilus influenzae*; however, *Streptococcus pyogenes*, *Staphylococcus aureus*, and anerobes of the upper respiratory tract (including β-lactamase producers) must also be considered. In uncomplicated sinus disease, amoxicillin is the drug of choice. β-lactamase producers are resistant to amoxicillin, but amoxicillin can be combined with potassium clavulanate to overcome such resistance and also provide coverage for many anerobes.

Alternative drugs to consider are erythromycin-sulfisoxazole and sulfamethoxazole-trimethoprim, although resistance to group A streptococcus and *S. pneumoniae* may occur. Newer cephalosporins (cefadroxil monohydrate and cefuroxime axetil) are excellent agents. Both are resistant to β-lactamase producers and are given twice daily. In particularly refractory cases in which anerobes are highly suspect, clindamycin and metronidazole may be added.

Although no adequate studies on the length of treatment have been performed, a 2-week course for acute sinusitis is needed. For chronic sinusitis, 4 to 6 weeks may be necessary, and in any child in whom surgery is being contemplated, a 6- to 12-week course should be given.

Useful adjunctive treatment consists of a saline nasal spray, which may improve mucociliary clearance. In cases of extreme nasal mucosal edema, topical decongestants such as oxymetazoline given 10 minutes before administration of an intranasal steroid spray, may improve delivery. However, topical decongestants should not be used for more than 3 to 5 days because of the danger of rebound or rhinitis medicamentosa.

A short course of oral corticosteroids may be indicated if marked nasal occlusion is present. The long-term use of α-adrenergic decongestants remains controversial, but these may provide some benefit early in the treatment. Antihistamines may be helpful for allergic patients but are otherwise not indicated. Although intranasal steroids have not been conclusively shown to be of benefit in sinusitis, they can theoretically decrease inflammation and therefore promote drainage as well as decrease symptoms secondary to allergy.

Although our patient did not require surgical intervention, there are patients in whom medical therapy fails. A CT scan is obtained after antimicrobial treatment to assess the site and degree of residual sinus disease. Surgery is indicated if significant diseased tissue is still present. Functional endoscopic sinus surgery should be performed only by surgeons with extensive experience in the technique in children. Adenoidectomy may also be indicated in some patients with such symptoms as nasal obstruction, snoring, persistent mouth breathing, and chronic middle ear disease.

RESULTS

After the 4-week course of antibiotics, the child's cough and nasal congestion resolved. Dust mite precautions were instituted (Box 16-1) and she was subsequently able to discontinue the intranasal steroids as well as the inhaled sodium cromolyn. In the following spring, before the onset of the tree and grass season, intranasal sodium cromolyn was begun, and the child remained essentially asymptomatic. Follow-up pulmonary function test results were normal.

As can be seen from the above case, an adequate length of antibiotic therapy and the removal of potential allergens are important factors in this disease. Too often, limited (7- to 10-day) courses of antibiotics are given that may suppress symptoms only to have them return in a short time. In addition, causative organisms may become resistent if an antibiotic is given for an inadequate period of time or in suboptimal dose. If allergic factors are not addressed, symptoms may return once medical therapy is discontinued. In some patients, immunotherapy with appropriate allergens may be indicated. Another important

BOX 16-1

Dust Mite Precautions

1. Impermeable covers should be placed on pillows, boxspring, and mattress
2. Drapes and blinds should be removed from the bedroom; replace with shades
3. Remove rugs and clutter from the bedroom
4. Stuffed animals should be removed if not washable
5. Sheets, pillow cases, blankets, and stuffed animals should be washed in hot water (>130° F) every 2 weeks
6. A humidity gauge should be obtained (ideal 40%-50%); humidity >50% promotes the replication of dust mite
7. If possible, cleaning should be performed by someone else, and the allergic person should be out of the house for 4 hours after cleaning is done
8. If any cleaning is done, a dust mask should be worn
9. Exhaust filter and double-thickness vacuum cleaner bags should be obtained
10. Filters should be installed and cleaned regularly on heating and air conditioning units.

BOX 16-2

Proposed Mechanisms Linking Upper Airway Disease and Asthma

Reflex bronchospasm produced by nasal stimulation
Postnasal drip of inflammatory material into the lower airways
Delivery of inflammatory products to the lower airways from the paranasal sinuses via the systemic circulation
Nasal obstruction resulting in mouth breathing of cold air
Reduction of β-adrenergic responsiveness

From Coven J, Rachelefsky GS: Interrelationship between sinusitis and asthma, *Immunol Allergy Clin North Am* 14:1, 1994.

issue raised in our example is the relationship between asthma and sinus disease. Addressing this issue specifically in children, many studies have documented significant improvement in asthma after appropriate management of sinusitis. One study by Rachelefsky and colleagues[6] showed that 70% of 48 children no longer required bronchodilators once their sinusitis had been treated. In addition, pulmonary function test results returned to normal in 67% of those with pretreatment abnormalities. In Box 16-2 the proposed mechanisms explaining the relationship between sinusitis and asthma are presented.

DISCUSSION

Our case has illustrated several critical factors that must be addressed in any evaluation and treatment of a child with sinusitis and asthma. Several pitfalls to avoid are listed below.

1. Failure to treat for an adequate length of time and with appropriate antibiotics.
2. Failure to address underlying contributing factors, particularly allergic phenomena where environmental controls may potentially eliminate recurrence.
3. Failure to consider that cough may be caused not only by postnasal drip but by several other factors, including underlying hyperactive airway disease.
4. Failure to maximize use of adjunctive therapies: intranasal steroids, saline nasal spray, and decongestants where indicated.
5. Failure to treat the upper and lower airway with antiinflammatory therapy and relying solely on symptomatic treatment. Often, when antiinflammatory therapy has been instituted, the necessity of using these drugs daily, as opposed to "as needed," is not appropriately emphasized.
6. Relying on negative plain films to rule out sinus disease, since disease in the ethmoid sinuses may be missed. If clinically indicated, empiric antimicrobial treatment should be instituted. Only if the patient is unresponsive and surgical intervention is being contemplated should a CT scan be performed.

Upper and lower airway disease is one of the most common problems seen by the primary care physician. Proper management and successful outcome can be achieved by proper attention to detail and by utilizing the expertise of appropriate specialists, including allergists and otolaryngologists, in a team approach.

REFERENCES

1. Gottleib MJ: Relation of intranasal disease in the production of bronchial asthma, *JAMA* 85, 1925.
2. Virant FS, Shapiro GG: *Evaluation of the child with chronic cough and/or wheezing.* In Tinkelman DG, Naspitz CK, editors: *Childhood Asthma, pathophysiology and treatment,* New York, 1987, Marcel Dekker.
3. Slavin RG, Piphorn U, McFadden ER Jr: Pathophysiological interaction of the upper and lower airway, *J Respir Dis* 12:59, 1991.
4. Wald ER: Chronic sinusitis in children, *J Pediatr* 127:339, 1995.
5. Bierman CW, Pearlman DS, Shapiro GG, Busse WW: *Allergy, asthma and immunology from infancy* to adulthood, ed 3, Philadelphia, 1996, WB Saunders.
6. Rachelefsky GS, Katz RM, Siegel SC: Chronic sinus disease with associated reactive airway disease in children, *Pediatrics* 73:526, 1984.

SUGGESTED READINGS

Ellis EF: *Asthma in infancy and childhood.* In Middleton E, Reed CE, Ellis EF, et al, editors: *Allergy principles and practice*, ed 4, St. Louis, 1993, Mosby–Year Book.

Very comprehensive and practical.

Friedman WH, Slavin RG: Diagnosis and medical and surgical treatment of sinusitis in adults, *Clin Rev Allergy* 2:409, 1984.

Hannaway PT, Hoffer DK: Cough variant asthma in children, *JAMA* 246:206, 1982.

Virant FS: Chronic sinus disease, *Immunol Allergy Clin North Am* 14:1, 1994.

Excellent comprehensive reference that covers in 12 chapters the essential concepts in evaluation and management of sinus disease in adults and children (both medical and surgical treatments).

CHAPTER 17

Management of Recurrent Maxillary Sinus Disease by Caldwell-Luc

Andrew Blitzer

PROBLEM

A 70-year-old man presented with a several-year history of foul drainage from the nose and a "bad taste" in his mouth.

MEDICAL HISTORY

The patient had an extraction of a second maxillary molar about 5 years before presentation. One year previously he was found to have a small oroantral fistula and sinusitis. He was placed on antibiotics and then underwent an endoscopic middle meatal antrotomy and sinus irrigation. An oral surgeon also performed several procedures, using a buccal mucosal advancement flap to close the fistula. Despite these operative procedures, the patient continued to have drainage and facial pain.

PHYSICAL AND RADIOGRAPHIC EXAMINATION

On examination, he was found to have some tenderness over the right maxillary sinus as well as a small pinhole fistula through the maxillary alveolar ridge that extended into the sinus. When the fistula was probed, purulent material expressed itself from the sinus into the oral cavity. A culture was taken and revealed a mixed flora. A computed tomographic (CT) scan showed a bony dehiscence in the area of the fistula as well as evidence of persistent chronic maxillary sinusitis (Figs. 17-1 to 17-3).

TREATMENT

It was suggested to the patient that simply opening a wide middle meatal antrotomy and closing the oral mucosa was not enough. The persistence of the fistula with purulent drainage despite long courses of antibiotics, endoscopic surgery, and oral closure of the fistula was suggestive of a persistent nidus of infection such as a foreign body or osteomyelitis. A Caldwell-Luc approach with an anterior antrotomy is better able to reach and visualize the interstices of the sinus. It also allows for the removal of all infected soft tissues within the maxillary antrum. At the time of surgery an area of necrotic bone was found in the area of the maxillary alveolar ridge. In combination with an oral incision the bony sequestrum was removed and the bone was trimmed back to healthy, bleeding bone. All the granulation tissue was removed using the oral cavity and through an antrotomy. When the area was totally clean, the buccal flap was trimmed, released, and advanced to allow for closure of the fistula. The middle meatal antrotomy was opened widely. The patient was kept on antibiotics for several weeks. The flap healed without incident and the sinus remained free of disease.

DISCUSSION

This case demonstrates that despite the advent of endoscopy and changes in paranasal sinus surgery, some patients still have conditions that require the greater visualization and access provided by the Caldwell-Luc operation.

Early sinus surgery, particularly in the preantibiotic era, was designed to establish ventilation and drainage from the sinuses. At first, various techniques were used to puncture the antrum in order to permit irrigation. It next

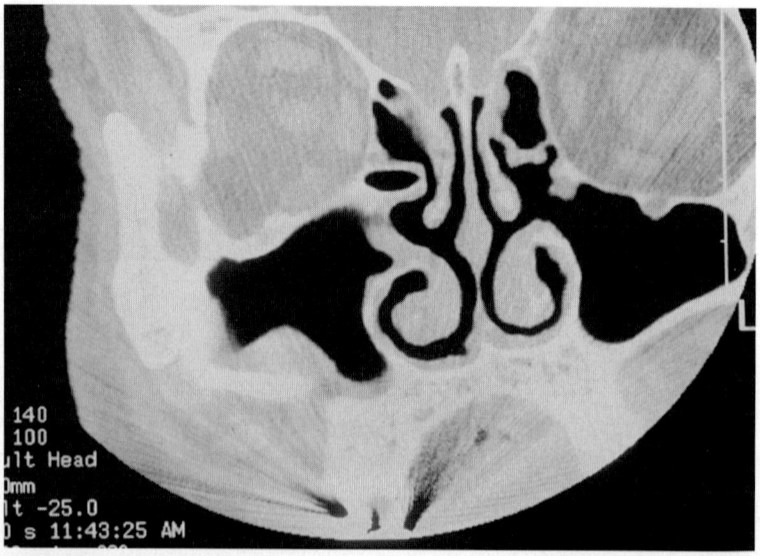

Fig. 17-1. Coronal computed tomography (CT) of the maxillary sinuses showing a dehiscence in the maxillary alveolar bone as well as soft tissue swelling in the floor of the right maxillary antrum.

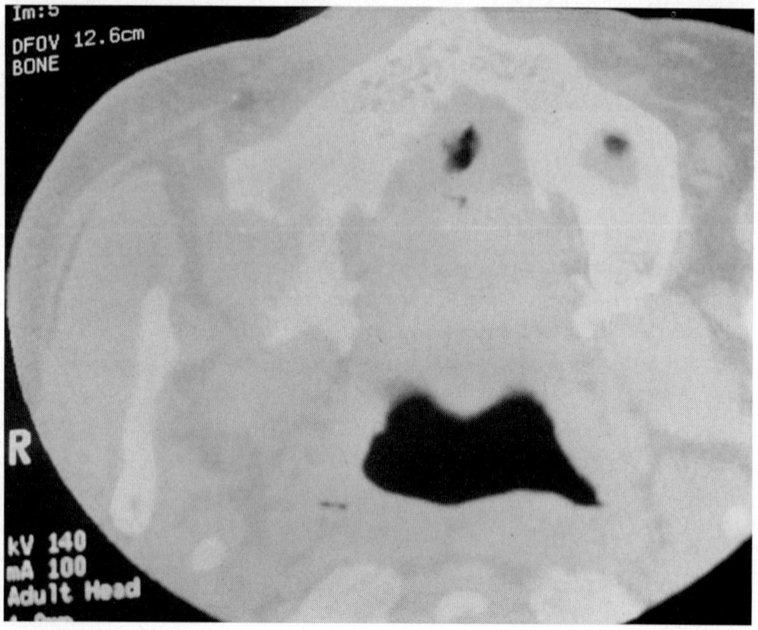

Fig. 17-2. Axial CT through the maxillary alveolar structures showing loss of bone on the right.

became recognized that a larger opening was needed to allow continued drainage, facilitate repeat sinus irrigations, permit inspection of the antrum, and allow the removal of polypoid or necrotic tissue from the cavity. Sluder (1919) advocated removal of the entire medial wall of the antrum. However, despite the creation of these large openings, chronic sinusitis persisted due to infected polypoid mucosa present within the sinus. In 1893, George Caldwell described a procedure that made a temporary opening in the canine fossa to reach the sinus for the removal of the mucous membranes, and combined this with a large nasal antrostomy. In 1894, Guy Luc reported a similar procedure. This operation has since become known eponymously as the Caldwell-Luc procedure in the United States and the Luc-Caldwell in Europe.[1-4]

The Caldwell-Luc procedure has become a standard approach for the management of antral disease as well as an operative route to reach such sites as the pterygomaxillary space, orbit, ethmoid labyrinth, and medial skull base.[5] New antibiotic therapy has obviated the need of the original Caldwell-Luc procedure to remove all the infected polypoid mucosa of the maxillary antrum. Technologic advances have led to the development of endoscopic sinus surgery. Surgery using video cameras and endoscopes with angled views and magnification have changed, and continue to change, many of the indications for the Caldwell-Luc procedure. It is no longer necessary

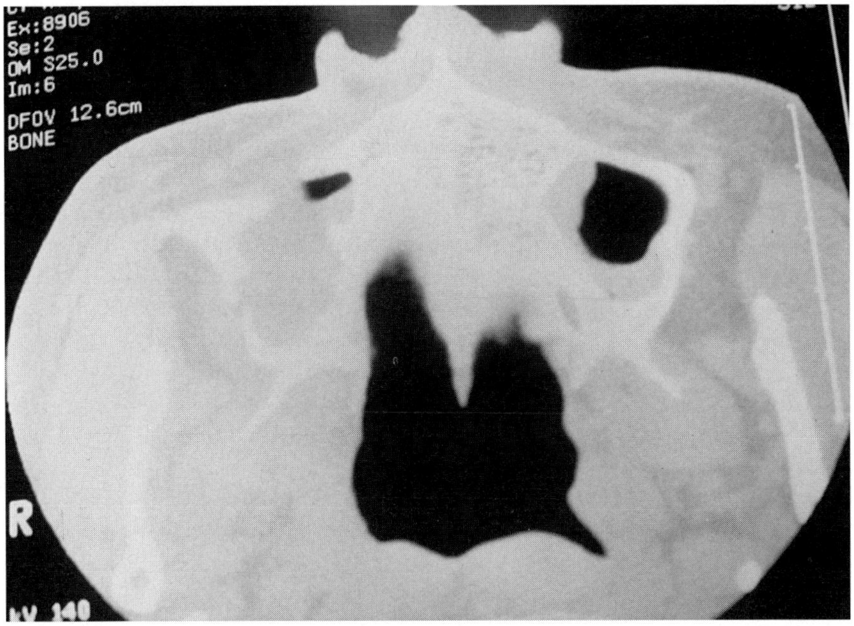

Fig. 17-3. Axial CT at a higher level through the maxillary sinus showing opacification with soft tissue of the right maxillary antrum, as well as a dehiscence in the lateral antral wall and evidence of previous anterior antrotomy.

to violate the anterior wall of the antrum to remove a polyp or cyst, to obtain a biopsy, to remove most foreign bodies, or to establish drainage of the sinus. Messerklinger and colleagues also reestablished the work of McKenzie in defining the important role of the middle meatus, and developed an endoscopic middle meatal antrotomy.[6,7] There still remain, however, situations in which the wide anterior exposure provided by the Caldwell-Luc procedure is beneficial to the treatment of disease. With new modifications, the procedure can be performed with relatively few side effects.[8,9,10,11]

One such instance is orbital decompression of significant malignant exophthalmos in patients with Graves' disease (Fig. 17-1). Over the years, several procedures have been employed in an attempt to create additional space for the increased orbital volume resulting from the swelling of the extraocular muscles. The Krönlein[1] procedure removed the lateral orbital rim, permitting expansion of the orbital contents into the temporal fossa. Naffziger[1] reported removing the orbital roof to allow expansion of the orbital contents into the anterior cranial fossa. This later procedure was complicated by the transmission of dural pulsations to the globe. Hirsch[12] described removal of the orbital floor, while Sewall[13] reported resection of the lamina papyracea to decompress the orbit medially. Walsh and Ogura[14] combined the Hirsch and Sewall procedures to achieve wide exposure and maximal decompression. Others have used the endoscopic approach to perform a decompression, but the exposure for removal of the posterior and lateral areas of the orbital floor is limited. Therefore, a wide anterior approach gives better access with less risk of damage to the neural and vascular structures.

Walsh and Ogura believed that their procedure was indicated in patients with Graves' ophthalmopathy in whom were loss of visual acuity, changes on the corneal epithelium, progressive loss of extraocular function, conjunctival chemosis, orbital edema, or cosmetic disfigurement was found. Briefly, the Walsh and Ogura procedure is performed through a wide anterior wall antrotomy. A transantral ethmoidectomy is performed by way of the maxilloethmoidal plate. The thin bone of the orbital floor (including the entire canal of the infraorbital nerve) and the lamina papyracea is removed, exposing the periosteum. At this point, parallel incisions are made through the periosteum with a sickle knife to allow herniation of orbital fat. The number and extent of periosteal incisions are determined by observation of the eyes to ascertain the adequacy and symmetry of reduction. Poor reduction of volume in severe cases endangers vision; consequently, only procedures yielding maximal exposure and safety to the eye, as well as maximal decompression, should be advocated for this disorder.[15]

Another use of the Caldwell-Luc procedure is for surgical access of the pterygomaxillary space. In 1928 Seiffert[16] first reported the transantral approach to the pterygopalatine fossa for ligation of the internal maxillary artery (IMA) to treat epistaxis. Other authors, including Gergely,[17] Hirsch,[18] Davis,[19] and Chandler and Serrins,[20] also advocated this approach for IMA ligation. Sewall[21] described the transantral approach for sphenopalatine ganglion resection. Resection of the second division of the fifth cranial nerve or sphenopalatine ganglion for trigeminal or sphenopalatine neuralgia, respectively, and resection of the vidian nerve for chronic vasomotor rhinitis by way of a transantral approach have also been reported.[22-24] With the increased use of the operating microscope and the availability of smaller instruments, the technique may be performed through a smaller anterior antrotomy with excellent visualization and control of the structures of the pterygomaxillary space. The transantral approach to the IMA has the advantage of permitting ligation of the distal branches as well as the main trunk, for more complete hemostasis of the nasal cavity. The use of new instruments such as vascular clip appliers and telescopes allow for smaller antrotomies with a decreased risk of complications.[25] Neel[26] reviewed the use of the transantral approach to the pterygomaxillary space, in combination with other approaches (e.g., transnasal, transpalatal, facial degloving), for the resection of vascular tumors such as juvenile angiofibromas (Fig. 17-2).

The transantral approach is also occasionally employed in cases of facial trauma. The sublabial incision allows access to fractures of the malar bone, nasomaxillary complex, and orbital floor. With an unstable malar fracture, the antrum can be filled with a balloon or gauze pack for support. With comminution of the orbital floor and prolapse and/or entrapment of the orbital contents, a combined infraorbital-transantral approach permits reduction under direct vision; an antral pack can also be placed to buttress the bony fragments.[27] The anterior or degloving approach also allows for placement of plate or wire fixation.

The Caldwell-Luc procedure offers maximal exposure for the removal of foreign bodies that may be large or in a very anterior, posterior, or lateral position, making endoscopic removal difficult. The foreign bodies may have concomitant inflammatory tissues in the sinus or may be associated with underlying dental disease. Materials such as root fragments after exodontics, supernumerary teeth, sinoliths, displaced dental materials, and embedded projectiles have all been successfully treated via the Caldwell-Luc procedure.[1,28-31]

This approach is often necessary to repair oroantral fistulas. Most such fistulas arise as a consequence of dental extraction. In patients with normal sinus function, these fistulas often close spontaneously or can be repaired with a local flap. The refractory cases are those with preexisting sinus abnormalities, in which chronic inflammatory disease in the antrum interferes with the healing of the dental socket. These cases should be treated from above and below to ensure permanent closure of the fistula. The Caldwell-Luc technique provides access for the removal of polyps, granulation tissue, dental fragments or filling materials, and osteitic bone and also supplies sinus ventilation.[32-34]

The Caldwell-Luc procedure is also excellent for the management of maxillary osteomyelitis or osteoradionecrosis. It may be necessary to resect necrotic bone back to the zygomatic process, orbital apex, or pterygoid plates. Such an extensive resection is best and most safely performed through a direct approach.[35]

The Caldwell-Luc approach also offers a wide exposure for the removal of a variety of odontogenic lesions, including cysts and benign tumors (Fig. 17-3).[36] These lesions are often related to the roots of erupted teeth and the crowns of unerupted teeth. Pathologic conditions of the dentoalveolar portion of the maxilla are best removed through a sublabial approach by means of a gingival flap that also permits closure of the oroantral communication.[37] Other benign tumors that may invade the maxillary sinus include inverting papillomas,[38,39] ossifying fibromas, odontogenic keratocysts,[40] osteomas, fibrous dysplasia,[41] myxomas, giant cell tumors, fibromas, and hemangiomas. They are more readily enucleated with the wide exposure achieved via the Caldwell-Luc approach.[42] Some medial skull base tumors can be treated through a transmaxilloethmoidosphenoidal approach,[43] which has also been used to reach the clivus.[44]

Finally, the Caldwell-Luc procedure is necessary in patients in whom there has been irreversible scarring and metaplasia of the sinus mucosa with failure of the mucociliary apparatus. These patients do poorly with inferior or middle meatal antrotomies because there is often little or no propulsion of the mucous blanket, and stasis leads to chronic infection. These are the cases that require revision after comprehensive endoscopic nasal surgery, including complete ethmoidectomy via intranasal, external, or transantral approaches.[45,46] The failed endoscopic procedures often involve polypoid and scarred mucosa, despite a widely patent middle meatus. Failure is due not to poor ventilation or residual ethmoidal disease, but to irreversible mucosal changes.[1,47-51]

CONCLUSION

The Caldwell-Luc procedure has been the mainstay of maxillary sinus surgery over the past century. Its role dramatically changed in the face of new technology, just as laparotomy has become less often employed with the advent of the laparoscope. However, the Caldwell-Luc approach still has a limited role in providing wide access for the performance of other procedures; for the removal of foreign bodies or benign tumors; and for the management of chronic, refractory sinus disease.

REFERENCES

1. Blitzer A: *Surgery for infection and benign disease of the maxillary sinus*. In Blitzer A, Lawson W, Friedman WH, editors: *Surgery of the Paranasal Sinuses*, ed 2, Philadelphia, 1991, WB Saunders, pp 277-287.
2. Buiter CT: *Nasalantrotomy*, *Rhinology* 26:5-18, 1988.
3. Caldwell GW: Diseases of the accessory sinuses of the nose, and improved method of treatment of suppression of the maxillary antrum, *NY Med J* 58:526, 1893.
4. Harle F: The history of maxillary sinus surgery from Leonardo da Vinci until today, *Bull Hist Dent* 40:79-84, 1992.
5. Tange RA: Some historical aspects of the surgical treatment of the infected maxillary sinus, *Rhinology* 29:155-162, 1991.

6. Messerklinger W: *Über die Drainage der Menschlichen Nasennebenho. Ohrenhelkunde und Laryngo-rhinogie*, Vienna, 1966, Verlag Urban and Schwartzenberg.
7. Messerklinger W: On the drainage of the normal frontal sinus of man, *Acta Otolaryngol* 63:176, 1967.
8. Stammberger H: Endoscopic endonasal surgery—concepts in the treatment of recurring rhinosinusitis. I. Anatomic and pathophysiologic considerations, *Otolaryngol Head Neck Surg* 94:143, 1986.
9. Wigand ME, Steiner W, Jaumann MP: Endonasal sinus surgery with endoscopic control: from radical operation to rehabilitation of the mucosa, *Endoscopy* 10:255, 1978.
10. Pradhan KA, Baser B: Caldwell-Luc operation without facial swelling, *Auris Nasus Larynx* 16:223-226, 1990.
11. Low WK: Complications of the Caldwell-Luc operation and how to avoid them, *Aust N Z J Surg* 65:582-584, 1995.
12. Hirsch O: Malignant exophthalmos, *Arch Otolaryngol* 51:325, 1950.
13. Sewall EC: Operative control of progressive exophthalmos, *JAMA* 112:37, 1939.
14. Walsh TE, Ogura JH: Transantral orbital decompression for malignant exophthalmos, *Laryngoscope* 65:544, 1957.
15. Lucente FE, Biller HF: Orbital decompression. In Blitzer A, Lawson W, Friedman WH, editors: *Surgery of the paranasal sinuses*, ed 2, Philadelphia, 1991, WB Saunders, pp 355-363.
16. Seiffert H: Ligature of the internal maxillary artery for epistaxis, *Z Hals Nasu Ohrenheilk* 22:323, 1928.
17. Gergely Z: Transmaxillary ligature of the artery maxillaris interna, *Acta Otolaryngol* 22:142, 1935.
18. Hirsch O: Ligation of the internal maxillary artery in patients with nasal hemorrhage, *Acta Otolaryngol* 24:589, 1936.
19. Davis EDD: Ligation of the internal maxillary artery through the antrum for uncontrollable epistaxis, *J Laryngol* 60:420, 1945.
20. Chandler JR, Serrins AJ: Transantral ligation of the internal maxillary artery for epistaxis, *Laryngoscope* 75:1151, 1965.
21. Sewall EC: An operation for the removal of sphenopalatine ganglion, *Ann Otol* 35:1, 1926.
22. Golding-Wood PH: Petrosal and vidian neurectomy in chronic vasomotor rhinitis, *J Laryngol Otol* 75:232, 1961.
23. Montgomery W: Analysis of pterygopalatine space surgery, *Laryngoscope* 80:1190, 1970.
24. Friedman WH: *Surgery of the pterygopalatine fossa.* In Blitzer A, Lawson W, Friedman WH, editors: *Surgery of the paranasal sinuses*, ed 2, Philadelphia, 1991, WB Saunders, pp 331-339.
25. Busch RF: A new vascular clip applier for internal maxillary and ethmoidal artery ligations, *Otolaryngol Head Neck Surg* 107:129-130, 1992.
26. Neel HB: *Juvenile angiofibroma.* In Blitzer A, Lawson W, Friedman WH, editors: *Surgery of the paranasal sinuses*, ed 2, Philadelphia, 1991, WB Saunders, pp 363-377.
27. Rowe NL: *Fractures of the zygomatic complex and orbit.* In Rowe NL, Williams JL, editors: *Maxillofacial injuries*, London, 1985, Churchill Livingstone, pp 506-522.
28. Bernstein L: *The Caldwell-Luc operation.* In English G, editor: *Otolaryngology*, Hagerstown, Md, 1989, Harper & Row.
29. Friedman WH, Katsantonis GP: The role of standard techniques in modern sinus surgery, *Otolaryngol Clin North Am* 22:759-775, 1989.
30. Fairbanks DFN, Barr NL: *Foreign bodies in the nose and paranasal sinuses.* In English GE, editor: *Otolaryngology*, Hagerstown, Md, 1989, Harper & Row, pp 1-7.
31. Di Felice R, Lombardi T: Ectopic third molar in the maxillary sinus. Case report, *Aust Dent J* 40:236-237, 1995.
32. Loscalzo LJ: *Treatment of chronic oroantral fistula.* In Blitzer A, Lawson W, Friedman WH, editors: *Surgery of the paranasal sinuses*, ed 2, Philadelphia, 1991, WB Saunders, pp 289-297.
33. Montgomery WW, Cheney ML, Turner PA: *External sinus surgery.* In Pillsbury HC, Goldsmith MM, editors: *Operative challenges in otolaryngology–head and neck surgery*, St. Louis, 1990, Mosby–Year Book, pp 258-264.
34. Jerome CE: Maxillary molar root fragment caused by sinus surgery: case report, *Endodont Dent Traumatol* 10:286-288, 1994.
35. Fairbanks DNF, Vanderveen TS, Bordley JE: *Intracranial complications of sinusitis.* In English GE, editor: *Otolaryngology*, Philadelphia, 1989, Harper and Row, pp 5-12.
36. Lee CY, Mohammadi H, Mostofi R, Habibi A: Calcifying epithelial odontogenic tumor of the maxillary sinus, *J Oral Maxillofac Surg* 50:1326-1328, 1992.
37. McClatchey KD: *Odontogenic lesions—tumors and cysts.* In Batsakis JG, editor: *Tumors of the head and neck*, (Baltimore, 1979, Williams & Wilkins, pp 531-561.
38. Benninger MS, Lavertu P, Levine H, Tucker HM: Conservation surgery for inverted papillomas, *Head Neck Surg* 13:442-445, 1991.
39. Dolgin SR, Zaveri VD, Casiano RR, Maniglia AJ: *Different options for treatment of inverting papilloma of the nose and paranasal sinus: a report of 41 cases*, *Laryngoscope* 102:231-236, 1992.
40. Absi EG, Sim RL: Odontogenic keratocyst involving the maxillary sinus: report of two cases, *Dento-Maxillo-Facial Radiol* 23:226-229, 1994.
41. Kearns D, McGill T, Potsic W: Fibrous dysplasia, *Head Neck* 14:510-512, 1992.
42. Yanagisawa E, Yanagisawa K, Fortgang P: Endoscopic excision of a large benign antral lesion via a modified ("mini") Caldwell-Luc procedure, *Ear Nose Throat J* 74:620-621, 1995.
43. Fraioli B, Esposito V, Santoro A, et al: Transmaxillosphenoidal approach to tumors invading the medical compartment of the cavernous sinus, *J Neurosurg* 82:63-69, 1995.
44. Rabadan A, Conesa H: Transmaxillary-transnasal approach to the anterior clivus: a microsurgical anatomical model, *Neurosurgery* 30:473-481, 1992.
45. Malotte MJ, Petti GH, Chonkich GD, Rowe RP: Transantral sphenoethmoidectomy: a procedure for the 1990's?, *Otolaryngol Head Neck Surg* 104:358-361, 1991.
46. Loury MC, Hinkley DK, Wong W: Endoscopic transantral antrochoanal polypectomy: an alternative to the transantral approach, *South Med J* 86:18-22, 1993.
47. Ng M, Rice DH: Revision sinus surgery, *Ear Nose Throat J* 73:44-46, 1994.
48. Forsgren K, Fukami M, Penttila M, et al: Endoscopic and Caldwell-Luc approaches in chronic maxillary sinusitis: a comparative histopathologic study on preoperative and postoperative mucosal morphology, *Ann Otol Rhinol Laryngol* 104:350-357, 1995.
49. Lund VJ, Neijens HJ, Clement PA, et al: The treatment of chronic sinusitis: a controversial issue, *Int J Pediatr Otorhinolaryngol* 32 suppl:S21-35, 1995.
50. Hyams VJ: *Pathology of the nose and paranasal sinuses.* In English G, editor: *Otolaryngology*, Hagerstown, Md, 1989, Harper & Row, pp 11-13.
51. Blitzer A, Lawson WL: The Caldwell-Luc procedure in 1991, *Otolaryngol Head Neck Surg* 105:717-723, 1991.

CHAPTER

18

The Intranasal Sphenoethmoidectomy

William Lawson
Anthony J. Reino

PROBLEM

A 34-year-old man complains of 10 years of green, mucoid drainage from both nostrils and midfacial pain. He notes that he averages three to five such episodes of purulent rhinorrhea per year, which require antibiotic treatment. He now finds each such episode is slower to respond to antibiotics and requires longer durations of treatment. Previous evaluation by his general physician included plain film x-rays of the face, which were said to show sinusitis.

Historically, the first account of surgery performed on the ethmoidal labyrinth was by Hippocrates (460-370 BC), who avulsed nasal polyps and adjacent ethmoidal cells using a sponge attached to traction strings.[1] This was used in conjunction with an instrument that resembled today's polyp snare. Much to the patient's dismay, bleeding was controlled with a hot iron cautery. These simple avulsion techniques for nasal polypectomy were considered the standard of care until 1884, when Jansen[2] reported the first transantral ethmoidectomy. This marked the true beginning of the planned operative removal of ethmoidal sinus disease.

In 1912, Mosher[3] presented a method of intranasal extirpation of the ethmoidal sinus based on his anatomic studies. In his technique, the labyrinth was widely exenterated and the middle turbinate totally resected. Yankauer[4] described the complete exenteration of the ethmoids and removal of the anterior wall of the sphenoid in a stepwise procedure that he termed *sphenoethmoidectomy*.

After delineation of the anatomy of the ethmoidal labyrinth and its relationship to contiguous structures, transnasal ethmoidectomy has evolved from the classic or conventional method performed with a headlight to the use of such optical adjuncts as the microscope and endoscope. The procedure may encompass a portion or the whole of the accessible ethmoidal sinus.

Partial ethmoidectomy, or ostiomeatal resection, is performed in patients with limited anterior ethmoidal disease. This makes up a small portion of the authors' practice. With diffuse and scattered disease within the labyrinth, total ethmoidectomy is performed, generally in conjunction with a sphenoid sinusotomy. The marsupialized sphenoid ostium is used as a critical landmark to the posterior limit of dissection and for the removal of intracavitary disease. In patients with extensive nasal polyposis, with or without asthma, a total sphenoethmoidectomy is invariably performed.

The operative technique uses both the coaxial headlight and endoscopes, for reasons to be cited, combining the advantages of both methods. The authors' methods differ from the purely endoscopic approach in that the resection is initially carried anterior to posterior in the manner of Yankauer[5] and then retrograde along the ethmoidal roof endoscopically in a manner similar to that of Wigand and Hosemann.[6] The middle turbinate is partially resected to obtain improved operative access and wider patency of the middle meatus postoperatively. Removal of the ground lamella of the middle turbinate destabilizes it and favors synechiae formation, occasionally requiring revision surgery. We have not found any instance of atrophic rhinitis after its resection at our institution in several thousand cases.

Most cases are performed with the patient under general anesthesia without increased blood loss, with greater patient comfort and compliance, and with virtually the complete elimination of asthmatic attacks intraoperatively.

In patients experiencing increased bleeding from advanced disease in which sequential endoscopic removal is difficult or impossible, surgical debulking with the headlight has reduced operative time considerably and has made complete ethmoidectomy feasible.

The operative management of ethmoidal sinus disease has been controversial since its inception in the early part of the twentieth century. The various schools of intranasal, transantral, external, and endoscopic ethmoidectomy have had their proponents according to the relative advantages and disadvantages of each method. However, for reasons that will soon become apparent, the ethmoidal sinus remains a minefield for both the experienced and novice sinus surgeon despite much-improved instrumentation and technology.

INDICATIONS FOR SURGERY

Candidates for intranasal ethmoidectomy are those individuals with chronic recurrent sinusitis who have been refractory to medical management and who show radiographic evidence of a pathologic sinusal condition. Surgery on the ethmoidal sinuses is directed not only toward the extirpation of disease in the labyrinth, but also to the reversal of mucosal changes in the adjacent maxillary, frontal, and sphenoid sinuses by the widening of their ostia and ventilation of their cavities.

The clinical diagnosis of sinusitis is made on a tripartite basis, involving symptoms, rhinoscopy, and radiographic findings. Many signs and symptoms such as purulent rhinorrhea, facial and dental pain, nasal odor, and fetid breath are highly suggestive of a suppurative inflammatory process, but others such as nasal congestion, headache, postnasal discharge, and aural fullness are not.

Advocates of endoscopy cite its value in diagnosing sinus disease by permitting thorough examination of the nasal cavity, and detecting the presence of edematous and polypoid mucosa and purulent secretions in the recesses of the lateral wall, indicating an active disease process. They also cite the demonstration by telescopic rhinoscopy of such anatomic structures as a hypertrophic uncinate process, or bulla ethmoidalis (secondary to increased pneumatization), and an enlarged or paradoxically bent middle turbinate as predisposing factors to sinusitis by causing obstruction of the middle meatus.

Radiographic studies by Zinreich and colleagues[7–8] employing serial coronal computed tomographic (CT) scans have demonstrated the strategic position of excessively aerated agger nasi and Haller's cells producing infundibular narrowing and obstructing frontal and maxillary sinus drainage, creating a high potential for chronic inflammatory disease. However, in the comparative CT study of Bolger and colleagues[9] of 166 patients with chronic sinusitis and 36 patients lacking them, the incidence of Haller's cells, pneumatization of the middle turbinate, and the paradoxically bent middle turbinate was the same in both groups. Extensive differences exist in the development of the ethmoidal complex, producing what should be correctly termed anatomic variations rather than anatomic abnormalities, signifying a high probability of occult sinus disease. These anatomic variations should not be considered an indication for surgery (Fig. 18-1). Calhoun and associates[10] also found on a CT study of 100 sinusitis patients compared with 82 controls that the incidence of a paradoxically bent middle

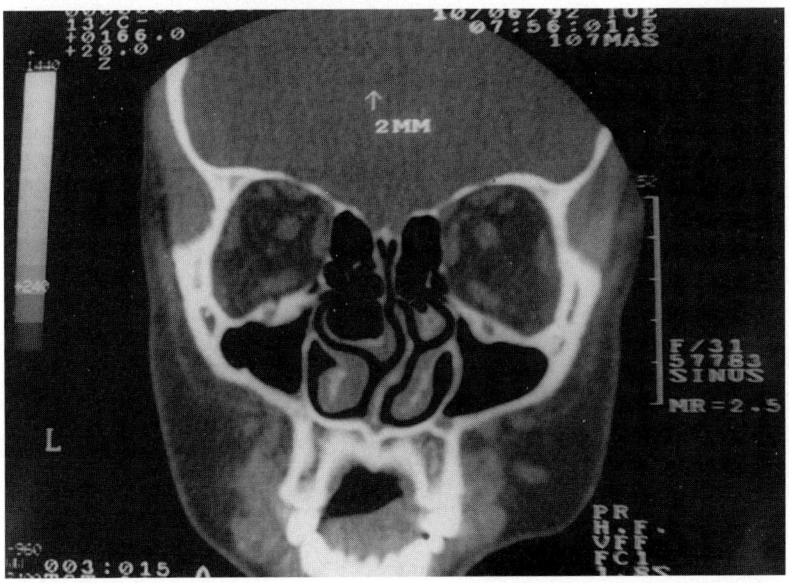

Fig. 18-1. Large concha bullosa with normal sinuses.

turbinate was the same in both groups (12%). Furthermore, the studies by Bolger[9] and Havas[11] and their colleagues revealed a 42% incidence of mucosal abnormalities detected by CT in one or more of the paranasal sinuses in patients without sinus complaints. Glasier[12] and Diamant[13] and their associates noted CT evidence of mucosal disease in 70% of asymptomatic infants under 1 year of age and 50% of children under 12 years of age. It is the authors' opinion that surgery should rarely be performed in patients with a normal CT result (Fig. 18-2). Surgery is indicated for chronic sinusitis that is diagnosed by the above three cited parameters and has been refractory to adequate medical management.

Another major surgical group of patients are those with nasal polyps, with or without asthma, or established atopy. While the predominant symptom is that of nasal obstruction, there generally is also a component of secondary infection resulting from stasis of the secretions.

Some workers[14,15] have extended its applications to the decompression of sinus mucoceles. Kennedy and colleagues[14] reported successful endoscopic marsupialization of frontal sinus mucoceles in nine of 11 patients. However, the longest follow-up in the series was 39 months, with most cases evaluated in less than 2 years. With marsupialization procedures of the frontal sinus, long-term follow-up is essential before success can be claimed. It is well recognized that even the external frontoethmoidectomy, with prolonged stenting and mucosal resurfacing of the neoduct, is subject to stenosis with time. Representative of this situation is the series of cases of Neel and associates,[15] who reported a failure rate of 7% after 3 years that climbed to 20% at 10 years. The series of Kennedy and colleagues[14] included marsupialization of mucopyoceles of the frontal sinus with posterior table erosion and dural exposure. This is a very controversial subject because of the danger of retrograde infection with the development of an intracranial complication in such cases. These workers also reported decompressing ethmoidal mucoceles endoscopically. Wigand[16] employed a combined endoscopic and limited external approach to the removal of polyps, foreign bodies, mucoceles, and benign tumors of the frontal sinus. It is technically feasible to decompress frontal and ethmoidal mucoceles endonasally, but the weight of clinical experiences points to the external approaches (external frontoethmoidectomy, osteoplastic flap) as yielding the best results over time.[17,18]

Contraindications to intranasal ethmoidectomy are radiographic evidence of a bony defect of the lamina papyracea, fovea ethmoidalis, or the cribriform plate (Fig. 18-3). These may be due to congenital absence, previous trauma, or surgery. A relative contraindication is the absence of the middle turbinate with revision surgery. Other contraindications to intranasal surgery are an orbital abscess or an intracranial complication of sinusitis. However, Stammberger[18] favors endoscopic management of orbital complications of sinusitis and considers only intracranial extension of disease a limitation to its application. As stated earlier, we favor the external approach for the management of orbital infections, as it accomplishes surgical drainage, widefield ethmoidal exenteration, and orbital decompression, if needed.

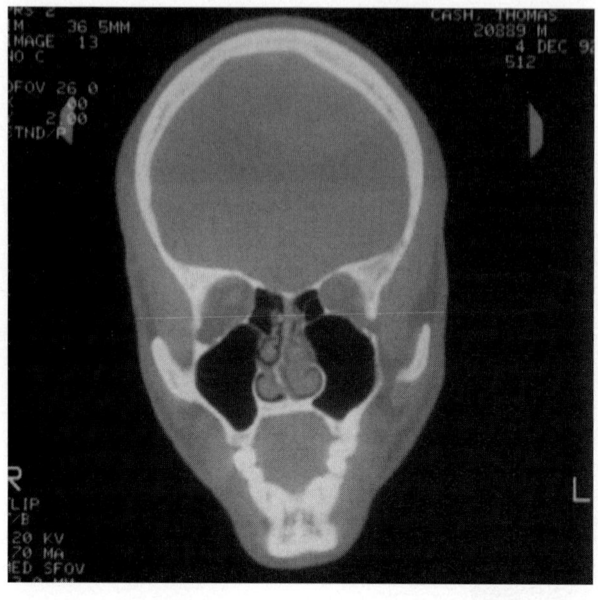

Fig. 18-2. Blocked ostiomeatal unit with normal maxillary and ethmoidal sinuses.

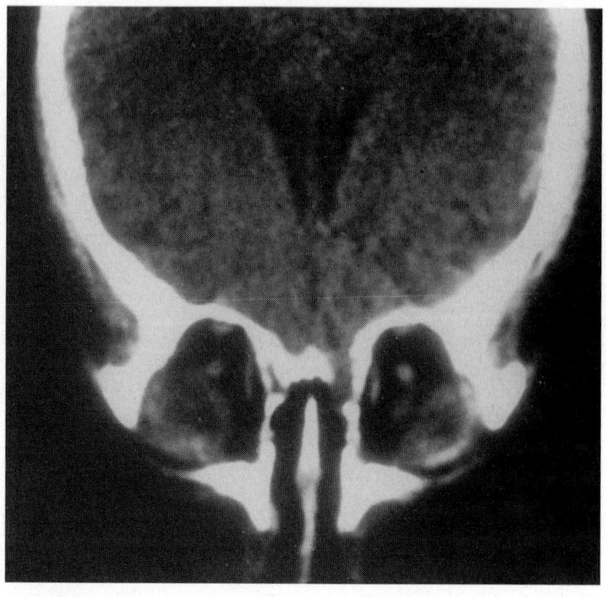

Fig. 18-3. Anatomic defect of the cribriform plate, a contraindication to intranasal ethmoidectomy.

OPERATIVE TECHNIQUE

The procedure is performed using both local and general anesthesia. The latter is preferred because of greater patient compliance, an increased ability to control the blood pressure, and the ability to provide bronchial dilation in severe asthmatics with appropriate inhalant agents. In both instances the nasal cavity is vasoconstricted with topical application of 4% cocaine and infiltration of 1% lidocaine (Xylocaine) and epinephrine 1:100,000 into the nasal septum and lateral nasal walls. The patient is placed in the seated position. This serves to reduce venous pressure, but more important, it places the roof of the nasal cavity parallel to the floor of the room, making inadvertent injury to the fovea ethmoidalis less likely (Fig. 18-4). The procedure is performed with a coaxial headlight and endoscopes. The former provides a panoramic perspective of the entire ethmoidal labyrinth relative to key operative landmarks. The endoscopes are used to evaluate certain areas such as the fovea ethmoidalis and frontal recess. Both are used interchangeably throughout the procedure. While the endoscopes provide magnification and angled vision, they suffer from a narrow, nonstereoscopic, and somewhat distorted optical perspective. This is compensated for by the headlight, which transmits a more three-dimensional view. Video display is of importance primarily for teaching purposes, for in the final analysis it reinforces two-dimensional operative visualization. We believe tactile sense to be a more important factor in performing this type of surgery, which in essence is the serial removal of bony septa surrounded by other thin bony lamellae separating the ethmoidal sinus from the orbit and intracranial cavity.

If there is a significant deviation of the nasal septum, it is corrected to improve access to and exposure of the middle meatus. The middle turbinate is initially preserved to provide protection of the cribriform plate medially, unless it is markedly hypertrophic, pneumatized, or polypoid, restricting visibility of the ethmoidal labyrinth.

The middle turbinate is medially displaced with a long, narrow speculum. We choose to enter the labyrinth through the bulla to avoid inadvertent injury to the lacrimal bone from a hypoplastic uncinate process. Upon entering the ethmoidal sinus, polyps and septa are removed. A blunt, olive-tipped suction device is used as a sound to fracture the septa between cells and to confirm that there is no dehiscence in the medial orbital wall. Light grasping forceps are used principally to remove polyps and bony fragments, similarly relying on tactile sensation. Punch forceps and curettes are avoided. The dissection is carried in a retrograde fashion to open uncinate and agger nasi cells. The dissection is next carried posteriorly through the basal lamina of the middle turbinate, opening and debulking most of the labyrinth.

The middle turbinate is now partially resected, holding the scissors blades horizontally to preserve the superior half of the turbinate, with the plane of division inclined downward following the path of insertion of the turbinate. The posterior ethmoidal cells that abut the sphenoid face are opened by sweeping away the soft tissue and septa of these cells with a Freer elevator.

The sphenoid ostium is cannulated with a beaded probe. The position of the ostium 7 cm and 30 degrees from the nares is a relatively constant relationship. Before the ostium is enlarged, it is sounded with a specially designed bayoneted, small, right-angle (4-mm) probe. While

A

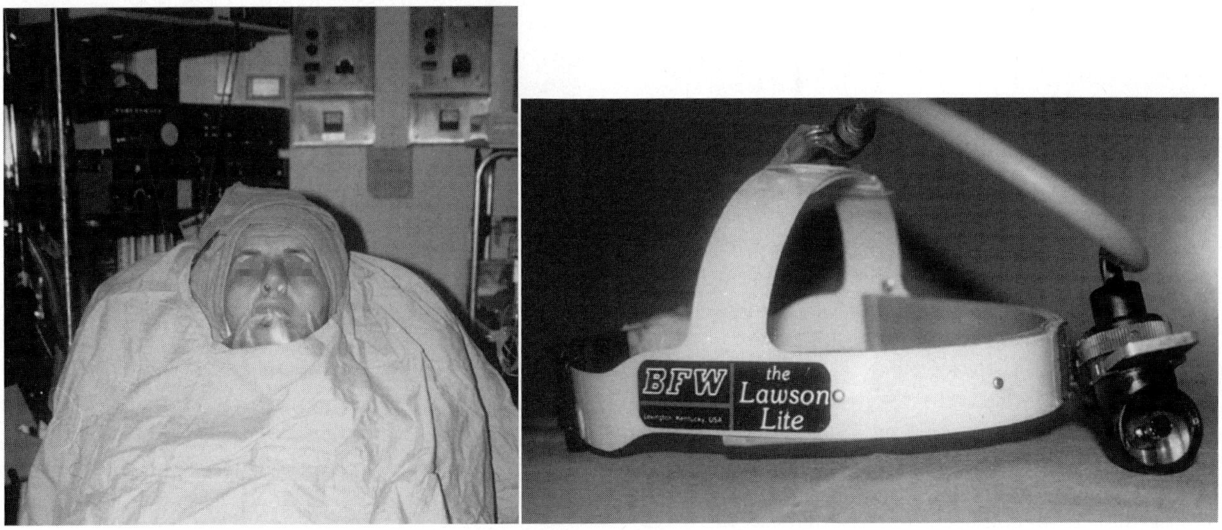

B

Fig. 18-4. **A,** Proper positioning of the patient in the semisitting position. **B,** Coaxial fiberoptic headlight used in conjunction with the 0- and 30-degree sinus endoscopes.

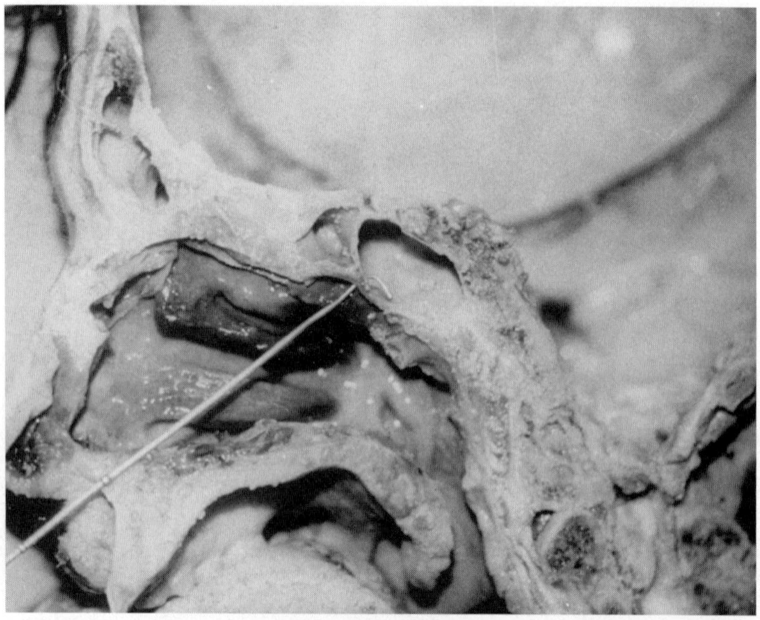

Fig. 18-5. Demonstration of the use of the right-angle probe to identify the sphenoid sinus ostium.

the sphenoid ostium is generally a few millimeters from the nasal septum, an unsuspected deflection of the septum may inadvertently place the beaded probe into a posterior ethmoidal cell, where instrumentation would be hazardous. When the right-angle probe is in the sphenoid sinus and hooked downward, it remains locked in position; the walls of posterior ethmoidal cells are thinner and will break from the pull upon the probe (Fig. 18-5). The ostium is widened with a small right-angle punch forceps laterally, superiorly, and medially. Dissection is limited inferiorly to prevent injury to the sphenopalatine artery.

Should it not be possible to cannulate the sphenoid ostium by this method, it is approached transseptally. Occasionally, it is cannulated on the contralateral side, and the intersinal septum and posterior portion of the nasal bony septum are removed by biting across the midline to eliminate the obstructing plate of bone. However, the sphenoid sinus is never manipulated or instrumented without knowledge of its anatomy and the extent of pneumatization based on preoperative CT scanning (Fig. 18-6).

Polypoid mucosa over the sphenoid face beneath the ostium is electrocauterized rather than avulsed to reduce the risk of an arterial injury. The posterior cut end of the middle turbinate is also cauterized to prevent bleeding from the lateral branch of the sphenopalatine artery. Dissection is never performed in posterior ethmoidal cells present behind the face of the sphenoid sinus, to prevent injury to the optic nerve and to lessen the risk of intracranial injury. The roof of the sphenoid sinus is the upper plane of the ethmoidectomy. The dissection of the entire ethmoidal labyrinth is now completed, working anteriorly along the fovea ethmoidalis, using angled, 30-degree endoscopes. Opening the superiormost group of anterior cells serves to

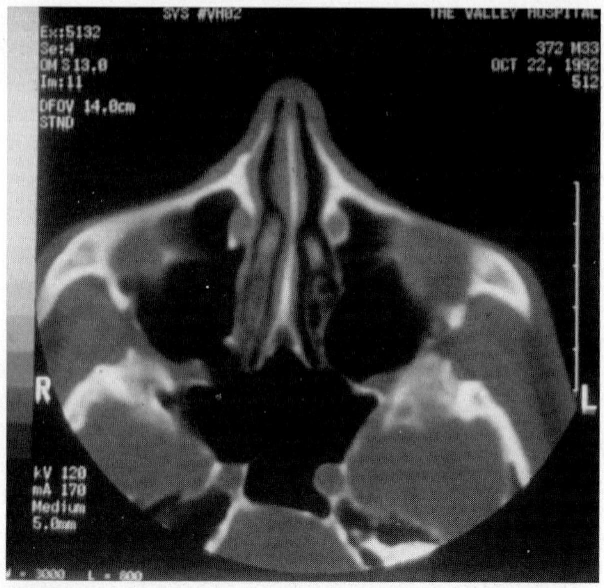

Fig. 18-6. Dehiscence of the lateral wall of the sphenoid sinus showing the exposed carotid artery.

marsupialize the frontal recess and promote drainage of the frontal sinus. This is performed only if there is radiographic evidence of frontal sinus disease in symptomatic patients.

The middle meatal antrostomy is performed by enlarging the natural ostium with punch forceps under endoscopic control. Grossly polypoid tissue is removed from the antrum with angled grasping forceps. The antrostomy, similar to the uncinectomy, should not be carried too far anteriorly, to avoid injury to the nasolacrimal duct. Bleeding points are controlled by suction

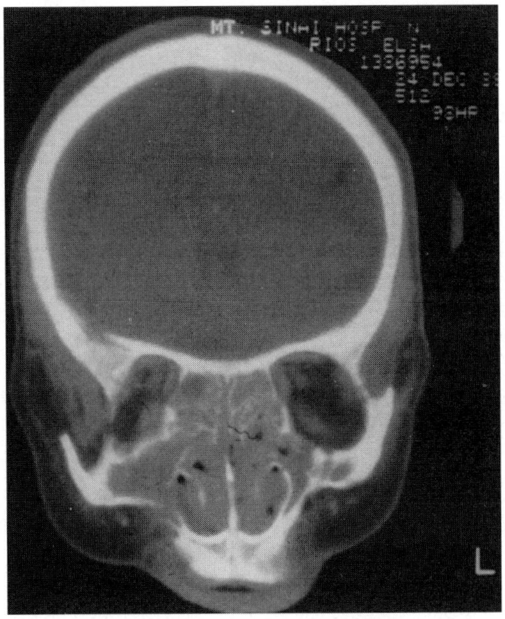

Fig. 18-7. Preoperative computed tomographic (CT) scan of a patient with Samter's syndrome: a triad of asthma, aspirin sensitivity, and nasal polyposis.

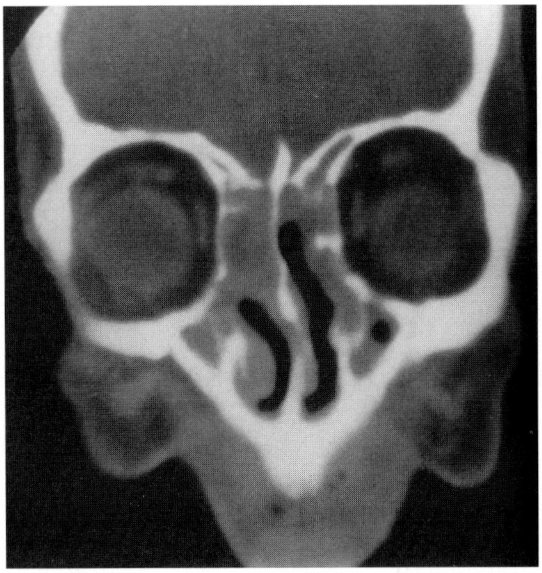

Fig. 18-8. Postoperative CT scan 1 year after complete sphenoethmoidectomy showing extensive recurrence of sinus disease.

electrocautery. A small amount of petrolatum-impregnated gauze is placed into the ethmoidal cavity and antrostomy opening and is left only overnight.

SUCCESS RATE

It is virtually impossible to interpret or compare the reported results of intranasal ethmoidectomy. This is because of the lack of a uniform system of classification and staging, which quantifies the type (infection vs. polyp) and extent (focal vs. diffuse) of disease, as well as specifying the presence or absence of such important systemic modifying factors as atopy, asthma, and aspirin sensitivity (Figs. 18-7 and 18-8). Moreover, many patients are cited as undergoing functional endoscopic sinus surgery, which implies limited ostiomeatal resection rather than total sphenoethmoidectomy. Also, the criteria for success differ widely, ranging from symptomatic relief of airway obstruction or rhinorrhea to the total absence of disease with a rhinologically normal nose. Subjective evaluation by the patient may be misleading because most receive adjunctive medical treatment with antibiotics, steroids, mucolytics, decongestants, and antihistamines, which greatly influences their symptoms. Objective parameters are rarely used as an end point. Finally, prolonged follow-up, which is essential for determining the efficacy of surgery, is often unavailable. Success rates of 80% to over 90% have been reported by several authors,[19–21] but the duration of follow-up of these cases has generally been under 2 years.

There are very few series of cases with follow-up of more than 3 years after intranasal ethmoidectomy. Among the 236 ethmoidectomies performed by Eichel[22] over a 12-year period, 46 patients were available for evaluation 3 to 8 years postoperatively. The success rate was 83% in this group. However, of the 10 patients coming to revision surgery, seven were asthmatics; three of the seven also had aspirin sensitivity. The largest series of cases (146) is that of Sogg,[23] who reported a success rate of 69% after an interval of 6 to 13 years. However, Jantti-Alanko and colleagues[24] reported a 34% success rate for 85 patients followed for 4 years. Of extreme interest is the study of Wigand and Hosemann[6] of 220 cases followed for an unspecified period. Of the 220 patients, 82% claimed symptomatic improvement, but only 24% were totally symptom free and only 52% had a normal nasal mucosal lining.

In the study by the senior author, a subset of 90 patients undergoing 166 procedures and followed for an average of 3.5 years revealed the overall success rate to be 73%. However, when analyzed by type and extent of disease and as to whether asthma was present, the latter became the most significant factor. While the recurrence rate for both focal and diffuse polyp and infectious disease was 12% in nonasthmatics, it rose to 50% in patients with asthma. The number of cases is relatively small, but this is the second largest reported series with follow-up of more than 3 years. Prolonged follow-up is essential, as the mean interval to the development of recurrences in this author's series was 30 months.

BOX 18-1

Classification of Complications of Intranasal Ethmoidectomy

I. Orbital
- Orbital hematoma
- Orbital cellulitis
- Periorbital ecchymosis
- Periorbital emphysema
- Extraocular muscle injury
- Optic nerve injury

II. Intracranial
- Cerebrospinal fluid leak
- Meningitis
- Pneumocephalus
- Brain laceration
- Carotid artery injury
- Carotid-cavernous fistula

III. Sinonasal
- Nasofrontal duct injury
- Frontal mucocele
- Frontal sinusitis
- Nasolacrimal duct injury
- Anosmia
- Ozena
- Ostium closure
- Synechiae
- Hemorrhage

IV. Other
- Neuralgias
- Asthma attack
- Anesthetic reaction

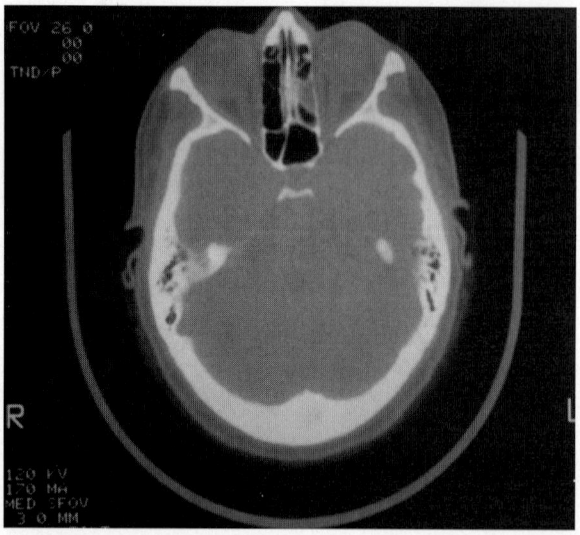

Fig. 18-9. Dangerous, shallow anatomic variation of the ethmoidal labyrinth showing lack of widening posteriorly.

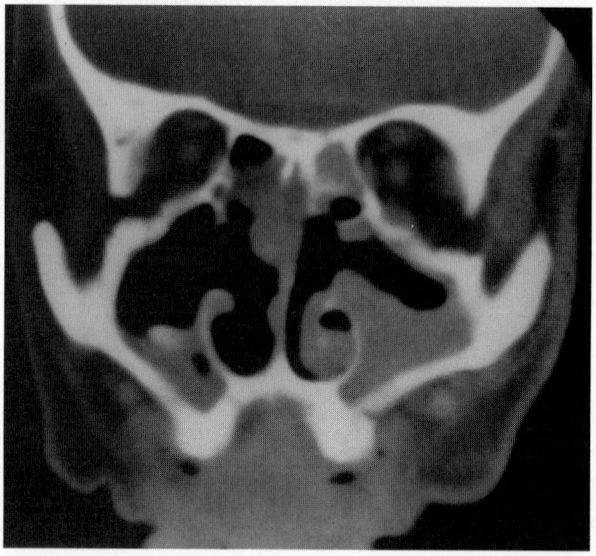

Fig. 18-10. Absence of normal landmarks after previous procedures.

In attempting to establish a prognosis, it is important to distinguish between scattered sporadic sinus involvement (usually unilateral, or focal infundibular), presumably secondary to obstructive disease, and diffuse multisinus disease, which represents a biochemical or local immunologic mucosal abnormality. The former is highly curable operatively and accounts for the excellent reported cure rates, but surgery for the latter often results in limited success, with rapid and frequent recurrences and occasional worsening of the condition.

COMPLICATIONS

Complications of intranasal sphenoethmoidectomy can be broadly subdivided into orbital, intracranial, sinonasal, and other problems (Box 18-1). The orbital complications include orbital hematoma, orbital cellulitis, periorbital ecchymosis and emphysema, extraocular muscle injury, and optic nerve damage. The intracranial consist of cerebrospinal fluid leak, meningitis, pneumocephalus, brain laceration and hemorrhage, carotid artery injury, and carotid-cavernous sinus fistula. Sinonasal complications are nasofrontal and nasolacrimal duct injuries, frontal mucocele, frontal sinusitis, anosmia, ozena, ostium closure, synechiae, and hemorrhage. The remaining other complications are postoperative neuralgias, asthmatic attacks, and anesthetic reactions.

The complications of intranasal ethmoidectomy are related to multiple factors, including the anatomic complexities of the ethmoidal labyrinth, the type and extent of disease, previous surgery, and the experience of the operator

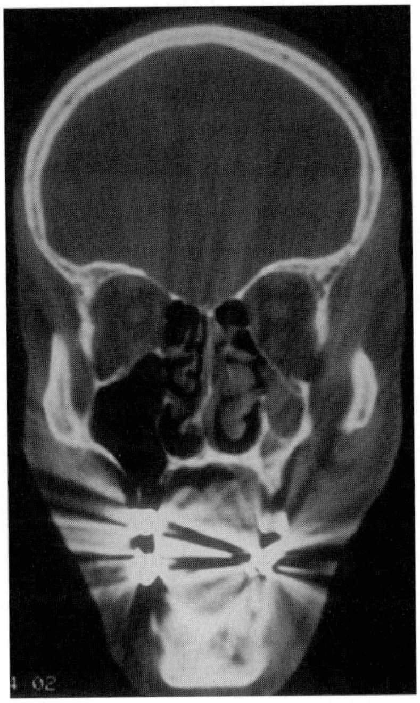

Fig. 18-11. Paradoxically bent middle turbinate with normal maxillary sinus. Also note the left hypoplastic maxilla with its diseased sinus, a consistent entity that is not uncommon.

(Figs. 18-9 to 18-11). A comparative study of the various methods of intranasal surgery revealed that the conventional, endoscopic, and microscopic techniques involve a relatively similar incidence of major complications, averaging 1% to 3% in the large reported series.[5] Instances in which it is extremely high, with reported rates of 8% to 29%,[19,25-27] represent smaller series involving surgical inexperience, attempts to perform total ethmoidectomy for advanced disease, or a combination of both.

Reports of series of 2500 and 4000 cases performed endoscopically[28] and microscopically,[29] respectively, without any complications, are anomalous and difficult to explain in light of the fact that, early in the learning curve, mishaps commonly occur in all fields of surgery. It must also be recognized that even the most experienced surgeons are not exempt from incurring major complications.

Factors that favor complications include (1) revision surgery, (2) an absent middle turbinate, (3) bleeding, (4) chronic infection, (5) right-sided surgery, and (6) inexperience. Factors serving to reduce the incidence of complications include (1) proper illumination, (2) use of the seated position, (3) measures to reduce bleeding, (4) increased access by septal and turbinate surgery, (5) surveillance of landmarks, and (6) monitoring of the eyes.

An advantage of the so-called conventional method of intranasal ethmoidectomy by its macroscopic nature is that it permits rapid visual surveillance of landmarks to maintain operative orientation. These include the sphenoid face with its enlarged ostium, the middle turbinate remnant, and the membranous portion of the middle meatus for a three-dimensional perspective of the ethmoidal labyrinth. It is essential to monitor the eyes, as perforation of the lamina papyracea may occur and go unrecognized endonasally. When instrumentation is used in the ethmoidal labyrinth, the eyes should be uncovered and constantly observed for any evidence of motion. In this regard, use of suction preliminary to the application of forceps will act as a sound and elicit movement of the eye if the medial orbital wall has been violated. This can be done rapidly and frequently by the conventional technique, by minor movement of the operator's eyes and head, as compared with procedures done through an optical system or from a television screen.

To achieve maximal operative access to the middle meatus and sphenoid face, the middle turbinate is partially resected. This also permits easy cleansing of the opened sinus cavities postoperatively and eliminates closure of the middle meatus by synechia formation. No instance of ozena was observed in these authors' total operative experience after middle turbinate resection if a normal inferior turbinate was also present. The rarity of the development of atrophic rhinitis after middle turbinate resection has also been noted by Friedman and Katsantonis.[30]

REFERENCES

1. Harrison DFN: Surgery in allergic sinusitis, *Otolaryngol Clin North Am* 4:83, 1971.
2. Jansen A: Zur Eriffung der Nebenhohlen der Nase bei Chronischer Eiterung, *Arch Laryngol Rhinol* 1:35-58, 1884.
3. Mosher H: The applied anatomy and the intranasal surgery of the ethmoid labyrinth, *Trans Am Laryngol Assoc* 34:25-39, 1912.
4. Yankauer S: Demonstration of intranasal surgery on wet specimens, *Laryngoscope* 40:642-654, 1930.
5. Yankauer S: The complete sphenoethmoid operation, *Laryngoscope* 31:831–842, 1921.
6. Wigand ME, Hosemann W: Microsurgical treatment of recurrent nasal polyposis, *Rhinology* 8(suppl):25-30, 1989.
7. Zinreich SJ, Kennedy DW, Rosenbaum AE, et al: Paranasal sinuses: CT imaging requirements for endoscopic surgery, *Radiology* 163:769-775, 1987.
8. Zinreich SJ, Kennedy DW, Gayler BW: Computer tomography of the nasal cavity and paranasal sinuses: an evaluation of anatomy for endoscopic sinus surgery, *Clear Images* 1:2-10, 1988.
9. Bolger WE, Butzin CA, Parsons DS: Paranasal sinus bony anatomic variations and mucosal abnormalities: CT analysis for endoscopic sinus surgery, *Laryngoscope* 101:56-64, 1991.
10. Calhoun KH, Waggenspack GA, Simpson CB, et al: CT evaluation of the paranasal sinuses in symptomatic and asymptomatic populations, *Otolaryngol Head Neck Surg* 104:480-483, 1991.
11. Havas TE, Motbey JA, Gullane PJ: Prevalence of incidental abnormalities on computed tomographic scans of the paranasal sinuses, *Arch Otolaryngol Head Neck Surg* 114:856-859, 1988.
12. Glasier CM, Mallory GB, Steele RW: Significance of opacification of the maxillary and ethmoid sinuses in infants, *J Pediatr* 114:45-50, 1989.
13. Diamant MJ, Senac MO, Gilsanz V, et al: Prevalence of incidental paranasal sinuses opacification in pediatric patients: a CT study, *J Comput Assist Tomogr* 11:426-431, 1987.

14. Kennedy DW, Josephson JS, Zinreich J, et al: Endoscopic sinus surgery for mucoceles: a viable alternative, *Laryngoscope* 99:885-895, 1989.

15. Neel HB, McDonald TJ, Facer GW: Modified Lynch procedure for chronic frontal sinus disease: rationale, technique, and long-term results, *Laryngoscope* 97:1274-1279, 1987.

16. Wigand ME: *Endoscopic surgery of the paranasal sinuses and anterior skull base*, New York, 1990, G Thieme.

17. Lawson W: *The frontal sinus.* In Blitzer A, Lawson W, Friedman W, editors: *Surgery of the paranasal sinuses*, Philadelphia, 1985, WB Saunders, pp 120-144.

18. Stammberger H: Endoscopic surgery for mycotic and chronic recurring sinusitis, *Ann Otol* 94(suppl 119):1-11, 1985.

19. Schaefer SD: Endoscopic total sphenoethmoidectomy, *Otolaryngol Clin North Am* 22:723-732, 1989.

20. Toeffel PH, Aroesty DJ, Weimann RH: Secure endoscopic sinus surgery as an adjunct to functional nasal surgery, *Arch Otolaryngol Head Neck Surg* 115:822-825, 1989.

21. Rice DH: Endoscopic sinus surgery results at 2-year follow-up, *Otolaryngol Head Neck Surg* 101:476-479, 1989.

22. Eichel BS: The intranasal ethmoidectomy: a 12 year perspective, *Otolaryngol Head Neck Surg* 90:540-543, 1982.

23. Sogg A: Long-term results of ethmoid surgery, *Ann Otol Rhinol Laryngol* 98:699-701, 1989.

24. Jantti-Alanko S, Holopainen E, Malmberg H: Recurrence of nasal polyps after surgical treatment, *Rhinology* 8(suppl):59-64, 1989.

25. Silverstein H, McDonald AB: *Microsurgical sphenoethmoidectomy.* In Goldman JL, editor: *The principles and practice of rhinology*, New York, 1987, John Wiley, pp 435-442.

26. Stankiewicz JA: Complications of endoscopic intranasal ethmoidectomy, *Laryngoscope* 97:1270-1273, 1987.

27. Stankiewicz JA: Complications in endoscopic intranasal ethmoidectomy: an update, *Laryngoscope* 99:686-690, 1989.

28. Stammberger H: Endoscopic endonasal surgery—concepts in treatment of recurrent rhinosinusitis. Part II, *Otolaryngol Head Neck Surg* 94:147-156, 1986.

29. Hiermann J, Neves D: Intranasal microsurgery of all paranasal sinuses, the septum, and the lacrimal sac with hypotensive anesthesia: 25 years' experience, *Ann Otol* 95:631-637, 1986.

30. Friedman WH, Katsantonis GS: The role of standard techniques in modern sinus surgery, *Otolaryngol Clin North Am* 22:759-775, 1989.

C H A P T E R
19

Transnasal Sphenoethmoidectomy

George P. Katsantonis
William H. Friedman

PROBLEM

A 46-year-old man was referred to the office because of a 4-month history of nasal congestion, intermittent nasal obstruction, excessive postnasal discharge associated with chronic cough, and recurrent episodes of paroxysmal coughing spells. Before the referral he had been treated with several courses of broad-spectrum antibiotics, antihistamines, decongestants, steroidal nasal and oral sprays, bronchodilator sprays, and bursts of systemic steroids, but there was only partial and temporary improvement of the symptoms. He underwent an allergy evaluation, which was negative, and computed tomography (CT) of the paranasal sinuses, which revealed a multifocal but not contiguous thickening of the paranasal sinus mucosa in the ethmoidal, maxillary, and frontal sinuses.

This brief presentation illustrates a typical case of chronic rhinosinusitis associated with reflex bronchospasm. Because of the history of unresponsiveness of symptoms despite aggressive conservative measures and the findings of "patchy" pansinusitis, a transnasal sphenoethmoidectomy (TSE) was recommended. The patient's asthmatic condition was not considered a contraindication to surgery. On the contrary, it was thought that surgical intervention would interrupt the reflex mechanism producing the coughing spells (nasopulmonary reflex) and that a complete eradication of diseased mucosa would offer the best hope in controlling the sinusitis.

The indications for TSE have expanded considerably in the last few decades (Box 19-1). The operation introduced by Yankauer in 1921 was primarily designed to provide adequate decompression and drainage for acute and subacute bacterial sinusitis.[1,2] Original indications for the procedure were therefore advanced infectious sinusitis and recurrent nasal polyposis. Because of the widespread use of broad-spectrum antibiotics, the characteristics of inflammatory sinus disease have changed significantly, and chronic hyperplastic rhinosinusitis (CHR) has replaced infectious acute or subacute sinusitis as the prevalent inflammatory paranasal sinus condition. The histopathologic spectrum of CHR includes polypoid, fibrous, cystic, follicular, and papillary changes.[3]

These changes are usually irreversible and surgical extirpation is therefore the treatment of choice, particularly when they produce obstruction of pathways of egress of sinus secretions, which in turn further exacerbates the infectious process perpetuating the vicious cycle of hyperplasia-infection-hyperplasia. The use of CT in the evaluation of sinus disease has led to the unveiling of such mucosal changes in early or occult stages, broadening the indications for TSE. Additional indications for TSE are frequent recurrent bouts of purulent pansinusitis and sinobronchial syndrome caused by persistent sinusitis. Recurrent nasal polyposis is another indication for TSE, and although most such patients display an inexorable tendency toward regrowth of hyperplastic tissue, complete disease removal and wide opening of all sinuses can ensure longer disease-free intervals than limited approaches.

The functional importance of the infundibular region has been well understood and remains the focal point of functional endoscopic sinus surgery (FESS).[4,5] Obstruction of the sinus outflow by disease process in this area potentially affects most of the paranasal sinuses, and surgical intervention usually results in reversion of the process. Nevertheless, chronic sinusitis may originate in areas other than the infundibulum and is frequently characterized by multifocal involvement. In such cases, FESS is not as effective as TSE in controlling chronic sinusitis.

MEDICAL HISTORY

Unlike the case reported here, many patients with CHR do not have reflex bronchospasm or asthma. In fact, asthmatics constitute a minority among CHR patients. The classic symptoms of CHR are nasal congestion, anterior and posterior nasal discharge, and intermittent or continuous nasal obstruction. Less frequently, dull facial and head pain, disturbance of sense of smell, chronic cough, and nonspecific ear complaints (such as a sensation of pressure, fullness, or fluid) are also present. Many patients display periodic exacerbations of these symptoms; others have repeated frequent bouts of acute sinusitis with intervals relatively free of symptoms.

RADIOGRAPHIC ASSESSMENT AND STAGING

Undoubtedly, CT has proved a superb method of evaluating chronic sinusitis and paranasal sinus pathology in general.[6] The high-resolution, three-dimensional imaging provides valuable information for accurate assessment of the extent of disease, and is extremely helpful in the selection of the appropriate surgical procedure. CT is almost indispensable in confirming the diagnosis of early chronic sinusitis, because routine radiography usually fails to identify early or intermediate mucosal changes.[7]

The superior imaging of sinus pathology provided by CT has also generated the impetus for the development of a staging system for chronic rhinosinusitis. The need for a standardized method of classifying sinusitis and evaluating its treatment has been driven by the high interest in paranasal sinus surgery coupled with the recognition that sinusitis is now the most common medical diagnosis.

Publications, presentations, and discussions on the subject until 1990 were lacking uniformity in assessing the severity of sinusitis and quantifying treatment outcomes according to disease extent.[8] A reliable staging system for

BOX 19-1

Indications for Transnasal Sphenoethmoidectomy

1. Chronic hyperplastic rhinosinusitis
2. Persistent infectious pansinusitis refractory to antibiotic therapy
3. Frequent episodes of acute sinusitis
4. Recurrent nasal polyposis
5. Sinobronchial syndrome with evidence of chronic sinusitis

A

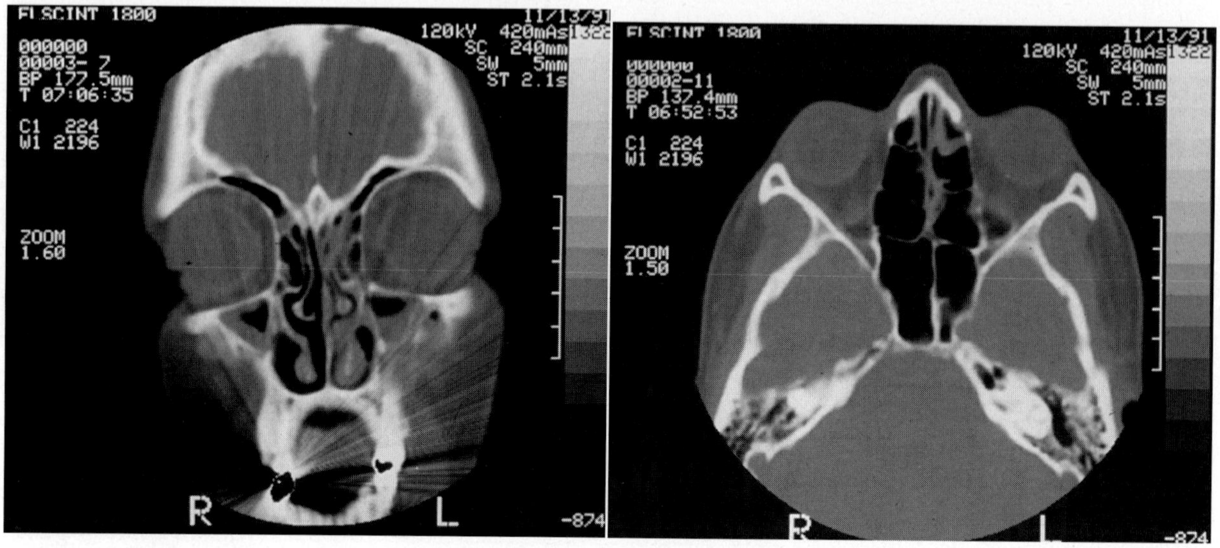

B

Fig. 19-1. **A** and **B,** Coronal and axial computed tomographic (CT) scans of a patient with stage II disease. Note the multifocal but not contiguous hyperplastic disease throughout the ethmoidal and maxillary sinuses.

chronic sinusitis was thought to be of crucial importance not only as a means of communication among otolaryngologists for reporting scientific data but also as a meaningful and simple method for accurately assessing and classifying disease extent, outlining treatment plans, and predicting outcomes. Several staging systems based solely on information gained by CT have been proposed.[9-12] In 1989, Friedman and colleagues proposed a staging system based on CT as well as clinical response to a standardized medical regimen consisting of a 3-week course of broad-spectrum antibiotics, a short course of systemic steroids; steroid nasal sprays; and a combination of oral antihistamines, decongestants, and expectorants.[13] CT is performed immediately after completion of the medical regimen. The staging system includes four stages: stage I, radiographic evidence of single focus disease, either unilateral or bilateral; stage II, radiographic evidence of multifocal noncontiguous or "patchy" areas of disease (Fig. 19-1); stage III, contiguous disease throughout the ethmoidal labyrinth, with or without involvement of other major sinuses and symptomatic response to the medical therapy (Fig. 19-2); and stage IV, contiguous hyperplastic disease usually involving all sinuses with no symptomatic response to medication (Fig. 19-3)(Box 19-2). Distribu-

A

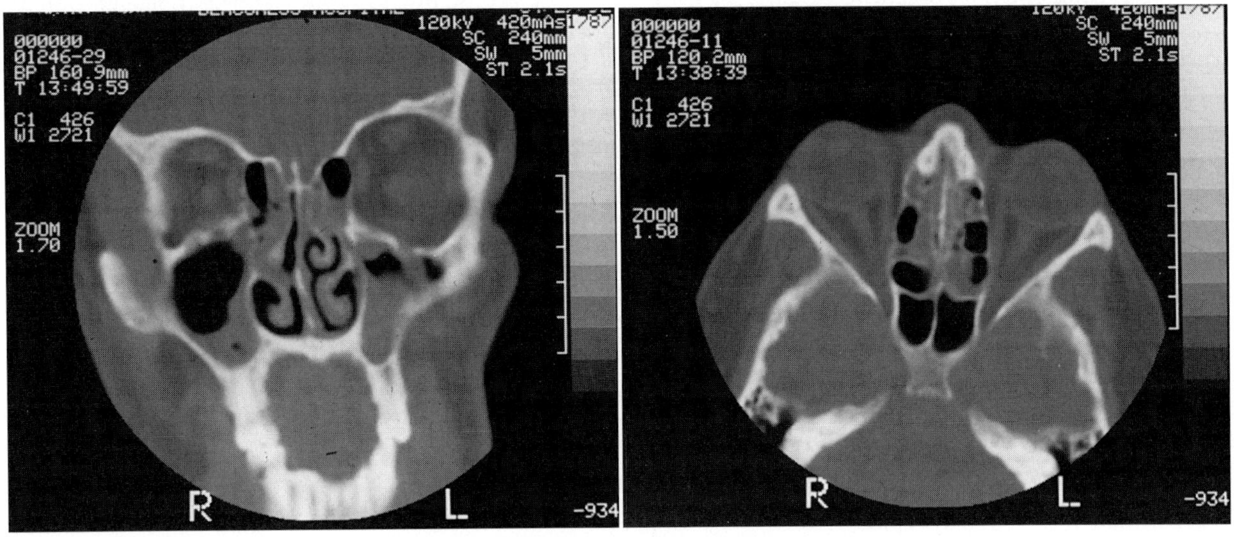

B

Fig. 19-2. **A** and **B**, Coronal and axial CT scans of a patient with stage III disease. Note the contiguous hyperplastic mucosal changes throughout the ethmoidal and maxillary sinuses.

A

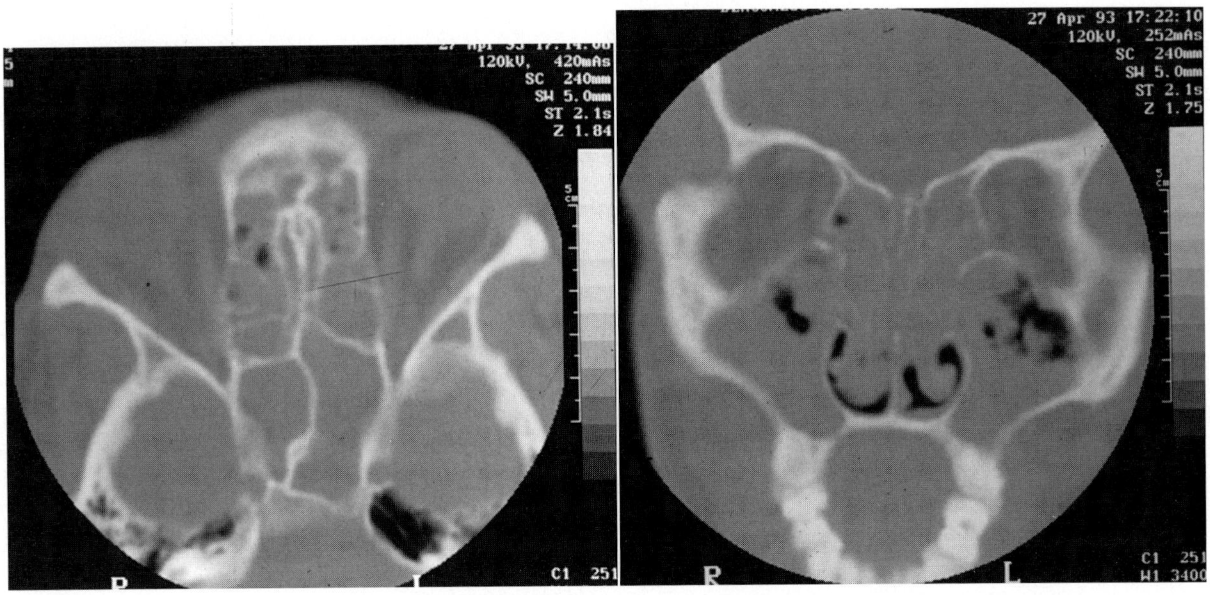

B

Fig. 19-3. **A** and **B**, Coronal and axial CT scans of a patient with stage IV disease. Note the complete whiteout with contiguous hyperplastic disease throughout all the paranasal sinuses.

tion of the number of patients per stage in a series of 2058 patients with chronic sinusitis is seen in Table 19-1.

Central to the classification and staging of chronic sinusitis is the definition of this entity. Besides the described symptoms of chronic sinusitis, there should be radiographic (CT) evidence of irreversible sinus mucosal changes. From this perspective, chronic sinusitis should be defined as "radiographic evidence of mucosal hyperplasia of the paranasal sinuses following adequate medical therapy for prolonged or recurrent symptoms of sinusitis." It is hoped that the medical protocol used here, in addition to assisting classification into stages, provides elimination of acute or subacute sinusitis changes before CT scanning. The length of treatment required for acute changes to recede remains controversial.[14] In the authors' series, frequent and early recurrence after initial medical therapy was noted in all or most patients with stages II to IV, and therefore lengthy intervals between medical therapy and CT are not advocated. In fact, the arbitrary 3-week interval selected here has assumed an early response to therapy, and reduced patient symptoms and acute radiographic changes to levels that enable CT evaluation of chronic disease in a clinically efficient time frame.

To evaluate the usefulness of this staging system in developing treatment strategies, a retrospective study was carried out in which recurrence rates of chronic sinusitis were analyzed according to various treatment modalities per stage. A fairly satisfactory control of disease was noted in stage I patients treated medically (30% recurrence rate). Conversely, most stage II patients treated conservatively recurred either immediately or shortly after completion of the medical regimen (59%). Patients with advanced sinusitis (stages III and IV) had either a transient response or no response to any medical therapy. Recurrence rates for patients with stages II, III and IV disease treated surgically (primarily with TSE) were 8.9%, 16.1%, and 25%, respectively.[13] The results of this study suggested that TSE should be the treatment of choice for stages II, III, and IV disease, while medical therapy is appropriate for stage I patients. Recurrent or persistent disease in stage I patients after conservative management is treated with a limited surgical approach to the focus of the disease.

BOX 19-2

The Staging System

Stage I	Single focus disease, unilateral or bilateral (single sinus mucosal thickening; unilateral polyp; cloudy ethmoidal, sphenoid, or maxillary sinus).
Stage II	Multifocal, noncontiguous mucosal thickening or polyps, unilateral or bilateral (may include one or more dependent sinuses).
Stage III	Diffuse contiguous disease throughout the ethmoids with or without involvement of any dependent sinuses, partially responsive to medication.
Stage IV	Diffuse, contiguous disease; throughout the ethmoidal sinuses, and most or all other sinuses, nonresponsive to medication.

OPERATIVE TECHNIQUE

The technique described here is essentially based on the one reported by Yankauer,[1] but many refinements and modifications have been added to the original operation. Preferably the procedure is performed using local anesthesia with sedation and monitoring provided by the anesthetist. After surface mucosal anesthetization and vasoconstriction with 10% cocaine, local regional anesthesia is administered (2% lidocaine [Xylocaine] with 1:50,000 epinephrine) to the septal, middle turbinate, and nasal vault mucosa as well as to the sphenopalatine ganglion via the greater palatine foramen.

Although the procedure can be carried strictly endoscopically, conventional illumination is used while endoscopes serve as adjunctive tools. Illumination is provided by monocular coaxial lighting such as the Good-Lite (Good-Lite Company, Forest Park, Ill) or the Lawson fiberoptic light (Luxtec Company, Sturbridge, Mass). Endoscopes of 0, 25, and 70 degrees are used to visualize or remove disease from areas that are difficult to expose by conventional means (infundibular and frontal recess cells, middle meatal antrostomy, maxillary sinus mucosa, nasofrontal duct). The surgical armamentarium also includes a universal handle with various attachments (right and left Holmes scissors, Myles forceps, Wilde ethmoidal forceps, Watson-Williams 45-degree ethmoid punch, backbiting forceps) and an assortment of Blakesley forceps (0, 45, and 90 degrees). At the outset a submucous resection of the nasal septum is performed even in cases of relatively minor septal deflections, to ensure adequate access into the nasal vaults during surgery and ease at tending the cavities postoperatively. The middle turbinate is removed at its attachment to the cribriform

Table 19-1. Chronic sinusitis distribution by stage

Stage I	294 (14.3%)
Stage II	885 (43.0%)
Stage III	563 (27.4%)
Stage IV	316 (15.4%)
Total	2058

plate with Holmes scissors, leaving only a small ridge (Fig. 19-4). The ground lamella is then transected with Wilde forceps and the posterior ethmoidal cells are removed completely, exposing widely the face of the sphenoid. The sphenoid sinus is entered through its ostium or by punching an opening through the bony wall with the Wilde forceps. This opening is enlarged until the contents of the sphenoid sinuses are well visualized (Fig. 19-5). Using the imaginary anterior projections of the lateral and superior sphenoid sinus walls as landmarks, the remainder of the posterior ethmoidal cells are resected. A 0-degree endoscope is introduced to ensure adequate resection of all cells, because occasionally some cells are located laterally and superior to the sphenoid sinus (Onodi cells). Attention is then directed to the anterior ethmoidal cells. The uncinate process is removed with the 45-degree Blakesley forceps, and the nasofrontal duct is visualized with a 70-degree endoscope. The first and second basal lamellae are resected to ensure opening of the duct and the frontal recess. At the anterosuperior end of the uncinate process, the agger nasi cells are identified easily if present and are removed with the 45-degree Blakesley forceps (Fig. 19-6).

A blunt curved rasp is applied through the posterior fontanel into the maxillary sinus. The antrostomy is first widened posteriorly by removing the medial wall of the maxillary sinus between the inferior turbinate and the ethmoidal crest with straight and 45-degree Blakesley forceps. The perpendicular plate of the palatine bone is also resected up to the ethmoidal crest, with care taken not to transgress the sphenopalatine foramen and sphenopalatine artery. Bleeding from the sphenopalatine artery is rare and has not been a major problem in the author's experience. The antrostomy is then enlarged in an anterior direction under direct visualization with a 30-degree scope, backbiting forceps, and 90-degree Blakesley forceps to the

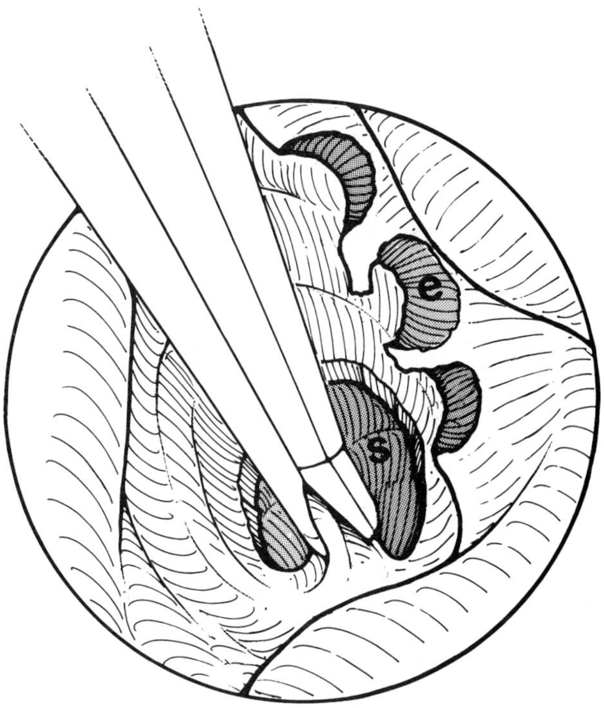

Fig. 19-5. The posterior ethmoidal cells *(e)* have been completely resected. The sphenoid sinus *(s)* is widely open.

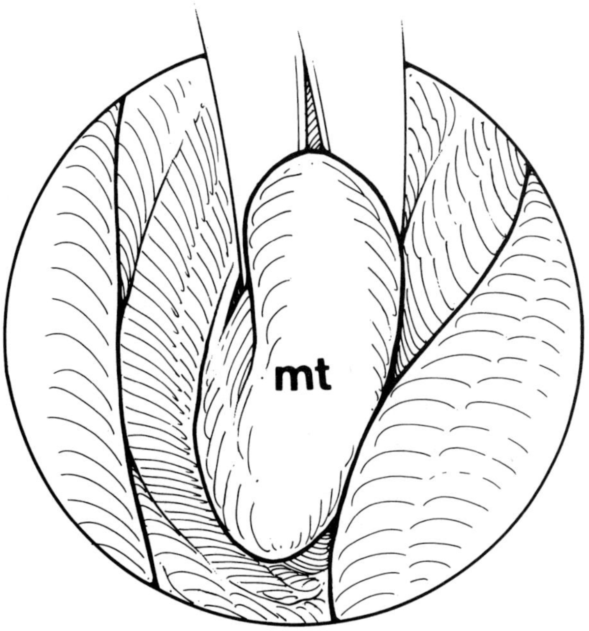

Fig. 19-4. The middle turbinate *(mt)* is resected at its attachment to the cribriform plate with Holmes scissors.

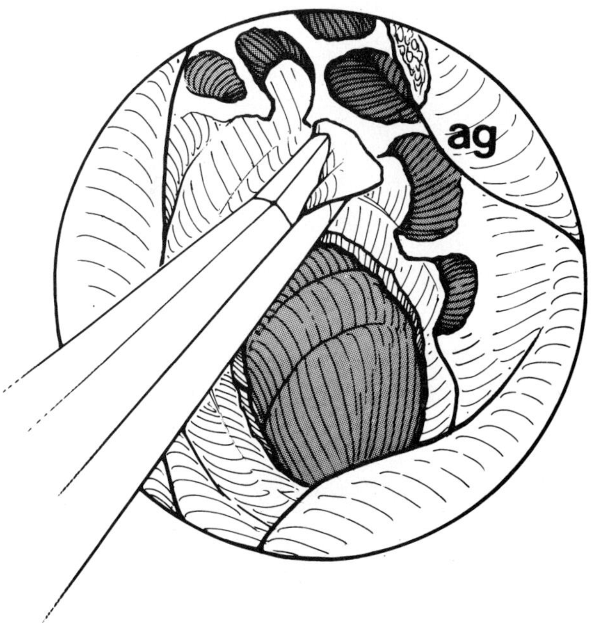

Fig. 19-6. The agger nasi cells *(ag)* are resected to gain access into the infundibulum.

bony ridge just posterior to the nasal lacrimal duct orifice. If there is hyperplastic disease in the maxillary sinuses, it is removed under direct visualization with a 30-degree scope and an assortment of Blakesley forceps. Through the widely open antrostomy the inferior and medial orbital walls are easily outlined, and any ethmoidal cells that might have remained because of the proximity of the orbital wall are now safely opened (Haller cells) (Fig. 19-7). Particular care is taken to adequately remove hyperplastic disease from areas with narrowed bony confines such as the anterior ethmoidal region. Nasal packing is usually not required unless a submucous resection is performed or there is persistent oozing (seen occasionally in revision surgery). At the completion of the operation the entire ethmoidal labyrinth, sphenoid, and maxillary sinuses are widely opened into the nasal vault, hence, the term *marsupialization*.

RESULTS

Overall an 85% cure rate of CHR was achieved in 3140 sphenoethmoidectomies performed in 1812 patients by the authors in a 20-year span. Most of these patients were followed for at least 2 years after surgery (follow-up time ranged from 1 to 18; mean follow-up, 38 months). The criteria for diagnosis of recurrent disease are similar to those of chronic rhinosinusitis: (1) persistent symptoms of chronic sinusitis with evidence of regrowth of hyperplastic mucosa, purulent discharge, or recurrent polyps; (2) recurrent purulent sinusitis (more than four episodes annually); and (3) CT evidence of hyperplastic disease. The recurrence rates for stages II, III, and IV disease were 8.9%, 16.1%, and 25%, respectively (Table 19-2). There was an almost perfect linear correlation between recurrence rate and stage of disease. Multiple regression analysis resulted in a correlation coefficient of 0.91 (Fig. 19-8). The recurrence rates for stage I disease were almost identical to those for stage II. However, only a few stage I patients underwent TSE in this series. Most patients with stage I disease either received conservative therapy or underwent limited endoscopic procedures. Recurrence rates for asthmatic patients were significantly higher than those observed in nonasthmatics in this series, particularly in cases of advanced disease (Table 19-3).

There was an overall 1.94% complication rate in this series of TSE procedures. Complications were classified into major and minor (Table 19-4). In the major group seven patients had a cerebrospinal fluid (CSF) leak, three had orbital hematoma, two developed pneumoencephalos, and one developed a frontal mucocele several months after the initial procedure. The rate of major complications was 0.4%. In the group of patients with minor complications, 18 suffered asthmatic attacks intraoperatively or early postoperatively. Twelve developed early or delayed postoperative epistaxis that required packing or surgical intervention for control of bleeding, and eight had persistent crusting. Six patients complained of anosmia

Table 19-2. Transnasal sphenoethmoidectomy: recurrence rates per stage

STAGE	PATIENTS	PROCEDURES	RECURRENCE
I	48	52	4 (7.7%)
II	885	1378	123 (8.9%)
III	563	1108	178 (16.1%)
IV	316	602	154 (25%)
Total	1812	3140	459 (14.6%)

Table 19-3. Sphenoethmoidectomy recurrence (1988/1992)

	ASTHMA			NONASTHMA		
	REC	TSE	%	REC	TSE	%
STAGE I	3	20	15%	1	34	2.94%
STAGE II	54	283	19.08%	69	1094	6.3%
STAGE III	59	272	21.61%	19	835	14.25%
STAGE IV	101	295	34.23%	53	307	17.26%
Total	217	870	24.91%	142	2270	6.25%

after surgery, four developed periorbital edema, and two had periorbital subcutaneous emphysema. The minor complication rate was 1.34% (Table 19-4).

DISCUSSION

Many of the controversies surrounding surgery for chronic rhinosinusitis have been resolved since the mid-1980s. Intranasal sinus surgery has become the standard, and the issue of conventional versus endoscopic techniques has been resolved in favor of the latter, particularly among the younger otolaryngologists who have been trained in this new era of sinus surgery. However, significant controversy remains in other areas, and in some there is still a virtual standoff. Although there is a consensus that the treatment of advanced sinusitis justifies extensive intranasal surgery, there is considerable debate concerning the management of intermediate disease. The authors' rationale of treating stage II disease with TSE is supported by observations of CT results in patients with early disease, as well as a retrospective analysis of a group of patients undergoing various treatments for stage II rhinosinusitis. Early sinusitis appears to be multifocal disease in most patients, with pathologic mucosa arising or existing simultaneously in many regions of the paranasal sinuses.[13] Recurrence rates of stage II disease treated conservatively or with limited surgical procedures such as FESS were significantly higher than the ones observed after TSE.[15] Because TSE (at least in this series) carries no greater morbidity than functional endoscopic sinus surgery, it is considered the procedure of choice for intermediate and advanced sinusitis (stages II, III, and IV).

There have been differences in opinion about the importance of the middle turbinate since the early days of sinus surgery, and the fate of this structure during intranasal surgery remains the focus of major controversy.[16-18] Proponents of turbinate preservation maintain

Table 19-4. Transnasal sphenoethmoidectomy complications (no. of procedures, 1340)

MAJOR		MINOR	
Cerebrospinal fluid leak	7	Asthma	18
Orbital hematoma	3	Epistaxis	12
Pneumoencephalos	2	Anosmia	6
Frontal mucocele	1	Crusting	6
Total	13 (0.4%)	Periorbital edema	4
		Periorbital emphysema	2
		Total	48 (1.52%)

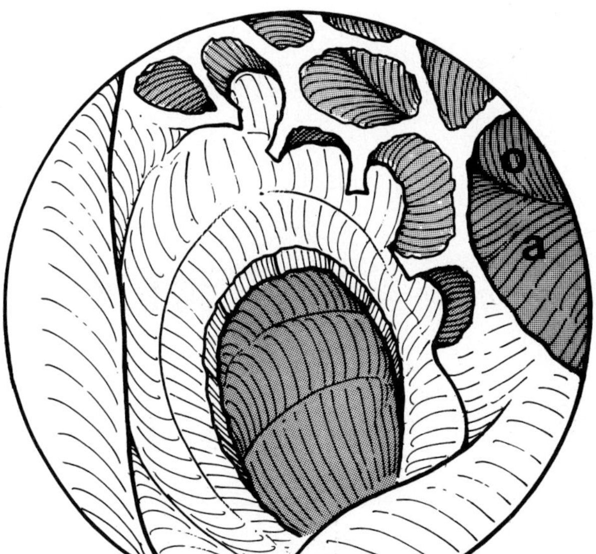

Fig. 19-7. The maxillary ethmoidal and sphenoid sinus have been completely marsupialized into the nasal cavity. Note the outlining of the medial and inferior walls of the orbit *(o)* visible through the wide antrostomy *(a)*.

that this is a physiologically important structure contributing to olfaction and that its removal usually results in atrophic rhinitis. On the other hand, advocates of middle turbinate resection contend that its removal provides excellent visualization of the entire nasal vault during surgery and renders it easily accessible for debridement and suctioning in the postoperative period, thus improving cure rates of CHR. Additionally, they point out that the middle turbinate is frequently pneumatized to a degree that impedes adequate exposure and may obstruct individual sinus ostia, or in certain cases is even involved with hyperplastic disease.[19-21]

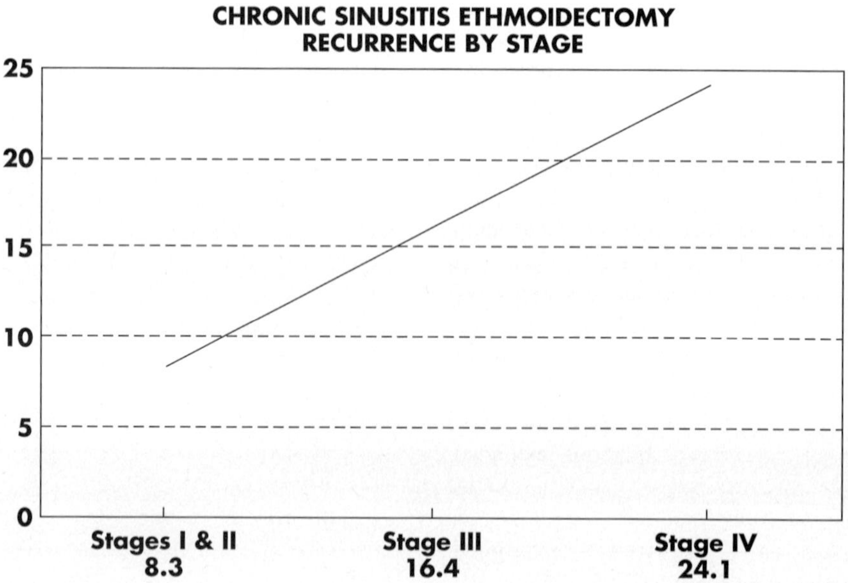

Fig. 19-8. Linear correlation of recurrence rate and stage (correlation coefficient, 0.9).

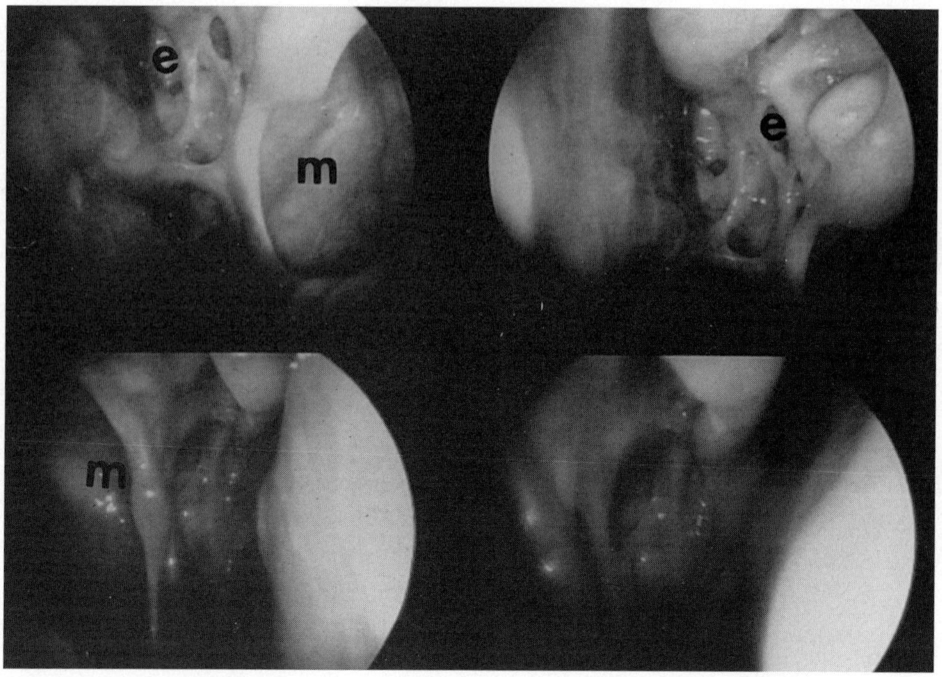

Fig. 19-9. Endoscopic view of the nasal vaults 3 months after sphenoethmoidectomy. Note the complete marsupialization of the paranasal sinus into the nasal cavity. *e*, Ethmoid cells; *m*, maxillary sinus.

Another point of controversy is whether the sphenoid sinus should be opened if not involved with disease. According to the classic description of the sphenoethmoidectomy operation, the wide opening of the sphenoid sinus provides orientation for the surgical dissection because the extension of the roof and lateral wall of the sphenoid sinus anteriorly corresponds with the roof of the ethmoid and the lamina papyracea.[22] Certainly in cases of advanced sinusitis these landmarks are obscured, and a widely opened sphenoid sinus can provide valuable guidance. Although carotid artery and optic nerve injuries have been reported in association with surgical manipulations within the sphenoid sinus, caution and improved illumination can preclude such occurrences. In this series of more than 3100 sphenoethmoidectomies during which the sphenoid sinuses were widely opened, no such complications were documented.

The term *ethmoidal marsupialization* was first proposed by Friedman and colleagues[23] to emphasize that complete removal of disease mucosa and wide opening of the sphenoid, ethmoid, and maxillary sinuses into the nasal cavity are crucial in improving cure rates for CHR (Figs. 19-9 and 19-10). Several modifications (extended middle meatal antrostomy, removal of agger nasi cells, wide opening of the infundibulum, use of endoscopes) described in this chapter have been added to the original operation of intranasal sphenoethmoidectomy for the purpose of obtaining a more complete marsupialization of the paranasal sinuses. These refinements are thought to be responsible for a gradual decrease in recurrence rates observed by the authors in several consecutive series of patients treated since the mid-1970s.[24]

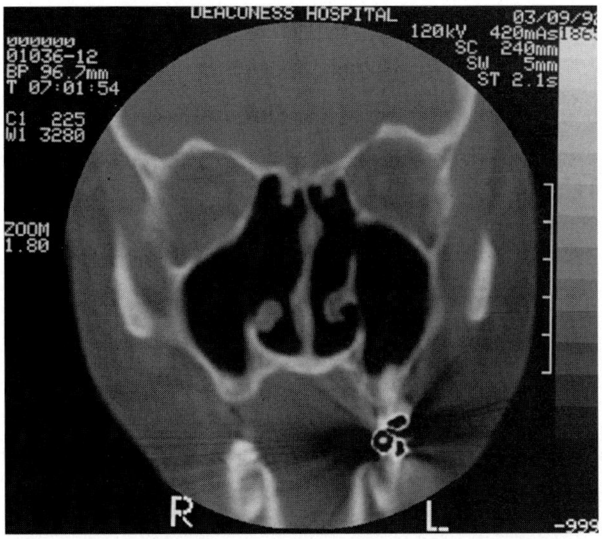

Fig. 19-10. Coronal CT scan of the patient in Fig. 19-9 depicting complete marsupialization of the ethmoidal and maxillary sinuses into the nasal cavity.

The concept for staging chronic sinusitis has played a crucial role in our understanding of the natural history of this disease and communicating this understanding to others. Staging allows accurate assessment of the extent of disease and has been helpful in outlining treatment strategies and predicting outcomes. A valid staging system should be easily remembered, simple to use, comprehensive (encompassing all variations of disease extent), and (most important) predictive of outcomes; in other words, there should be a linear correlation between stage and outcome. The staging system proposed here has satisfied these criteria and has been used successfully in staging approximately 2500 patients.

Although intranasal ethmoidectomy performed conventionally or endoscopically remains the most frequently litigated procedure in our specialty, and once it was characterized by one of its founders as "an easy way in which you could kill somebody," its morbidity in this series was very low and in accordance with complication rates observed by other experienced intranasal surgeons.[25,26] A transient increase in complication rates of endoscopic sinus surgery in general was reported early in the era of endoscopic sinus surgery.[27] This observation could be justified by the fact that a learning curve is inevitable with the introduction of a new procedure, and that aggressive marketing and the widespread availability of new instruments has resulted in an explosive increase of the popularity of sinus surgery, and thus attracted many novices.[28]

CSF leakage is usually caused by iatrogenic penetration of the floor of the anterior cranial fossa, and appears to be the most common serious complication not only in this series but in general. Occasionally, CSF leakage occurs without penetration of the skull base because the olfactory branches or anterior ethmoid artery may communicate directly with the subarachanoid space.[29] Although other, more serious intracranial complications such as meningitis or intracerebral injury by penetration have been reported, no such complications were observed in this series.[30]

Atrophic rhinitis and persistent crusting has been portrayed by many usual opponents of middle turbinate resection as a potential complication after TSE. However, its incidence in this series was negligible. Undoubtedly, in the preantibiotic era, uncontrolled postoperative infection frequently followed any nasal surgery, the result of bony exposure in a contaminated field with supervening osteitis. One of the major refinements in the postoperative management of these patients has been the use of broad-spectrum antibiotics for as long as 6 weeks after surgery. This, along with meticulous postoperative local care using frequent nasal debridement and suctioning, has almost eliminated persistent nasal crusting. Patients are followed in weekly intervals for approximately 6 weeks, and the marsupialized sinus cavities and nasal vaults are easily tended with conventional or endoscopic illumination in the office. Diligent postoperative local care and the use of broad-spectrum antibiotics has not only reduced the rate of postoperative complications but also augmented the cure rates of CHR.

SUMMARY

CHR has become the most common inflammatory sinus condition otolaryngologists are faced with today. Persistent and/or partially treated infection constitutes the primary cause of this condition. However, other factors such as allergies, hereditary predisposition, anatomic abnormalities, environmental pollution, hormonal imbalance, and emotional problems play a significant role. The pathologic changes of CHR are usually multifocal and irreversible.

Improved methods of radiographic imaging illumination and magnification have brought about dramatic changes in the diagnosis, assessment, and management of CHR. Staging systems for CHR have improved communication among otolaryngologists in reporting the extent of disease, and treatment outcomes are helpful in assessing prognosis and have contributed significantly to a better understanding of the natural history of CHR.

The intranasal or transnasal sphenoethmoidectomy is a time-honored procedure for the treatment of intermediate or advanced infectious and hyperplastic rhinosinusitis. The operation involves complete removal of hyperplastic disease, and although many authors have characterized it as radical, it offers superior control of CHR and carries an extremely low rate of morbidity.

REFERENCES

1. Yankauer S: The complete sphenoethmoidectomy operation, *Laryngoscope* 31:831-842, 1921.
2. Mosher HP: The surgical anatomy of the ethmoid labyrinth, *Ann Otol Rhinol Laryngol* 38:869-901, 1929.
3. Davidson FW: Hyperplastic sinusitis: a five year study, *Ann Otol Rhinol Laryngol* 72:462-474, 1963.
4. Messerklinger W: The ethmoidal infundibulum. Inflammatory illnesses, *Arch Otolaryngol* 222:11-22, 1979.
5. Kennedy DW: Functional endoscopic sinus surgery, *Archiv Otolaryngol* 111:643-649, 1985.
6. Som PM, Lawson W, Biller HF, et al: Ethmoid sinus disease: CT evaluation in 400 cases. Part I. Nonsurgical patients, *Radiology* 159:591-597, 1986.
7. Katsantonis GP, Maas C, Cusumano J, et al: Comparison of accuracy of CT and routine radiography in chronic hyperplastic rhinosinusitis, *Am J Rhinol* 6:173-177, 1992.
8. Lawson W: The intranasal ethmoidectomy: an experience with 1,077 procedures, *Laryngoscope* 101:367-371, 1991.
9. Kennedy DW: Prognostic factors, outcomes, and staging in ethmoid sinus surgery. Part II, *Laryngoscope* 102:1-18, 1992.
10. May M: Personal communication, 1994.
11. Mackey I, Lund V: Personal communication, 1994.
12. Levine HL: Functional endoscopic sinus surgery/evaluation, surgery, and follow-up of 250 patients, *Laryngoscope* 100:79-84, 1990.
13. Friedman WH, Katsantonis GP, Sivore M, et al: Computed tomography staging of the paranasal sinuses in chronic hyperplastic rhinosinusitis, *Laryngoscope* 100:1161-1165, 1990.
14. Lepold DA: Pollution: the nose and sinuses, *Otolaryngol Head Neck Surg* 106:713-719, 1992.
15. Friedman EH, Katsantonis GP: Staging systems for chronic sinus disease, *Ear Nose Throat J* 73:480-484, 1994.
16. Mosher HP: The applied anatomy in the intranasal surgery of the ethmoid labyrinth, *The American Laryngological Association* 34:25-39, 1912.
17. Pratt J: The present status of the intranasal ethmoid operation, *Arch Otolaryngol* 1:42-50, 1925.
18. Skillern RH: Observations on the ethmoid problem, *Ann Otol Rhinol Laryngol* 37:173-181, 1978.
19. Morgenstein KM, Kreger MK: Experiences in middle turbinectomy, *Laryngoscope* 90:1596-1603, 1980.
20. Friedman WH, Katsantonis GP, Rosenblum BN, et al: Sphenoethmoidectomy: the case of ethmoid marsupialization, *Laryngoscope* 96:743-749, 1986.
21. Bolger WG, Butzin DA, Parsons DS: Paranasal sinus bony anatomic abnormalities: CT analysis for endoscopic sinus surgery, *Laryngoscope* 101:56-64, 1991.
22. Goldman JL, editor: *Intranasal sphenoethmoidectomy and antrostomy: the principles and practice of rhinology*, New York, 1987, John Wiley.
23. Friedman WH, Katsantonis GP, Rosenblum BN, et al: Sphenoethmoidectomy: the case of ethmoid marsupialization, *Laryngoscope* 90:473-479, 1986.
24. Katsantonis GP, Friedman WH, Bruns M: Intranasal sphenoethmoidectomy: an evolution of technique, *Otolaryngol Head Neck Surg* 111:781-786, 1994.
25. Friedman WH, Katsantonis GP: Intranasal and transantral ethmoidectomy: a 20 year experience, *Laryngoscope* 100:343-348, 1990.
26. Freedman HM, Kern EB: Complications of intranasal ethmoidectomy: a review of 1,000 consecutive operations, *Laryngoscope* 89:421-434, 1979.
27. Stankiewicz JA: Complications of endoscopic intranasal ethmoidectomy, *Laryngoscope* 97:1270-1273, 1983.
28. Stankiewicz JA: Complications in endoscopic intranasal ethmoidectomy: an update, *Laryngoscope* 99:686-690, 1989.
29. Lawson W: The intranasal ethmoidectomy: evaluation and assessment of the procedure. Part II, *Laryngoscope* suppl 64:104-106, 1994.
30. Maniglia AJ: Fatal and major complications secondary to nasal and sinus surgery, *Laryngoscope* 99:276-283, 1989.

CHAPTER

20

Endoscopic Sphenoethmoidectomy (P to A)

Andreas R. Gunkel
Wolfgang Freysinger
Walter F. Thumfart

PROBLEM

A 38-year-old man presented with a long-standing history of chronic rhinitis with secretion from the nose and, more recently, complete blockage of both nasal pathways. For at least 2 years he has noticed complete anosmia. He underwent two local polypectomies and a septal correction elsewhere. Previous treatment with antihistamines and decongestive spray and several courses of oral antibiotics were unsuccessful. An aspirin intolerance syndrome is suspected. Allergy testing for common allergens was negative. Apart from polyposis, he presented with no other disorders.

One of the main problems in endonasal sinus surgery is recurrent and chronic polyposis of the paranasal sinuses. These patients require surgery if intensive conservative medical treatment is unsuccessful.

Considering the long-lasting history of this patient with unsuccessful previous intensive conservative medical treatment and two local polypectomies, we recommended a complete sphenoethmoidectomy (CSE). From the clinical point of view, it was obvious that an extensive endonasal clearance of polyps was necessary for therapy to be successful.

The patient underwent a complete sphenoethmoidectomy posterior to anterior as outlined below. The application of a three-dimensional (3D) navigation systems for improvement of intraoperative anatomic orientation is especially useful in patients who have had one or more previous operations.

MEDICAL HISTORY

When performing the anamnesis, the physician should carefully account for possible factors that could prolong a chronic sinusitis, such as allergy or toxic agents in the environment. In younger patients with massive and recurrent polyposis, mucoviscidosis should always be ruled out. Many patients scheduled for CSE need revision surgery after earlier local polypectomies, simple fenestration of the maxillary sinus, or partial ethmoidectomy. In our patient, an aspirin intolerance syndrome was suspected but could not be proved. Intensive conservative drug treatment with antibiotics, decongestive spray, local cortisone application, and antihistamines had not significantly improved the amount of polyposis or the symptoms. Apart from the chronic sinusitis, the patient was in normal health.

PHYSICAL EXAMINATION

At the first examination he presented with massive bilateral polyposis completely blocking the nasal cavity. On the right side the polyps were almost protruding outside the nasal cavity at the nostril. The polyps showed a very solid consistency, almost resembling fleshy tissue. At this time a complete anosmia was detected.

An endoscopic inspection of the whole nasal cavity, particularly the region of the middle meatus, is mandatory to evaluate the amount of disease. Frequently, large polyps are hanging down freely from the ethmoid into the nasal cavity. Application of a decongestive packing (gauze with solution of cocaine 10%) before inspection improves the view into regions that play a crucial role in the ventilation of the different sinuses (e.g., middle meatus, frontal recess). However, some patients do not show free polyps during endoscopic examination but nevertheless have a considerable amount of polyposis involving nearly all paranasal sinuses. Diagnosis of polyposis is not complete without radiologic imaging.

RADIOGRAPHIC EXAMINATION

Every patient with significant chronic sinusitis should undergo a computed tomographic (CT) scan of the paranasal sinuses if an endoscopic sinus procedure is discussed or planned. A conventional radiograph is often not sufficient. Normally, axial scans are taken, and sometimes coronal slices also, depending on the individual anatomy or the special indication. In cases of revision surgery, sometimes a coronal view is necessary to evaluate the exact relationship of the lamina cribrosa to the roof of the ethmoid or to the frontal recess. If previous operations are suspected to have violated the bony skull base, a coronal projection is strictly indicated. A CT scan is necessary to reveal the relationship of the individual anatomy of the paranasal sinuses to structures that might be put at risk during the operation (orbit, internal carotid artery, skull base with dura and frontal lobe of brain). Abnormalities in the course of the internal carotid artery, a medial protrusion of the lamina papyracea, or a low roof of the ethmoid and the lamina cribrosa cannot exactly be verified in the conventional x-ray film. Therefore, preoperative CT is mandatory even for the experienced surgeon. Radiologic imaging should reflect the long-term condition of the disease. Scans performed at the time of or shortly after treatment with cortisone may lead to a misgrading of the disease, as may scans taken at the time of an acute exacerbation of minor polyposis. If there is a discrepancy among the symptoms, the clinical endoscopic findings, and the CT results, a second scan may be necessary.

Radiologic CT imaging of our patient showed massive bilateral polyposis involving all paranasal sinuses (Fig. 20-1). The CT scans showed a complete opacification of the whole paranasal sinus system. Nevertheless, the bony structures at the ethmoidal roof and toward the orbit were intact, as judged from the radiologic aspect.

For the use of 3D navigation intraoperatively an axial CT scan has to be performed, taken according to a special protocol to allow an adequate 3D reconstruction. Thin bony structures such as the lamina papyracea, cribriform plate, or orbit need to be interpreted very carefully, since the integrity can be checked reliably only in coronal projections. Possible reformatting capacities of the 3D navigation system to generate coronal projections from axial ones need to be used with caution.

LABORATORY EXAMINATION

Standard laboratory blood tests normally do not show any specific changes in patients with chronic sinusitis. If an operation is planned, the regular blood parameters (blood cell count, electrolytes, and especially the coagulation parameters) should be tested.

A

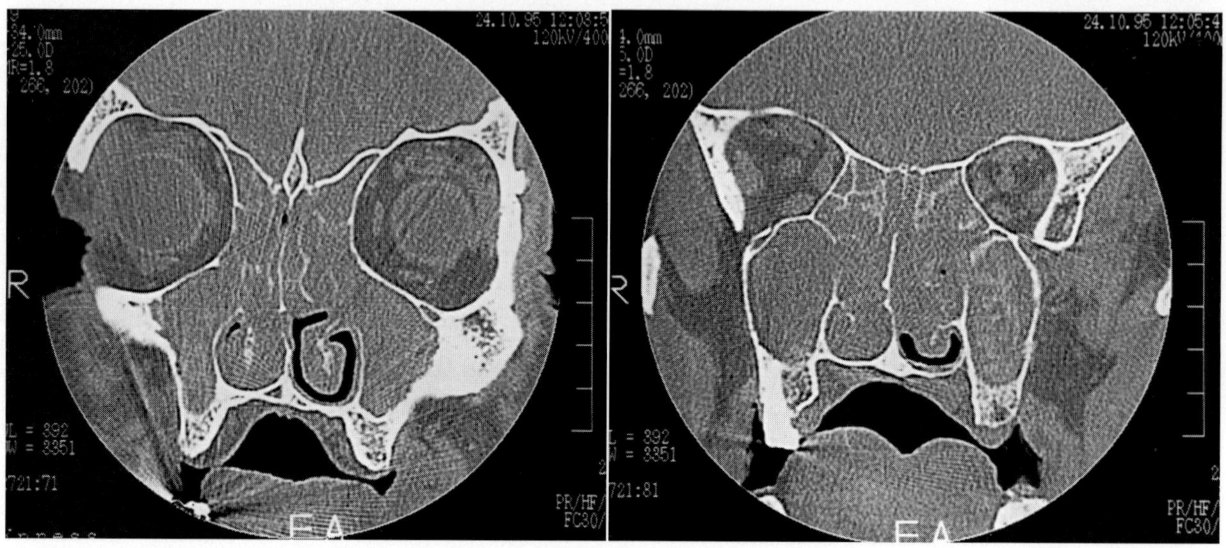

B

Fig. 20-1. Coronal computed tomographic (CT) scan of a patient with bilateral massive polyposis of all paranasal sinuses and the nasal cavity. Note the blockage of the middle meatus by the polyps. **A,** Scan crossing the anterior ethmoid and the maxillary sinus. **B,** Scan through the posterior ethmoid.

TREATMENT: COMPLETE SPHENOETHMOIDECTOMY

Indication

Patients with chronic polyposis of the sinuses resistant to long-term local or systemic drug therapy are frequently treated by endonasal operations, such as partial ethmoidectomy or CSE, depending on the amount of polyposis. The CSE from posterior to anterior is typically performed in patients with extensive disease. In these patients, several or all paranasal sinuses are normally affected, either unilaterally or bilaterally. A CSE was also performed in our patient.

Technique

M.E. Wigand developed endoscopic sinus surgery into CSE. On the basis of studies of the function of the nasal and paranasal mucosa in healthy individuals and in patients with chronic sinusitis, the aim of this technique is to achieve reventilation of obstructed sinuses.[1-7] Together with his colleagues, Wigand also introduced the suction-irrigation endoscope into endonasal sinus surgery.[8] This provided the surgeon with a far better view of the operating site than before. This is especially important in cases of heavy bleeding blurring the lens.

Patient positioning, operating room set-up. The surgeon normally stands on the right side of the patient looking into his or her face. The head of the patient is slightly elevated; it should not be reclined too much, because this forms a straight line to the frontal skull base, putting it at higher risk. The nurse with the instrumenting table stands on the right side of or opposite to the surgeon so that the surgeon can pick up and change the instruments easily with little changing of the upright position and without turning the head or neck. The best position of the light source and the videoendocamera system is close to the head of the patient. If used, the 3D navigation system is best set parallel to the video monitor. This allows the surgeon to watch the video monitor directly and helps to keep the endoscope steady and therefore fairly clean (Fig. 20-2). After the patient's face is cleaned and the sterile dressing applied, the suction-

A

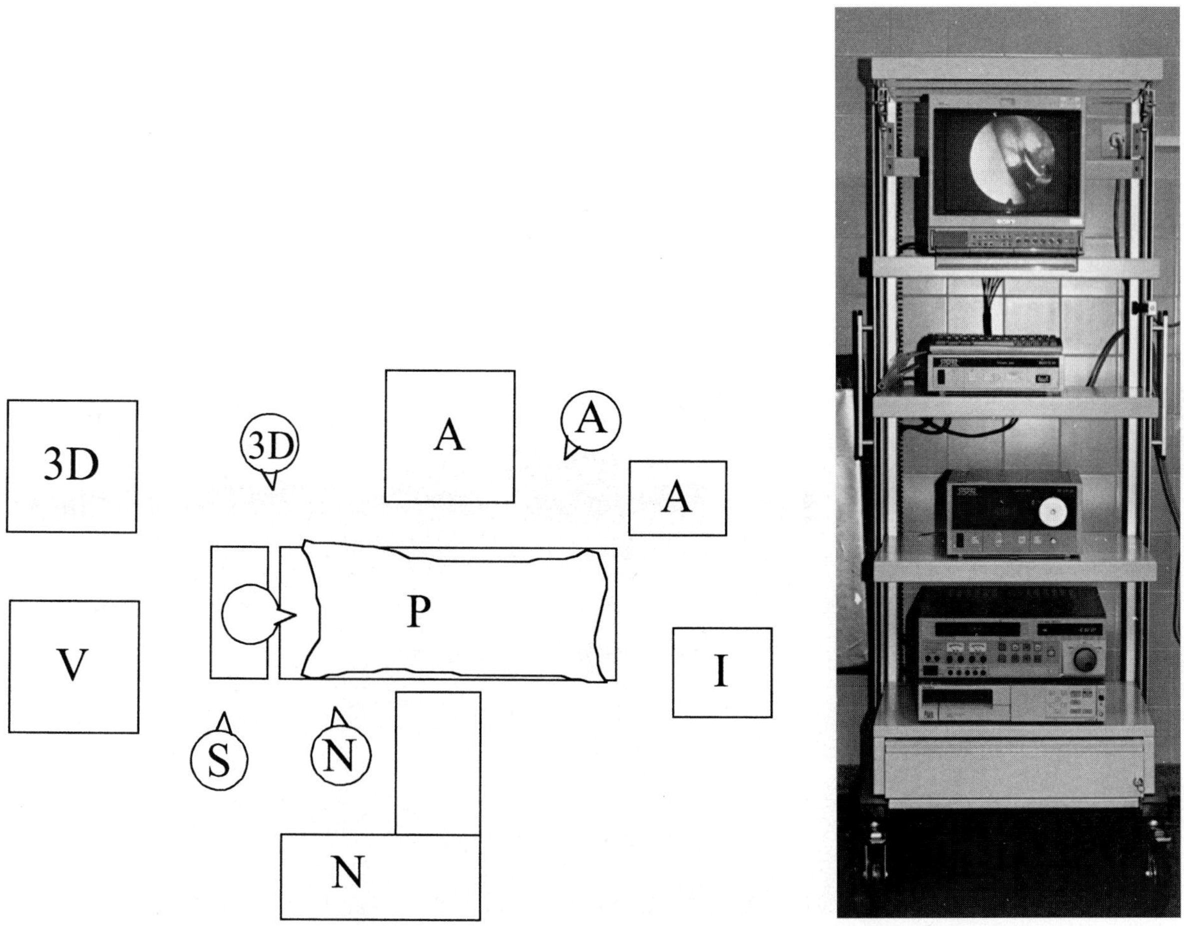

B

Fig. 20-2. Intraoperative set-up. **A**, Sketch of the complete set-up. *P*, Patients; *S*, surgeon; *N*, nurse and instrument table; *V*, video equipment; *3D*, three-dimensional navigation unit and operator; *A*, anesthetist and equipment; *I*, adjustable irrigation unit. **B**, Videoendoscope system, *from top to bottom*: monitor, camera, light source, videorecorder, videoprinter.

irrigation endoscope mounted with a chip-endocamera is laid onto the patient's thorax, fixed with clamps in such a way that it can easily be moved.

We do not regularly operate with the patient in a condition of artificial arterial hypotonia as some otorhinolaryngologic surgeons recommend. To a large extent, the amount of bleeding depends on the individual operation technique. A minimal invasive technique under videoendoscopic control helps the surgeon to recognize arterial vessels before they are touched and before they can be the source of excessive bleeding. The eyes of the patient must always be visible so that a possible orbital complication is detected immediately. Inspection of the size of the pupils before and during the operation is mandatory. The onset of anisocoria is an alarming symptom. Any suspicion of orbital complications needs immediate consultation with the ophthalmologist.

Suction-irrigation endoscope. We have extended the functions of the suction-irrigation endoscope (Fig. 20-3) by using a device to warm the irrigation saline solution (0.9%) to about 40°C and to flush the lens of the scope and the operating site with adjustable pressure. This provides a better cleaning effect, and the hyperthermic saline lowers the tendency toward bleeding (Fig. 20-4). We have modified the device—originally developed for transplantation surgery—for the necessities of otorhinolaryngology. Practical use showed an impressive improvement of the function of the suction-irrigation endoscope compared with a conventional infusion system. The warmed saline solution protects the lens in the tip of the endoscope from blurring too soon.

Instruments. Our instruments for the endonasal procedures are a set of different blunt forceps (straight or angled, 45- or 90-degree), punch and backbiting forceps, rongeurs, and a set of curved forceps to gain access even to remote areas of the paranasal system (lateral part or floor of the maxillary sinus, frontal sinus). In our experience, most of the sphenoethmoidectomy can be performed simply with a middle-sized 45-degree Blakesley forceps. Gentle manipulation of the instruments, particularly in dangerous areas, rarely leads to serious iatrogenic trauma.

Operative procedure

The operation is started by packing the nose with gauze soaked with a 10% solution of cocaine, enlarging the work space inside the nose. A significant septal deviation hindering the entrance into the posterior area of the nose and the ethmoid is corrected before the CSE. This eases postoperative care and follow-up for both surgeon and patient.

The first step in CSE is the medialization of the middle turbinate to obtain access to the middle meatus, to the posterior ethmoid, and to the anterior wall of the sphenoid cavity. Often the middle turbinate is hyperplastic and pneumatized (concha bullosa) or its mucosa is changed by the polyps. The posteroinferior part of the middle turbinate is resected with scissors. It is important to preserve the upper part of the middle turbinate, especially the medial surface with the olfactory epithelium. Stabilization of the concha is maintained by resecting the posteroinferior part of the turbinate only, preserving the insertion to the roof of the ethmoid. The cutting line should run close to the far posterior end, so that the cut segment can be pulled off easily (Fig. 20-5). Tearing off an incompletely cut segment frequently leads to heavy bleeding of branches of the sphenopalatine artery. Sometimes it is easier to grasp the cut lower segment with the Blakesley forceps and push it posteriorly before actually removing it. Large polyps, hanging freely into the lumen

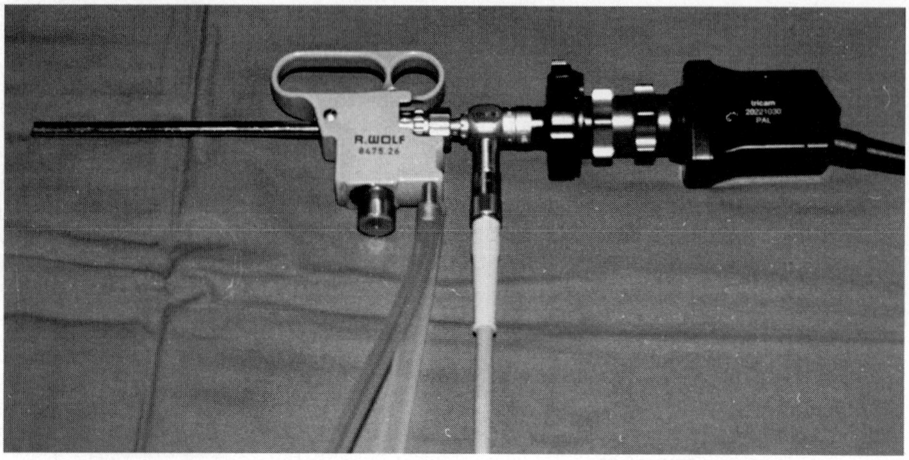

Fig. 20-3. Suction-irrigation endoscope with 25-degree Panoview optic (R. Wolf, Germany), mounted with a three-chip videocamera (K. Storz, Germany). The endoscope is inserted in a shaft and the handle; the lines for irrigation, suction, and the light cable are in place.

I

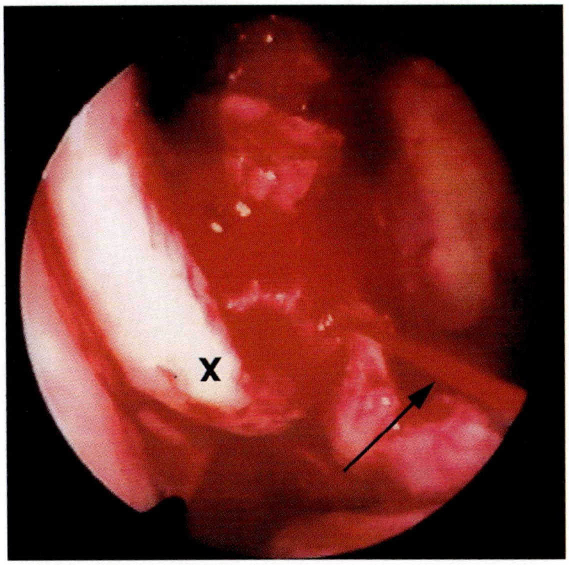

II

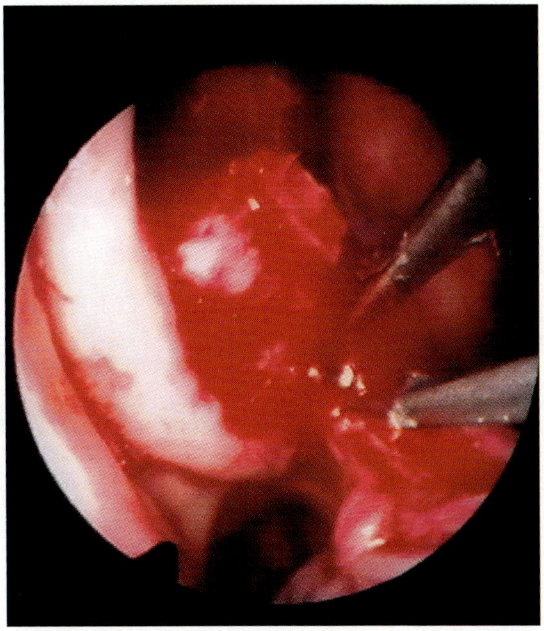

Color Plates I and II. Management of bleeding from the sphenopalatine artery. **I,** Strong arterial bleeding *(arrow)* just from the posterior end of the middle turbinate (*x*). **II,** Bleeding stopped by bipolar coagulation under videoendoscopic view.

of the nasal cavity, must be removed to view the middle turbinate. One should avoid pulling too strongly on polyps hanging down medially to the middle turbinate from the olfactory rim. This might cause cerebrospinal fluid (CSF) leakage from the lamina cribrosa, because the fila olfactoria might stick to the polyps and be torn off and out of the lamina.

The second step is the identification of the anterior wall of the sphenoid cavity with its natural ostium. The anatomic landmarks are the choana and the region just medial to the resection line of the posterior end of the middle turbinate. The sphenoid ostium is normally about 1 to 1.5 cm superior and medial to the highest point of the upper rim of the choana. If the location of the sphenoid is uncertain, one should keep the instrument closer to the nasal septum rather than to the lateral nasal wall. The area adjacent to the lateral nasal wall hides vital structures, such as the internal carotid artery or the optic nerve, which can be violated. Polyps are often protruding out of the natural sphenoid ostium that has been enlarged by the long-standing pressure exerted by the polyps. The CT scan gives exact information about the anatomy of the sphenoid cavity and its relationship to the optic canal and internal carotid artery. Once identified, the natural ostium of the sphenoid is widened with a Blakesley forceps or a rongeur (Fig. 20-6). Alternatively, the anterior wall is penetrated with a blunt forceps, or often, simply with a straight suction probe. Penetration of the bony wall has to be done extremely carefully, and the hand leading the in-

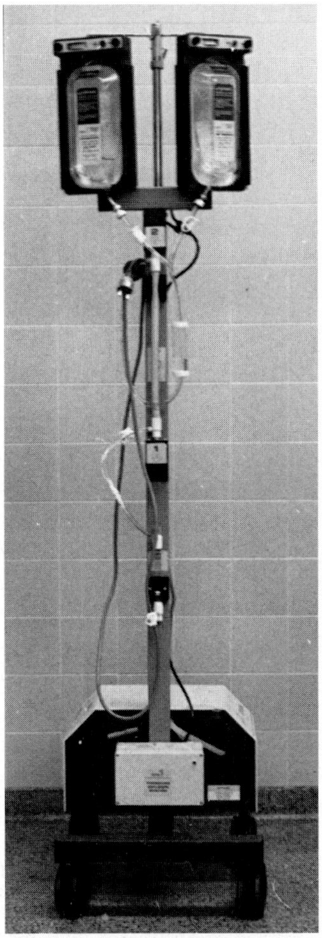

Fig. 20-4. Device for warming saline solution and adjusting the pressure of the irrigation fluid (Level 1 Technologies Inc., Rockland, Mass).

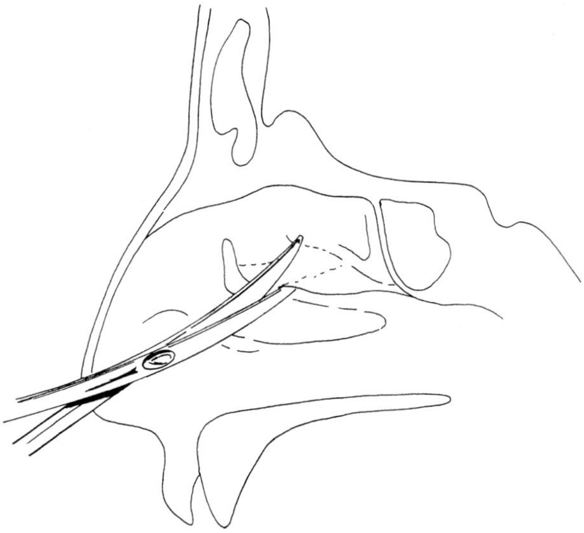

Fig. 20-5. Medialization and partial or subtotal resection of the middle turbinate with a pair of curved scissors.

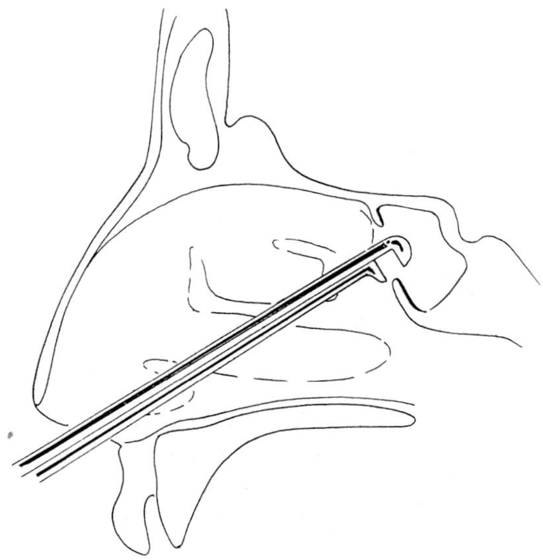

Fig. 20-6. Penetration and opening of the anterior wall of the sphenoid cavity. The opening is enlarged with a rongeur.

strument should lie on the upper lip of the patient. This gives enough support for a very controlled penetration into the sphenoid with little risk of iatrogenic trauma. Many patients have large posterior ethmoidal cells that may be mistaken for the sphenoid cavity. A simple but very useful rule of thumb to keep proper anatomic orientation is as follows: the distance from the columella to the posterior wall of the nasopharynx (columella-nasopharynx distance [CND]) nearly always equals the distance from the columella to the posterior wall of the sphenoid cavity (columella-sphenoid distance [CSD]). With a straight suction probe the CND is measured and correlated to the distance to the back of the opened (but not positively identified) cavity or posterior ethmoidal cell. If it is a posterior ethmoidal cell, this distance is shorter than the CND; if the sphenoid is opened, this distance is just as long as the CND (CND = CSD). One should never proceed further than the CND into a cavity in order not to inadvertently penetrate the skull base. Significant asymmetry of the sphenoid cavities or the intersphenoidal septum may mean that the surgeon enters the contralateral sphenoid via the intersphenoidal septum.

The anterior wall of the sphenoid, sometimes nearly the whole anterior wall, is removed until a sufficiently large opening is created. We regularly use a 90-degree rongeur to enlarge the opening; with this instrument, it is possible to feel and easily remove the rim of bone around the natural or created opening of the sphenoid sinus. Free polyps are removed, but healthy mucosa should be left in place. Caution is necessary when grasping at the lateral wall of the sphenoid cavity, because the internal carotid artery and the optic nerve can run through the lumen

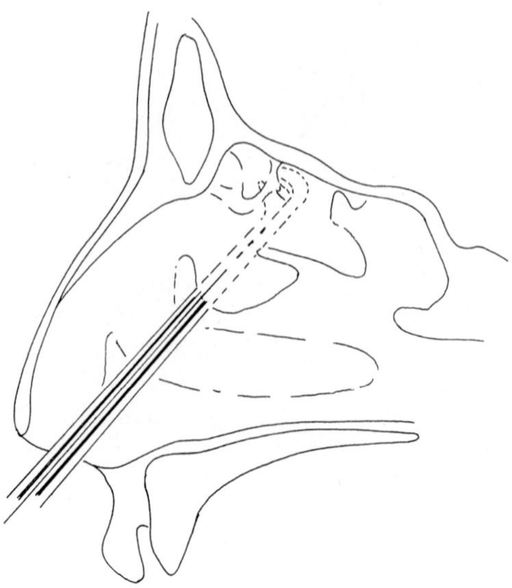

Fig. 20-7. Removal of the ethmoidal cells from posterior to anterior along the frontal skull base. Care must be taken not to penetrate through the ethmoidal roof.

without any bony covering. In the lateral inferior aspect of the anterior wall the sphenopalatine artery enters the nasal cavity from posterior, and this is sometimes opened while bone is removed in this area. Arterial bleeding is easily seen with the endoscope and can be stopped by packing or bipolar coagulation.

The third step is to remove the ethmoidal cells, starting posteriorly and working anteriorly, following the ethmoidal roof. Polyps and the bony septa of the posterior, middle, and anterior ethmoid are removed step by step along the roof of the ethmoid. The laterally located lamina papyracea can be felt as a thin and elastic resistance, when touching it with the Blakesley forceps. The skull base is recognized by its typical color, which is smooth and more yellowish than the bony lamellae separating the different groups of ethmoidal cells (Fig. 20-7). The posterior and anterior ethmoidal arteries cross the operating field transversely just below the ethmoidal roof. They run in separate bony canals that can mostly be detected with the endoscope before they are opened inadvertently. Most of the work is performed with the 45-degree Blakesley forceps, allowing comfortable working close to the skull base, around the tip of the endoscope. It is crucial that all instruments be handled gently in the vicinity of the skull base. All polyps or bony septa should be *taken away* from the roof of the ethmoid and thus from the skull base. The working direction should never go into the depth of the operating field, but always along the slightly curved surface of the ethmoidal roof.

After the anterior ethmoid has been almost completely opened, the entrance to the frontal nasal duct comes into view. It is located only a few millimeters behind the anterior insertion of the middle turbinate. Typically the agger nasi cells are located around the opening into the frontal recess. To obtain a full view into the opening to the frontal sinus, one can switch from the 25-degree to the 70-degree optic. With a bent suction probe, a bent forceps, or a microdebriding device, polyps obstructing the duct are removed (Fig. 20-8). It is crucial not to traumatize too much of the mucosal lining of the opening of the frontal nasal duct, to avoid postoperative swelling and scarring resulting in obstruction of the small entrance to the frontal sinus. If the approach to the frontal sinus is extremely tight owing to the individual anatomy, it can be extended by the punching forceps or a drill. If removal of bone around the frontal recess is necessary, it should be done anterior to the ostium because the risk of violating the frontal skull base and dura is considerably lower here, rather than posterior to the opening, especially in patients with a so-called, "dangerous" frontal sinus. In these cases the floor of the anterior cranial fossa declines from posterior to anterior. The surgeon can violate the skull base, even if the level of the middle and posterior ethmoid has not yet been reached, where the floor of the anterior cranial fossa lies higher than anteriorly.

The final step is to create a wide supraturbinal opening into the maxillary sinus. If the bulla ethmoidalis has not been opened completely it is done at this stage of the operation. Thereafter, the thin medial wall of the maxillary sinus is removed by penetrating it with the 45-degree Blakesley forceps or the bent suction probe in the region of its natural ostium. Together with the uncinate process, the lateral nasal wall, down to the upper rim of the inferior turbinate, is removed. The opening is enlarged with the backbiting forceps anteriorly until the maxillary sinus can be totally inspected (Fig. 20-9). With the 70-degree lens one can look down to the inferior recess and remove polyps or cysts based there.

Practice has shown that it is advantageous to put a temporary packing of gauze with cocaine solution into the completely opened operating field for a few minutes to stop diffuse bleeding. This helps detect polyps that have been missed before. If an initial septal correction has been performed, the incision is closed and Silastic sheets are fixed with two nonresorbable transseptal mattress sutures. Thereafter, a packing of gauze or self-expanding Merocel is inserted into the nasal cavity and left in place for 1 or 2 days.

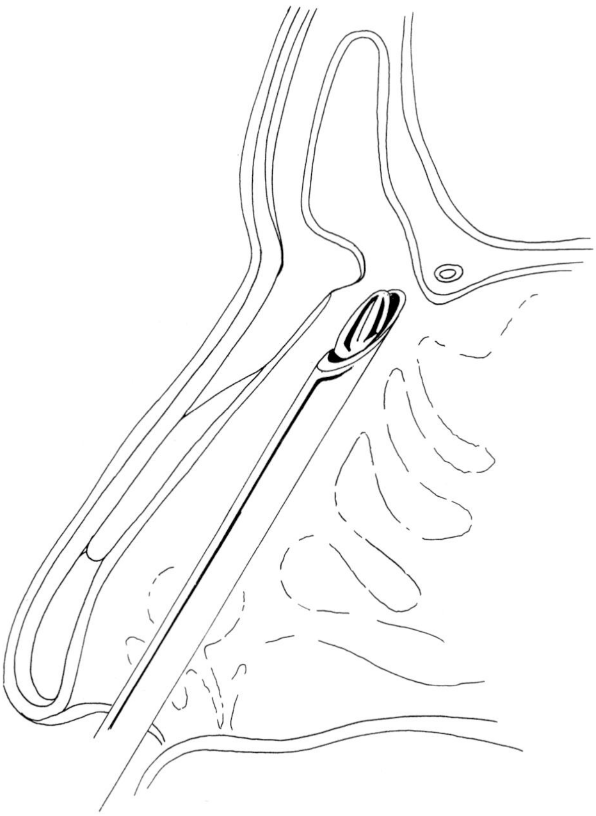

Fig. 20-8. Removal of polyps obstructing the entrance to the nasofrontal duct. Schematically, the use of a microdebriding device is shown.

COMPLICATIONS

The close proximity of vital and delicate anatomic structures to the surgical field may lead to life-threatening lesions (Fig. 20-10). Bleeding, trauma of the skull base with consecutive CSF leakage, and trauma to the orbit and contained structures are the main serious complications. Trauma to the internal carotid artery, the anterior cerebral artery, the frontal lobe of the brain, or even the brainstem after penetration of the clivus can also happen but are fortunately rare. The latter complications lead to severe damage of brain function or even to the death of the patient. For understandable reasons, reports about such tragic cases are rare. A serious complication is more often caused by a less experienced surgeon, but clinical practice has shown that under certain conditions they can happen even to a surgeon with great experience in endonasal surgery.

Bleeding from the ethmoidal arteries is caused if their bony canal is opened while the surgeon is working close to the roof of the ethmoid. Bleeding from the sphenopalatine artery happens mostly while resecting the posterior end of the middle turbinate or during the removal of the anterior wall of the sphenoid. Intranasal blood control is achieved by packing with a strip of gauze moistened with cocaine 10% or by bipolar coagulation. In our experience, the suction-irrigation endoscope provides a good view of the site of bleeding, and in most cases the stump of the artery squirting blood inside the nasal cavity can be identified and easily coagulated

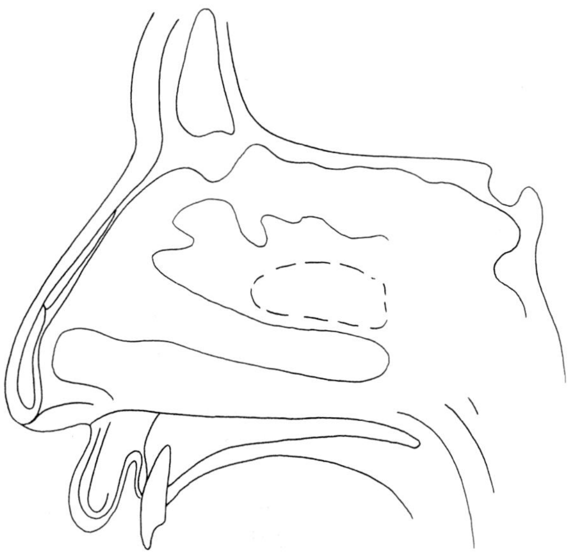

Fig. 20-9. Sphenoethmoidectomy is completed. All paranasal sinuses are opened, and finally a large supraturbinal window *(dashed line)* to the maxillary sinus is created. For the sake of orientation, some bone is left at the entrance to the frontal sinus.

A

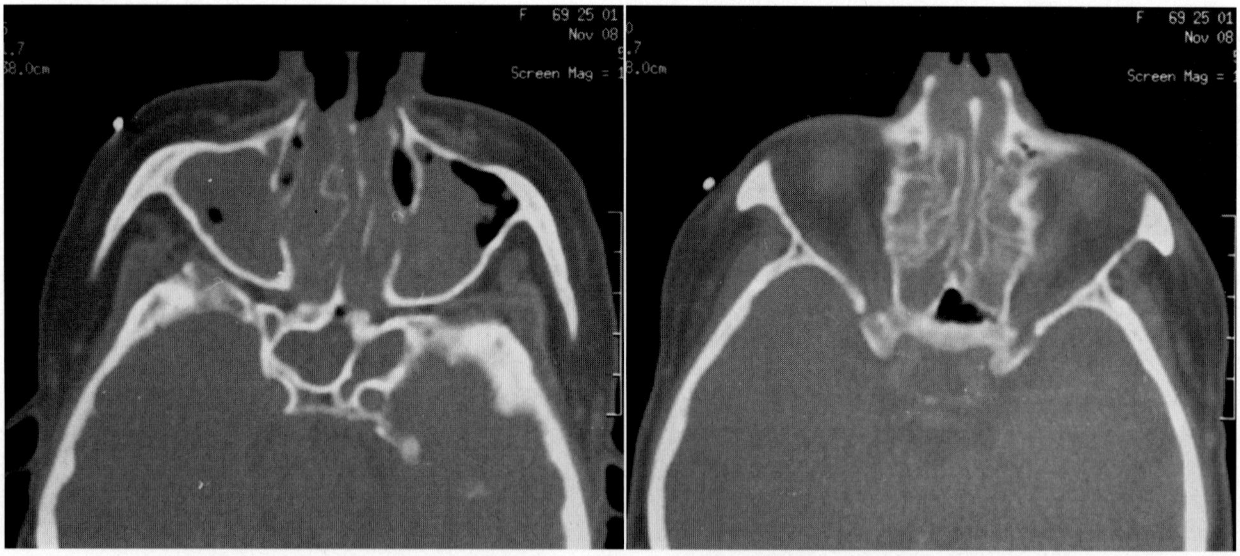

B

Fig. 20-10. Axial CT scans of a patient with massive polyposis, taken for 3D navigation. Note the intimate neighborhood of the sphenoid cavity, the carotid canal, and the posterior orbit with the optic nerve. On the skin over the zygoma, one of the radiopaque fiducial markers is visible. **A**, Scan through the maxillary sinus and the sphenoid cavity. **B**, Scan through the upper part of the ethmoid and the apex of the orbit.

(see Color Plates I and II). The patient's eyes should be controlled for signs of possible orbital complications (e.g., anisocoria, protrusio bulbi). This happens mostly if the proximal end of the ethmoidal artery retracts into the orbit and immediately leads to a massive intraorbital hematoma with increasing pressure to the delicate orbital structures. If an orbital bleeding is detected or an impairment of the optic nerve is suspected, the operation should be interrupted and an ophthalmologist contacted at once. An endonasal decompression of the orbit with opening of the periorbital fascia is the emergency procedure of choice in this situation. This emphasizes that extensive endonasal surgery, like CSE, bears the risk of serious complications and should therefore be performed only by a surgeon who is also trained in handling possible complications.

THREE-DIMENSIONAL NAVIGATION

The development of modern computer-assisted intraoperative 3D navigation and orientation systems indicates important progress for endoscopic surgery to the endonasal sinuses and the anterior skull base. 3D navigation opens up a new possibility to reduce the complication rate due to trauma to structures that the surgeon should not have touched or penetrated. One of the reasons for a lack of anatomic orientation is the absence of surgical landmarks, for example, in revision surgery. After one or several endonasal procedures, the middle turbinate is sometimes subtotally resected or the whole natural anatomy is lost because of scarring.[9-12] To overcome these problems, we have started to use several computer-assisted orientation systems as a support during endonasal sinus surgery and other operative procedures near to vital structures at the frontal skull base and the orbit. Today we use the Viewing Wand (ISG, Canada) routinely in complete sphenoethmoidectomy and other endonasal procedures (Fig. 20-11). This system has proved safe and reliable and we are able to achieve an intraoperative accuracy of 1 to 3 mm. We are testing and developing another 3D navigation system based on Interventional Video Tomography (IVT). The ARTMA Virtual Patient system allows an interactive, real-time correlation of the life endoscopic video image with CT data or other imaging modalities. Pathways and structures of interest can be generated and marked, respectively, in either the CT scan or the video at the same time (Fig. 20-12). Changes of the structures in one image modality are simultaneously updated in the others. This greatly enhances the possibilities of intraoperative 3D navigation. Additional information about these systems can be found elsewhere.[13-15]

RESULTS

The endoscopic sinus procedure in our patient led to a significant improvement of symptoms. The patient noticed free ventilation of the nose, and the feeling of pressure in the region of the maxillary and frontal sinus and the orbit completely disappeared. Also, after 6 weeks he noticed a return of his smell function, which could be

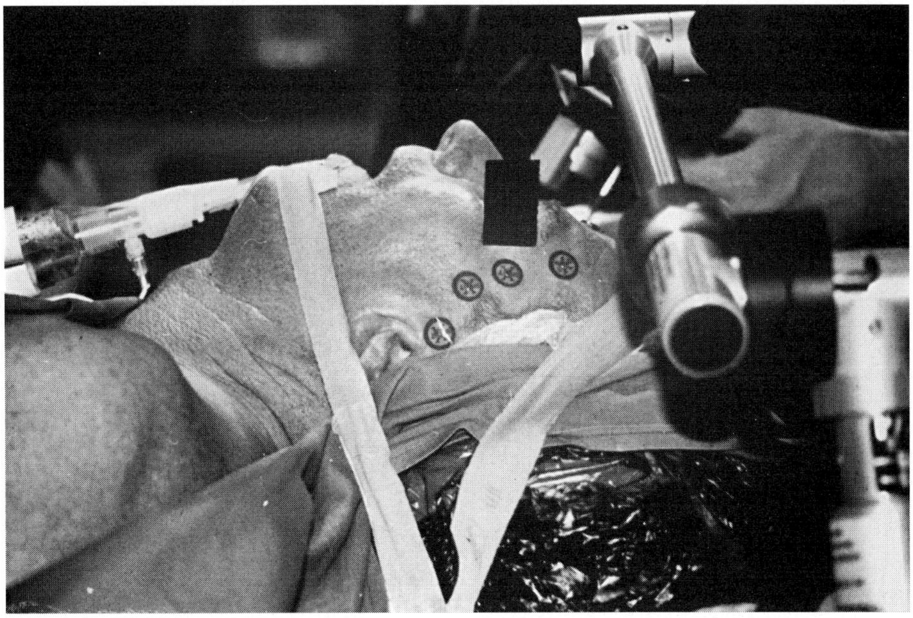

Fig. 20-11. Intraoperative set-up of the Viewing Wand 3D navigation system. The high-precision mechanical arm is fixed to the operating table; the patient shows fiducial markers on the skin. Patient fixation is satisfactorily achieved with surgical tape.

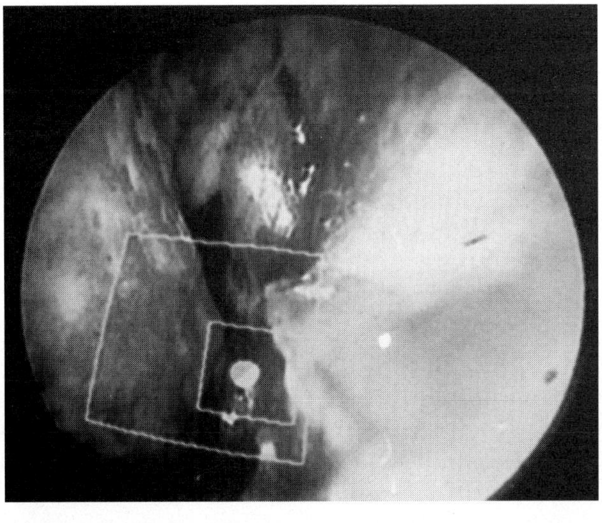

Fig. 20-12. Intraoperative screenshot of a surgery performed with the ARTMA Virtual Patient system. The pathway *(rectangles)* interactively integrated in the live endoscopic video screen view leads the surgeon to defined anatomic structures *(dot)*.

quantified by olfactory tests. Additionally, the amount of watery secretion from the nose was significantly reduced. The postoperative follow-up with regular nasal endoscopy showed satisfactory wound healing and little scarring, if any, particularly in the region of the frontal infundibulum. Despite the scarring, sufficient ventilation of both frontal sinuses was achieved. To suppress postoperative swelling and recurrent development of polyps, we prescribed a topical corticosteroid for 6 weeks. The patient was instructed to perform regular nasal irrigation with saline solution at least twice a day.

DISCUSSION

Endonasal operative procedures for the treatment of chronic sinusitis were first tried unsuccessfully at the beginning of the twentieth century. The lack of suitable instruments, particularly videoendoscopes with different viewing angles, frequently caused serious complications and a considerable rate of mortality.[16-18] Therefore, these techniques were abandoned in favor of sinus surgery via various external approaches. The increase of knowledge about the underlying causes of chronic sinusitis, and the achievement of milestones in technical development such as the Hopkins optics and powerful video cameras, led to a revival of endonasal operation techniques. This opened up the possibility for conservative endonasal surgical procedures, different from the radical therapy via the external route. Today, further developments of endonasal operation techniques make it possible to operate on most patients via the endonasal route, at the same time limiting the procedure to only what is absolutely necessary. This technique can truly be termed *minimal invasive surgery*. However, some patients still require extensive surgery via the endonasal approach. In these cases, CSE has to be performed. The main indication for CSE is massive polyposis of the paranasal sinuses. However, a total endonasal opening of the ethmoid, the sphenoid, and the maxillary sinus is an approach to the skull base or the orbit, too, for example, in cases of severe endocrine orbitopathy demanding an endonasal orbital decompression or for endoscopic closure of CSF leaks after skull base trauma.

Today, endoscopic endonasal operations for chronic polyposis have become a daily routine in ENT surgery, and the number of operative procedures on the paranasal sinuses performed via external approaches has decreased. Modern suction-irrigation endoscopes, combined with a high-performance endocamera (chip camera), provide a clear vision of the operating field. This allows the surgeon to work safely inside the nose, the paranasal sinuses, and the frontal skull base and close to the posterior part of the orbit. Working under videoendoscopic control is safer, especially for the less experienced surgeon, because it is easier to supervise every step of the operation. Permanent videoendoscopic control is routinely used in our clinic today.

CSE is performed close to delicate and vital anatomic structures that should not be violated at all. It is therefore not a beginner's operation but should be done by an experienced surgeon. To minimize the risk of harming vital anatomic structures, 3D navigation techniques have been developed. Two of these systems are routinely used in our clinic today, especially if the special conditions of the patient and his or her anatomy are likely to cause problems in the intraoperative orientation near to delicate anatomic structures. 3D navigation will certainly open up new possibilities in endonasal surgery, guiding the surgeon in areas close to vital and vulnerable structures.

As the indications for an endonasal operative approach (e.g., CSE) steadily increase, the indications for an external approach decrease proportionally. Meanwhile, massive polyposis is nearly always primarily treated endonasally using the Wigand technique.

Surgeons performing CSE should be aware of the possible complications, although it has become a daily routine operation. Finally, one should remember that an endonasal operation alone, even one as extensive as CSE, is only part of the treatment of chronic mucosal disease. Other factors causing the onset of polyposis have to be detected and treated also.

ACKNOWLEDGMENT

We thank Mr. Peter Bauer for providing us with Figs. 20-5 to 20-9.

REFERENCES

1. Messerklinger W: Über die Drainage der menschlichen Nasennebenhöhlen unter normalen und pathologischen Bedingungen. 1. Mitteilung, *Mschr Ohrenheilk* 100:56-68, 1966.
2. Messerklinger W: Das Infundibulum ethmoidale und seine entzündlichen Erkrankungen, *Arch Otolaryngol* 222:11-22, 1979.
3. Wigand ME: Transnasale, endoskopische Chirurgie der Nasennebenhöhlen bei chronischer Sinusitis. I. Ein biomechanisches Konzept der Schleimhautchirurgie, *HNO* 29:215-221, 1981.
4. Wigand ME: Transnasale, endoskopische Chirurgie der Nasennebenhöhlen bei chronischer Sinusitis. II. Die endonasale Kieferhöhlen-Operation, *HNO* 29:263-269, 1981.
5. Wigand ME: Transnasale, endoskopische Chirurgie der Nasennebenhöhlen bei chronischer Sinusitis. III. Die endonasale Siebbeinausräumung, *HNO* 29:287-293, 1981.
6. Wigand ME: Transnasal ethmoidectomy under endoscopical control, *Rhinology* 19:7-15, 1981.
7. Wigand ME: *Endoscopic surgery of the paranasal sinuses and anterior skull base,* New York, 1990, Thieme.
8. Wigand ME: Ein Saug-Spül-Endoskop für die transnasale Chirurgie der Nasennebenhöhlen und der Schädelbasis, *HNO* 29:102-103, 1981.
9. Anon JB, Lipman SP, Oppenheim D, Halt RA: Computer-assisted endoscopic sinus surgery, *Laryngoscope* 104:901-905, 1994.
10. Mösges R, Klimek L, Krückels G, Irion K: Die Integration von endoskopischer Bildinformation und dreidimensioinaler radiologischer Bildgebung, *Eur Arch Otorhinolaryngol Suppl* 2:63-64, 1992.
11. Schlöndorff G, Mösges R, Meyer-Ebrecht D, et al: CAS (computer assisted surgery): ein neuartiges Verfahren in der Kopf-Halschirurgie, *HNO* 37:187-190, 1989.
12. Zinreich SJ, Tebo SA, Long DM, et al: Frameless stereotactic integration of CT imaging data: accuracy and initial applications, *Radiology* 188:735-742, 1993.
13. Gunkel AR, Freysinger W, Thumfart WF, Truppe MJ: Application of the ARTMA image guided navigation system to endonasal sinus surgery. Proceedings of the 9th International Congress of Computer Assisted Radiology, June 21-24, 1995. Berlin, 1995, Springer.
14. Thumfart WF, Gunkel AR, Freysinger W: Endoscopic approach to the anterior skull base, *Op Tech Otolaryngol Head Neck Surg* 6:213-216, 1995.
15. Gunkel AR, Freysinger W, Thumfart WF, Pototschnig C: Complete sphenoethmoidectomy and computer-assisted surgery, *Acta Otorhinolaryngol Belg* 49:257-261, 1995.
16. Hajek M: Zur Diagnose und intranasalen chirurgischen Behandlung der Eiterungen der Keilbeinhöhle, *Arch Laryngol* 16:195-108, 1904.
17. Halle M: Externe oder interne Operation der Nebenhöhleneiterungen, *Berl Klin Wschr* 43:1369-1372, 1404-1407, 1906.
18. Mosher P: The applied anatomy and the intranasal surgery of the ethmoid labyrinth, *Trans Am Laryngeal Assoc* 34:25-45, 1912.

CHAPTER

21

Endoscopic Ethmoidectomy

Peter H. Hwang
David W. Kennedy

PROBLEM
A 38-year-old woman presents with a 2-year history of recurrent sinus infections that have been partially responsive to antibiotic therapy.

HISTORY OF PRESENT ILLNESS

The patient has a history of frequent symptomatic episodes characterized by bilateral nasal obstruction, purulent nasal discharge, fatigue, and facial pressure. The patient also reports some decreased sense of smell and complains of some pain that localizes to the medial canthal regions bilaterally. Her symptoms have persisted over 2 years. In addition to being given topical nasal steroids, she has been treated with multiple 10- to 14-day courses and one longer 4- to 6-week course of broad-spectrum antibiotics such as cefuroxime axetil, amoxicillin-clavulanate, and trimethoprim-sulfa. She has experienced fairly good symptomatic improvement while on antibiotics, but she relapses quickly after completing a treatment course. A course of oral steroids has also been tried with improvement, but she experienced early symptom relapse after the therapy. The patient was significantly troubled by some psychological changes while taking the oral steroids.

First, a thorough history regarding the character and chronicity of symptoms must be obtained. A diagnosis of true sinusitis should be distinguished from other rhinologic diagnoses such as allergic rhinitis, vasomotor rhinitis, and other noninfectious rhinitides. The American Academy of Otolaryngology–Head and Neck Surgery has developed symptom-based criteria for defining acute and chronic sinusitis, as well as temporal criteria for distinguishing acute, subacute, recurrent acute, and chronic sinusitis. Response to previous antibiotics can help guide their future selection.

Nasal congestion and nasal obstruction are the most common symptoms of early chronic sinusitis. Classically, ethmoidal sinusitis discomfort presents in the region of the orbit or medial canthus, although patterns of radiation may be variable, particularly when the dependent maxillary or frontal sinuses are involved. This patient's history of present illness suggests a diagnosis of chronic sinusitis, with likely involvement of the ethmoidal sinuses.

MEDICAL HISTORY

The patient denies any history of systemic medical illness. She has had no previous operations. Apart from topical nasal steroids, she uses no other medications regularly. She developed a rash when last placed on cephalosporins and has trouble tolerating macrolides. She had allergies and asthma in childhood. This was treated with desensitization, and she has had no seasonal symptoms or asthma since her early teens. More recently, she has undergone repeat skin testing for environmental allergies because she felt that her current symptoms might be related to allergy, but this demonstrated only mild reactions to dust and molds. However, the patient now believes that she is allergic to cigarette smoke, dust, and perfumes. Temperature changes also often worsen her nasal obstruction. She does not smoke or drink. She notes that her mother and an uncle have been treated for chronic sinusitis. Her aunt and her daughter have asthma.

A complete medical history should be obtained, including information regarding asthma or other evidence of upper respiratory tract hyperreactivity; environmental allergy; systemic illnesses such as diabetes or ischemic heart disease; and bleeding disorders. Allergies to medications may provide important clinical information; for example, aspirin sensitivity may be a predisposing factor toward more aggressive disease and perhaps less favorable surgical outcomes. More frequently, however, a patient may report a history of IgE-mediated allergy in childhood, with recent allergy testing showing only mild perennial reactions. However, the patient frequently notices that the symptoms are exacerbated by multiple environmental irritants and even environmental temperature change, and may interpret this as allergy to factors. A positive family history is commonly identified in patients with chronic sinusitis and suggests that there may be a genetic predisposition toward mucosal hyperreactivity and susceptibility to infection.

Tobacco use is strongly discouraged. In our practice, any patient with chronic sinus symptoms who actively smokes is not considered for elective surgery owing to the risk of granulation tissue formation and poor healing over exposed bone. In some patients, alcohol consumption, particularly of red wine or beer, may trigger marked mucosal congestion and thereby exacerbate symptoms.

PHYSICAL EXAMINATION

Anterior nasal endoscopy using a rigid 30-degree endoscope shows moist nasal mucosa, with edema of the left middle meatus. The left uncinate is perforated and a small stream of mucopus is observed in the left middle meatal region. The ethmoidal bulla also shows edematous change. The left sphenoethmoid recess is clear. The right middle meatus shows a similar degree of mucosal thickening as on the left side, but no mucopus is seen. There is an accessory ostium in the posterior fontanel on the right. The right sphenoethmoidal recess is clear, as is the nasopharynx. The remainder of the complete head and neck examination is normal.

A complete head and neck examination is a requisite part of the initial evaluation. The nasal endoscopy is the most critical aspect of the examination, and a systematic endoscopic technique ensures a thorough and consistent examination. We favor a three-pass technique using a 30-degree endoscope. The first pass of the endoscope is made along the floor of the nose, inspecting the inferior turbinate, inferior meatus, and nasopharynx. The endoscope is then withdrawn. The second pass is made between the inferior and middle turbinate to examine the inferior aspect of the middle meatus. The uncinate process is inspected for edema, displacement, or other structural abnormality. The findings in this patient of a perforated uncinate process and an accessory ostium are consistent with a history of sinusitis. The second pass is extended posteriorly and medially to the region of the sphenoethmoidal recess, where the mucosa of the sphenoid sinus ostium can be examined.

The final pass is executed on withdrawal of the endoscope after the second pass and is aimed at more careful inspection of the structures of the middle meatus. Gentle displacement of the middle turbinate medially may be required to visualize the ethmoidal bulla. The infundibular mucosa may sometimes be assessed by gentle lateral pressure against the uncinate process. If there is significant edema of the infundibulum, the mucosa will prolapse medially into view.

If mucopus is identified on endoscopic examination, attempts should be made to follow its course retrograde to determine its origin. In addition, endoscopic cultures obtained with either a calcium alginate swab or a suction trap can prove useful in guiding antimicrobial therapy.

RADIOLOGIC STUDIES

The patient underwent a computed tomographic (CT) scan of the sinuses after 6 weeks of culture-directed antibiotic therapy and continuation with topical nasal steroids. The scan revealed bilateral anterior and posterior ethmoid opacification with mucosal thickening in the ostiomeatal complexes bilaterally (Fig. 21-1). There was minimal mucosal thickening in the maxillary sinuses and in the floor of the frontal sinuses. The sphenoid sinuses were clear bilaterally.

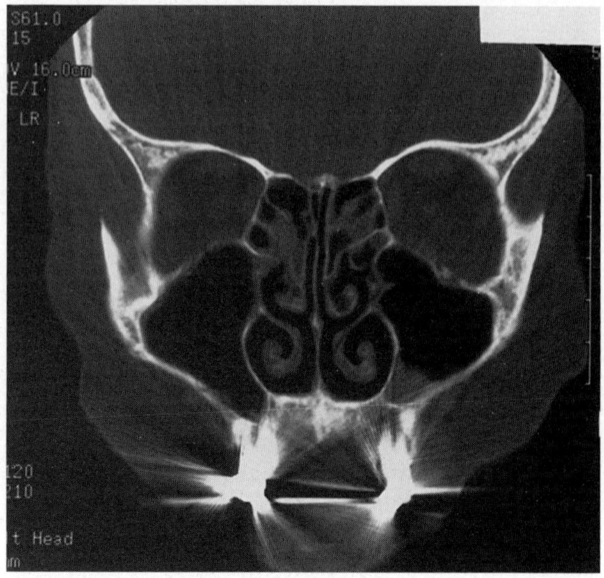

Fig. 21-1. Coronal computed tomographic (CT) scan taken after completion of extended medical therapy demonstrates persistent posterior ethmoid sinus disease. The patient also showed bilateral anterior ethmoid disease.

The imaging study of choice in chronic sinusitis is the 3.0-mm coronal CT scan. Ideally the images are obtained in a direct coronal plane with bone windowing. Axial images can be helpful in planning sphenoid sinus surgery but alone are inadequate to completely assess all sinuses. Contrast is not required for routine imaging but should be considered if there is concern regarding orbital or intracranial complications. Some centers offer a limited study at significantly reduced cost. These limited studies may have value in screening patients, but a complete study should be performed in any patient who will be undergoing surgery.

In obtaining CT scans for diagnosis of chronic sinus disease, timing is of critical importance. To avoid overestimating the extent of disease, the study should be performed only after the patient has completed an intensive course of medical therapy lasting at least 4 to 6 weeks, including antibiotics, topical nasal steroids, and oral steroids if indicated. Furthermore, any previous studies should be carefully reviewed in light of the medical therapy completed at the time of the scan.

CT scans should be studied carefully not only to determine the extent of sinus opacification, but also to evaluate anatomic features that may have surgical relevance. Specifically, every scan should at least be examined for the structure and/or atelectasis of the uncinate process, shape and integrity of the skull base, bony integrity of the medial orbital walls, relative height of the ethmoidal labyrinth, and presence of sphenoethmoid (Onodi) air cells.

With the increasing use of intraoperative CT guidance during surgery, consideration should also be given as to whether the initial sinus CT scan in a patient who may be a candidate for surgery should be performed in such a way to enable the subsequent use of intraoperative imaging. This requires the use of a suitable protocol and appropriate reference points or reference headset, thereby allowing the subsequent use of intraoperative imaging from the data obtained from the initial scan.

TREATMENT

The patient underwent bilateral endoscopic anterior and posterior ethmoidectomy for chronic ethmoid sinusitis refractory to extensive medical therapy. Significant mucosal thickening was found in the area of the maxillary sinus ostia, and middle meatal antrostomies were performed.

Surgical intervention should be contemplated only after the patient has clearly failed to show significant improvement with broad, intensive medical therapy. Patients should understand that although their need for medical therapy may be reduced postoperatively, it may be necessary to continue such therapy in order to achieve a long-term successful surgical outcome.

Preoperatively, all patients are counseled regarding the nature of the surgical procedure and its attendant risks and potential complications. These risks include, but are not limited to, orbital injury, blindness, cerebrospinal fluid leakage, brain injury, and alteration or loss of smell or taste. Patients are also warned that revision surgery may be required. The importance of compliance with follow-up visits for postoperative care is also stressed. Patients whose preoperative nasal endoscopy indicates marked mucosal hyperreactivity or extensive polyposis may benefit from a preoperative course of steroids and/or antibiotics. Septoplasty is planned concurrently if a septal deviation precludes access to the narrow side with a 4-mm telescope. When required, the septal correction is typically performed endoscopically after the ethmoidal sinus on the wider side has been exenterated. The septal incision is always made on the previously operated side, to avoid the possibility of blood contamination of the endoscope during surgery on the second side.

Endoscopic ethmoidectomy may be performed with equal ease using either general anesthesia or local anesthesia with sedation. In either case, the nasal mucosa is prepared with topical phenylephrine or oxymetazoline. This is followed by additional topical decongestion with cocaine powder applied slowly and cautiously on cotton applicators. The lateral wall of the nose is infiltrated submucosally with 1% lidocaine with 1:100,000 epinephrine, and greater palatine foramen blocks are also employed when entry in the posterior ethmoid is to be performed. The 0-degree endoscope is the telescope of choice for ethmoidectomy.

After adequate time has been allowed for decongestion and anesthesia to take effect, the uncinate process is identified, incised with a sickle knife, and removed with Blakesley forceps. If the uncinate process is markedly atelectatic, the uncinate may be approached from a posterior to anterior direction to avoid potential injury to the orbit. A ball-tipped seeker may be used to identify the posterior edge of the atelectatic uncinate, and the uncinate may then be removed with a backbiting forceps. With either approach, care should be taken to ensure complete removal of the uncinate; the maxillary sinus ostium should be identifiable with a 30-degree endoscope after complete uncinectomy.

Removal of the uncinate process should reveal the ethmoidal bulla, the anteriormost of the anterior ethmoidal air cells. The bulla may be entered and removed with standard Blakesley forceps, but thereafter the ethmoidectomy is best completed with through-cutting forceps to optimize mucosal preservation. The medial orbital wall should be identified early in the procedure to serve as a landmark for dissection more posteriorly.

Removal of the ethmoidal bulla and one or two additional anterior ethmoidal air cells usually reveals the basal lamella. The latter, which represents the lateral insertion of the middle turbinate on the medial orbit, divides the ethmoidal labyrinth into anterior and posterior compartments. The basal lamella can be identified intraoperatively by following the structure medially and confirming its continuity with the lateral surface of the middle turbinate. After its identity is confirmed, the basal lamella may then be entered to reach the posterior ethmoid labyrinth. Owing to the downsloping nature of the anterior skull base, the vertical height of the ethmoidal sinus drops as one proceeds more posteriorly. Therefore, the basal lamella should generally be entered at its inferior aspect to minimize the potential for injury to the skull base.

After entering the posterior ethmoid, one should continue with meticulous through-cutting dissection technique. Alternatively, the dissection may be performed with powered instrumentation. The latter helps in mucosal preservation but does not provide the same "feel" during the dissection as is given by hand instruments. The medial orbital wall should be skeletonized and should continue to serve as a landmark for dissection. Again, while dissecting within the posterior ethmoid, it is preferable to maintain an inferior course as one proceeds posteriorly, to avoid inadvertent violation of the skull base. Any residual partitions that remain superiorly should be left alone for the time being, as these can be easily and more safely removed once the skull base has been positively identified. The posterior most ethmoidal air cell serves as a useful surgical landmark for identification of the skull base. It can usually be identified by its pyramidal shape and its confluence with the skull base superiorly. The insertion of the superior turbinate should also be visible once the posterior most ethmoidal air cell has been opened. Care should be taken to review the patient's CT scan to rule out a sphenoethmoid (Onodi) air cell, which if present may be manifested as an exposed optic nerve or carotid artery within the posterior ethmoidal cavity. Should disease be found in the posterior ethmoid, a sphenoidotomy is performed by identifying the superior meatus medially from within the ethmoidal sinus, sharply resecting the most inferior aspect of the superior turbinate with through-cutting forceps, and then widening the ostium until the entire anterior wall of the sinus is removed. The sphenoid sinus ostium provides the safest access to the sphenoid sinus and can be reliably identified just medial to the superior turbinate posteriorly, after resection of its inferior aspect.

The total ethmoidectomy is completed by skeletonizing the skull base from a posterior to anterior direction to remove any remaining intercellular bony partitions that are left along the superior aspect of the ethmoid. Fine, upbiting, through-cutting forceps are preferred for this aspect of the procedure, and care is always taken to feel behind the bony partitions before they are removed. As the dissection continues anteriorly, the skull base will continue to slope upward, approaching the frontal recess. If no frontal sinus surgery is planned, instrumentation should stop here, and the procedure is thereby completed.

After adequate hemostasis is determined, the ethmoidal cavity is packed with a Merocel sponge. Suture tails attached to the packing are securely taped to the cheek using benzoin and adhesive surgical tapes.

POSTOPERATIVE CARE

The patient was discharged on the day of surgery and returned the next morning for removal of the packing. She returned on weekly visits for examination and debridement of the ethmoidal cavity. She was maintained on antibiotics until all areas of exposed bone were reepithelialized, and was restarted on topical steroids in the early postoperative period. Now 3 months postoperatively, the patient's sinus symptoms are significantly improved. She returns intermittently during the first postoperative year to ensure that the mucosa within the sinuses remains stable.

Postoperative care for endoscopic ethmoidectomy shares equal importance with the surgical procedure itself in determining a successful surgical outcome. Careful, regular surveillance of the ethmoidectomy cavity can prevent synechia formation, detect ongoing or new inflammation or infection, and allow a general assessment of the status of mucosal healing within the surgical cavity.

This close surveillance begins on postoperative day 1, when packing is removed. A formal nasal endoscopy is performed at this time. Any loose fragments of mucosa and bone are removed, and clots are gently debrided. The patient is started on a saline nasal spray and is instructed to refrain from nose blowing; heavy exercise; or any form of bending, lifting, or straining.

At the first postoperative visit, nasal endoscopy is again performed. The presence or absence of mucosal thickening is noted, as are any areas of exposed bone or early synechia formation. Exposed bone that appears markedly osteitic may require debridement or curettage at a subsequent visit if poor healing is seen in the area of concern. Typically, topical nasal steroids are reinitiated within the first few days postoperatively.

The patient thereafter returns for weekly nasal endoscopic examinations until a widely patent, noninflamed, mucosalized cavity is achieved. On average, four to six weekly visits are required, although the postoperative care plan is highly individualized and does not adhere to a fixed schedule. In addition to weekly visits, antibiotics and (frequently) oral steroids are administered in the postoperative period. The dosage and duration of therapy are adjusted weekly on the basis of endoscopic findings. Significant crusting that persists despite careful debridement may be alleviated by adjunctive irrigations using mupirocin ointment dissolved in normal saline at a concentration of 7.5 g/L.

Once a satisfactorily healed surgical cavity has been attained, maintenance visits continue every few months. The interval between visits is gradually lengthened once the stability of the sinal cavity has been determined.

SUMMARY

The achievement of successful outcomes in endoscopic ethmoidal surgery requires careful planning and consideration at all stages:

Preoperative

- Candidates for surgery must be selected carefully and rigorously. The surgeon should make sure that medical options have been exhausted before contemplating surgery.
- Radiologic studies should be obtained only after completion of an extended course of medical therapy. Any previous "positive" studies not ordered by the operating surgeon should be reviewed with respect to the nature of any medical therapy ongoing or completed at the time of the study.
- The sinus CT scan must be studied intently before surgery. Preoperative recognition of anatomic variations or quiescent complications can prepare the surgeon for more complex intraoperative dissections and thereby reduce the risk of surgical complications.

Intraoperative

- To avoid injury to the orbit, the medial orbital wall should be identified as early as possible during the dissection and should be used as a surgical landmark for completion of the ethmoidectomy.
- To avoid injury to the skull base, the ethmoidal dissection should be carried out inferiorly until the skull base can be clearly defined at the level of the posteriormost ethmoidal cell. Thereafter, the ethmoidectomy can be completed safely by working retrograde along the skull base to clear residual partitions superiorly.
- Mucosal preservation techniques in ethmoidectomy permit more rapid healing of the sinus cavity. More important, mucosal preservation is critical to maintaining optimal long-term sinus function and reducing the risk of stenosis and of the development of postoperative osteitis or osteomyelitis. Ultrastructural studies have demonstrated that mucosa that has regenerated after being stripped lacks a functional ciliated epithelium, whereas mucosa that has been preserved retains its normal ciliary structure and function.

Postoperative

- Postoperative care is performed meticulously and frequently.
- Medical therapy is adjusted on a weekly basis in the early postoperative period according to the findings on endoscopic examination. Medical therapy continues in the long term, even after healing is complete, until it is clear that the mucosa has stabilized. Subsequent therapy, if required, is primarily based on objective evaluation of the sinus mucosa, rather than waiting for the reemergence of symptoms. The latter often occurs significantly later than the objective signs of persistent or recurrent disease.
- Medical therapy remains the primary mode of treatment for all surgical patients.

REFERENCES

1. Bolger WE, Butzin CA, Parsons DS: Paranasal sinus bony anatomic variations and mucosal abnormalities: CT analysis for endoscopic sinus surgery, *Laryngoscope* 101:56-64, 1991.
2. Kennedy DW: Prognostic factors, outcomes, and staging in ethmoid sinus surgery, *Laryngoscope* 102 (suppl 57):1, 1992.
3. Kennedy DW, Zinreich SJ: The functional endoscopic approach to inflammatory sinus disease, *Am J Rhinol* 2:89, 1988.
4. Kennedy DW, Zinreich SJ, Shaalan H, et al: Endoscopic middle meatal antrostomy: theory, technique, and patency, *Laryngoscope* 97(suppl 43):1, 1987.
5. Lanza DC, Kennedy DW: Adult rhinosinusitis defined. Part 2, *Otolaryngol Head Neck Surg* 117:1, 1997.
6. Moriyama H, Yanagi K, Ohtori N, et al: Healing process of sinus mucosa after endoscopic sinus surgery, *Am J Rhinol* 2:97, 1996.
7. Schaefer SD, Manning S, Close LG: Endoscopic paranasal sinus surgery: indications and considerations, *Laryngoscope* 99:1, 1989.
8. Stammberger H, Pasawetz W: Functional endoscopic sinus surgery: concept, indications and results of the Messerklinger technique, *Eur Arch Otorhinolaryngol* 247:63, 1990.

CHAPTER 22

Minimizing Complications in Endoscopic Endonasal Sinus Surgery

Sam J. Marzo
James A. Stankiewicz

PROBLEM

The patient is a 50-year-old machine-tool operator with a 5-year history of chronic facial headaches, nasal pressure, nasal congestion, and intermittent rhinorrhea. He was diagnosed as having chronic sinusitis and nasal polyposis and underwent endonasal sinus surgery (ENSS) at an outside institution 2 years previously. His postoperative course was complicated by decreased vision and transient diplopia, both of which resolved with medical therapy and observation. He now presents to this office for evaluation. Physical examination and computed tomography (CT) show pansinusitis and nasal polyposis.

The management of this patient is complex in that he has suffered an intraorbital complication of ENSS; furthermore, he is symptomatic. Our goal is to elucidate which one or two nasal complaints trouble him the most and then focus on these. After a complete history taking and thorough head and neck examination have been performed, imaging studies are reviewed. Next, medical management is instituted. If this fails to improve the symptoms, revision endoscopic surgery is discussed.

MEDICAL HISTORY

Of the symptoms of facial headache, nasal pressure, nasal congestion, and intermittent rhinorrhea, the headaches and nasal congestion trouble this patient the most. It is often helpful to have patients quantitate their complaints on a 10-point scale. We also have all our new patients with sinus problems complete a simple 2-page questionnaire (Fig. 22-1) before the physician enters the room. The physician can then briefly skim the questionnaire with the patient and focus on key areas. This ensures that all relevant questions are answered.

Other important points in the history are previous medical treatments (listings of antibiotics and treatment duration), previous nasal surgeries (e.g., septoplasty, ENSS), and history of allergies (asthma, animal danders, work and home environments). Next, any risk factors for bleeding are identified: for example, hypertension, recent aspirin or nonsteroidal antiinflammatory drug use, and history of bleeding with surgery. As this patient had undergone earlier surgery, we would try to obtain copies of the operative reports and details of the treatment of any postoperative complications.

PHYSICAL EXAMINATION

After the history is completed, a thorough head and neck examination is performed. In this patient the otologic, oral cavity, and neck examination results were unremarkable. We generally examine the nasal cavity at the end of the examination, first with a nasal speculum and then with a fiberoptic endoscope. We also allow the patient and the family to view the nasal examination as it occurs on a television camera coupled to the nasal endoscope. In

Sinus questionnaire

1. Who referred you to us?
2. Allergies:
3. Medications:
4. Previous nasal/sinus surgeries:
5. Previous CT scans of sinus:
6. Which one or two symptoms trouble you the most?
7. What outcome do you expect of your treatment here?
8. On a scale of 0 (none) to 10 (terrible), please rank your symptoms:

   Nasal congestion: 0 1 2 3 4 5 6 7 8 9 10
   Nasal drainage: 0 1 2 3 4 5 6 7 8 9 10
   Postnasal drip: 0 1 2 3 4 5 6 7 8 9 10
   Bad breath: 0 1 2 3 4 5 6 7 8 9 10
   Visual problems: 0 1 2 3 4 5 6 7 8 9 10
   Ear congestion: 0 1 2 3 4 5 6 7 8 9 10
   Cough: 0 1 2 3 4 5 6 7 8 9 10
   Facial pain: 0 1 2 3 4 5 6 7 8 9 10
   Where is the pain?
   How often do you get the pain?
   Describe the type of pain:
   What makes it better?
   Headache: 0 1 2 3 4 5 6 7 8 9 10
   What is the headache like?
   What makes it better?
   Any nausea? yes no Vomiting? yes no
   Have you seen a neurologist? yes no Name:
9. Please rate how you feel today: 0 1 2 3 4 5 6 7 8 9 10
10. Have you been tested for allergies? yes no
    If yes, date: Name of allergist:
    What are you allergic to?
11. What kind of treatment do you take for your allergies?
12. Are you a smoker? yes no How many packs per day:
13. Do you have any of these health problems? Circle all that apply:
    Diabetes Bleeding disorder
    Heart trouble Cancer
    High blood pressure Asthma
    Ulcers Aspirin sensitivity
14. Is there anything else that you would like to tell us?

Fig. 22-1. Sinus questionnaire.

the patient this revealed moderate bilateral polyposis, pale and edematous middle turbinates, and a significant right nasal septal deviation.

A thorough flexible fiberoptic nasal examination is critical and should be performed in a structured manor. We first examine the inferior meatus and inferior turbinate, and then the middle meatus and turbinate, trying to determine which surgical landmarks remain. Next the maxillary ostia, frontal recess, anterior and posterior ethmoids, and sphenoid ostia are examined.

The patient was found to have significant bilateral polyposis, residual uncinate processes, and intact middle turbinates. None of the sinus ostia were patent. There was also a moderate right nasal septal deviation.

It is also important to perform an ophthalmologic examination. Vision can be assessed with a Snellen eye chart. Pupils are checked for symmetry and reactivity. Extraocular muscles are evaluated for entrapment. As the patient also had an orbital complication of endoscopic surgery, we would most likely have an ophthalmologist evaluate him in case further surgery was required. The eye examination in the patient proved unremarkable.

RADIOGRAPHIC EXAMINATION

Next, any previous sinus imaging studies are reviewed. We obtain a new baseline CT scan of the paranasal sinuses on the day of the patient's visit if necessary. The CT scan in the patient revealed a significant soft tissue thickening involving all sinuses, as well as a right nasal septal deviation (Fig. 22-2). Both middle turbinates were preserved and remnants of the uncinate processes could be seen bilaterally. No defects in the fovea ethmoidalis or lamina papyracea could be seen.

LABORATORY EXAMINATION

This is tailored to the patient. Any significant bleeding history is evaluated with a complete blood count, prothrombin time and partial thromboplastin time, and bleeding time. Patients with allergic symptoms who have not previously been evaluated undergo a serum radioallergosorbent test (RAST), which screens for the most common inhalant allergies in our geographic area. The patient's laboratory examination was normal.

TREATMENT

Patients with documented chronic sinusitis (such as J.H.) first undergo a trail of intense medical therapy. Our first choices for antibiotics are amoxicillin-clavulanate (Augmentin) or cefuroxime axetil (Ceftin) clarithromycin (Biaxin) if penicillin allergic). Treatment durations are generally 3 to 4 weeks. If there are no contraindications to oral steroids, a short 5- to 6-day burst of prednisone (20 mg orally tid for 3 or 4 days, then 20 mg orally bid for 2 or 3 days) is prescribed for several days. Oxymetazoline (Afrin) is begun on an 8-day cycle (5 days on, 3 days off). Beclomethasone (Vancenase or Beconase) is also added to the armamentarium. With the addition of budesamide (Rhinocort) and dexamethasone (Dexacort) topical sprays, enhanced treatment of nasal polyps is available.

Patients are then seen in follow-up after 3 to 4 weeks. If the symptoms are considerably improved, the nasal steroids are continued and patients are observed. If the symptoms are moderately improved, antibiotics and nasal steroids are continued for several weeks. We then obtain a posttreatment CT scan to assess response to therapy if there is no change or improvement. Patients with good clinical responses to antibiotic and steroid therapy are followed periodically in the clinic. Those with minimal or no response to medical management and with documented disease are offered surgical therapy.

Patients who have undergone previous surgery and then develop recurrent nasal polyps are less responsive to intense medical therapy, as noted above. It should be offered as an alternative, but they will most likely need surgical treatment. Postoperative chronic medical therapy is most important in these patients to control polyp regrowth. A plan for management should be developed preoperatively and may involve oral and topical steroids.

The patient received little benefit from medical management; his history of recurrent nasal polyposis and septal deviation was probably a factor. He was then offered surgical therapy. The surgical procedure, risks, and possible complications were discussed at length and documented in the chart. Alternatives to surgery, such as continued medical therapy or no surgery, were also discussed along with their risks and complications. Not every conceivable complication of ENSS need be discussed (Box 22-1), but one should generally include infection, bleeding (possibly requiring transfusion), injury to the eye (resulting in temporary or permanent blindness or double vision), and cerebrospinal fluid leakage with possible meningitis or brain injury, as well as the possible need for further surgery. Although patients may be somewhat frightened by this disclosure, it often helps to add a statement about the surgeon's experience, such as "In over 2000 cases we have not had a patient lose his vision, nor had a brain injury."

The patient was later taken to surgery. In the preoperative holding area, his nose was decongested with Afrin nasal spray. In the operating room, he received a general anesthetic, since his procedure would be prolonged. Heightened awareness on the part of the surgeon to landmarks and location is most important when general anesthesia is used. The CT scan was mounted in the operating room and again reviewed. Cocaine (10%) on nasal cotton pledgets was inserted into each nasal cavity, and the turbinates and septum were vasoconstricted further with injected 1% lidocaine with 1/100,000 epinephrine. Preoperative treatment with Afrin may help lessen systemic absorption of cocaine. An alternative for patients with significant cardiac histories is topical application of

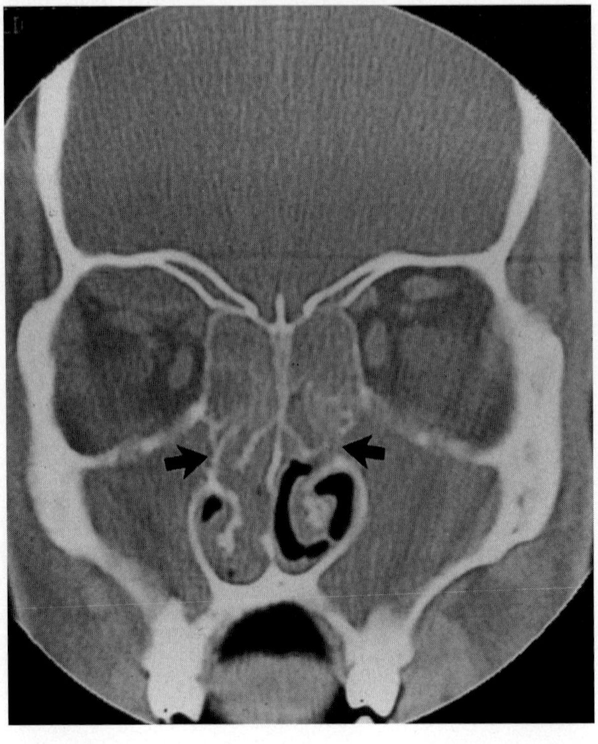

Fig. 22-2. Paranasal sinus computed tomographic (CT) scan of the patient. Notice the mucosal thickening involving all sinuses. Remnants of the uncinate processes are seen bilaterally *(arrows)*.

BOX 22-1

Possible Complications of Endoscopic Sinus Surgery

Nasal
- Bleeding
- Infection/toxic shock
- Synechiae[8]
- Nasal lacrimal duct injury[1,9]
- Mucocele
- Change in sense of smell[10]
- Neuroma[2]

Orbital
- Periorbital ecchymosis[11]
- Periorbital emphysema[11]
- Extraocular muscle injury/diplopia[12]
- Orbital cellulitis/abscess
- Intraorbital/retroorbital hematoma[5]
- Optic nerve injury/neuritis[13]

Intracranial
- Cerebrospinal fluid leak/meningitis[14]
- Pneumocephalus
- Vascular injury[15]
- Encephalocele[14]

tetracaine (Pontocaine) with ephedrine. For patients with limited or unilateral disease requiring less than 2 hours of operative time, a local anesthetic or sedation by the anesthesiologist is preferred.

We have found that the safest way to perform revision sinus surgery is to proceed from one landmark to the next. Using a 0-degree telescope, the nasal cavities were inspected. We approached the left nasal cavity first, as this was more patent than the right because of the septal deviation. The arthroscopic microdebrider is useful for polyp removal in that it is safe and quick and seems to decrease bleeding. Next, the middle turbinate was reflected medially with a Freer elevator, and an uncinectomy was performed using a backbiting forceps (a sickle knife can also be used, but it is easier to penetrate the orbit with forceps). The eye is palpated while the residual lamina papyracea is inspected to ensure that no entrance into the orbit has occurred.

If the natural maxillary ostia is not visualized, a 30-degree telescope is used. A curved probe can help identify and enlarge the ostia. It is further enlarged posteriorly with a straight punch, and anterioinferiorly with a backbiting or downbiting punch. One should not dissect anteriorly to the anterior margin of the middle turbinate, to prevent injury to the nasal lacrimal duct.[1] There are also reports of trigeminal neuroma resulting from a vigorous posterior enlargement.[2] Identifying the maxillary ostia is key, since the medial wall of the maxillary sinus is contiguous superiorly with the lamina papyracea. In patients with nasal polyps and pansinusitis, a larger than usual antrostomy is performed.

Next the bulla ethmoidalis is opened with a straight-biting forceps or punch. Polypoid tissue can be removed with the microdebrider. If diseased tissue is encountered, a beaded probe or other measuring device is used to measure the basal lamella, and this is next entered. The beaded probe has marks at 5, 7, and 9 cm, corresponding to the average adult distance from the nasal vestibule to the bulla ethmoidalis, anterior wall of sphenoid, and posterior wall of sphenoid, respectively. Medial bony walls are removed, leaving as much mucosa as possible laterally and superiorly. The microdebrider, as a mucosa-sparing instrument with real-time suction, is helpful in this regard.

If the sphenoid shows disease on the CT scan (as in this case), the ostia is probed with a beaded probe. It can usually be found medial to the superior turbinate. The approach to the sphenoid can be either medial or lateral to the middle turbinate. A small straight Fraser-tip suction is then used to enlarge the ostia. This is then extended inferiorly and medially with a universal sphenoid punch, or the microdebrider. The finding of the sphenoid sinus establishes the posterior landmark with the skull base.

Next, a curved suction is used as a "cell seeker" to identify any diseased superoposterior ethmoidal cells. The tissue is then removed with a right-angle or upward forceps (Fig. 22-3). Dissection proceeds anteriorly into the anterior ethmoids with the same technique. At all times the landmarks of the maxillary ostia, sphenoid ostia, middle turbinate, and skull base are maintained.

For significant frontal sinus disease, the frontal ostia is sought with a 30-degree telescope and a Kuhn probe. Giraffe forceps or frontal sinus curettes can be used to re-

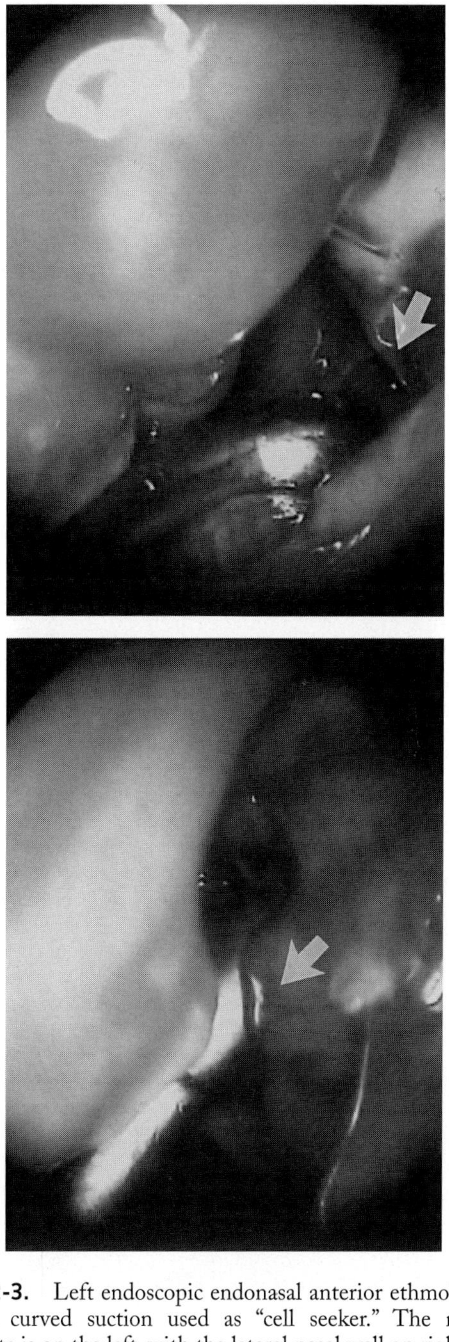

Fig. 22-3. Left endoscopic endonasal anterior ethmoid dissection curved suction used as "cell seeker." The middle turbinate is on the left, with the lateral nasal wall on right. Arrow in top panel points to the anterior ethmoidal cell. In the lower panel the cell is dissected with curved suction, so that it can then be safely removed with a right-angle forceps.

move diseased tissue from this area. The microdebrider is also useful in removing polypoid tissue obstruction from the frontal recess. An S-shaped suction can also be used to irrigate the sinus, if necessary. It is important to minimize trauma to the frontal sinus ostia, as it can easily scar and stenose. Lastly, any remnants of the uncinate process and agger nasi cells are opened and removed. Occasionally a trephination or Lothrop inferior frontal sinusotomy is used to help control frontal sinus disease. An osteoplastic flap is reserved for these failures.

The middle turbinate is examined for stability. If it is floppy or flaccid, it is partly resected with a straight punch, leaving a superior remnant as a landmark to prevent lateralization. The mucosal edges of the middle turbinate are then cauterized to prevent postoperative bleeding. Large, obstructing conchae bullosae are approached by vertical bisection with a sickle knife and curved scissors, and then the lateral portion is removed with a straightbiting punch forceps. A small Telfa pack is then placed lateral to the middle turbinate for hemostasis.

The contralateral side is next approached. In the case of this patient, a septal deviation prevented adequate visualization, and a septoplasty was performed. For severe nasal septal deviations, we find it best to operate on the most patent nasal cavity first, then perform the septoplasty, and then the contralateral ENSS. When the septoplasty is performed first, septal edema and bleeding make both sides of the ENSS more difficult. For limited septal deviations, an endoscopic septoplasty is a convenient and quick technique.[3] Upon finishing the septoplasty, the contralateral endoscopic sinus surgery is then completed as described above.

Postoperative care is performed 4 days postoperatively when ethmoid Telfa or Telfa/Merocel packs are removed. No patient is sent home after surgery with lower packs, even after septoplasty. Further visits occur at 7- to 10-day intervals. Loose debris is removed; fixed debris acts as a biologic dressing. The frontal recesses especially are cleaned of debris to prevent scarring. Patients usually show signs of satisfactory cavity healing by 4 to 6 weeks, with the frontal recesses taking up to 8 weeks to heal.

A few notes about technique follow. During the case, we generally leave the eyelids undraped and in the field. Small pieces of $^1/_2$-inch paper tape placed laterally over the eyelids prevent scleral exposure. Keeping the eyes in the surgical field allows intermittent finger palpation to assess for dehiscent areas of the lamina papyracea (Fig. 22-4). With this technique, a dehiscence was noted in the patient's left anterior ethmoidal cells, and further injury was averted. Covering or protecting the eyes with goggles or towel drapes is mentioned only to be condemned; there have been documented cases of blindness noted after surgery when the goggles or drapes were removed.[4]

It is easier to identify possible orbital injury in patients given a local anesthetic, as they often complain of pain when the lamina is breached and/or orbital fat is grasped. All specimens from the patient are also placed in a half-filled saline cup, and the scrub nurse is instructed to check for floating debris (which may be orbital fat). If an orbital injury occurs, the procedure is terminated. The patient is awakened to assess visual acuity. Small venous orbital hematomas with intact vision can be managed medically with steroids, diuretics, and orbital massage. Blindness or a "rock-hard eye" from arterial orbital hematoma requires an immediate orbital decompression and ophthalmologic consultation.[5]

We always operate with the patient supine and the surgeon in a sitting position, on the patient's right side.

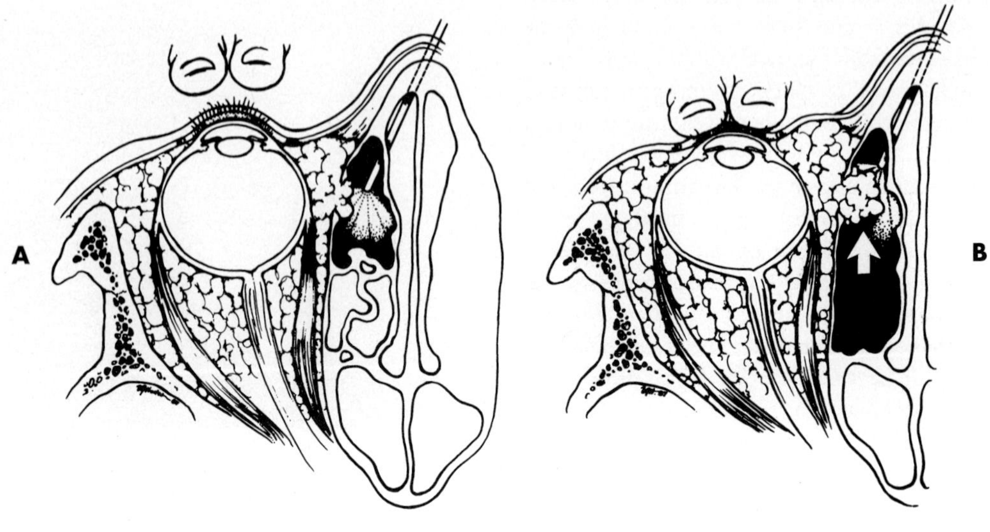

Fig. 22-4. **A** and **B** Orbital palpation to detect dehiscent lamina papyracea. This shows the effect of gentle manual palpation on the globe, causing intraorbital fat prolapsing into the anterior ethmoidal compartment *(arrow)*.

The surgery is also televised for the benefit of the anesthesiologist, nurses, and medical students. We operate through the telescope rather than "off the television screen." The relationship of the surgeon, telescope, and patient's nasal cavity is thus constantly maintained, and we believe this provides another area of control. The benefits of one or the other use of the telescope are debatable.

Another extremely important area in ENSS is proper documentation. Informed consent is mandatory. We also include a brief preoperative note in the patient's chart stating the indications for surgery and the anticipated risks. Immediately after the procedure is performed and the patient is safely awakened, the operative note is dictated. An "operative findings" section summarizes the main areas of disease and treatment. If a less than complete procedure was performed because of a patient's labile blood pressure or significant epistaxis, this is also included. These steps improve postoperative care, since documentation is available to remind the surgeon of difficult anatomic areas or surgical problems. Furthermore, since endoscopic ENSS is a leading area of otolaryngology–head and neck surgery malpractice suits, this documentation is the surgeon's main defense should a lawsuit arise later.[6]

RESULTS

The senior author has performed over 3000 endoscopic sinus surgeries over a 10-year endoscopic career. As expected, complication rates have decreased with further operative experience.[7] To date, no orbital complications resulting in blindness or double vision have occurred. No intracranial complications arose, but seven intraoperative or postoperative cerebrospinal fluid fistulas were endoscopically repaired. Thus far, there has been no operative mortality.

DISCUSSION

Chronic sinusitis is an enormous health care problem. First-line treatment consists of intensive medical therapy. Surgical therapy is reserved for infectious complications or persistent symptomatic disease. Endoscopic ENSS has revolutionized the surgical treatment of sinus disease but is clearly not without risks. It is not for the novice surgeon, and it requires diligence and a thorough knowledge of surgical nasal cavity anatomy. Informed patient consent and thorough documentation are mandatory. Aggressive postoperative care is extremely important to obtain good results.

In this chapter, we have presented our management scheme for patients with sinus disease and have emphasized how to minimize complications. We do not propose that our philosophy be adopted by all, but rather that the reader select any helpful techniques or suggestions, which we have mostly learned by trial and error.

REFERENCES

1. Bolger WE, et al: Lacrimal drainage system injury in functional endoscopic sinus surgery: incidence, analysis, and prevention, *Arch Otolaryngol Head Neck Surg* 118:1179-1184, 1992.
2. McGrew RN: Trigeminal traumatic neuroma, a previously unreported complication of sinus surgery: nerve exposure and traumatic neuroma of V_2 secondary to maxillary antrostomy, *Am J Rhinol* 7:273-279, 1993.
3. Giles WC: Endoscopic septoplasty, *Laryngoscope* 104:1507-1509, 1994.
4. Stankiewicz JA: Blindness and intranasal ethmoidectomy: prevention and management, *Otolaryngol Head Neck Surg* 101:320-329, 1989.
5. Sacks SH, et al: Surgical treatment of blindness secondary to intraorbital hemorrhage, *Arch Otolaryngol Head Neck Surg* 114:801-803, 1988.
6. Schuring AG: The operative report, *Am J Otol* 11:71-73, 1990.
7. Stankiewicz JA: Complications of endoscopic intranasal ethmoidectomy: an update, *Laryngoscope* 97:1270-1273, 1987.
8. Stammberger H, Posavetz W: Functional endoscopic sinus surgery, *Eur Arch Otorhinolaryngol*: 247(2) 63-76, 1990.
9. Serdahl CL, et al: Nasolacrimal duct obstruction after endoscopic sinus surgery, *Arch Ophthalmol* 108:391-392, 1990.
10. Hosemann W, et al: Olfaction after endoscopic endonasal ethmoidectomy, *Am J Rhinol* 7:11-15, 1993.
11. Schaitkin B, et al: Orbital penetration and endoscopic sinus surgery, *Am J Rhinol* 7:49-52, 1993.
12. Neuhaus RW: Orbital complications secondary to endoscopic sinus surgery, *Ophthalmology* 97:1512-1518, 1990.
13. Johnson PJ: Optic neuritis following endoscopic sinus surgery, *Am J Rhinol* 7:247-255, 1993.
14. Kane WJ, et al: Endoscopic intranasal ethmoidectomy complicated by CSF rhinorrhea and maxillary sinus encephalocele, *Am J Rhinol* 6:129-132, 1992.
15. Maniglia AJ: Fatal and other major complications of endoscopic sinus surgery, *Laryngoscope* 101:349-354, 1991.

CHAPTER
23

Endoscopic Frontal Sinusotomy

Steven D. Schaefer

PROBLEM

A 40-year-old male physician presents with a 20-year history of facial pain, and more recently, after multiple intranasal sinus surgeries, tenderness over the frontal sinus and purulent rhinorrhea.

The advent of intranasal endoscopic frontal sinusotomy is the most unique aspect of endoscopic paranasal sinus surgery.[1,2] The methods of patient selection and application of surgical techniques continue to evolve. One approach to surgical selection is illustrated in the algorithm in Fig. 23-1.

MEDICAL HISTORY

The classic triad of frontal sinusitis is frontoethmoid pain, tenderness over this site, and purulent rhinorrhea. In reality, any combination or lack of any one of these specific symptoms may be present in acute and chronic relapsing frontal sinusitis. Many patients initially present complaining of headaches with a vague history of other symptoms of sinusitis. Others note the onset of their frontal sinus symptoms after sinus surgery. This latter group in my experience appears to be increasing.

The patient presented above had undergone a left antrostomy 20 years earlier. Although he continued to have symptoms of bilateral ethmoidal and maxillary sinusitis, he remained relatively well for the subsequent 16 years. He then underwent a series of three separate surgical procedures consisting of various forms of intranasal ethmoidectomies, antrostomies, and sphenoidotomies for purulent sinusitis and polyps. Despite nearly continuous treatment with broad-spectrum oral antibiotics, the purulent rhinorrhea and frontal headaches only worsened over the next 2 years. Other than the above history, the patient was in good health without evidence of bronchopulmonary complications from the chronic sinusitis.

PHYSICAL EXAMINATION

As the nose and sinuses are elements of the larger upper aerodigestive tract, examination of this region should be performed in the context of a complete physical examination. The use of topical vasoconstrictive and anesthetic agents is recommended to enhance visualization of the nose. Otoscopy and examination of the other regions of the head and neck can be performed while allowing several minutes for the topical agents to enhance the nasal examination. Visualization of the nose should be performed with a rigid 0- and 30-degree endoscope. A flexible nasolaryngoscope can be a useful substitute for a 30-degree rigid endoscope to examine the frontal recess. The nose should be systematically examined, with a division into three regions. The inferior examination consists of passing a 0-degree endoscope along the floor of the nose to visualize the orifice of the nasolacrimal duct, inferolateral nasal wall, eustachian tube orifice, and nasopharynx.[3] The second passage should be at approximately a 30-degree angle from the floor of the nose to examine the sphenoethmoid recess, middle meatus, and sphenoid ostium. The superior passage should be directed toward the frontal recess to examine these cells, the attachment of the middle turbinate, and the superior recess between the middle turbinate and nasal septum. In patients who have undergone previous sinus surgery, the examination should be directed toward determining the patency of the communication of the frontal sinus with the nose and evaluating the health of the frontal sinus. Purulent secretions in the frontal recess or frontal sinus cavity, or polyps at these sites, suggest a dysfunctional sinus. Dense green

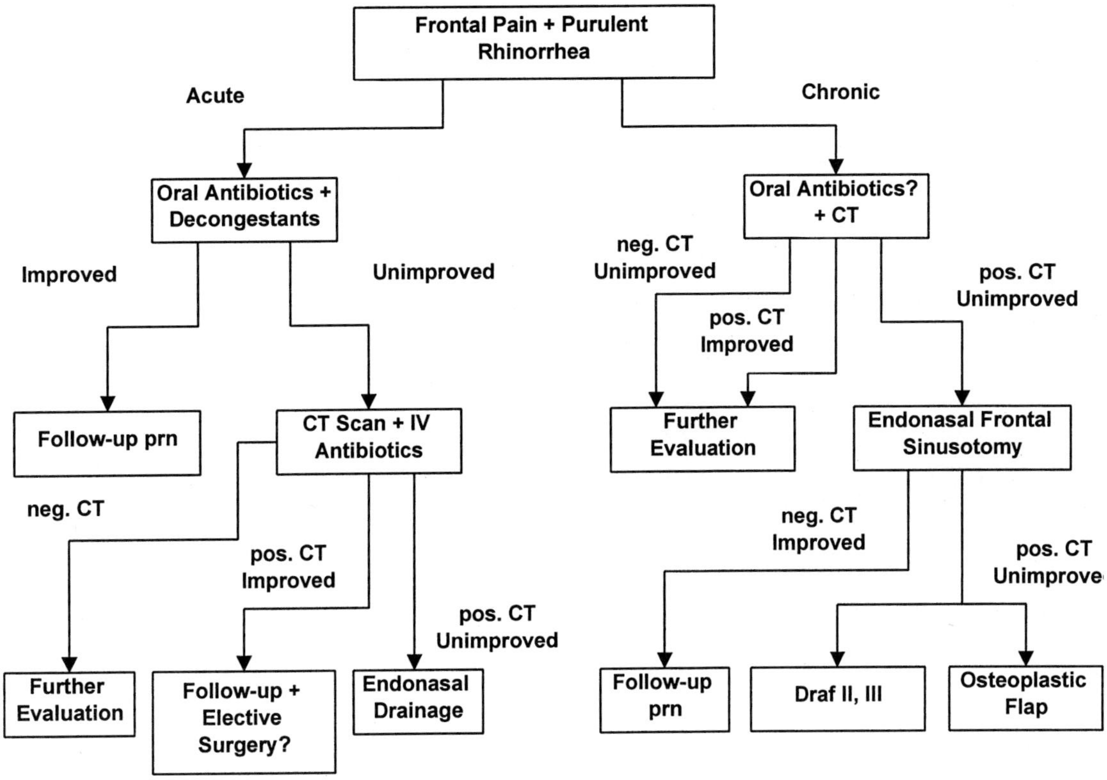

Fig. 23-1. Algorithm for surgical management of chronic frontal sinusitis.

or brown secretions, often accompanied by polyps, are indicative of allergic fungal sinusitis.

In this patient, examination of the nose revealed only a remnant of both middle turbinates at their insertion on the agger nasi, bilateral middle meatus antrostomies, stenosis of both sphenoidotomies, and residual right anterior ethmoidal cells. Polyps and fibrotic mucous membrane obliterated both frontal recesses.

RADIOGRAPHIC EXAMINATION

Routine radiographic evaluation of the frontal sinus should consist of axial and coronal computed tomographic (CT) imaging. With the advent of helical scanners, images in one projection can be digitally reconstructed to produce high-quality images in other projections. Sagittal reconstructions are useful to examine anatomic variants and obstructions of the frontal recess, frontal sinus ostium, and frontal sinus. Such digital imaging information can also be transferred to a computer work station in the operating room to provide three-dimensional displays for image-guided surgery. This technology is particularly helpful in identifying the ostium of the frontal sinus and in approaching disease within the cavity of this sinus (Fig. 23-2).

TREATMENT

Indications

Acute frontal sinusitis unresponsive to antibiotic therapy is classically first treated by drainage of the infected sinus via trephination through an infra-brow incision. An alternative to external drainage is an endoscopic intranasal anterior ethmoidectomy and frontal sinusotomy. A 4-mm Silastic drain can be placed intranasally for postoperative irrigation of the frontal sinus (Fig. 23-3).[1] Chronic frontal sinusitis is surgically managed in patients who are refractive to repeated trials of medical management and who radiographically exhibit persistent sinusitis. The physical examination may also offer clues to those patients who will require surgical treatment. Such findings include obstruction of the frontal recess by polyps, a lateralized middle turbinate, or fibrosis after previous surgery.

Surgical technique

Anterior ethmoidectomy is recommended as the first step to maximize exposure to the frontal recess. The plane of this procedure proceeds from inferior to superior using a 0-degree endoscope, with each level of the dissection completed before proceeding superiorly. Residual superior cells, mucous membrane, and polyps are re-

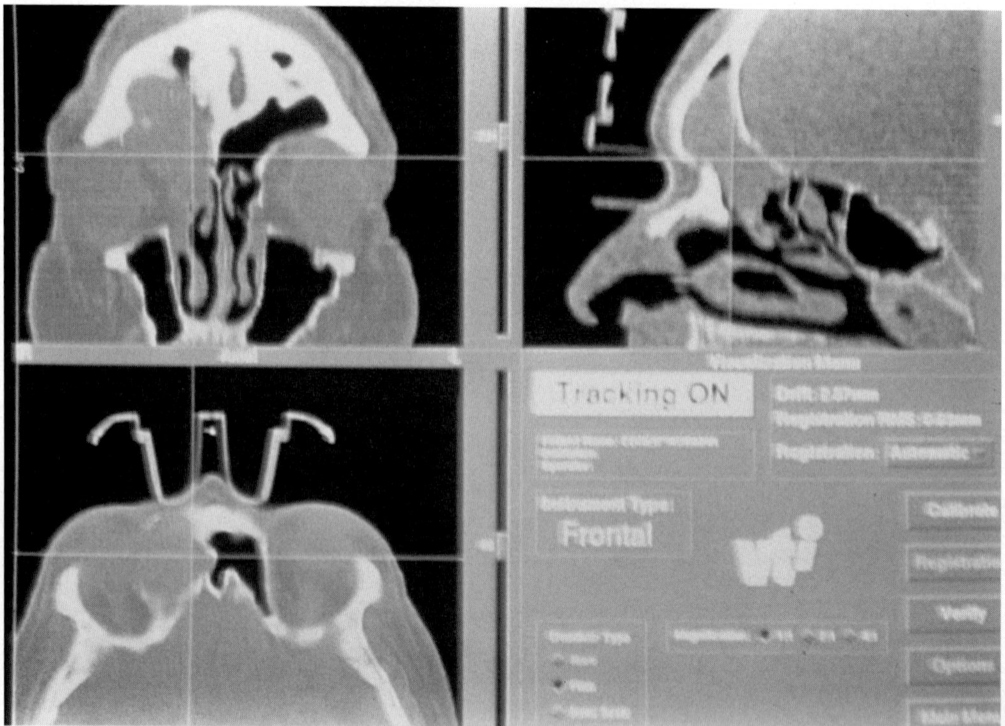

A

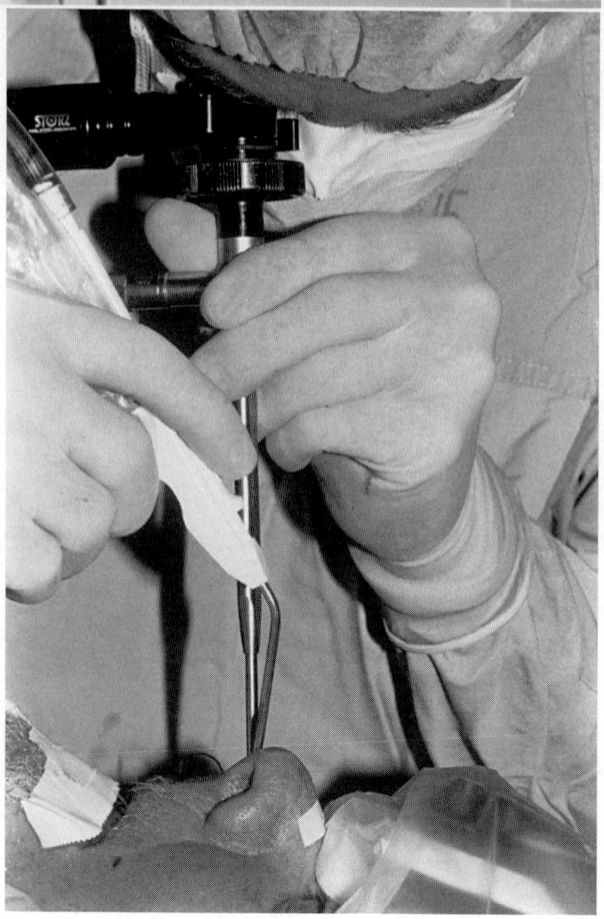

B

Fig. 23-2. Computer-guided surgery. **A,** Three-dimensional computer display showing a computer-guided probe in the frontal sinus. **B,** Head set or radio receiver on a patient undergoing frontal sinus surgery. The suction device held by the surgeon emits a radiofrequency that is localized in space by the three-plane receiver in the head set (Visualization Technology, Inc., Boston, Mass).

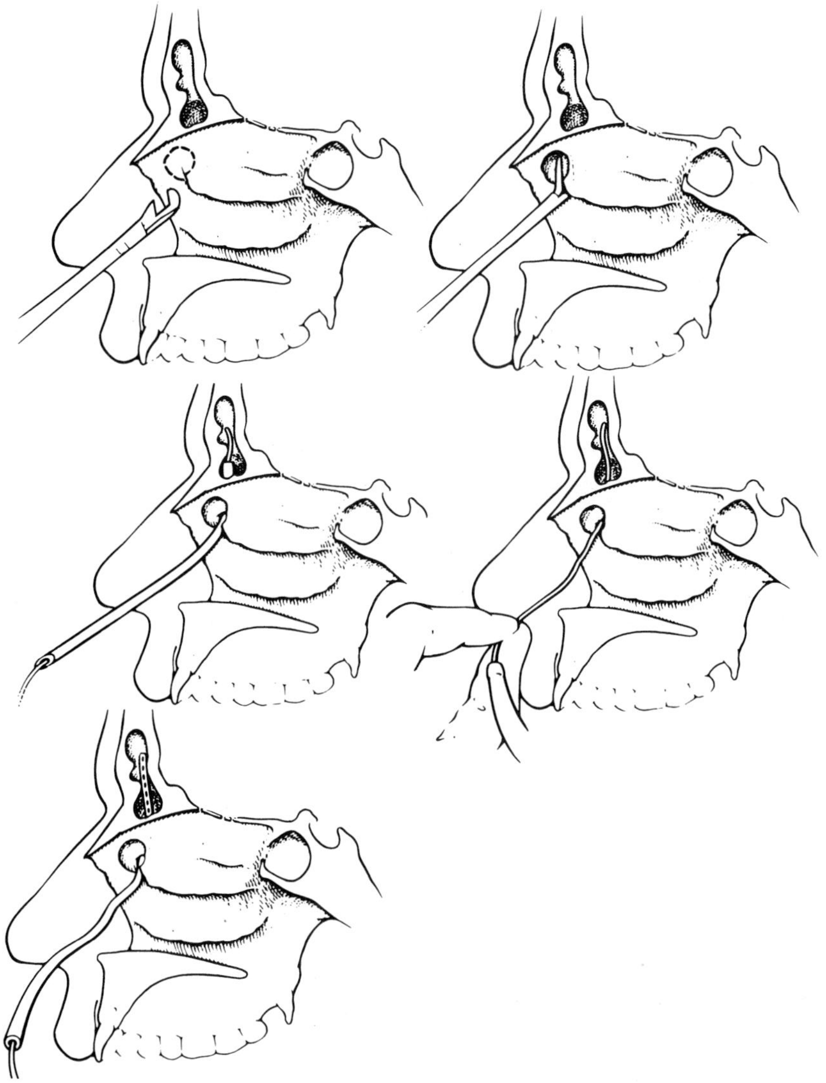

Fig. 23-3. Endoscopic drainage of the frontal sinus as an alternative to trephination in acute sinusitis refractive to medical therapy. *Top left,* Agger nasi and frontal recess cells are removed to improve access to the frontal recess (represented by the circle). *Top right,* The frontal recess cells and mucous membrane are removed with a combination of upturned forceps, frontal sinus curettes, and frontal sinus forceps. Care is taken to minimize trauma to normal mucous membrane and to the frontal sinus ostium. *Middle left,* A 4-mm bent suction device can be placed into the frontal sinus, and the Silastic obturator from a suction bovie cautery is threaded through the suction. *Middle right,* The suction is removed, leaving the obturator in the frontal sinus. *Bottom,* A 4-mm Silastic tube is placed over the obturator and guided into the frontal sinus. The tube is sutured to the columella. (From Schaefer SD: Endoscopic management of frontal sinus disease, *Laryngoscope* 100:155-159, 1990.)

moved under direct visualization using a 30-degree endoscope. The superior dissection is conducted both posteriorly to anteriorly and anteriorly to posteriorly, to maximize exposure of the frontal sinus. Visualization is enhanced by removing the ethmoidal infundibular cells, which are superior to the agger nasi. These cells have been referred to as either the agger nasi or frontal recess cells; they arise from ethmoidal infundibular cells that have migrated across the infundibulum. Since the strict definition of the agger nasi is of an eminence at the anterior insertion of the middle turbinate, there is some confusion over which cells are to be removed. Those cells in this eminence, which is created by the pneumatization of the lacrimal bone, are not disturbed. As the uncinate process is key to exposing the frontal recess, care must be taken to follow this structure superiorly and to remove the entire uncinate. This maneuver is best performed by removing the uncinate to expose the frontal ostium from medial to lateral using a frontal sinus curette. This step has been likened by Stammberger to uncapping an egg, as each egg cap is curetted inferiorly to expose the frontal sinus ostium.

The significance of the variations of the uncinate are discussed later in this chapter. In many individuals the ostium of the frontal sinus is seen as a paramedian hiatus between the anterior insertion of the middle turbinate and anterior ethmoid artery. Lateral to the frontal sinus ostium is the ostium of the supraorbital ethmoids, which are extensions of the infundibular cells. The latter ostium is often confused with the frontal sinus ostium. If the frontal sinus ostium is not apparent, a frontal sinus probe (available from such manufacturers as K. Storz, R. Wolf, or Xomed) is useful for palpating the ostium. Such probing is particularly problematic with fibrosis from previous surgery. Once the ostium is identified, the goal of the surgery is to perform the minimal procedure that restores drainage of the frontal sinus. Such a procedure can range from removing frontal recess cells that are adjacent to the frontal ostium to excising mucous membrane obstructing the outflow of the sinus. If the frontal ostium is more than 4 mm in diameter and if all the mucous membrane is circumferentially intact, experience suggests that the ostium should remain patent. The goal should be to do nothing to the frontal ostium. However, smaller ostia, or those with disrupted mucosa, rarely may be enlarged through the removal of the anterior bony plate of the sinus floor known as the "beak."[6] I have found that such ostia must be enlarged through the removal of their anterior bony wall to approximately 1.5 cm in diameter to remain patent. Such enlargement is difficult and requires the use of either drills or rasps designed for this specific purpose (Fig. 23-4). The mucosa covering the posterior aspect of the ostium should be left intact to help reduce postoperative scarring of the ostium. Although significant reduction in the final ostium is anticipated, it has been found that stents are an inadequate alternative to widely opening the ostium, and I have abandoned their use.

DISCUSSION

Endoscopic endonasal management of frontal sinus disease remains an evolving procedure. This process reflects the increasing cumulative experience of surgeons with this procedure, inadequate consensus on the criteria for endoscopic surgical management, improving imaging techniques, difficulty in performing such surgery, improving instrumentation, and significant variation in surgical skill.

The attractiveness of endoscopic frontal sinus surgery is the potential minimally invasive nature of this approach. As more surgeons gain experience with this procedure, certain common observations emerge. First, most chronic frontal sinusitis is due to obstruction of the outflow of the sinus by the uncinate process and/or the anterior ethmoidal cells that make up the frontal recess and infundibular cells of the ethmoid. Removal of these cells without disturbing the ostium or cavity of the frontal sinus is frequently sufficient to restore aeration of this sinus.[1] The importance of these ethmoidal cells in the development of frontal sinusitis is not a concept new to endoscopic surgery; rather it dates to various reports, including the anatomic dissections of J. Parsons Schaeffer.[7] Schaeffer rightly regarded the frontal sinus as an outgrowth of the ethmoidal sinus. He also recognized that more than one cell may pneumatize the frontal bone and communicate independently with the frontal recess. Such cells have been called accessory frontal sinus cells or

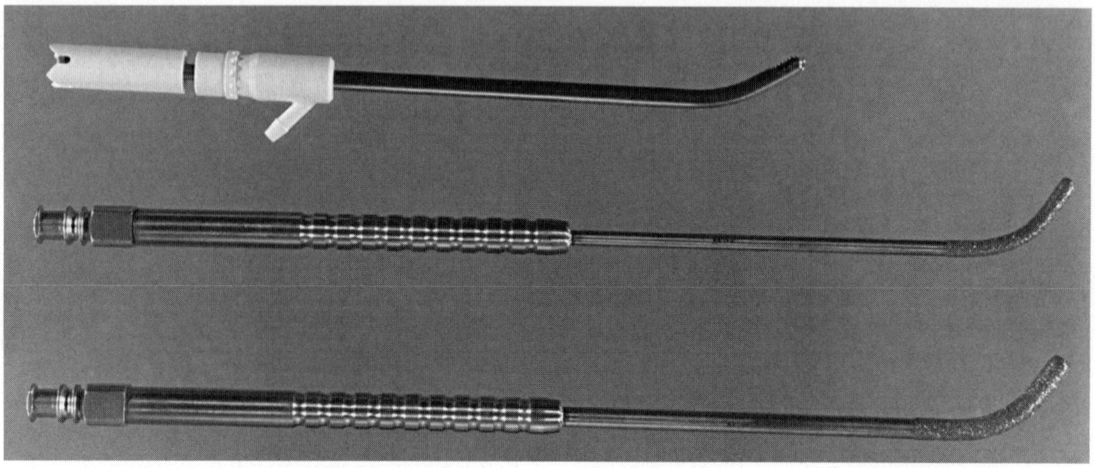

Fig. 23-4. Frontal sinus instruments for enlarging the bony ostium of the sinus: Schaefer frontal sinus rasps and a Xomed frontal sinus drill.

frontal cells.[8] These cells have been described by Kuhn as potential sources of obstruction of the outflow of the frontal sinus, who proposed a classification.[9] This classification is useful because it helps to focus the physician's efforts at surgery on the removal of these cells in the treatment of frontal sinus obstruction.

In this classification, cells are divided into either single or multiple cells between the agger nasi and the frontal sinus (types I and II, respectively) and those that either pneumatize cephalad into or arise within the frontal sinus (types III and IV, respectively). Second, endonasal frontal sinus surgery is characterized by the principle that "minimal surgery is best." The goal of surgery should be confined to the removal of only that disease necessary to restore outflow of the sinus. If the ostium must be enlarged as previously discussed, as little normal mucosa as possible should be disturbed. Third, the increasing incidence of iatrogenic frontal sinusitis in the preoperatively normal sinus reflects both the difficulty in operating on this sinus and the practice of surgically altering the frontal recess and infundibular ethmoidal cells. As more surgeons recognize the role of this process in the pathogenesis of iatrogenic frontal sinusitis, it is anticipated that this problem will decrease. Fourth, an increasing understanding of the role of normal and variants in anatomy in the etiology of frontal sinusitis is leading to improvements in surgical management.

One example of improving surgical skill through a better understanding of normal anatomy is seen in the ability to differentiate the ostium of the frontal sinus from the opening of supraorbital ethmoids into the frontal recess. The latter is lateral to the medial frontal sinus ostium. However, the ethmoidal ostium is frequently confused with the frontal sinus ostium, resulting in inadequate drainage of the frontal sinus. An example of an important and highly variable structure is the uncinate (from the Latin word *uncus*, a hook) process. Variations include the uncinate coursing superolaterally to insert on the lamina papyracea. This forms a blind pouch known as the *sinus terminalis*, and the communication of the frontal recess with the middle meatus is medial to the ethmoidal infundibulum. If the uncinate process courses to the skull base or fuses with the medial aspect of the middle turbinate, the ethmoidal infundibulum may pass superiorly into the frontal recess.[10] Another variation is extensive pneumatization of the uncinate process, which potentially obstructs the outflow of the frontal sinus.[4]

A consensus on the endonasal versus external approach for the management of frontal sinus disease has yet to evolve. Current positions are as extreme as "one should manage all frontal sinus disease by an external approach" to the exact opposite. I believe that the location of the disease, the pathogenesis of the disease process, and the surgeon's experience and results should determine the approach. For example, mucosal disease or polyps in the extreme lateral aspect of the frontal sinus is inaccessible by an endonasal route. Such access can be improved by combining an infra-brow approach to the floor of the sinus with an endonasal procedure. However, if the disease process is so diffuse that it cannot be encompassed by such an approach or marsupialize into the nose, then recurrence of this process is likely.[1]

Improvements in computed imaging should further the intelligent application of endonasal frontal sinus surgery and in turn produce improved surgical results. First, with the advent of helical CT scanners the frontal recess can be preoperatively evaluated in the coronal, axial, and sagittal planes. Such imaging permits the anatomy of the obstruction of the outflow of the frontal sinus to be better understood. Surgeons over time should be able to review their results after extensive removal of retained ethmoidal cells, diffuse fibrosis, or bone to determine which process is treatable by an endonasal route. Second, the selective use of magnetic resonance imaging (MRI) permits identification of such processes as epidural extension of sinus disease. Other selective MRI applications include the use of fat saturation techniques to identify mucoceles. Third, computer-guided imaging in the operating room is progressing and enhances the accurate intraoperative identification of surgical landmarks. Such imaging also permits the localization required to find or confirm the disease process, such as mucocele, for which the procedure is being performed.

The advent of specific instrumentation has significantly improved endonasal frontal sinus surgery. Since 1990, there have been modifications to curettes, ostial probes, forceps, rasps, and drills. These instruments are important because they assist the surgeon in better locating the frontal sinus and in removing mucous membrane and bone that obstruct the outflow of the sinus.

As the learning curve of endonasal frontal sinusotomy is very long, I would strongly question the universality of this procedure. I believe our own failure rate, as defined by the need for further frontal sinus surgery since the mid-1980s, is approximately 10% in all patients. Most of our patients have undergone at least one previous procedure that involved or obstructed the frontal sinus. Our failure rate is much lower if we are the first surgeon. This experience begs several questions. Is endonasal endoscopic surgery a technique that should be routinely employed by all otolaryngologists? This is a difficult question to answer, because training and professional experience varies greatly. Opposing trends further complicate the answer to this question: improved training in residency programs versus the likelihood of fewer patients undergoing such surgery by any one surgeon owing to improved medical therapy and restrictions on surgery by third-party payers. Sadly, this question may be resolved by the "business of medicine" rather than by such traditional criteria as specialization certification and surgical skill.[11]

REFERENCES

1. Schaefer SD, Close, LG: Endoscopic management of frontal sinus disease, *Laryngoscope* 100:155-159, 1990.
2. Wigand ME: *Endoscopic surgery of the paranasal sinuses and anterior skull base*, New York, 1990, Thieme.
3. Kennedy DW, Zinreich J, Johns ME: Functional endoscopic sinus surgery, *Arch Otolaryngol* 111:576-582, 1985.
4. Rice DH, Schaefer SD: *Endoscopic paranasal sinus surgery*, ed 2, New York, 1992, Raven Press.
5. Manning SC, Mabry RL, Schaefer SD, Close LG: Evidence of IgE mediated hypersensitivity in allergic fungal sinusitis, *Laryngoscope* 103:717-721, 1993.
6. May M: Frontal sinus surgery: endonasal endoscopic ostioplasty rather than external ostioplasty, *Op Tech Otolaryngol* 2:247-256, 1991.
7. Schaeffer, JP: The genesis, development, and adult anatomy of the nasofrontal region in man, *Am J Anat* 20:125-143, 1916.
8. van Alyea OE: Frontal cells: an anatomic study of these cells with consideration of their clinical significance, *Arch Otol* 34:11-23, 1941.
9. Bent JP, Cuilty-Siller C, Kuhn FA: The frontal cell as a cause of frontal sinus obstruction, *Am J Rhinol* 8:185-191, 1994.
10. Stammberger HR, Clement PAR, Hosemann W, et al: Paranasal sinuses: anatomic terminology and nomenclature, *Ann Otol Rhinol Laryngol* 104:suppl 167, 1995.
11. Schaefer SD: Is there a role for educators in health care?, *Arch Otolaryngol* 120:585-586, 1994.

CHAPTER

24

Endoscopic Frontal Sinusotomy (Lothrop Procedure)

Charles W. Gross
William E. Gross
Daniel G. Becker

PROBLEM

A 54-year-old woman presented with a history of persistent chronic sinusitis manifested by purulent discharge, nasal obstruction, and headache.

MEDICAL HISTORY

The patient had a history of increasingly severe sinusitis over the past several years, had been very aggressively treated medically for some time, and then underwent sinus surgery. After this, the infections persisted and increased in severity; the symptoms of frontal sinusitis in particular worsened. She was referred to a university service and underwent frontal sinus trephinations with attempted repair of the nasal frontal duct. The patient continued not to do well, developing severe pansinusitis, and was hospitalized for intravenous antibiotics. She responded, only to have a relapse later. She was then referred to us for a third opinion. When seen by us her cultures showed *Staphylococcus aureus* and *Haemophilus influenzae.* She responded again to medical therapy. The sinusitis responded well except for persistent frontal sinus disease. An endoscopic examination was then relatively normal except for scarring and stenosis in the frontal recess area. Upon completion of an additional 2-month course of antibiotics, the patient developed recent recurrent symptoms of the chronic frontal sinusitis. Consequently, she underwent a modified intranasal Lothrop procedure (frontal drillout). Since that time she has done well, with occasional mild infections, which have responded readily to antibiotic therapy without persistence. When she was last seen the frontal sinus region was widely patent and there was no evidence of active infection.

Most cases of chronic frontal sinusitis requiring surgery respond to functional endonasal endoscopic techniques.[1-4] There remains, however, a small subset of patients with this condition who require additional procedures. The "gold standard" for such cases has been the osteoplastic procedure described by Hardy and Montgomery,[5] although the Lynch-Howarth frontoethmoidectomy still has many proponents.[6-8]

The endonasal endoscopic approach for severe chronic frontal sinusitis is an area of great interest at this time. With the advent of computed tomography (CT), endoscopic techniques, and advanced drill technology, several centers around the world have developed a renewed interest in reestablishing drainage pathways from the frontal sinus using the basic tenet of Lothrop's procedure.[9-12] Several authors have reported their experience.[10-12] At the 1994 meeting of the American Academy of Otolaryngology–Head and Neck Surgery, we presented our early experience with the modified transnasal endoscopic Lothrop procedure (frontal drillout) as an alternative to an osteoplastic procedure. We continue to use this procedure and find it quite acceptable.[13-15] Its theoretical advantages over frontal sinus obliteration include decreased morbidity, the ability to endoscopically evaluate postoperative patients for recurrent disease, and improved cosmesis. In our institution (University of Virginia), this is the current procedure of choice for persistent chronic sinusitis in patients who have failed functional endoscopic surgery. It is recognized that perhaps some patients may not respond to this approach because of extensive advanced disease and that the osteoplastic procedure may still be required. Although long-term follow-up (5 to 10 years) is not yet available, the preliminary results are encouraging. To date, we have had no significant complications from this procedure such as cerebrospinal fluid (CSF) rhinorrhea, restenosis, or persistent frontal sinusitis. This chapter reviews the history of the development of endonasal surgical approaches to the frontal sinus. It then focuses on the modified transnasal Lothrop procedure, with a discussion of the underlying basic principles, patient selection, operative technique, and a brief review of results.

HISTORY

Reestablishment of drainage pathways from the frontal sinus has been of long-standing interest in the history of sinus surgery. The significant history of this approach dates back to 1914, when Lothrop[9] reported removing the intersinus septum along with the superior nasal septum and nasal floor of the frontal sinus to join the two nasofrontal ducts into a common opening. This was a combined approach using transnasal drilling while visualizing through the defect afforded by external frontoethmoidectomy. His procedure was abandoned or not duplicated by other surgeons.

Lothrop's technique as described in 1914[9] consisted of an intranasal ethmoidectomy followed by an external Lynch-type approach with resection of the medial frontal sinus floor, superior nasal septum, and intersinus septum, creating a large frontonasal communication. Lothrop reported that an intranasal approach to his procedure was too dangerous because of lack of adequate visualization. However, the external approach often allowed medial collapse of orbital soft tissue and subsequent stenosis of the nasofrontal communication.

Embryology and anatomy

Embryologic studies provided a clearer understanding of the development and anatomy of the frontal sinus and frontal recess. Kasper described evidence seen in the embryo at the end of the third or early part of the fourth month of a beginning extension forward and upward of the middle nasal meatus.[16] This early extension was thought to be the forerunner of the frontal recess and, strictly speaking, the first step in the formation of the frontal sinus and certain of the anterior group of ethmoidal cells. Onodi,[17] Schaeffer,[18,19] and others also recognized that the recessus frontalis is demonstrable as early as the fourth fetal month. Schaeffer[18,19] also made valuable contributions to our understanding of frontal sinus and frontal recess development (Table 24-1).

Kasper's[16] important study of 100 adult nasofrontal connections suggested five different developmental pathways:

1. In 57% by expansion of a frontal anterior ethmoidal cell or cells in the frontal recess.
2. In 34% by expansion of an infundibular anterior ethmoidal cell or cells in the ethmoidal infundibulum.
3. In 4% by direct expansion of the ethmoidal infundibulum.
4. In 3% by direct extension of the frontal recess.
5. In 2% by expansion of a cell or furrow in the suprabullar area.

More recently, Stammberger has provided an elegant description of the nasofrontal connection and its variations.[20]

Intranasal approaches: early experience

Intranasal drainage of the frontal sinus was attempted early in the history of sinus surgery. Van Alyea[21] noted in 1946 that cells that tend to encroach on the frontal area are often broken down by the mere passage of a cannula,

Table 24-1. Developmental anatomy of frontal sinuses: measurements in a series of specimens

	VENTRODORSAL LENGTH (MM)	CEPHALOCAUDAL HEIGHT (MM)	MEDIOLATERAL WIDTH (MM)
6-12 mo	3.5	2	3.5
1-2 yr	4-5	5	5
3-4 yr	4.5-5.5	5-7	7.5
5-6 yr	6	7-8	7
7-8 yr	7-8.5	13-15	20

(From Schaeffer JP: *The genesis, development, and adult anatomy of the nasofrontal region in man: a genetic, developmental, and anatomicophysiological consideration,* Philadelphia, 1920, P Blakiston's & Son.)

and a permanent improvement in the drainage channels is established forthwith. In his experience with the removal of such structural barriers, acute attacks of frontal sinusitis tended to subside quickly because of the ample size of the ostium and because of its location in the most dependent portion of the sinus floor.

Van Alyea recognized that the sinus membranes typically showed no other changes than those of chronic inflammation. Microscopically, they presented every characteristic of being able to repair themselves in due course when favorable conditions were provided, the most potent being the establishment of a functional drainage pathway. He considered that the alternative to reestablishing drainage, a radical procedure, offered little more and also took with it the last hopes of a cure of the disease by restoration of sinus function.

Nonetheless, these early efforts often resulted in surgical complications and treatment failures.

External approaches

The large number of external approaches described in the literature attests to the fact that none has been entirely satisfactory. External procedures for frontal sinus drainage include the well-known Lynch-Howarth frontoethmoidectomy.[6-8] This approach has been cited as producing a high rate of recurrence (30%) and postoperative complications.[3] During the external approach the bony scaffolding laterally overlying the frontal recess is removed, allowing soft tissue to collapse in and restenose the area, thus often leading to recurrent sinusitis.

While no one procedure has met with universal acceptance, the osteoplastic flap with fat obliteration has emerged as a "gold standard" of treatment in the United States. This procedure, albeit formidable, has survived the test of time because it is relatively safe, is familiar to most otolaryngologist–head and neck surgeons, usually results in little cosmetic deformity, and has an acceptable success rate.[5] When residual or recurrent inflammatory disease occurs, however, evaluation of the patient after obliteration can be extremely difficult.

Problems related to the obliterative approach include an inability to visualize the operative area after surgery and the difficulty of interpreting a radiographic image after an obliteration.[2] Obliterative procedures can also involve significant morbidity. Intraoperative CSF leaks, persistent forehead neuralgia or numbness, the need for revision, and poor cosmesis have all been reported. Hardy and Montgomery's[5] series of 250 consecutive osteoplastic procedures for frontal sinus disease reported a 19% rate of operative complications, with a 2.8% rate of CSF leaks. Twenty of 208 (9%) required revision surgery, with follow-up of at least 3 years in 83% of patients. Furthermore, 6% had persistent frontal headache (moderate to severe) without evidence of disease.[5]

Endoscopic techniques

Currently, functional endoscopic sinus surgery can be used in most cases to remove disease from the frontal recess of the ethmoid, thereby relieving the blockage of drainage of the frontal sinus.[1-4,10] When frontal recess exploration has failed to relieve obstruction of the frontal sinus, external procedures are often resorted to.

With the advent of CT scans and endoscopic techniques, several centers around the world have developed a renewed interest in reestablishing drainage pathways from the frontal sinus. Several authors have described using a drill transnasally to enlarge frontal sinus drainage.[4,10-15,22] In the endoscopic era, Draf[11] first reported the use of a drill transnasally to address the frontal sinus. In a series of 387 patients requiring frontal sinus surgery, 12 cases required "median drainage," which appears to be very similar to a transnasal Lothrop procedure, the main difference being in Draf's use of the microscope and his occasional combination of a combined transnasal and external approach. Draf described the use of this procedure in cases of revision surgery, mucocele formation, and orbital and intracranial complications of sinusitis. With a 5- to 8-years follow-up, Draf reported a closure rate of approximately 20% with the median drainage procedure (April 1995, Rhinologic Society Spring Meeting, Palm Desert, Calif). His overall long-term success rate using an endonasal approach (including 191 cases with "simple drainage," which appears to be an aggressive frontal recess opening; 186 cases of extended drainage," which involves unilateral resection of the floor of the frontal sinus; and 12 cases of "median drainage") has been reported as 90% (November 1994, 2nd International Symposium on Endonasal Endoscopic Surgery for Inflammatory Diseases of the Paranasal Sinuses, Pittsburgh).

May and Schaitkin[10] reported a 67% success rate in six patients who underwent the median drainage procedure with a 6-month to 4-year follow-up. The two patients with persisting symptoms underwent an external osteoplastic obliterative procedure.

Wigand and Hoseman[12] reported follow-up on 126 procedures of endoscopic frontal sinus surgery with the use of a drill to enlarge the frontal "infundibulum." This series included 20 operations within the frontal sinus, some with a combined external approach. They reported a 0% surgical complication rate, but in 30% of these procedures scar proliferation resulted in a loss of probe patency.

Close and associates[22] reported a frontal drillout procedure. In their description, a bridge of bone was left intact posteriorly between the fenestration and the natural frontal sinus ostia. They believed that this reduced the likelihood of injury to the posterior frontal sinus wall mucosa and bone, consequently decreasing the likelihood of a circumferential mucosal defect of the ostia area and subsequent stenosis, and also decreasing the possibility of dural injury and CSF leakage. These authors used a conventional cutting burr to drill away the floor of the frontal sinus in 11 patients. Five patients required a small infrabrow incision and frontal sinusotomy. One CSF leak was reported in this series.

The availability of advanced drill technology with a protective sheath and suction at the surgical site has been instrumental in allowing a reassessment of the intranasal techniques. At our institution, it was believed reasonable to reassess the basic tenet of the Lothrop procedure (i.e., removal of the intersinus septum, superior nasal septum, and nasal floor of the frontal sinus), thereby creating a large frontonasal communication that would essentially marsupialize the frontal sinus.

A modification to Lothrop's procedure in which the approach is entirely intranasal has the advantage of preserving the lateral bony walls and avoiding medial collapse of soft tissue. The posterior sinus–frontal recess mucosa is largely preserved. Advanced drill technology and endoscopic techniques have allowed this procedure to be performed safely and expeditiously in our hands.

The theoretical advantages of this procedure over frontal sinus obliteration include decreased morbidity, improved cosmesis, and the ability to endoscopically evaluate postoperative patients for recurrent disease. We have also shown that this approach is less expensive.

At our institution, this modification was first studied in cadavers to quantify the potential size of the frontonasal opening. Subsequently, we pursued this approach in appropriate clinical candidates. Previously we relied primarily on frontal sinus of obliteration with fat via an osteoplastic approach to treat most patients with medically refractive, chronic sinusitis who had undergone unsuccessful endoscopic frontal sinusotomy. As described elsewhere, we now primarily use the modified transnasal Lothrop procedure for surgical management of patients with disease similar to that previously treated with an osteoplastic flap approach.[15]

Cadaver dissection. Two cadaver heads were dissected from above to determine the size of the opening that could be created by removing the structures mentioned above. In both these dissections an opening of 2 cm in lateral dimension by 1 cm anterosuperior dimension was created. The superior septum was also resected. The opening was semicircular to crescentic in shape (Fig. 24-1).[6]

Also, the modified transnasal endoscopic Lothrop procedure using drills was performed in two fresh cadavers.[6] The technique used in these cadavers and subsequently in the clinical setting is described below.

Animal studies. The cat has become a well-established animal model for frontal sinus surgery.[23-25] In their reports on the anterior osteoplastic frontal sinus obliteration, Montgomery and Pierce described their early clinical results as well as animal studies.[23] Montgomery performed this operation in cats and sacrificed them after 6 months, at which time he examined their sinuses and also

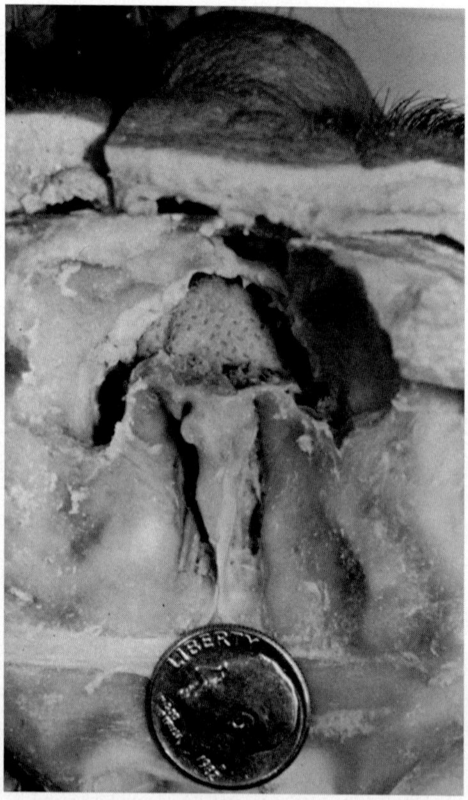

Fig. 24-1. Cadaver dissection from above reveals a 2 × 1 cm opening in the floor of the frontal sinus after drilling.

obtained histologic and serial sections for examination and review. Donald and Fenton and colleagues performed further studies using the cat model of the frontal sinus.[24]

Six cats whose frontal sinuses had been assessed for size and patency by three-dimensional (3D) CT scan underwent a modified Lothrop procedure. 3D CT was undertaken 6 months later, at which time the animals were sacrificed and the sinus cavities opened and examined. All cats had widely patent sinuses and normal mucosa at 6 months (Becker and colleagues, unpublished data submitted for publication).

OPERATIVE TECHNIQUE

Patient selection

The modified transnasal Lothrop procedure is performed primarily in patients with chronic recurrent frontal sinus disease that has been refractory both to aggressive medical therapy and to surgical correction via endoscopic frontal recess surgery.

In addition, in selected patients with frontal sinus trauma, we have performed a modified frontal drillout after direct visualization via an osteoplastic flap. Patients

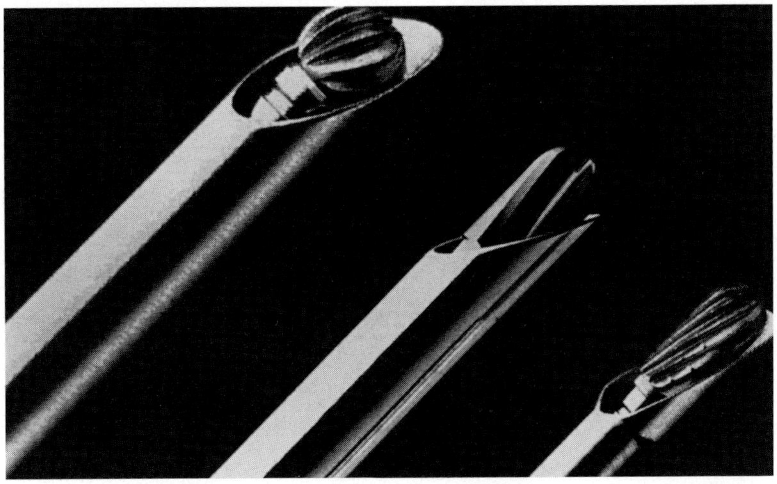

Fig. 24-2. The advanced bone-cutting drills have a beveled sheath that guards the "back" side of the burr. Suction is applied through the sheath so that material can be suctioned free at the site of the burr.

with frontal sinus trauma involving the nasofrontal duct may not require obliteration. Pope[27] and Goode[26] have described the use of septectomy in cases of unilateral nasofrontal injury. Similarly, an osteoplastic flap approach allows exploration of the sinus to ensure the status of the posterior table. The frontal opening may then be drilled from above and via the intranasal approach. Partial ethmoidectomy with removal of agger nasi cells endoscopically usually ensures adequate postoperative endoscopic visualization of the frontal opening.

The frontal drillout has also been used in selected patients who, despite an obliteration procedure, have persistent symptoms and endoscopic and CT findings of consistent frontal sinusitis. In these cases an endoscopic and external approach via the previous osteoplastic flap is often employed, with the goal of reestablishing endonasal drainage pathways.

Equipment

We use standard 4-mm rigid 0- and 30-degree endoscopes and standard endoscopic equipment, as described below. K wires of 5-mm gauge are used to mark the location of the frontal recess once it has been identified. We currently use the Apex Universal Drive System (Linvatec Corporation, Largo, Fla). Rotational speeds used range from 1000 to 6000 rpm. The footswitch has variable sensitivity control that can be adjusted to the surgeon's preference. There are two handpieces. The Microjoint handpiece is for the smaller drills (2 to 3.5 mm). Generally, we use the standard handpiece, which is for the larger drills (3.5 to 8 mm) and weighs 385.5 g. The cross-sectional shape of both handpieces is "teardrop."

The soft tissue shaving and bone-cutting burrs have a wide range in diameter. The ones designed for the Microjoint handpiece are 2 to 3.5 mm in diameter and 8.9 cm in length; the ones designed for the standard handpiece are 3.5 to 8 mm in diameter and 13.3 cm in length. The soft tissue cannulas have a blunt cannula tip and a lateral port. An oscillating or rotating inner cannula with a similar lateral port cuts and extracts soft tissue as it is suctioned through the side port of the cannula.

The proximal and distal edges of the aperture are smooth; the lateral aspects are smooth or serrated. The inner blade cuts and extracts soft tissue as it is suctioned into the side port; this inner blade can oscillate or can rotate in forward or reverse. In oscillate mode the blade rotates one 360-degree arc in one direction before rotating in the opposite direction. Some of the soft tissue blades can be bent from 0 to 30 degrees in any direction by the surgeon at the operating table.

The cutting burrs (Fig. 24-2) consist of a burr affixed to a shaft either 8.9 or 13.3 cm in length. The burrs are available in spherical, tapered, or oval shapes. The shaft of the burr is protected by a sheath. The end of the sheath is beveled so that the "back" side of the burr is protected or guarded. As with the soft tissue shavers, suction is applied through the sheath so that material can be suctioned free at the site of the burr. This enables the surgeon to adequately visualize the precise drilling site and keep the field clear of debris.

Modified transnasal Lothrop procedure

The modified transnasal Lothrop procedure is performed with the patient under general anesthesia. The nose is injected and topicalized with local anesthetic (lidocaine and epinephrine) in the usual fashion. The patient is positioned as for a conventional functional sinus surgery using endoscopes. The patient's CT scan is always in the room for reference. In addition to the standard coronal views, we now routinely obtain axial CT cuts to assess the depth of the frontal sinus and the location and integrity of the posterior sinus wall.

Step 1: Resect agger nasi, superior uncinate, and anterior ethmoidal cells. If agger nasi, superior uncinate, or anterior ethmoidal cells are present, they are removed using conventional endoscopic instrumentation to enlarge

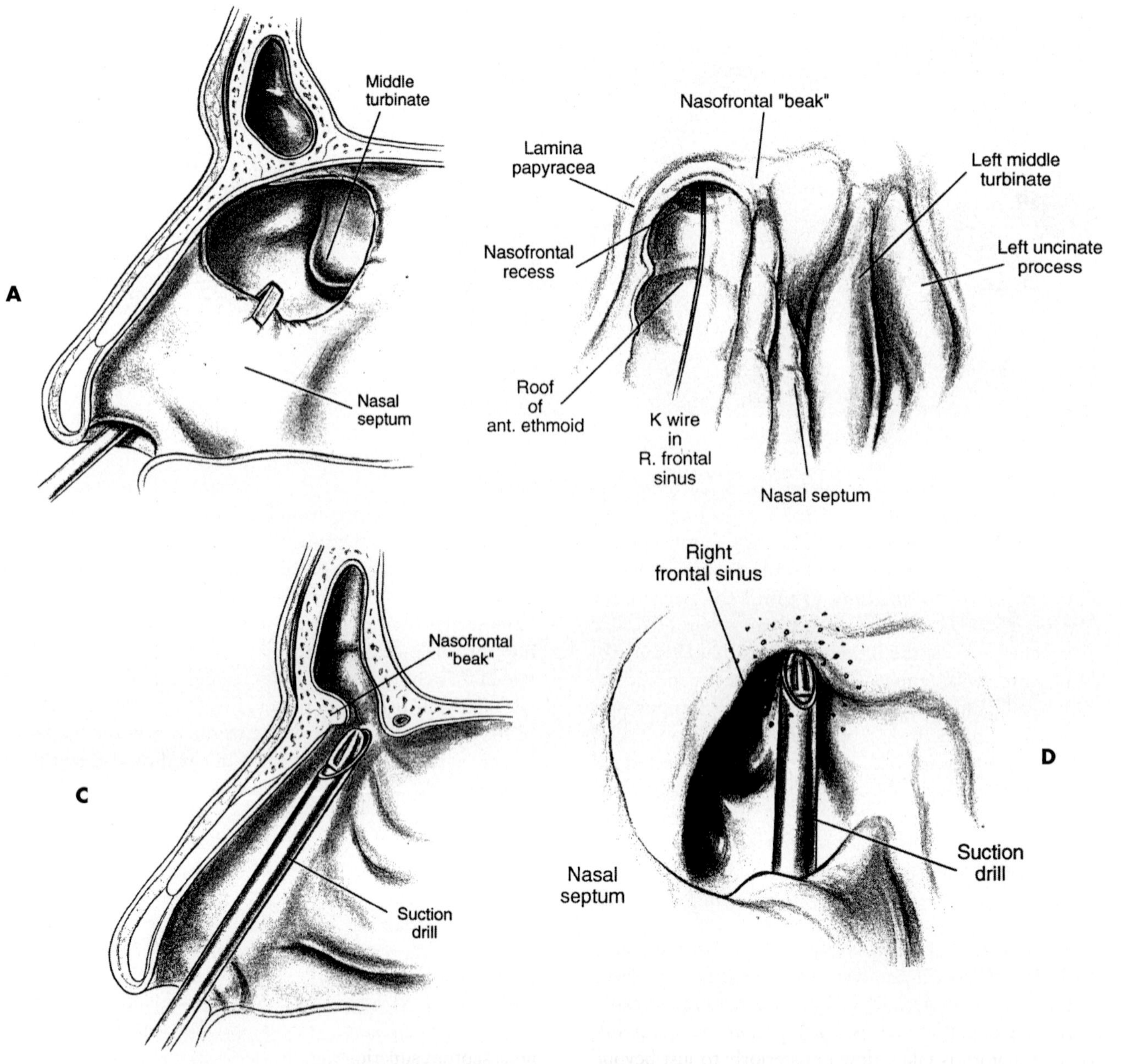

Fig. 24-3. Step-by-step operative technique. **A,** The anterosuperior nasal septum is resected. **B,** View after removal of the anterosuperior nasal septum. Both nasofrontal regions are visible. A K wire has been placed in the right frontal recess. **C,** Sagittal view. The nasofrontal "beak" of bone is drilled. The beveled shaft protects the posterior wall. Suction is applied through the shaft, providing a clear surgical field. **D,** Endoscopic view through the left nostril. The drill was inserted through the right nostril. Drilling began on the right in this patient and proceeded toward the midline.

Continued

access to the frontal recess. Any other revision endoscopic work that is necessary may be accomplished at this time.

Step 2: Locate the frontal recess. The frontal recess on one side is located if possible. The procedure is typically bilateral, so the easiest frontal recess is chosen. When landmarks are obscured in these cases, we employ the C arm to increase the surgeon's confidence in the exact identity of the frontal recess area. Alternatively, direct visualization from above through a small external incision and frontal trephine may be considered, although we have not found this necessary in our series to date.

Step 3: Takedown of anterosuperior nasal septum. The superior septum in the region between the two frontal recesses, anterior to the nasofrontal isthmus, is resected (Fig. 24-3, *A*). This is accomplished early in the procedure, as it greatly increases exposure and provides a

E

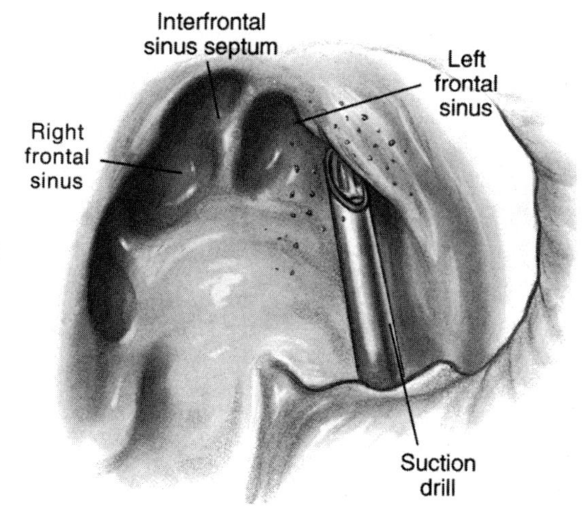

F

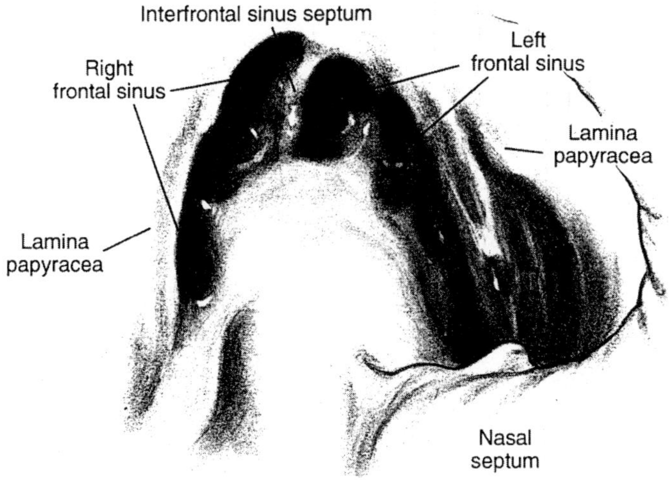

G

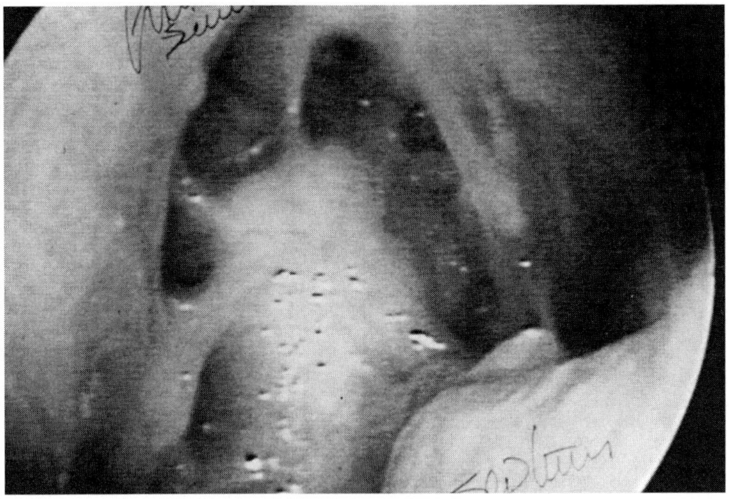

Fig. 24-3, cont'd **E,** Endoscopic view through the right nostril. As drilling proceeds past the midline, the endoscope can be placed in the right nostril to allow continued drilling via the left nostril. **F,** Endoscopic view through the right nostril of completed drillout. This labeled drawing corresponds to the postoperative photograph in **G.** (From Gross CW, Gross WE, Becker DG: Modified procedure: transnasal endoscopic frontal drillout, *Op tech Otolaryngol Head and Neck Surg* 6:193.-200, 1995.)

window to work through so that the endoscope placed through one nostril can visualize the drill tip placed through the opposite nostril. This produces broad exposure of the operative area and also greater maneuverability. The septum is taken down posteriorly to just beyond the anterior aspect of the middle turbinate. Experience has shown that when the septum is not taken down inferiorly enough, crusts or sinus drainage may catch on the superior surface of the remaining septum.

Septal takedown begins with mucosal takedown on both sides of the septum using the soft tissue shaver tip. This minimizes avulsion of the mucous membrane, which is particularly important with regard to the olfactory region posterosuperiorly. We typically use the 4.2-mm soft tissue shaver, although a smaller cannula may occasionally be necessary.

Bony and cartilaginous septa are taken down using conventional straight and backbiting forceps. Once the septum has been adequately taken down, one can visualize both frontal recess areas and the intranasal floor of the frontal sinus.

Step 4: Preparation of frontal sinus floor for drilling. Using the endonasal soft tissue shaver, mucosa is removed from the area of the frontal sinus floor between the two frontal recesses. The white remnant of cartilaginous septum superiorly and just posteriorly to the area of drilling serves as a midline marker.

Step 5: Placement of K wire. A wire probe is placed through the nasofrontal isthmus into the frontal sinus to assist in anatomic orientation and to protect posterior structures (e.g., the anterior ethmoid artery) (Fig. 24-3, *B*). Frequently the K wire is omitted when the anatomy is such that the surgeon feels it is necessary. As mentioned previously, we now use the C-arm before drilling if needed to help identify the exact location of the frontal recess. Image guided surgery is also helpful when precise guidance is needed.

Step 6: Frontal Drillout. The endonasal bone-cutting drill is used to remove bone from the anterior face of the frontal recess on one side, taking care to stay anterior to the probe within the frontal recess (Fig. 24-3, *C* to *E*). This bone that is removed constitutes part of what is known as the nasofrontal "beak" of bone. The endonasal drill is used to enter the floor of the frontal sinus anteriorly and just medially to the frontonasal isthmus, in an area named by Lothrop as the nasal crest. The nasal crest is removed and the frontal sinus progressively opened. With the posterior table under direct visualization, drilling proceeds to the midline and beyond. Drilling continues until the contralateral frontal recess and isthmus are opened and in communication with the frontonasal opening. The 4.5-mm bone-cutting drill is typically used at the outset, although a smaller drill may occasionally be necessary at first; as the drillout is widened, a 5-mm or larger drill bit may be used. An irrigation system such as Endoscrub (Xomed, Jacksonville, Fla) is used to provide irrigation at the site of drilling and to maintain a clean endoscope. This procedure is best approached by identifying both nasofrontal recesses and drilling from both sides, although we have also drilled from one frontal recess across the midline to the opposite one in some patients.

As much bone as possible is removed anteriorly, until there remains only a thin bony shell around the frontonasal communication at the glabellar area. Once the floor of the frontal sinus is removed, the interfrontal sinus septum and any other bony obstructions are removed as far superiorly into the frontal sinus as convenient. Mucosa of the posterior table and posterior nasofrontal duct mucosa are preserved, and a single common frontal opening is created that includes both nasofrontal ducts and the floor of the frontal sinus. With angled scopes, the entire contents of the frontal sinus can be visualized. The opening is typically semicircular or crescentic in shape (Fig. 24-3, *F* and *G*).

Postoperative care

Frequent office visits for postoperative care are required to ensure the patency of the opening. This may require removal of clots, crusts, polyps, and granulation tissue. Postoperative care is similar to that with standard functional endoscopic sinus surgery.[28]

RESULTS

We have reported the results of the modified transnasal Lothrop procedure performed in 20 patients with persisting severe frontal sinus disease from October 1993 until April 1995 (Zachmann, Becker, Gross, and colleagues, National Meeting AAOHNS, September 1995, New Orleans).[13-15] Three procedures were performed by one of the authors (WEG) at an outside institution; the remaining 17 were performed at the University of Virginia. Since then, many additional procedures have been performed without complication. All patients had a history of previous sinus surgery. All had failed aggressive medical therapy and showed persistent frontal sinus disease on coronal CT. All patients had undergone previous functional endoscopic sinus surgery addressing the frontal recess. All patients had frontal drainage obstruction on endoscopic examination and CT evaluation. The patients were aged 29 to 89, with an average age of 46 years.

All surgeries were performed using general anesthesia. None of the patients had significant complications. Specifically, there were no cases of CSF leakage, meningitis, visual loss, or diplopia. Thirteen of 20 procedures were performed on an outpatient basis. Two early patients were admitted overnight for observation only. Another patient was admitted overnight for blurry vision that resolved by the first postoperative day. One patient undergoing inpatient treatment for acute frontal sinusitis remained for 2 days after the procedure. Certain other patients with significant medical histories were also admitted overnight for observation, including one with a significant seizure history; an 89-year-old patient with asthma, coronary artery disease, and diabetes; and a 66-year-old with severe asthma.

Follow-up ranges from 1 to 21 months, with a mean of 12 months. The status of patients' frontal sinus opening was recorded on their own individualized videotape at each outpatient visit.

Two patients had a history of a significant concurrent disease. One had sarcoidosis; she had a patent frontal sinus opening but with significant mucosal edema. Her 21-month course was marked by occasional headaches and purulence but was her most symptom-free period ever, by her description. The other patient with significant concurrent disease had widespread allergic fungal sinusitis and chronic pain. Follow-up revealed a widely patent frontal sinus, and his intermittent headaches and frontal pain decreased significantly in intensity, although they continued to persist.

The remaining 18 patients had patent frontal sinus openings and resolution of symptoms (Table 24-2). At their last follow-up, 13 had widely patent frontal openings with healthy-appearing mucosa. Four had patent frontal openings but with some mucosal edema. One patient had developed significant bilateral mucosal edema and narrowing of the frontal opening. She was treated with topical nasal steroids and a tapered oral steroid regimen, which markedly improved the frontal opening; it subsequently remained open on endoscopic examination. All patients expressed significant resolution of their symptoms, although six experienced intermittent frontal pain or occasional purulent drainage during postoperative follow-up.

The costs for the 17 patients in this series who underwent the frontal drillout at our institution were compared with those for all patients who underwent an osteoplastic flap procedure with fat obliteration of the frontal sinus at

Table 24-2. Patient profile

PT. NO.	AGE	PREOPERATIVE SX	DATE OF SURGERY	COMPLICATIONS	PATENCY/DATE LAST VISIT	SYMPTOMS
1	37	Frontal HA, drainage	10-11-93	No	Yes Sarcoidosis 12-95	Occasional HA
2	57	Frontal HA	10-29-93	No	Yes 5-17-95	None
3	36	Frontal HA	11-8-93	No	Yes 5-10-95	None
4	40	Frontal HA	12-10-93	No	Yes 1-18-95	None
5	30	Frontal HA	2-4-94	No	Yes Allergic fungal sinusitis 8-23-95	HA
6	42	Polyps	2-14-94	No	Yes 6-7-95	None
7	34	Frontal HA	2-21-94	No	Yes 3-1-95	None
8	35	Polyps	3-4-94	No	Yes 8-31-94	None
9	52	Frontal HA	4-29-94	No	Yes 7-26-95	None
10	38	Drainage	6-21-94	No	Yes 8-23-95	None
11	46	Frontal HA	6-27-94	No	Yes 7-12-95	None
12	66	Frontal HA	7-11-94	No	Yes 7-12-95	Minimal frontal pain
13	89	Drainage	7-29-94	No	Yes Severe asthma 8-1-95	None
14	48	Frontal HA	9-29-94	No	Yes 7-17-95	None
15	43	Frontal HA, drainage	10-21-94	No	Yes 5-24-95	None
16	45	Frontal HA	12-5-94	No	Yes 4-5-95	None
17	60	Frontal HA	1-13-95	No	Yes 5-31-95	None
18	34	Frontal HA	1-16-95	No	Yes 7-12-95	None
19	34	Frontal HA	4-11-95	No	Yes 10-95	None
20	57	Frontal HA	4-25-95	No	Yes 7-19-95	None

HA, Headache.

our institution during the same period (July 1993 to March 1995). Seven patients underwent an osteoplastic procedure; one was excluded from cost evaluation because he was a neurosurgical patient with a prolonged hospital stay related to the neurosurgical problems. The remaining six patients had inpatient stays of 2 to 6 days, with a mean of 3.7 days. Total inclusive costs of the modified Lothrop procedure have been approximately 20% less than those of the osteoplastic frontal procedure at our institution. We have not tabulated our experiences and results, since these 20 initial patients. However, we have now performed this procedure on more than 60 patients. We remain enthusiastic in the opinion that for selected patients who have failed lesser procedures, this procedure should be considered before having the patient undergo the osteoplastic procedure.

DISCUSSION

Our initial results indicate the efficacy of this procedure. All 20 patients have widely patent frontal sinuses. Endoscopic visualization is easily accomplished in the clinic, so early intervention is possible should it be necessary. We acknowledge that much longer follow-up will be required to demonstrate the ultimate efficacy of this procedure, but we are encouraged by our initial results.

We believe that this procedure provides many advantages over the osteoplastic frontal sinus obliteration for patients with severe persisting frontal sinusitis. The Lothrop procedure offers the patient a less invasive procedure with a shorter hospitalization (usually discharged the same day), less pain, less frontal and orbital edema, and improved cosmesis. It also offers the advantage of the ability to evaluate postoperatively for recurrent disease, thus avoiding the diagnostic dilemma of frontal pain after frontal sinus obliteration.

One possible limitation of this procedure would be for the treatment of diseased supraorbital cells, which could be inaccessible to this approach (Montgomery, personal communication, 1994). We have not encountered this problem to date. Another potential contraindication would be a frontal sinus that was pneumatized very high but was narrow in the anteroposterior dimension.

The mucociliary clearance of the normal frontal sinus has been described.[20] The frontal sinus has been described as the only sinus with active inward transport of mucus. Along the interfrontal septum, mucus is transported into the frontal sinus and then laterally along its roof and back medially via the floor and inferior portions of the posterior and anterior wall of the sinus. The secretion then exits the frontal sinus via the lateral aspect of its ostium. A whorl-like ciliary pattern that may be present in a shallow sulcus immediately above the frontal ostium, as well as inferior to it in the frontal recess, may cause an unspecified amount of mucus to come into contact with the inwardly directed transport and thus recycle through the sinus several times.[20]

The modified Lothrop procedure takes down the intersinus septum and widely opens the frontal recess and frontal opening. One would expect the "recycling" pattern of mucus transport to be eliminated. Whether the naturally occurring recycling pattern is of benefit or detrimental is not known. Similarly, it is not known whether the new mucocilary transport patterns in the new cavity are of benefit. The nature of mucociliary transport in these sinuses is the subject of current animal and clinical studies.

Because of the high incidence of delayed failures due to stenosis after the Lynch-Howarth frontoethmoidectomy[6] and other procedures that recreate frontal drainage, we have sought to develop an alternative procedure. We believe that the approach described in this chapter produces the largest opening anatomically possible. We sought to achieve a frontonasal communication that would be so large that if some scar contracture occurred it would not cause significant stenosis. Furthermore, ease of endoscopic follow-up in clinic allows intervention when necessary to prevent significant stenosis. Preservation of the mucosa of the posterior table and posterior nasofrontal duct, and avoidance of the loss of external skeletal support inherent in Lynch-type external procedures, should improve long-term patency. The procedure described in this chapter creates a uniquely large frontonasal communication. Our application of advanced drill technology has enabled us to perform this procedure safely and expeditiously. The drill system has built-in suction at the site of resection, which leads to improved visibility. A beveled sheath helps protect the posterior sinus wall and other important posterior structures from injury. As in otologic surgery, bone-cutting drills can allow better precision than provided by rongeurs or curettes. While long-term patency rates remain to be assessed, we are encouraged by our current results and are continuing to use this procedure as the need arises.

This approach allows for additional potential applications. The patient with frontal sinus trauma involving the nasofrontal duct may not require obliteration. Goode described the use of septectomy in cases of unilateral nasofrontal injury.[26] Similarly, a modified Lothrop procedure using an osteoplastic flap approach would allow exploration of the sinus to ensure the status of the posterior table; subsequent endoscopic follow-up could determine the patency of the frontal opening. The frontal opening could be drilled from above, while partial ethmoidectomy with removal of agger nasi cells endoscopically could ensure endoscopic visualization. This has been performed successfully in one patient at our institution. Also, the frontal drillout has been performed with success in several patients who had previously undergone frontal sinus obliteration. In these cases a combined approach using an osteoplastic flap and endoscopic technique was employed (Zachmann, Becker, Gross, and colleagues, submitted for publication).

As in otologic drilling, an irrigation system to moisten and cool the surgical field would be beneficial and is soon to be released on the market. Also, modifications of the current drill system continue. A bendable cutting burr is also currently under development. Modifications in burr size and shape and degree of exposure continue in order to optimize the surgeon's ability to drill precisely at any location in the nose and sinuses.

REFERENCES

1. Schaefer SD, Close LG: Endoscopic management of frontal sinus disease, *Laryngoscope* 100:155-160, 1990.
2. Kennedy DW, Josephson JS, Zinreich SJ, et al: Endoscopic sinus surgery for mucoceles: a viable alternative, *Laryngoscope* 99:885-895, 1989.

3. Rice DH: Chronic frontal sinus disease, *Otolaryngol Clin North Am* 26:619-622, 1993.

4. May M: Frontal sinus surgery: endonasal endoscopic ostioplasty rather than external osteoplasty, *Op Tech Otolaryngol Head Neck Surg* 2:247-256, 1991.

5. Hardy JM, Montgomery WW: Osteoplastic frontal sinusotomy: analysis of 250 operations, *Ann Otolaryngol* 85:523-532, 1976.

6. Rubin JS, Lund VJ, Salmon B: Frontoethmoidectomy in the treatment of mucoceles, *Arch Otolaryngol Head Neck Surg* 112:434-436, 1986.

7. Neel HB, McDonald TJ, Facer GW: Modified Lynch procedure for chronic frontal sinus disease: rationale, technique, and long-term results, *Laryngoscope* 99:885-895, 1989.

8. Johnson JT, Schaefer S: Treatment considerations in frontal sinus disease, *Op Tech Otolaryngol Head Neck Surg* 6:201-206, 1995.

9. Lothrop HA: Frontal sinus suppuration, *Ann Surg* 59:937-957, 1914.

10. May M, Schaitkin B: Frontal sinus surgery: endonasal drainage instead of an external osteoplastic approach, *Op Tech Otolaryngol Head Neck Surg* 6:184-192, 1995.

11. Draf W: Endonasal micro-endoscopic frontal sinus surgery: the Fulda concept, *Op Tech Otolaryngol Head Neck Surg* 2:234-240, 1991.

12. Wigand M, Hoseman W: Endoscopic surgery for frontal sinusitis and its complications, *Am J Rhinol* 5:85-89, 1991.

13. Gross WE, Gross CW, Becker DG, et al: Modified transnasal endoscopic Lothrop procedure as an alternative to frontal sinus obliteration, *Otolaryngol Head Neck Surg* 113:427-434, 1995.

14. Gross CW, Gross WE, Becker DG: Modified transnasal endoscopic Lothrop procedure: frontal drillout, *Op Tech Otolaryngol Head Neck Surg* 6:193-200, 1995.

15. Becker DG, Moore D, Lindsey WH, et al: Modified transnasal endoscopic Lothrop procedure: further considerations, *Laryngoscope* 105:1161-1166, 1995.

16. Kasper KA: Nasofrontal connections: a study based on one hundred consecutive dissections, *Arch Otolaryngol* 23:322-343, 1936.

17. Onodi A: *The accessory sinuses of the nose in children*, New York, 1910, Wood.

18. Schaeffer JP: *The genesis, development, and adult anatomy of the nasofrontal region in man: a genetic, developmental, and anatomicophysiological consideration, Philadelphia*, 1920, P Blakiston's & Son.

19. Schaeffer JP: The genesis, development, and adult anatomy of the nasofrontal region in man, *Am J Anat* 20:125-146, 1919.

20. Stammberger H: *Functional endoscopic sinus surgery: the Messerklinger technique*, St Louis, 1991, Mosby–Year Book.

21. Van Alyea OE: Frontal sinus drainage, *Ann Otol Rhinol Laryngol* 55:267-277, 1946.

22. Close LG, Lee NK, Leach JL, Manning SC: Endoscopic resection of the intranasal frontal sinus floor, *Ann Otol Rhinol Laryngol* 103:952-958, 1994.

23. Montgomery WW, Pierce DL: Anterior osteoplastic fat obliteration for frontal sinus: clinical experience and animal studies, *Tr Am Acad Ophthalmol Otol* 47:46-57, 1963.

24. Donald PJ: The tenacity of the frontal sinus mucosa, *Otolaryngol Head Neck Surg* 87:557-566, 1979.

25. Fenton WH, Donald PJ, Carlton W: The pressure exerted by mucoceles in the frontal sinus: an experimental study in the cat, *Arch Otolaryngol Head Neck Surg* 116:836-840, 1990.

26. Goode RL, Streslow V, Fee WE: Frontal sinus septectomy for chronic unilateral sinusitis, *Otolaryngol Head Neck Surg* 88:18-21, 1980.

27. Pope TH, Thompson WR: Treatment of chronic unilateral frontal sinusitis by removal of the interfrontal septum, *South Med J* 69:755, 1976.

28. Gross CW, Gross WE: Post-operative care for functional endoscopic sinus surgery, *Ear Nose Throat J* 73:476-479, 1994.

CHAPTER

25

Sinus Surgery in the Immunocompromised Patient

Gary D. Josephson
Jordon Stern

PROBLEM

A 25-year-old man presented with a 3-month history of nasal congestion, left ear congestion, and recurrent white coating of the oral cavity. He denied any significant medical history and was a nonsmoker and nondrinker.

Physical examination identified a generally healthy-appearing young man. Head and neck examination revealed serous otitis media (AS) of the left ear, and a retracted tympanic membrane (AD) of the right ear, adenoid hypertrophy, rhinosinusitis, and oral thrush. Medical management consisted of oral antibiotics and topical oral antifungal agents. Upon further hematologic investigation, human immunodeficiency virus (HIV) seropositivity was identified. The patient was subsequently given multiple courses of medical therapy. The sinusitis improved after endoscopic sinus surgery (ESS), adenoidectomy, and bilateral myringotomy and pressure equalizing tube insertion.

Rhinosinusitis is commonly diagnosed and treated by the primary care physician and otolaryngologist. In the immunocompromised patient, rhinosinusitis is a challenging problem that requires a team approach by the internist, infectious disease specialist, and otolaryngologist. The otolaryngologist is often the first to diagnose immunosuppression caused by HIV, because the head and neck manifestations of this disease are very common. On other occasions the primary care physician seeks otolaryngologic consultation for a patient with difficult-to-manage or unusual head and neck pathology that may lead to a diagnosis of HIV infection.

As with sinusitis in the immunocompetent host, sinusitis in the immunocompromised patient is a disease primarily managed by medical therapy.[1,2] Those cases unresponsive to medical therapy may require surgical intervention.[1,3] The immunocompromised patient is often plagued by sinusitis that is aggressive, or by unusual pathogens not traditionally infecting the sinuses.[1-10] In the patient discussed in this chapter the HIV infection was diagnosed after the initial presentation of sinus disease, as well as other suspicious pathology (adenoid hypertrophy with otitis media and thrush). The sinus disease progressed despite medical management, and required surgical intervention. Figs. 25-1 and 25-2 present two algorithms showing our treatment protocols for sinusitis in immunocompromised patients. Fig. 25-1 shows our treatment regimen for patients with immunosuppression secondary to chemotherapy. Like other authors,[11,12] we routinely obtain pretreatment computed tomographic (CT) scans in these patients. These offer an excellent baseline of sinus anatomy and pathology before immunosuppressive chemotherapy is begun.

Because of the permanent immunosuppressive state in patients with HIV infection and acquired immunodeficiency syndrome (AIDS), the course of the disease may differ somewhat from that in patients who are temporarily immunosuppressed by chemotherapy. Therefore, there must be a greater awareness of unusual pathogens[5-10] and tumors[13-16] that may occur in these patients, especially when the response to usual treatment is not as good as expected.

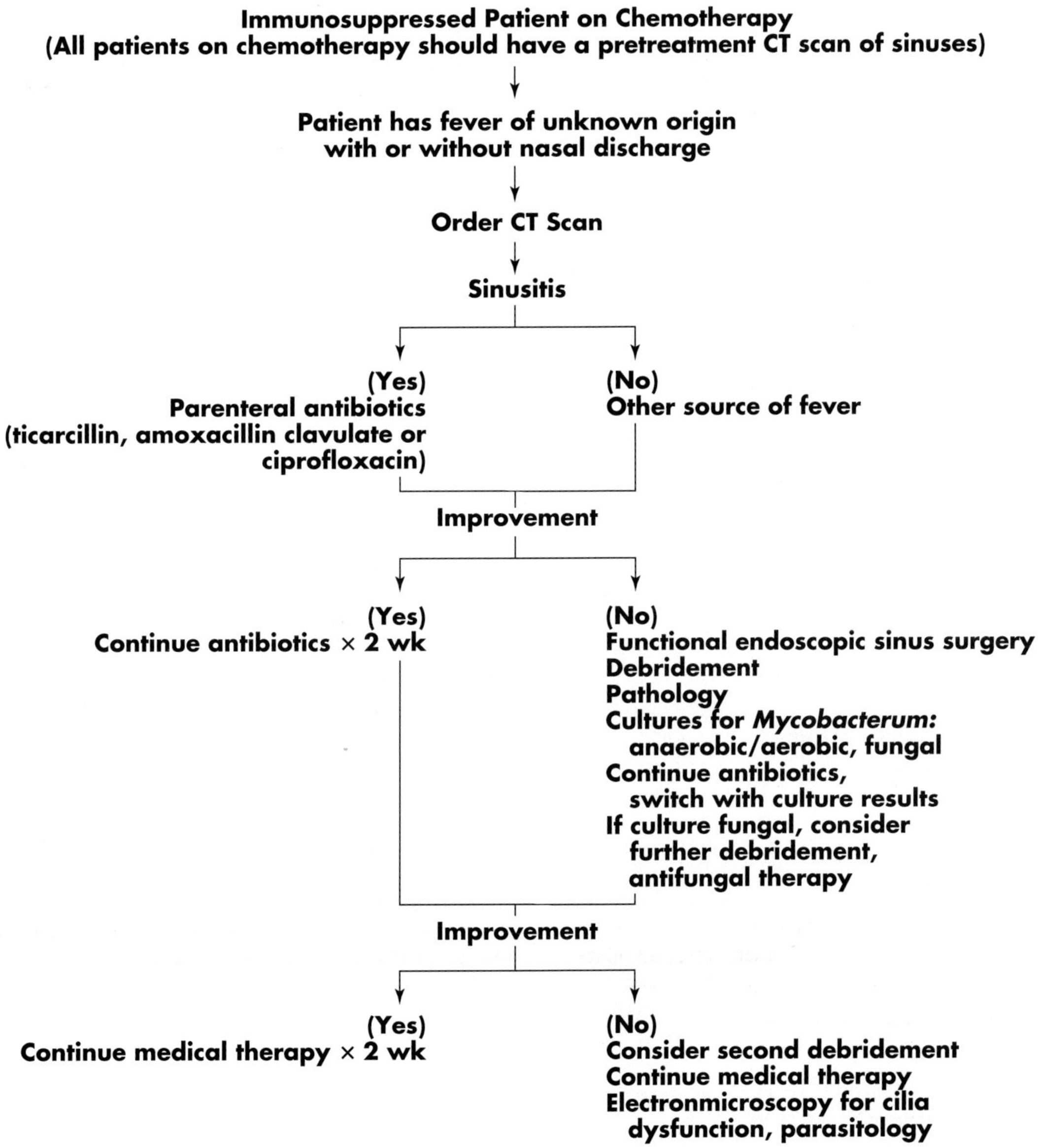

Fig. 25-1. Algorithm for an immunosuppressed patient on chemotherapy.

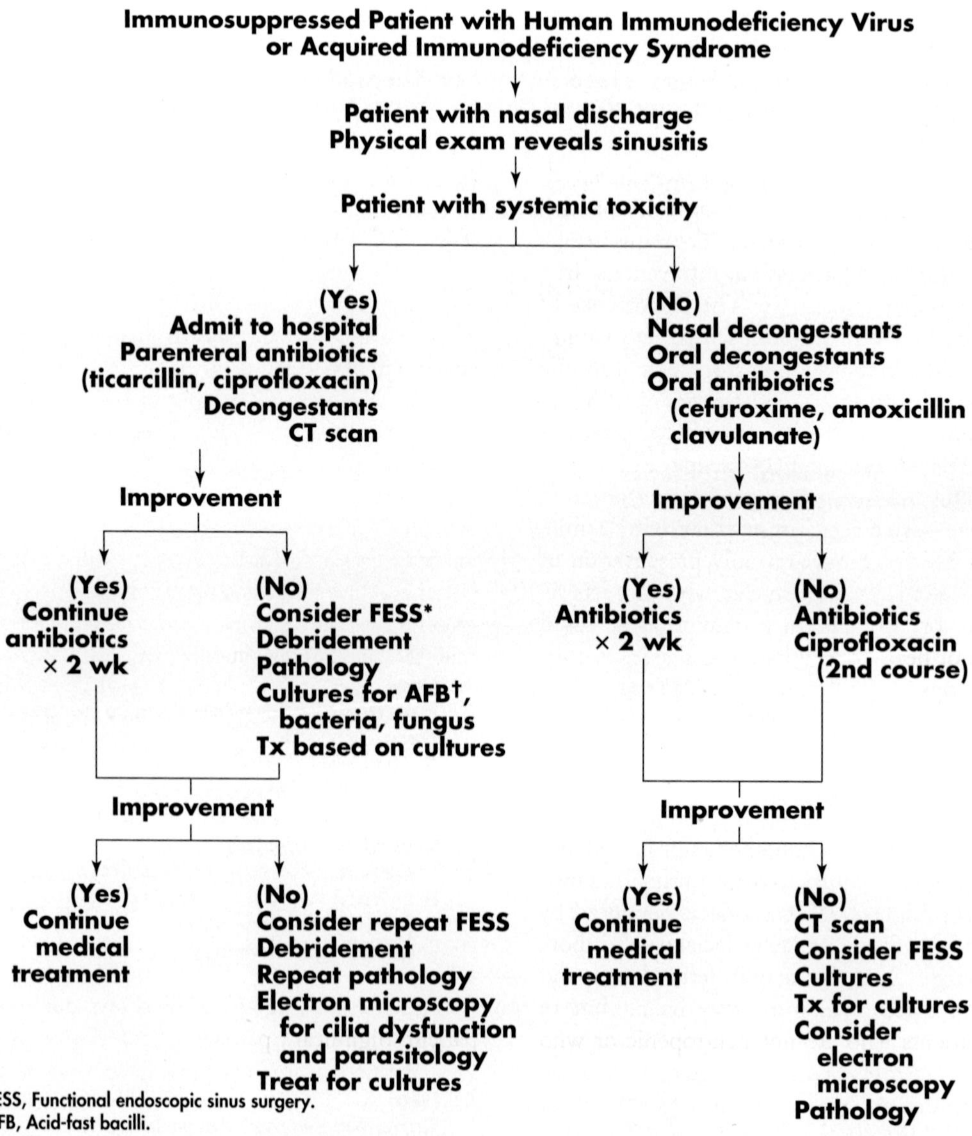

Fig. 25-2. Algorithm for an immunosuppressed patient with human immunodeficiency virus or acquired immunodeficiency syndrome.

MEDICAL HISTORY

Medical history in the evaluation of the immunocompromised patient is very important. Often the otolaryngologist is consulted to evaluate a patient with known immunosuppression, which prepares the clinician to be aware of the pathology that may affect these patients. However, many patients presenting to the otolaryngologist may be unaware of their HIV infection. The otolaryngologist may be the first to suspect this on the basis of characteristic findings in the head and neck examination. This was the case in the patient discussed here.

In areas of high risk for HIV, it is important to ask about risk factors for HIV disease, including sexual transmission, congenital transmission, intravenous drug use, and blood product transfusion. The importance of the history in the immunocompromised patient cannot be overemphasized. A thorough history can lead the physician to an early diagnosis and treatment of a potentially fatal sinus infection. This is because immunosuppressed patients who are neutropenic may not display the usual findings seen in sinusitis, such as nasal pus.[17] A history of deep-seated facial or eye pain or intermittent fevers may be the initial and only presentation of complicated sinusitis.[17,18] The clinician who suspects sinus disease by history alone in the immunocompromised patient should not hesitate to obtain a CT scan to confirm such suspicions.

PHYSICAL EXAMINATION

Physical examination in the immunocompromised patient may reveal findings similar to those in the immunocompetent patient. Signs and symptoms experienced by these patients include fever, headache, facial pain, rhinorrhea, postnasal drip, nasal obstruction, fetid breath, and nighttime cough. These symptoms may be present in HIV-positive patients who are not neutropenic or who have normal CD4 counts. The otolaryngologist treating an immunocompromised patient with vague physical findings must rule out the presence of aggressive disease.[11,17,18] Clinical symptoms are often subtle, but this should not detract from their possible significance.[17] Fever, chills, sweats, nasal mucosal edema, and/or facial pain in the immunocompromised host should prompt the physician to obtain a CT scan to assist in the evaluation. However, the clinician should recognize that radiographic findings may be misleading because of the impaired inflammatory response manifested by these individuals.[17] Aggressive disease can be overlooked by the unsuspecting clinician. Periorbital swelling or edema, exophthalmos, visual changes, meningeal signs, changes in mental status, and coma are obviously more severe physical findings with a graver prognosis.

Our patient presented with no knowledge of immunosuppression. Physical examination revealed multiple head and neck pathology that prompted further investigation. There was nasal inflammation, ostiomeatal obstruction, and nasal pus. Facial pain was present on palpation. Nasal endoscopy further revealed benign-appearing adenoid hypertrophy. There was bilateral serous otitis media and diffuse oral thrush. These findings did not change despite a 1-month course of antibiotics and decongestants. However, the oral thrush did improve with topical antifungal agents.

RADIOGRAPHIC EXAMINATION

Plain film radiographs with a four-view series is an inexpensive way to detect sinusitis in some patients, but with the advent of CT and magnetic resonance imaging (MRI), these have generally fallen out of favor. This is due to the well-documented difficulty of recognizing minimal sinus disease on plain radiography.[19] CT is the primary radiologic modality used for sinus imaging in the evaluation of sinusitis,[20] allowing for excellent delineation of bony anatomy and its pathology. MRI, on the other hand, can better evaluate soft tissue abnormalities and is best for differentiating tumors from retained secretions and inflammation. Magnetic resonance imaging is also excellent for the evaluation of the extent of aggressive disease and its soft tissue boundaries.[20] CT and MRI in patients with immunosuppression are complementary when used together and allow the clinician to better differentiate infectious from neoplastic disease of the paranasal sinuses. This is particularly important in patients with HIV infection and AIDS, who have an increased propensity to develop sinus tumors such as lymphoma.[13,14] However, as in immunocompetent patients, CT is still the "gold standard" for evaluating sinus disease.

The CT scan in Fig. 25-3 shows our representative patient. Significant paranasal sinus disease is a common finding among immunosuppressed patients with HIV infection. The correlation between the extent of sinus disease and CD4 counts in HIV-positive patients has been studied and identified as a determinant of severity of disease.[21] In our patient's CT scan, opacification of the anterior and posterior ethmoids is seen. Circumferential mucosal disease of the sphenoids with near-complete opacification is observed. Central stranding and bubbling are present, along with soft tissue opacification of the sphenoethmoidal recesses without expansion or destruction. Ostiomeatal unit and frontal recess opacification are further noted. A midline nasopharyngeal mass consistent with the adenoidal disease is identified.

Figs. 25-4 to 25-6 illustrate CT and MRI images of the appearance of other pathologic sinus conditions seen in immunocompromised patients.

Text continued on p. 230

A B C

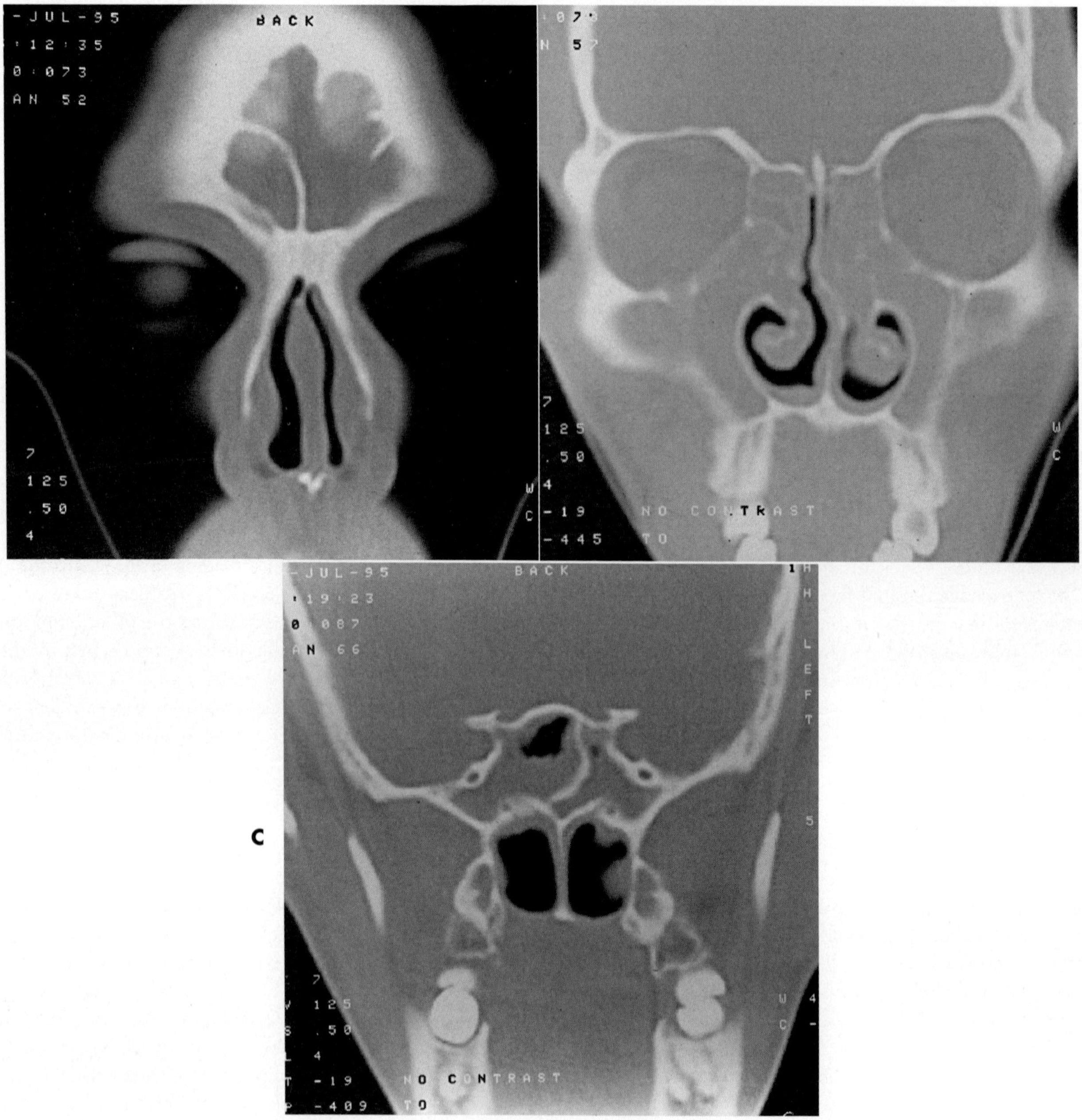

Fig. 25-3. Bacterial pansinusitis, coronal computed tomography (CT). **A,** Frontal sinus. **B,** Ostiomeatal unit. **C,** Sphenoid sinus. There is complete opacification of the frontal, ethmoidal, and maxillary sinuses and near-complete sphenoid opacification with a collection of thick secretions. All septations are intact.

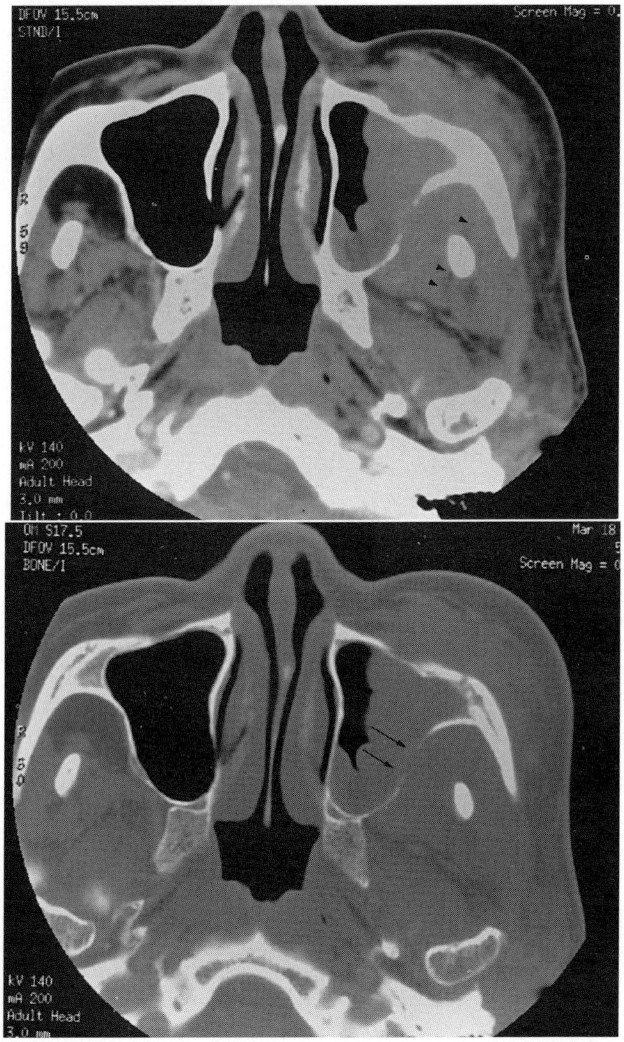

A

B

Fig. 25-4. CT of lymphoma. **A,** Soft tissue window. **B,** Bone window. There is a bulky soft tissue mass involving the left maxillary antrum, masticator space, and buccal tissue. The intervening bony plates remain in position, with permeative destruction of the posterior antral walls *(arrows)*. There is obliteration of fat planes in the retromaxillary space with infiltration of temporalis muscle *(arrowhead)*.

A

B

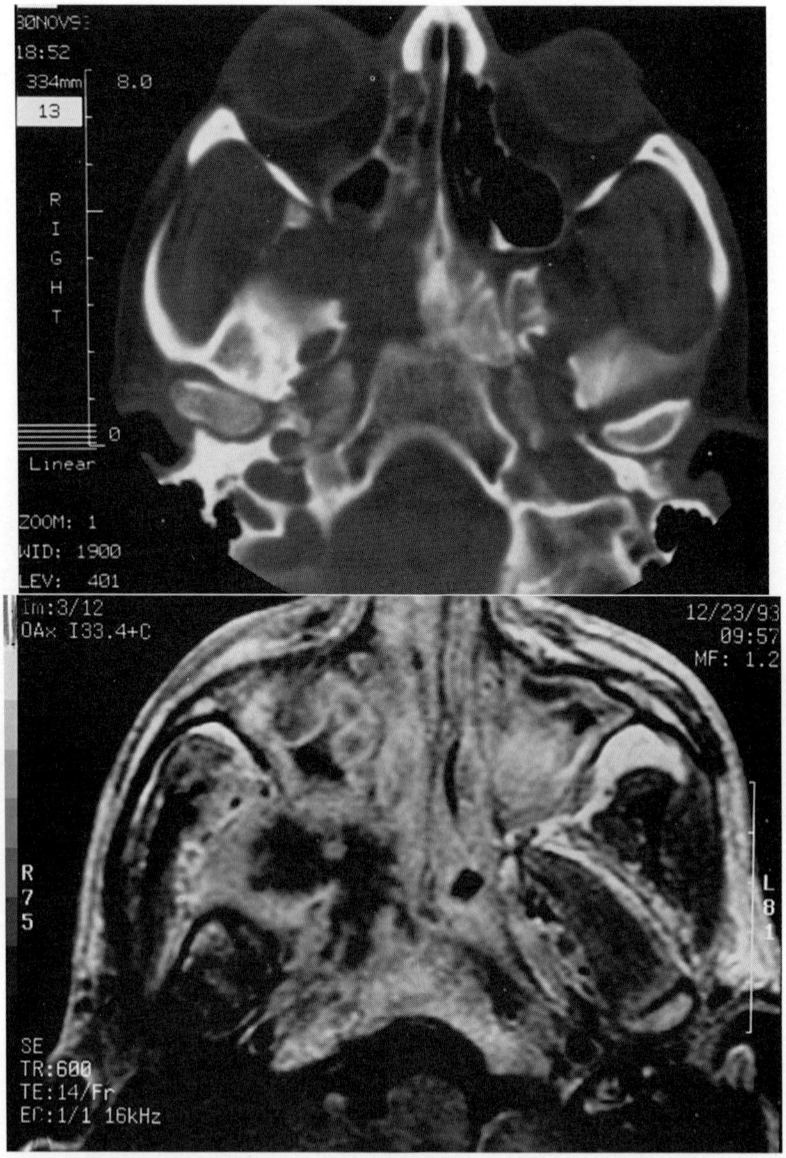

Fig. 25-5. *Aspergillus* infection. **A,** Axial CT of the skull base. **B,** Axial postcontrast T1-weighted magnetic resonance imaging (MRI) of the skull base. **A** and **B** show a destructive skull base lesion involving the basisphenoid and pterygoid process on the right side. There is dehiscence of the posterior antral wall at its apex. The foramen ovale is intact. There is a thick ring-enhancing lesion in the infratemporal fossa and into the nasopharynx. There is irregular heterogeneous disease in the right maxillary sinus.

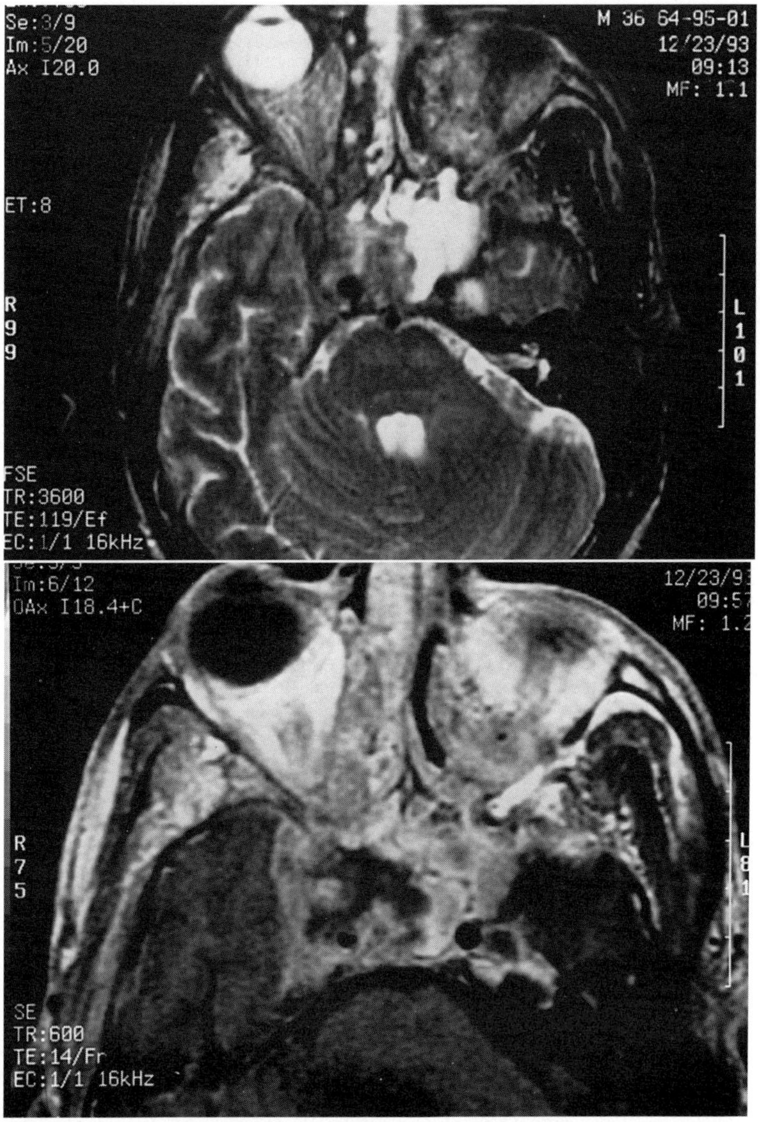

C

D

Fig. 25-5, cont'd. *Aspergillus* infection. **C,** Axial T2-weighted MRI of the sphenoid sinus. **D,** Axial postcontrast T1-weighted MRI of the sphenoid sinus. In **C,** superior extension of the lesion on T2-weighted MRI reveals irregular heterogeneous but predominantly isointense material in the right sphenoid. Note the more typical hyperintense inflammatory disease in the left sphenoid sinus. After contrast injection the right sphenoid contains a thick ring of enhancement with central low signal intensity. There is marked infiltration of the right cavernous sinus with encasement of the cavernous-carotid artery.

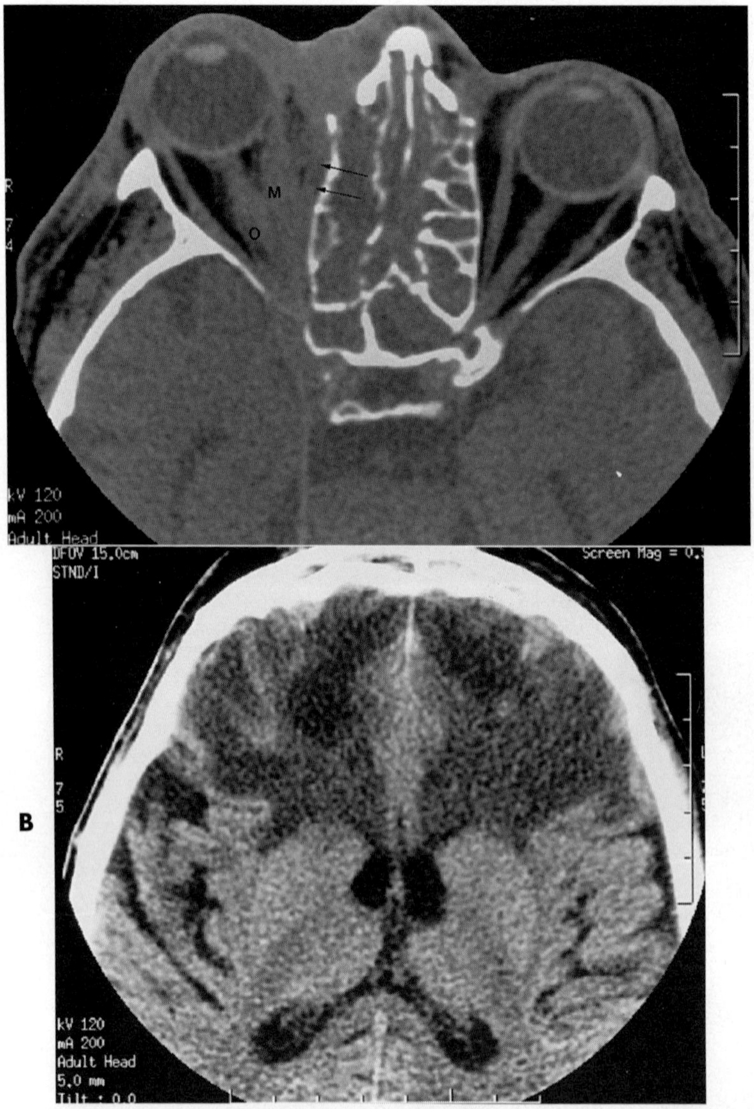

Fig. 25-6. Mucormycosis. **A,** Axial CT through the midorbit. **B,** Axial CT through the frontal lobes. There is complete opacification of the ethmoidal labyrinth and sphenoid sinus. Loss of septations is in part due to debridement. There is inflammatory infiltrate of the right orbit. The medial rectus muscle *(m)* and optic nerve *(o)* are enlarged, with ill-defined margins. There is a thin subperiosteal abscess *(arrows)* as well as an abscess in the lacrimal fossa. There is gross bony dehiscence of the anterior skull base *(not shown)*, with intracranial extension producing cerebritis.

LABORATORY EXAMINATION

Laboratory evaluation is also important in the evaluation of the immunosuppressed patient. For unsuspecting patients presenting with significant head and neck findings indicating immunosuppression, HIV testing is important. The presence or absence of HIV infection can help direct the physician toward the most appropriate treatment regimens. Furthermore, for seropositive patients, appropriate consultation can be obtained to help enroll the patient in treatment programs for psychological counseling and medical preventive measures. For patients with known immunosuppression, evaluation of the CD4 count is one of the current methods to help monitor the progression and stability of the disease.[22]

TREATMENT

Medical and Surgical Techniques

Rhinosinusitis is primarily a medical problem.[1,2] For those cases that fail medical therapy, surgical management can offer symptomatic relief as well as cure.[1,3] Treatment regimens are based on the physician's understanding of the pathogens involved. This has been clearly established in immunocompetent patients, but in immunocompromised patients, the physician must be cognizant of unusual pathogens. In addition, tumors affecting the sinuses (e.g., lymphoma and Kaposi's sarcoma) are more common in the immunocompromised host.

Empiric therapy for the usual organisms affecting the sinuses is begun in an outpatient setting and includes β-lactamase–stable antibiotics. Topical and systemic decongestants are also of value during therapy. In patients unresponsive to a 2-week course of β-lactamase–stable antibiotics cultures should be taken, and antibiotics that also cover *Pseudomonas* should be started. Sinus evaluation should be performed using endoscopes, which offer better visualization and enable adequate cultures to be taken from the middle meatus. Once culture results are obtained, antibiotic therapy should be instituted for 2 to 6 weeks. CT scans should be obtained for cases unresponsive after a course of medical treatment has been completed. CT must be performed before surgical therapy is instituted. Patients who remain symptomatic should be prepared for endoscopic sinus surgery. Repeated cultures for anaerobic and aerobic bacteria, acid-fast bacilli, and fungus should be obtained. Therapy is based on culture results. More than one isolate may be obtained from cultures in these patients, and therefore the physician should use broad-spectrum antibiotics that sufficiently treat these organisms.

ESS offers excellent visualization and directed biopsies of diseased tissue, and allows for mucosal debridement,[18,23,24] which is continued until normal healthy bleeding tissue is encountered. The normal sinus ostia are identified and opened widely to allow for good aeration and adequate drainage pathways. Extensive disease that extends past the normal sinal anatomic boundaries or that cannot be adequately debrided through the endoscope is additionally approached through external procedures. We have found this to be effective in our patients. Physicians less experienced with the use of endoscopes should not hasten to use an external approach to sinus disease.

All tissue obtained from the sinuses is sent for aerobic and anaerobic, acid-fast bacilli, fungal, and parasitic cultures as well as pathologic evaluation. Patients are placed on broad-spectrum antibiotics or antifungals according to the clinician's experience, judgment, and surgical findings. Our preference in medical therapy is indicated in Figs. 25-1 and 25-2. Consultation with an infectious disease clinician should be sought, as management and treatment of these patients is often difficult and requires a team approach.

Repeat endoscopy with cleaning is performed every 2 or 3 days after surgery until there is no evidence of mucosal disease or until resolution of disease is clear. Depending on the aggressiveness of the disease, further debridement may be necessary. This is performed in the clinic in a case of minimal infection; with more extensive disease, the patient is brought back to the operating room for additional debridement. Frequent evaluation of these patients is appropriate, especially in patients with severe neutropenia and/or low CD4 counts. Postoperative CT scans should be obtained, particularly in cases of recurrent disease,[18] to determine the results of treatment and successful resolution of disease.

RESULTS

Our patient improved after adenoidectomy and endoscopic sinus surgery. Culture results obtained during surgery grew *Streptococcus* and *Pseudomonas* organisms. Antibiotic therapy with broad-spectrum antibiotics that also covered *Pseudomonas* was successful in the treatment of this patient. Although *Pseudomonas* organisms are not common in immunocompetent patients, they have been found to be common pathogens in immunocompromised patients.[1,22,25] Physical findings pointed to the diagnosis of HIV disease in this patient and guided the choice of treatment.

In reviewing the results of other studies as well as data from our own patients, several factors are important for the management of HIV-positive patients with sinusitis. First, common pathogens infecting the sinuses of immunocompetent patients are also common among the immunocompromised.[1,4] Second, other pathogens such as *Pseudomonas* organisms and fungi *(Aspergillus)* were common in our patients as well as in other series in the literature.[1,11,17,18,22,25] Third, unusual pathogens, including *Candida* species, parasites (microsporidia),[10] and tumors (lymphoma),[13,14] must also be suspected. Fourth, patients with HIV appear to do well with endoscopic sinus surgery, keeping in mind the quantitative value of the CD4 count.[22,26] This is because the CD4 count is inversely proportional to the extent of the disease, and hence to the response to treatment.[21] It is therefore important to consider the CD4 count when planning ESS. Fifth, sinus endoscopy offers excellent visualization for directed biopsies of diseased tissue, and allows the surgeon to obtain cultures, as well as perform definitive surgical treatment.[18,23,24] External procedures are still indicated for aggressive invasive disease.

DISCUSSION

For many years, the otolaryngologist was confronted with the occasional immunocompromised patient on chemotherapy with bacterial or fungal sinusitis. However, the AIDS epidemic mandates an increased awareness by the otolaryngologist in the diagnosis and management of sinusitis in the immunocompromised host. The pathogens seen in this group were originally thought to be the same as those in the immunocompetent host, but it is becoming more apparent that the organisms involved either are more aggressive or are obscure pathogens not traditionally thought to infect the sinuses (Box 25-1). Unusual bacteria, invasive fungi, and even parasitic infections have been reported in these patients (Box 25-2). Other sinus pathology recognized in this group of patients includes malignancies such as lymphoma, Kaposi's sarcoma, and carcinoma. This makes the treatment of immunocompromised patients infected with HIV disease a challenge. Despite aggressive surgical management, many patients either succumb to their immunodeficiency-related diseases or have recurrent bouts of sinusitis. This often complicates the decision for surgical intervention in this group of patients.

This chapter focuses on the identification, management, and treatment of the rapidly growing population of patients with HIV disease seen in the physician's office. A brief overview is also presented on the management of chemotherapy-immunocompromised patients with sinusitis.

Sinusitis in the immunocompromised patient is becoming well recognized. Several mechanisms of anatomic or physiologic impairment have been hypothesized. Any one of these mechanisms, or a combination thereof, may contribute to or be the cause of the increasing incidence of sinusitis in these patients.

Immunologic factors have been investigated in the role of sinusitis in HIV-infected patients.[16,25,26] Patients with immunosuppression, whether from HIV disease or chemotherapy, become susceptible to infection during times of severe neutropenia. Granulocyte dysfunction is also observed in these patients.[25] This may be the basis for recurrent bacterial infections. CD4 counts of less than 200/mm^3 have been correlated with the incidence of sinusitis in several studies of HIV-infected patients.[21,25,26] Severe sinusitis involving both the anterior and posterior sinuses is more commonly seen and correlates with the longevity of a low CD4 count.[21] These patients also seem to respond incompletely to medical therapy.[21] Low CD4 lymphocyte counts are clinically manifested by infection with intracellular organisms and opportunistic infections.[25]

IgG subclass abnormalities have been investigated for their role of protection in immunocompromised patients. IgG1 and IgG3 antibodies tend to be elevated or unaffected. However, IgG2 and IgG4 subclasses have been recognized to be deficient in some AIDS patients.[27] This may explain the increased incidence of infection with encapsulated organisms such as in *H. influenzae* infection and streptococcal pneumonia.

Other humoral factors may predispose HIV patients to sinusitis. IgE levels seem to increase progressively in HIV-positive patients. Lucey and colleagues[28] showed an inverse relationship between CD4 counts and IgE levels. Allergic symptoms, histamine release, and nasal eosinophilia along with elevated IgE levels have all been identified in HIV-infected patients. It is possible that this hyperallergic state may contribute to the increase in frequency of sinusitis in these patients.[27]

In general, mucociliary clearance and cilia function are important for maintaining the protective function of the nose and sinuses. Alteration or impairment of this function can lead to nasal mucosal edema, mucous plugging, and ostiomeatal and sinus obstruction. Milgrim and colleagues[22] described prolonged mucociliary clearance among patients with HIV infection and AIDS. They also noted a direct correlation between mucociliary transit time and CD4 counts. Sisson and associates[29] described a derangement in mucociliary clearance with an increase in saccharin transit time in patients on immunosuppressive therapy. They found that when therapy was completed and immunosuppression had recovered, mucociliary transit time returned to normal. It therefore seems that immunosuppression causes impaired mucociliary clearance and hence an increased frequency of sinusitis. The abnormality at the ultrastructural level has not been clarified. Ciliary abnormalities, impairment of the pseudostratified columnar epithelium, or an irregularity within the nasal mucus blanket may be the inciting mechanism(s).

BOX 25-1

Common Pathogens Infecting the Sinuses of Immunocompromised Patients

Staphylococcus aureus
Streptococcus pneumoniae
Haemophilus influenzae
Pseudomonas aeruginosa
Aspergillus fumigatus
Cytomegalovirus
Phycomycetes
Mucormycosis

BOX 25-2

Uncommon Pathogens Infecting Immunocompromised Patients

Pathogen	Authors
Legionella pneumophila	Schlanger et al 19845
Acanthamoeba castellani	Gonzalez et al 19866
Alternaria alternata	Wiest et al 19877
Cryptococcus neoformans	Choi et al 19888
Candida albicans	Colmenero et al 19909
Microsporidia	Josephson et al 199610

In addition, impaired sinus drainage secondary to lymphoid hyperplasia has been suggested as one cause of the increased incidence of sinus disease.[26] Stern and colleagues[30] identified and reported adenoid hypertrophy causing nasal obstruction in HIV-positive patients. Biopsy revealed benign lymphoid hyperplasia in these cases. This further indicates that lymphoid hyperplasia may act as an additional mechanism in the cause of sinusitis in these patients.

Radiologic evaluation of the sinuses is an excellent modality to assist the clinician in the identification of sinusitis and help delineate the extent of the disease. CT is the "gold standard" for identifying sinus disease and delineating bony anatomic landmarks. MRI is an excellent adjuvant tool that may be used in conjunction with CT to better assess soft tissue pathology such as tumors within the sinuses, or meningeal and intracranial involvement.

Godofsky and associates[21] reviewed different radiographic imaging studies in HIV-infected patients and found an interesting correlation between the degree of immunosuppression and the extent of radiographic findings. Extensive disease involving more than four paranasal sinuses correlated well with a CD4 count of below $200/mm^3$. These authors also reported that most HIV-positive patients studied had more than 75% opacification of the sinuses on MRI and CT, indicating clinically significant disease.

Traditionally, sinus surgery was performed with Caldwell-Luc and intranasal sinus procedures using coaxial headlights and nasal specula. With the advent of ESS, more traditional approaches to the sinuses were replaced, leaving traditional techniques for special circumstances. ESS allows endoscopic visualization of all the paranasal sinuses, is less invasive than traditional approaches, and has achieved proven success.[23]

Sinus surgery is currently being evaluated for its success rates in the immunocompromised host. Patients with immunodeficiency secondary to chemotherapy appear to do well with ESS, depending on the organism causing the disease.[18] Invasive fungal or bacterial disease may be extremely aggressive, so that no surgical or medical modality can halt the disease process. However, ESS gives adequate visualization and exposure for surgical debridement of all the paranasal sinuses and is therefore an excellent surgical modality to assist the attempt to treat this disease.

The efficacy of ESS in HIV- or AIDS-infected individuals remains to be established. These patients not only have impaired immune systems, but also have deficiencies in wound healing as well as impaired platelet function that may lead to coagulopathies. This may sway some surgeons against any surgical intervention in view of the increased risk of postoperative morbidity and mortality. These factors must be considered during the evaluation of patients with this disease. Treatment regimen studies of sinusitis patients with HIV infection still need to be elicited. Patients infected by the HIV virus who do not have any systemic infections or AIDS, and who are not neutropenic and have near-normal CD4 counts, appear to have favorable results from ESS comparable with those in immunocompetent patients. Patients who have AIDS or are hospitalized with multisystem infections are likely to have a less favorable prognosis even with surgical intervention. However, ESS may be beneficial, as it offers excellent visualization of the sinuses, provides for directed biopsies and cultures of diseased tissue, and allows for debridement. Invasive and aggressive disease may require repeated endoscopic sinus procedures as well as traditional external approaches.

CONCLUSION

Sinusitis in the immunocompromised patient is becoming increasingly common with the greater incidence of HIV infection. Standard medical therapy is the first course of treatment for this disease as in the immunocompetent patient. Nasal cultures are important for guiding the clinician to the appropriate medical therapy. Axial and coronal noncontrast CT is an effective adjuvant modality for the diagnosis of sinus disease in these patients. MRI used in concert with CT may further delineate soft tissue pathology. Because of the paucity of fungal infections or malignant tumors, it is important to obtain a CT scan early in the treatment of these patients. Functional ESS is an effective surgical technique for treating patients not responsive to medical therapy. It offers nasal access with excellent visualization for directed biopsies and for surgical debridement. The surgeon must remember to send pathologic specimens for bacterial (anaerobic/aerobic), acid-fast bacillus, fungal, and parasitic cultures as well as pathologic examination, because the cause of the sinusitis in these patients may be unique or obscure. Medical therapy is further advised, depending on pathologic and culture results. The clinician must be aware of the frustrations in treating the immunocompromised host, as normal immune function is impaired or absent, and wound healing capability from surgical intervention may be compromised. Most important, a team approach among the general practitioners, otolaryngologists, and infectious disease specialists is crucial to patient care.

REFERENCES

1. Milgrim LM, Rubin JS, Rosenstreich DL, Small CB: Sinusitis in human immunodeficiency virus infection: typical and atypical organisms, *J Otolaryngol* 23:450-453, 1994.
2. Meiteles LZ, Lucente FE: Sinus and nasal manifestations of the acquired immunodeficiency syndrome, *Ear Nose Throat J* 69:454-459, 1990.

3. Poole MD, Postma D, Cohen MS: Pyogenic otorhinologic infections in acquired immune deficiency syndrome, *Arch Otolaryngol* 110:130-131, 1984.
4. Upadhyay S, Marks SC, Arden RL, et al: Bacteriology of sinusitis in human immunodeficiency virus-positive patients: implications for management, *Laryngoscope* 105:1058-1060, 1995.
5. Schlanger G, Lutwick LI, Kurzman M, et al: Sinusitis caused by *Legionella pneumophila* in a patient with the acquired immune deficiency syndrome, *Am J M* 77:957-960, 1984.
6. Gonzalez MM, Gould E, Dickinson G, et al: Acquired immunodeficiency syndrome associated with *Acanthamoeba* infection and other opportunistic organisms, *Arch Pathol Lab Med* 110:749-751, 1986.
7. Wiest PM, Wiese K, Jacobs MR, et al: *Alternaria* infection in a patient with acquired immunodeficiency syndrome: case report and review of invasive *Alternaria* infection, *Rev Infect Dis* 9:799-803, 1987.
8. Choi SS, Lawson W, Buttone EJ, et al: Cryptococcol sinusitis: a case report and review of literature, *Otolaryngol Head Neck Surg* 99:414-418, 1988.
9. Colmenero C, Monux A, Valencia E, Castro A: Successfully treated *Candida* sinusitis in an AIDS patient, *J Craniomaxillofac Surg* 18:175-178, 1990.
10. Josephson GD, Sarlin J, Reidy J, Pincus R: Microsporidial rhinosinusitis: is this the next pathogen to infect the sinuses of the immunocompromised host?, *Otolaryngol Head Neck Surg* 114:137-139, 1996.
11. Shaw GY, Panje WR, Corey JP, et al: Risk factors in the development of acute sinusitis in immunocompromised patients, *Am J Rhinol* 5:103-108, 1991.
12. Shibuya TY, Momin F, Abella E, et al: Sinus disease in the bone marrow transplant population: incidence, risk factors, and complications, *Otolaryngol Head Neck Surg* 113:705-711, 1995.
13. Goldberg JE, Moscatello AL, Babapour R, et al: AIDS related non-Hodgkin's lymphoma of the paranasal sinuses, *Am J Rhinol* 7:37-42, 1993.
14. Goldstein J, Rubin J, Becker N, et al: Lymphoma of the maxillary sinus in a patient infected with human immunodeficiency virus type 1, *Head Neck* 13:355-358, 1991.
15. Marcusen DC, Sooy CD: Otolaryngologic and head and neck manifestations of acquired immunodeficiency syndrome (AIDS), *Laryngoscope* 95:401-405, 1985.
16. Rosenberg RA, Schneider KL, Cohen NL: Head and neck presentations of acquired immunodeficiency syndrome, *Otolaryngol Head Neck Surg* 93:700-705, 1985.
17. Berlinger NT: Sinusitis in immunodeficient and immunosuppressed patients, *Laryngoscope* 95:29-33, 1985.
18. Wiatrak BJ, Willging P, Myer CM, Cotton RT: Functional endoscopic sinus surgery in the immunocompromised child, *Otolaryngol Head Neck Surg* 105:818-825, 1991.
19. Sarter E, et al: Radiographic evaluation of the paranasal sinuses, *Curr Probl Diagn Radiol* 14:27-39, 1985.
20. Zeifer B: *Sinus imaging*. In Baily BJ, editor: *Head and neck surgery–otolaryngology*, Philadelphia, 1993, JB Lippincott, pp 350-365.
21. Godofsky EW, Zinreich J, Armstrong M, et al: Sinusitis in HIV-infected patients: a clinical and radiographic review, *Am J Med* 93:163-170, 1992.
22. Milgrim LM, Rubin JS, Small CB: Mucociliary clearance abnormalities in the HIV-infected patient: a precursor to acute sinusitis, *Laryngoscope* 105:1202-1208, 1995.
23. Kennedy DW: Functional endoscopic sinus surgery: technique, *Arch Otolaryngol* 111:643-649, 1985.
24. Josephson JS, Balwally AN, Josephson GD: Complications of functional endoscopic sinus surgery, *Insights Otolaryngol* 7:1-8, 1992.
25. Rubin JS, Honigberg R: Sinusitis in patients with the acquired immunodeficiency syndrome, *Ear Nose Throat J* 69:460-463, 1990.
26. Zurlo JJ, Feuerstein IM, Lebovics R, Lane HC: Sinusitis in HIV-1 infection, *Am J Med* 93:157-162, 1992.
27. Small CB, Kaufman A, Armenaka M, Rosenstreich DL: Sinusitis and atopy in human immunodeficiency virus infection, *J Infect Dis* 167:283-290, 1993.
28. Lucey D, Zajac R, Melcher G, et al: Serum IgE levels vary with absolute CD4a lymphocyte counts in HIV persons (abstract ThBP 135). In Program and abstracts: Vth International Conference on AIDS, Montreal, Ottawa, 1989, International Development Research Centre, p 438.
29. Sisson J, Diamond J, Walter T, et al: Mucociliary transport is impaired during autologous bone marrow transplantation, *Am Rev Respir Dis* 147:A390, 1993.
30. Stern JC, Lin P, Lucente FE: Benign nasopharyngeal masses and human immunodeficiency virus infection, *Arch Otolaryngol Head Neck Surg* 116:206-208, 1990.

SECTION

FOUR

NEOPLASTIC DISEASE

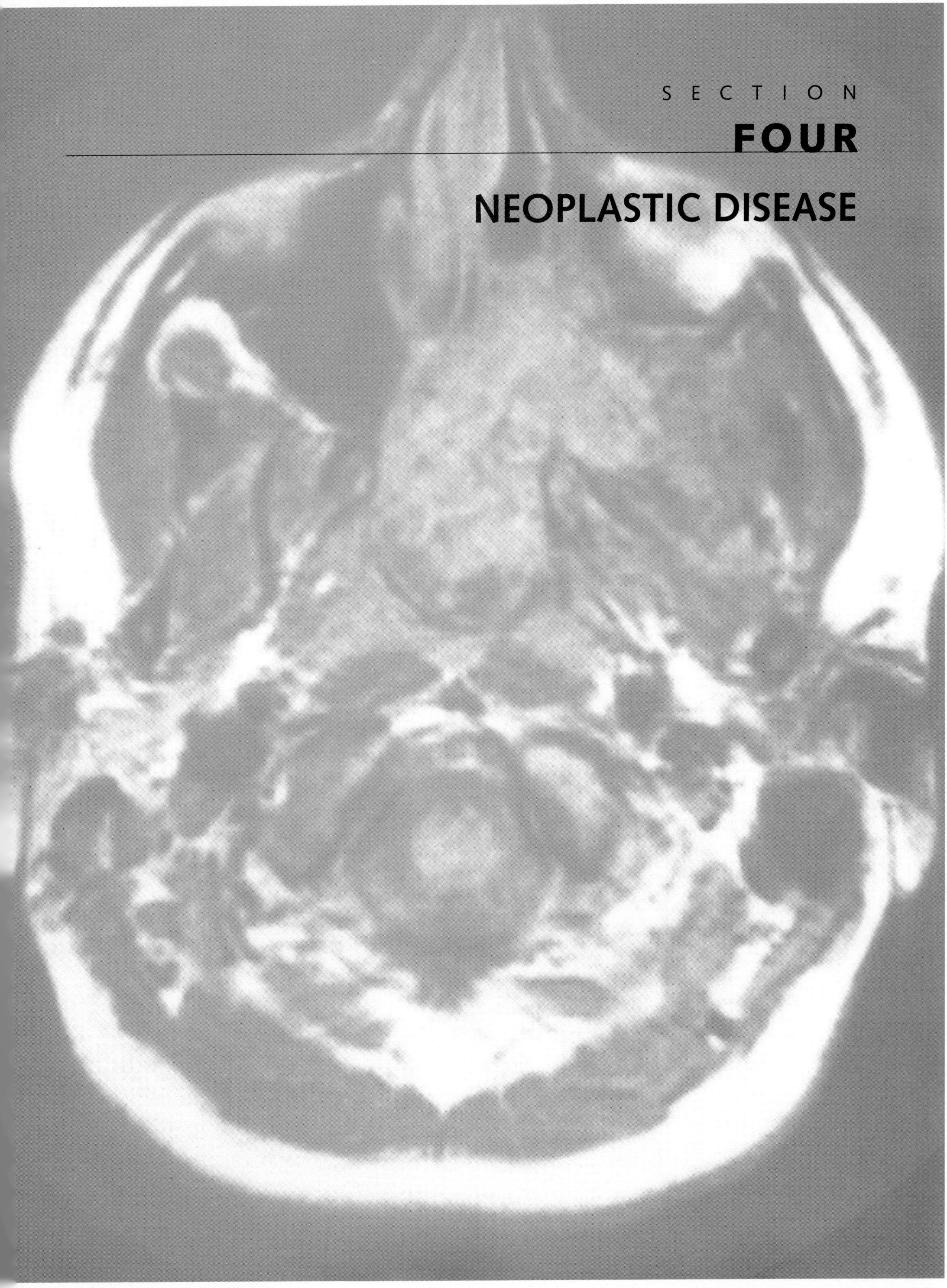

CHAPTER

26

Management of Angiofibromas

Thomas V. McCaffrey
H. Bryan Neel, III

PROBLEM

The patient is a 15-year-old male who has an occasional nosebleed and whose nose has become obstructed.

Angiofibroma is a benign tumor that predominantly affects male adolescents. The triad of nasal obstruction, nasopharyngeal mass, and recurrent epistaxis usually indicates an angiofibroma.

These tumors are aggressive and destructive. They are uncommon but still the most frequent *benign* tumor originating in the nasopharynx. They are rarely limited to the nasopharynx and usually extend into the nose, paranasal sinuses, pterygomaxillary fossa, infratemporal fossa, temporal fossa and cranium and even the neck; thus, the term *nasopharyngeal* angiofibroma is misleading and inaccurate. We prefer the term *angiofibroma* and no longer use the term *juvenile* because the neoplasm can occur in older patients.

Angiofibromas challenge the most experienced head and neck surgeons. Despite being classified as benign, they may grow considerably and cause significant structural and functional damage. We do not know why a histologically benign tumor should erode bone and push into and through regional structures. These tumors grow insidiously to a substantial size, sometimes into the cranium, before symptoms occur in most patients, and the symptoms may be attributed to more common problems (Fig. 26-1).

MEDICAL HISTORY

Nasal obstruction and epistaxis were the most common symptom and sign in the Mayo series,[1-3] occurring in more than 80% of patients. Table 26-1 lists the symptoms and signs of angiofibroma.

All the Mayo patients were white males whose ages ranged from 7 to 29 years. The median age at diagnosis was 15 years. The tumor occurred predominantly in adolescents. The tumor has not been found in individuals beyond the third decade of life or in females, and we have not found that the tumors are more aggressive or that the incidence of intracranial spread is higher in younger patients.

PHYSICAL EXAMINATION

The patient may have some bulging of the face or eye. Examination shows a pale, bluish smooth mass in the nasopharynx and often in the posterior aspect of the nose.

Diagnosis depends on a careful history and physical examination. The diagnosis of angiofibroma may be overlooked initially despite the heightened awareness of its existence in male adolescents. Patients have been observed for significant periods with diagnoses such as sinusitis, rhinitis, or antral choanal polyps. Since the mid-1970s, the duration of symptoms before treatment has decreased significantly from 20 months to about 6 months. This probably reflects an increased awareness of the tumor by physicians and improved diagnostic methods, such as endoscopy, that are now generally available to most practitioners.

In most patients the tumor is on one side of the nasopharynx. It sometimes fills the nasopharynx and is occasionally in the midline. The frequency of involvement of one side of the nose supports our view of the point of origin.

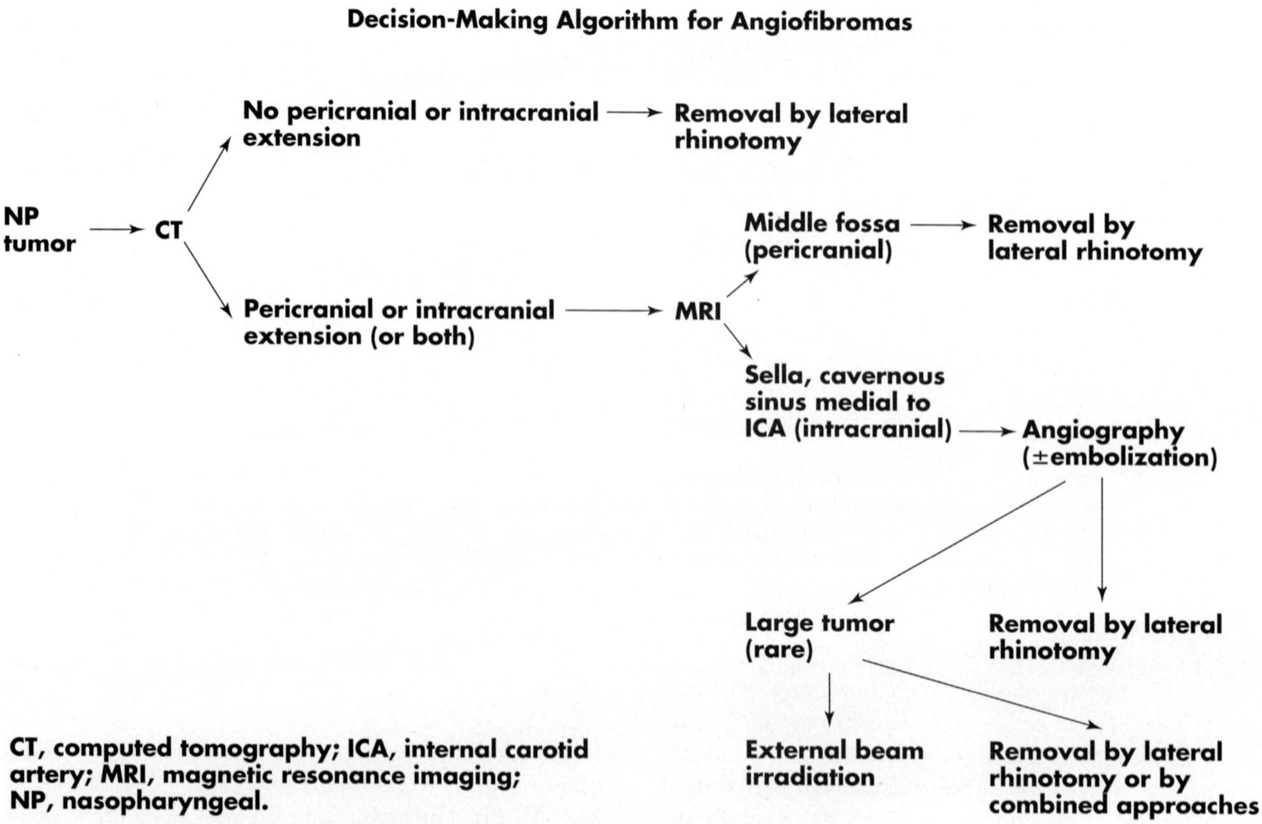

Fig. 26-1. Decision-making algorithm for angiofibromas.

Table 26-1. Symptoms and signs of angiofibroma in 150 patients, according to time of study

SYMPTOM OR SIGN	1972-1983 (N=30) NO. OF PATIENTS (%)	1945-1971 (N=120) NO. OF PATIENTS (%)
Epistaxis	26 (87)	84 (70)
Nasal obstruction	24 (80)	110 (92)
Nasal drainage	1 (3)	25 (21)
Facial deformity	4 (13)	23 (19)
Deafness, otitis	1 (3)	15 (13)
Bulging palate	1 (3)	12 (10)
Proptosis	4 (13)	10 (8)
Other*	6 (20)	24 (20)

* Other symptoms and signs, in one patient each, included breathing through the mouth, noisy sleeping, orbital pain, "allergy," "sinusitis," and female habitus.

For treatment planning, it is important to understand not only the point of origin of the tumor but also the pathways of extension. In a large surgical series the specific point of origin is documented to be at the posterolateral wall of the roof of the nose where the sphenoid process of the palatine bone meets the horizontal ala of the vomer and the root of the pterygoid process of the sphenoid bone (Fig. 26-2). This junction forms the superior margin of the sphenopalatine foramen, and the ethmoidal crest or attachment of the posterior end of the middle turbinate lies on or above the foramen. (This site is the approximate location of the attachment of the buccopharyngeal membrane in the embryo, which is the boundary between the stomodeal ectoderm and the foregut endoderm). From this point, the tumor may extend into the nose, nasopharynx,

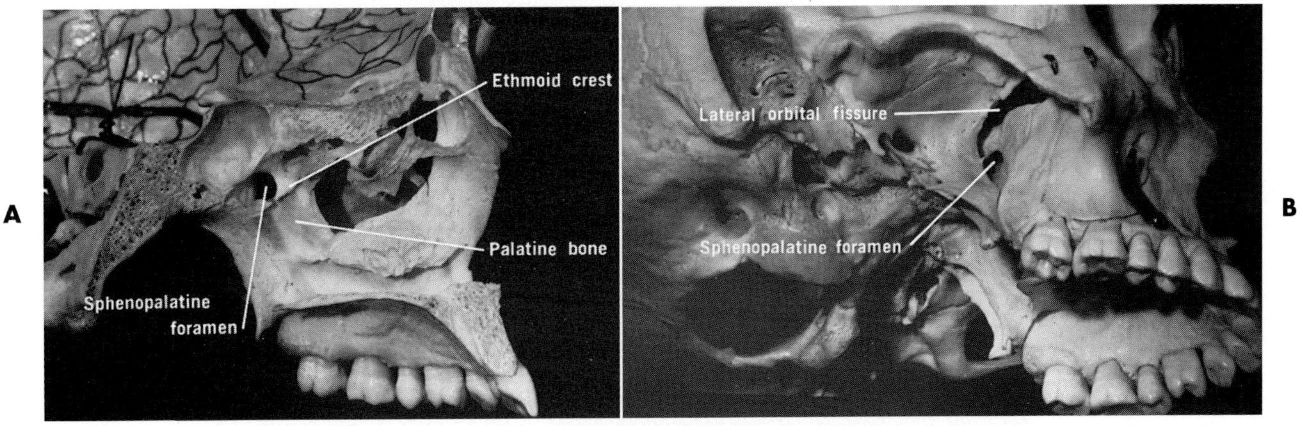

Fig. 26-2. A, The left nasal cavity shows the point of origin of the angiofibroma near the superior margin of the sphenopalatine foramen at the attachment of the posterior end of the middle turbinate. **B**, The right side of the skull shows infratemporal, temporal, and pterygomaxillary fossae and their relationships to the sphenopalatine foramen, pterygomaxillary fissure, and posterior wall of the maxillary antrum.

paranasal sinuses, temporal fossa, infratemporal fossa, and cranium. Because the tumor arises at or within the sphenopalatine foramen, the tumors are often characterized by a dumbbell appearance; the constriction at the sphenopalatine foramen and masses extends intranasally, with a secondary lobe extending laterally into the infratemporal fossa.

RADIOGRAPHIC EXAMINATION

The trend in the application of radiography for diagnosis has changed from plain sinus radiographs and sinus tomograms to computed tomographic (CT) scans and magnetic resonance imaging (MRI) of the head. CT is the preferred imaging modality for most tumors. Because of the high blood flow within the tumor, CT with contrast medium shows the enhancing lesion and clearly defines the bony architecture (Fig. 26-3). An enhancing nasal mass on the lateral nasal wall in an adolescent male can be considered diagnostic of an angiofibroma. Preoperative biopsy is contraindicated because of the risk of bleeding, and the characteristic appearance of angiofibroma on CT excludes essentially all other diagnostic possibilities. Because these tumors arise at or near the sphenopalatine foramen, the characteristic appearance of this lesion is bilobed with extension into the nose and into the infratemporal fossa, with a constriction at the sphenopalatine foramen (Fig. 26-4).

MRI may provide supplemental information if the CT appearance is not typical. On MRI, the large vascular channels within the angiofibroma show a typical "salt and pepper" appearance of flow voids within the tumor (Fig. 26-5). MRI also clearly demonstrates intracranial extension and is most useful for large tumors.

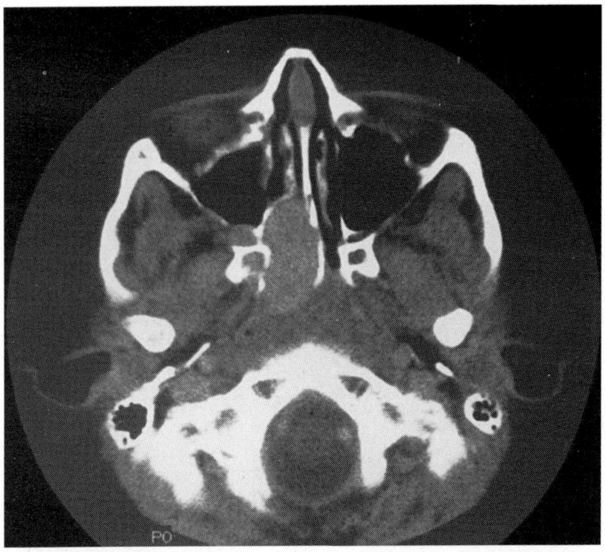

Fig. 26-3. Computed tomography (CT) demonstrates a nasopharyngeal angiofibroma in the typical location of the nasopharynx, with extension into the posterior nasal cavity. The lesion can be seen to be enhancing and centered on the sphenopalatine foramen. There was a small extension of the tumor into the infratemporal fossa through the sphenopalatine foramen and a bulging posterior wall of the antrum.

ANGIOGRAPHY

Because of the specificity and sensitivity of CT and MRI for angiofibromas, angiography is not usually necessary for the diagnosis of these lesions. However, angiography does provide information concerning the blood supply. The blood supply of the tumors is primarily from the sphenopalatine artery (Fig. 26-6), but as the tumors extend into the intratemporal fossa, blood supply from other sources may be acquired. Extension into the clivus

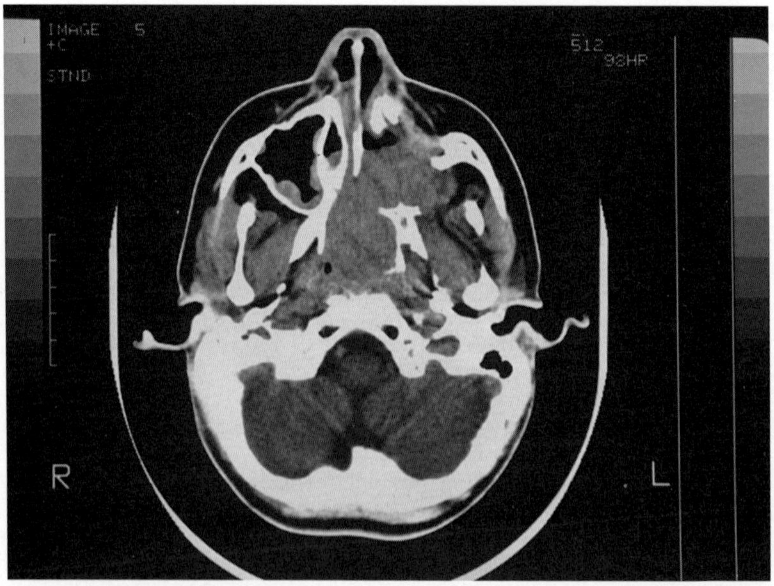

Fig. 26-4. Large nasopharyngeal angiofibroma with extension into the infratemporal fossa. There is a characteristic bilobed appearance with a constriction at the enlarged sphenopalatine foramen.

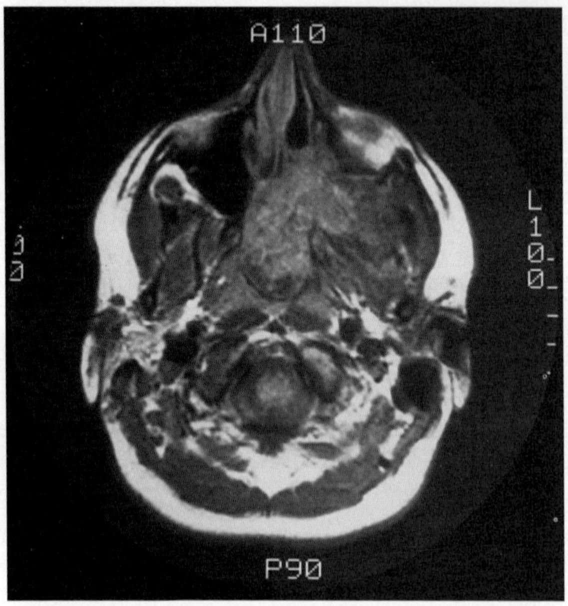

Fig. 26-5. Magnetic resonance imaging (MRI) demonstrates a bilobed nasopharyngeal angiofibroma. A "salt and pepper" appearance of the tumor is apparent. This is because the large vascular channels produce flow voids in the MRI scan.

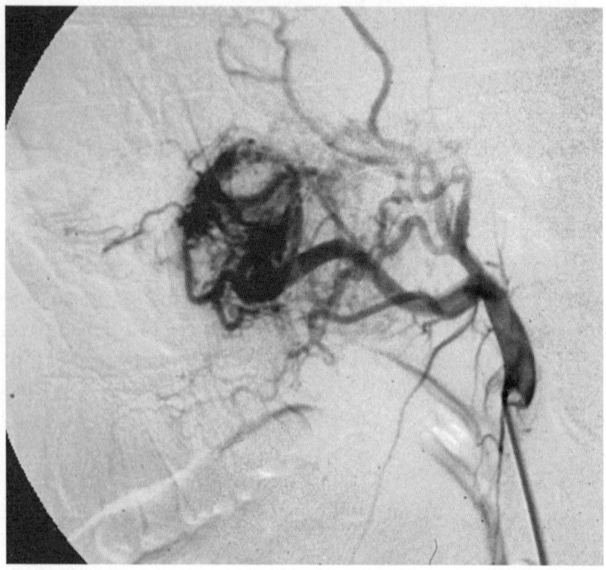

Fig. 26-6. Selective external carotid angiogram of a nasopharyngeal angiofibroma. The enlarged maxillary artery can be seen; the primary vascular supply is the sphenopalatine artery. Characteristic tumor enhancement of the angiofibroma is noted centered in the infratemporal fossa and nasopharynx.

and intracranial fossa results in blood supply arising from the internal carotid artery system. Knowledge of these vascular feeders aids in planning surgical excision of the tumor, because bleeding from the internal carotid system might not be easily controlled. In addition, angiography is necessary for planning embolization. At our institution, embolization is not used for all angiofibromas; however, large tumors and those with multiple feeding vessels may be embolized preoperatively to decrease operative blood loss.

LABORATORY EXAMINATION

Most patients are young males with good general health. Before operation a complete blood cell count and ABO/Rh typing are performed, because many of these patients require transfusions during surgery. They may make autologous blood donations, one unit every 7 to 14 days, to avoid the risk of bloodborne infectious diseases. Because the donated blood cells may be frozen, accumulation of 3 to 4 units is possible over several weeks before the operation.

TREATMENT

With an understanding of the point of origin of these tumors and after two major reviews of our outcomes, we believe that the lateral rhinotomy is the best approach to the tumor.[1-3] We rarely use radiation therapy. It should be clear that lateral rhinotomy is not an operation but rather an incision along the side of the nose. The incision can be extended down the center of the upper lip when lateral exposure is required beyond the infraorbital foramen (Fig. 26-7). This approach provides excellent surgical exposure of the tumor and its extension. An understanding of the several possible extensions may help the surgeon tailor the approach to the individual patient. As Neel and colleagues[3] noted in a detailed description of the surgical procedure, the tumor can be extracted from the pterygomaxillary fossa, infratemporal fossa, temporal fossa, sinuses, and middle fossa by pushing the tumor medially with packing. The middle fossa can also be approached through this incision. Most angiofibromas are *not* intracranial; rather, they are pericranial, having destroyed the bony floor of the middle cranial fossa. The tumor can be carefully removed from the middle fossa dura. Postoperatively, patients have healed well and cosmesis has been satisfactory, even in patients in whom the incision is used for reoperation.

Various other surgical approaches have been described: the facial degloving procedure and the combined intracranial and extracranial approaches. In most cases, facial degloving compromises exposure. A combined intracranial-extracranial approach has been necessary in only a few cases. The approach chosen may well depend on preoperative diagnostic studies and the surgeon's experience with a given technique. However, the lateral rhinotomy approach and its variations are the most direct routes to the body of the tumor and are versatile enough to reach all the extensions of the tumor. Other surgical approaches give limited, inadequate exposure.

The mean volume of blood replacement in our series was 1400 ml (range, 0 to 4000 ml). Comparison of our patient groups showed that little change has occurred in the requirement for blood transfusion since the mid-

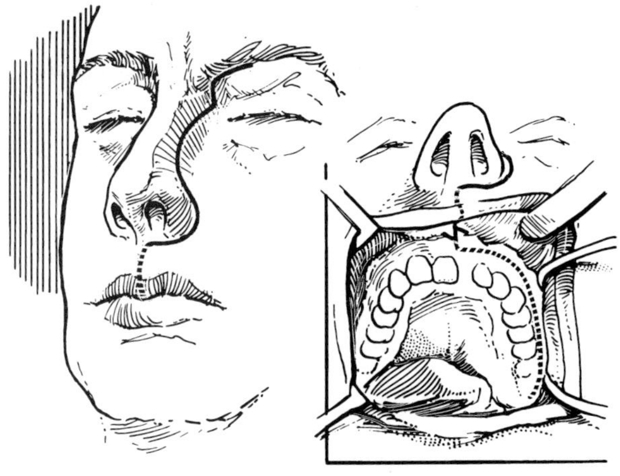

Fig. 26-7. Incision for the lateral rhinotomy approach, extending from the brow to the nasal ala along the lateral aspect of the nose. For cosmetic purposes it is not important to place the incision in the depths of the nasofacial groove. Additional exposure can be obtained by extensions through the midline of the upper lip and along the buccogingival sulcus. (From Bremer JW, Neel HB, DeSanto LW, Jones GC: Angiofibroma: treatment trends in 150 patients during 40 years, *Laryngoscope* 96:1325, 1986.)

1960s, and hypotensive anesthesia has not decreased the volume of blood transfusion.

Two techniques may decrease the need for blood replacement. One is the use of the "cell saver" at surgery. Our experience with this device has been somewhat limited, but it has been helpful in certain major head and neck cases. The other technique is intra-arterial embolization, which may decrease the vascularity of the angiofibroma.[4] Embolization has been used at our institution on a limited basis, usually in patients who have had epistaxis at some time after surgical resection, in whom no gross tumor is obvious at reexploration but a tumor blush is noted at angiography. It has been difficult to determine whether a decrease in intraoperative blood loss compared with previous experience was the result of preoperative embolization, careful surgical technique, or both. Gelfoam and other similar materials are absorbed. The development of vascular collaterals after embolization limits the effectiveness of this technique, so that it must be done during the perioperative period. We recognize that definite hazards are associated with embolization, especially in tumors supplied by the external and internal carotid arterial systems.

RESULTS

At the time we reported our most recent series of 29 patients treated with lateral rhinotomy, 27 were alive without disease and two were alive with known residual disease after lateral rhinotomy[1] (Table 26-2). None of the

Table 26-2. Outcome after lateral rhinotomy for angiofibroma in 86 patients, according to time of study

STATUS	1972-1983 (N=29) NO. OF PATIENTS (%)	1945-1971 (N=56) NO. OF PATIENTS (%)
Alive		
Without disease	27 (93)	45 (80)
With disease	2 (7)	5 (9)
Dead	0 (0)	5 (9)
Lost to follow-up	0 (0)	1 (2)
Total	29 (100)	56 (100)

Table 26-3. Tumor Stage (Sessions) and Recurrence, 1969-1984

STAGE	TUMORS NO. OF PATIENTS (%)	RECURRENCE NO. OF PATIENTS (%)
I	7 (17.5)	0 (0)
IIA	10 (25)	0 (0)
IIB	6 (15)	1 (17)
IIC	5 (12.5)	1 (20)
III	12 (30)	6 (50)

patients have died of their disease. In the previous surgical series of 56 patients who had lateral rhinotomies, 45 were alive without disease and five were alive with disease, and several of these patients seemed to have definite regression of small residual tumors.[3] Five patients died as a consequence of their disease, two during surgery and three postoperatively. All the postoperative deaths were in patients with extensive intracranial disease; two died of exsanguination at home, and one patient with tumor extension into the neck and trachea died of bronchopneumonia. The two surgical deaths were due to cardiac arrest, one of these presumably caused by hypovolemia.

The most common complication in the most recent series was nasal crusting (six patients). Other postoperative complications were nasolacrimal duct obstruction (four), hemorrhage requiring treatment (three), exotropia (one), mild proptosis (one), bifrontal headaches (one), facial asymmetry (one), and cheek numbness (one). None of the patients were dissatisfied with the appearance of the lateral rhinotomy incision. None had meningitis, diplopia, or cerebrospinal fluid leakage.

Various factors have contributed to the improved rates of surgical control reported in recent series: improved preoperative evaluation, better surgical supportive measures, various forms of adjunctive therapy, and a better understanding of the insidious nature of angiofibromas.

The natural history of this tumor, as determined by close follow-up after resection, indicates that regression of small residual tumors can occur. We have followed two patients with known residual tumor who have not required treatment and have shown no significant symptoms or signs of recurrence. In our earlier series, there were several such patients.

No clear relationship between the age of the patient and the clinical course has been observed.

DISCUSSION

Angiofibroma is a benign tumor that may impinge on several vital structures. It is usually highly vascular, and its natural history may lead to significant morbidity and mortality. The goal of treatment should be to relieve symptoms and not to totally remove every bit of tumor regardless of risk. Our usual indications for treatment are (1) hemorrhage, (2) nasal obstruction, and (3) orbital encroachment.

With extensive tumors, it is difficult to remove the tumor en bloc. However, adequate exposure and safe resection of these tumors, including the most extensive ones, can be achieved by variations of the lateral rhinotomy. All tumors, except those extending into the sella, can be removed this way. The proximity of the carotid artery to the sella precludes safe blunt dissection of tumor; however, extension through the sphenoid into the sella is rare. Almost all tumors are extradural and, if approached from below, can be safely dissected from dural attachments by progressive packing between dura and tumor, including the dura of the cavernous sinus.[2] Once the bulk of the tumor is removed and bleeding has ceased, tumor extensions are sought and removed from the sphenoid sinus.

Our overall recurrence rate of 20% for 40 tumors of all stages in a 15-year period is consistent with that reported in the literature for surgical management.[2] Our recurrence rate for tumors with intracranial extension was 50% (Table 26-3). There were no deaths.

The use of radiation as primary treatment is of much concern, especially in young patients, because thyroid carcinomas and radiation-induced sarcomas of bone and soft tissue are small but definite risks after radiation. Lifelong follow-up may be necessary. Radiation induces more profound local changes such as atrophic rhinitis and occasionally osteomyelitis or soft tissue necrosis. Radiation therapy may affect growth centers in the face, particularly in adolescents when rapid growth is occurring.

Currently, CT and MRI are used to establish the diagnosis, to define the extent of the tumor before biopsy, and to determine whether angiography is needed. In general, angiography and embolization have been used at our institution for the management of angiofibromas on a limited basis, usually in patients who have had epistaxis at some time after surgical resection.[4] We have had several patients with residual tumor who are asymptomatic; incomplete resection is not life threatening, and residual tumor can be treated expectantly.

REFERENCES

1. Bremer JW, Neel HB, DeSanto LW, Jones GC: Angiofibroma: treatment trends in 150 patients during 40 years, *Laryngoscope* 96:1321-1329, 1986.
2. Jones GC, DeSanto LW, Bremer JW, et al: Juvenile angiofibromas: behavior and treatment of extensive and residual tumors, *Arch Otolaryngol* 112:1191-1193, 1986.
3. Neel HB, Whicker JH, Devine KD, et al: Juvenile angiofibroma: review of 120 cases, *Am J Surg* 126:547-556, 1973.
4. Forbes G, Earnest F, Jackson IT, et al: Therapeutic embolization angiography for extra-axial lesions in the head, *Mayo Clin Proc* 61:427-441, 1986.

CHAPTER

27

Craniofacial Resection for Carcinoma of the Ethmoidal Sinus

Steven D. Schaefer
Raj Murali

PROBLEM

A 74-year-old man presents with a 4-month history of intermittent right nasal stuffiness and recent loss of vision in the right eye.

Neoplasms of the ethmoidal sinus and adjacent skull base have until recently been difficult to manage and almost uniformly fatal. After about 1980, various groups of otolaryngologists and neurosurgeons, in conjunction with other disciplines, began to form craniofacial teams to manage neoplasms that arose in either the visceral or neural cranium to involve the skull base. This chapter outlines through a case example the author's approach to one site which evolved over a period of 18 years.

MEDICAL HISTORY

Patients with neoplasms of the ethmoidal sinus and adjacent nasal vault often present with symptoms of epistaxis and nasal airway impairment. As the tumor enlarges, ophthalmic and neurologic symptoms become evident. As the dura is violated by the neoplasm and the frontal lobe infiltrated, the patient may exhibit loss of higher cognitive function to eventual altered consciousness.

In the present patient the history was rather benign until there was a rapid loss of vision over 1 month in the right eye. Immediately before the onset of the declining vision, the patient had been seen in an emergency room and diagnosed by computed tomography (CT) as having "severe sinusitis." Treatment then consisted of antibiotics. The patient was seen 10 days before his initial visit with us by another otolaryngologist who noted on nasal endoscopy an exophytic ulcerating mass in the right middle meatus. CT results were consistent with an ethmoidal neoplasm involving the skull base. The social history was of interest in that the patient was a professional carpenter and had a long history of woodworking.

PHYSICAL EXAMINATION

A complete head and neck, neurologic, and general examination should be performed. It is particularly valuable for both the otolaryngologist and neurosurgeon to be present during this examination to share observations and to plan subsequent treatment. Nasal endoscopy is employed to visualize the nasal component of the tumor, and for biopsy. Cranial nerve testing helps delineate the extent of the neoplasm, and particularly extraocular movement and visual abnormalities.

The present patient was a right-handed elderly man in no apparent distress. He was reasonably well oriented to person, place, and time. Recent and past memory were consistent with average intelligence and age. However, the patient was not aware that his right-sided vision was limited to light perception only. Pupillary reflexes were normal and extraocular movements appeared within normal range. Subsequent neuroophthalmologic consultation confirmed these findings. Sensory and motor testing of other cranial nerves was unremarkable. Nasal endoscopy showed an ulcerating mass replacing the ethmoidal bulla and the adjacent middle turbinate. Biopsy was performed intranasally of the nasal mass, revealing a histologic pattern and immunohistochemistry staining (S-100 and cytokeratin positivity) for a neuroendocrine neoplasm. These findings were most consistent with esthesioneuroblastoma.

RADIOGRAPHIC EXAMINATION

Imaging of tumors at the skull base should include both CT and magnetic resonance imaging (MRI). CT is necessary to delineate the hard tissue involvement of tumors, while MRI is superior for imaging brain and other soft tissue. MRI is also useful for differentiating opacification of a sinus on CT due to tumor from that secondary to obstruction of secretions. Such imaging should provide the location of the tumor, discern orbital involvement, and evaluate potential regional disease. Imaging of tumor location should include the extent of bony skull base destruction, extradural versus intradural tumor, and frontal lobe extension of tumor. Particular attention should be given to neoplasms that approximate the cavernous sinus, as invasion of this site may preclude successful surgical treatment. Such tumors may invade the dural sinus via anatomically weak points at the venous plexus around the superior orbital fissure, the medial wall around the pituitary body, and the dural pockets of the third and fifth cranial nerves.[1] Orbital evaluation should differentiate between tumor at or beyond the orbital septum, and identify extraocular muscle and optic nerve infiltration. As the ethmoidal and nasal cavity lymphatics drain to the retropharyngeal lymph nodes, imaging should include these regional sites along with the supraclavicular necks to rule out metastatic spread.

Magnetic resonance and helical CT angiography can provide noninvasive studies of tumor vascularity and blood supply. These forms of imaging continue to improve with developments in both hardware and software. For this reason, we now reserve invasive angiography for preoperative embolization of vascular tumors and/or assessment of collateral cerebral circulation. The latter has progressed from balloon occlusion of the internal carotid with clinical neurologic testing to selective vessel occlusion and measuring cerebral blood flow by single photon emission computed tomography (SPECT).[2] However, no form of preoperative assessment of cerebral circulation is 100% accurate, and a few patients experience postoperative strokes despite their presumed patent circle of Willis on angiography.

In the patient presented, CT showed an enhancing mass presumably arising from the right ethmoidal sinus extending into the anterior cranial fossa floor. The right orbital plate (lamina papyracea) was partially eroded, as was the entire roof of the right ethmoidal sinus and medial left ethmoidal sinus. MRI confirmed the CT findings and extension of tumor to both optic foramina. The right optic nerve was surrounded by tumor, and the left nerve was encroached medially by tumor. Neither optic nerve was obviously invaded by tumor. The dura was thickened and presumably invaded by tumor. There was questionable tumor in the subarachnoid space and frontal lobe. There was no penetration of tumor beyond the periorbita, or orbit proper. The inferior extent of the tumor was just superior to the right anterior lacrimal crest. The right maxillary sinus appeared opacified on CT, while MRI showed this opacification to be due to retained secretions (Fig. 27-1). On T2-weighted images the tumor was hypointense, and this finding was suggestive of a hypercellular matrix (Fig. 27-2). Differential diagnosis included esthesioneuroblastoma, lymphoma, and squamous cell carcinoma.

TREATMENT

Indications

Until the mid-1970s, treatment of ethmoid sinusal carcinomas involving the skull base was directed toward palliation. Such treatment primarily consisted of external beam radiation. As otolaryngologists and neurosurgeons began to approach such neoplasms jointly, the principles of surgical resectability were refined. These principles include (1) preservation of one functioning eye; (2) maintenance of the central nervous system's vascularity through collateral blood flow, preservation of vessels where collateral circulation is absent, or vascular bypass; (3) complete removal of neoplasms; (4) subtotal removal of benign tumors when total resection compromises life; (5) watertight closure of the dura to prevent cerebrospinal fluid (CSF) rhinorrhea and meningitis; and (6) returning a viable patient to as near a pre-disease state as possible. Radiation therapy is frequently administered to help control both local and regional disease. Postoperative radiation therapy is preferable to preoperative in order to reduce the likelihood of fistula formation and infection after surgery.[3] Adjuvant radiation and chemo-therapy in the treatmentof skull base malignancies is under investigation, with its role yet to be defined.[4]

Surgical technique

A combination of approaches can be used to resect tumors involving the ethmoidal sinus or superior nose and anterior cranial fossa floor. These approaches often combine a transfacial route with a frontal craniotomy. Such routes include lateral rhinotomy or an extension of the rhinotomy to permit direct visualization to the anterior cranial fossa floor. An alternative approach is to confine the procedure to the transcranial route and to avoid or minimize the use of facial incisions. This latter approach is attractive to the patient because it minimizes the po-

A

B

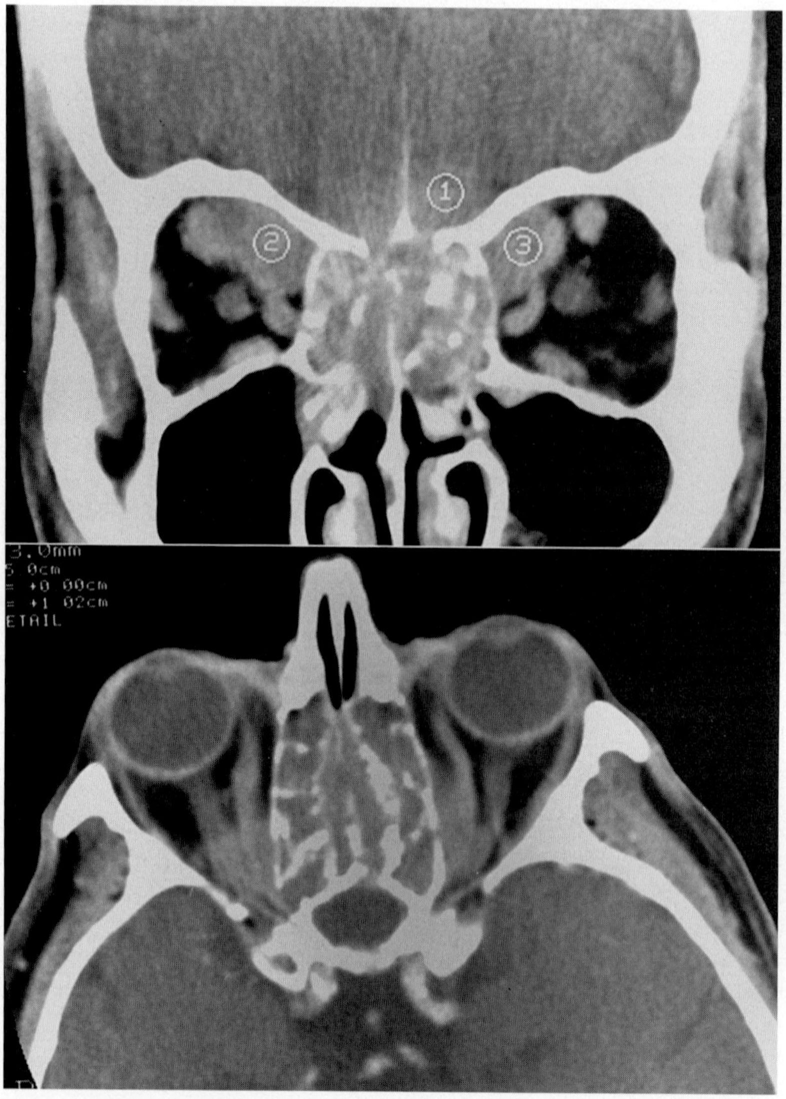

Fig. 27-1. **A,** Coronal and axial **B,** contrast computed tomography (CT) of the patient presented in this chapter before beginning radiation therapy. Note the erosion of the skull base and extension of tumor into the posterior orbit.

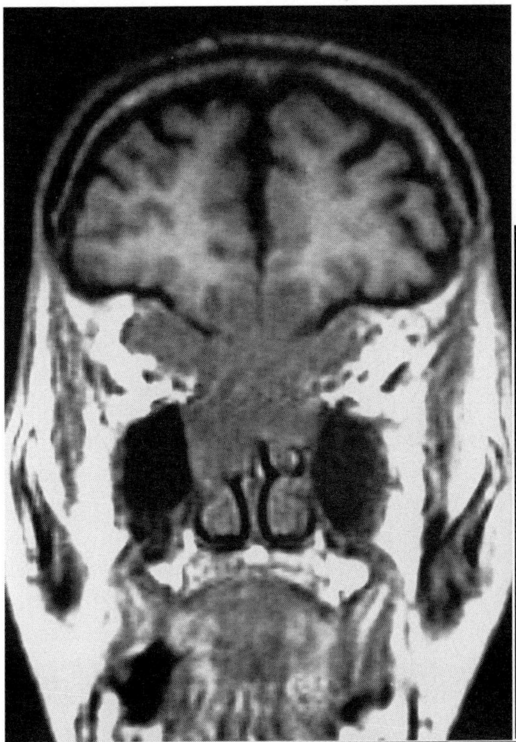

A

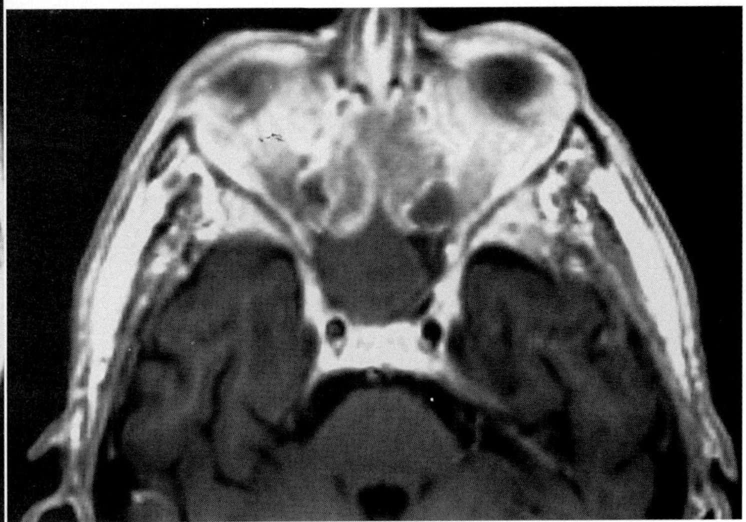

B

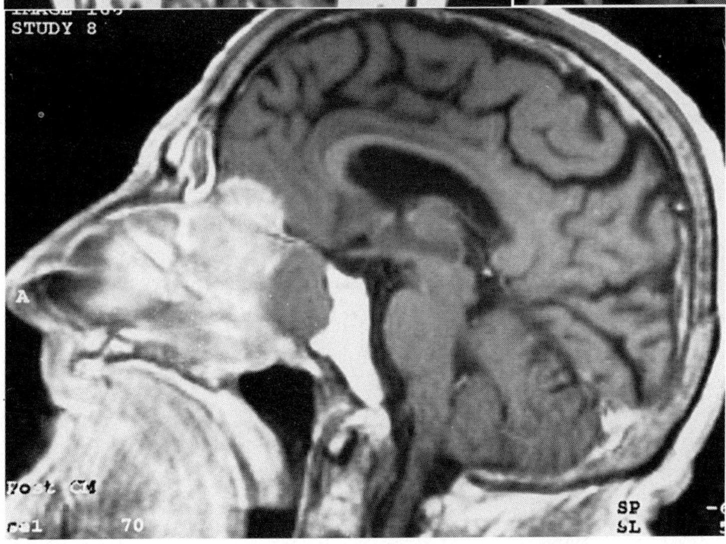

C

Fig. 27-2. **A,** Coronal axial **B,** and sagittal **C,** magnetic resonance imaging (MRI) of the patient in Fig. 27-1 before the beginning of treatment. Images show significant anterior cranial fossa dural thickening and enhancement, and extension of tumor to the optic canals.

tential cosmetic deformity after such surgery, but it can compromise the removal of the tumor. We have sought to refine this latter approach, as discussed later.

Resection of tumors begins with placement of a lumbar drain in the subarachnoid space. A closed drainage system is constructed using a commercially available epidural anesthesia kit. The drain is placed at the L3–L4 interspace using a 16-gauge Tuohy needle. The lumbar drain can exit the skin over the vertebrate or be tunneled to the midaxillary line. We prefer the latter because in our experience the drain is much less likely to become infected and more likely to function over several days. After intravenous administration of 80 mg gentamicin, 1 g vancomycin, and 100 mg phenytoin, a coronal incision is made and an inferiorly based flap elevated superficial to the galea. The galea-pericranium is incised posterior to the plane of the coronal incision and is separated inferiorly from the bone to beyond the supraorbital rim with careful preservation of the inferior blood supply. A bone flap is cut from immediately superior to the orbital rims inferiorly to 2 fingerbreadths anterior to the coronal suture line. After the bone flap is removed, the spinal drain is opened and the brain allowed to relax posteriorly. The dura is opened at the most anterior part of the sagittal sinus, and the falx is divided. Hemostasis is obtained and the anterior cranial fossa floor inspected. If the dura is involved with tumor, it is left in continuity with the tumor and a 1-cm margin of dura is included in the resection. If the orbit is not obviously involved with tumor, it is elevated from the anterior cranial fossa floor. The lateral margin of the resection is defined by identifying the lamina papyracea. This is performed by removing the medial orbital roof and creating a plane between the periorbita and lamina papyracea inferiorly to the orbital floor. If the periorbita appears to be invaded by tumor, a plane is developed between this membrane and the orbital contents. The use of this exposure of the medial orbit and further degloving of the midface by elevation of the coronal flap onto the nose and medial orbit permits complete resection of most neoplasms. The medial wall of the maxillary sinus can also be encompassed in the resection by degloving the face of the maxillae and lateral nose via a modified Caldwell-Luc technique. Once all margins of the tumor have been defined, the tumor is removed by performing anterior cranial fossa floor ostiotomies at the margins of the tumor resection. Additional osteotomies are then made as needed to complete the resection of the tumor. The dura is carefully reconstituted using pericranium (more correctly described as a galeopericranial flap), using great care to obtain a watertight seal. Particular care is taken to close the dura along the planum sphenoidale, which is the most dependent part of the closure and the most likely to fistualize. The vascularized pericranium is used as the second layer of the reconstruction of the anterior cranial fossa floor.[5,6] Autologous fibrin glue is used to fixate the pericranium to the skull base. As this flap is extended more posteriorly, the blood supply becomes more tenuous because the supraorbital and supratrochlear vessels are axial only in the proximal 20 to 70 mm of the flap.[7] For this reason, we utilize free flaps for massive reconstructions, especially in the presence of large soft tissue defects that create a large dead space. The procedure is completed with replacement of the frontal bone flap, drainage of the wound, and closure of the skin.

In the patient under discussion, initial treatment consisted of hyperfractionated radiation therapy rather than surgical resection. This was based on the combination of loss of vision in one eye and impending loss in the other, and possible invasion of the frontal lobe. Radiation therapy was begun within 2 days of the patient's first visit, and at 3000 Gy there was an improvement in vision in the right eye to finger counting. At 5000 Gy vision had stabilized, and MRI showed tumor confined to the ethmoidal sinuses and adjacent dura (Fig. 27-3). At this point the clinical impression was that the patient had had the maximal benefits of radiation therapy, and that the residual tumor was now resectable or otherwise would be fatal to the patient. Therefore, a bifrontal craniotomy was performed. A lumbar drain was used to permit removal of CSF, as discussed above. An en bloc resection encompassed lamina papyracea, ethmoidal sinuses, anterior cranial fossa floor and dura, nasal septum, anterior sphenoid bone, and posterior table of the frontal sinus. Both optic nerves were intracranially decompressed from their foramina into the orbit (Fig. 27-4). The inferior aspect of the resection was performed by a combination of an intracranial and degloving approach to the midface via the craniotomy flap. After complete removal of the tumor, the floor of the anterior cranial fossa was reconstructed using a pericranial graft to replace the resected dura and a pericranial flap. Immediately postoperatively the patient was moderately disoriented, which is frequently noted after such surgery and in the aged. Otherwise, he made an uneventful recovery. He has remained well and without recurrent tumor for the past 2 years (Fig. 27-5).

DISCUSSION

The evolution of craniofacial surgery for treatment of carcinomas and sarcomas has been well reviewed by O'Malley and Janecka,[8] who divide such treatment into three periods over a period of 40 years. The first period (1960–1970s) saw surgical treatment outcomes of approximately 50% for 5 years in neoplasms without intracranial or pterygopalatine extension. As surgical techniques improved in the 1970s to 1980s, more advanced tumors were also treated, with an overall slight increase in survival rates. In the last period (1980–1990s) the combi-

A

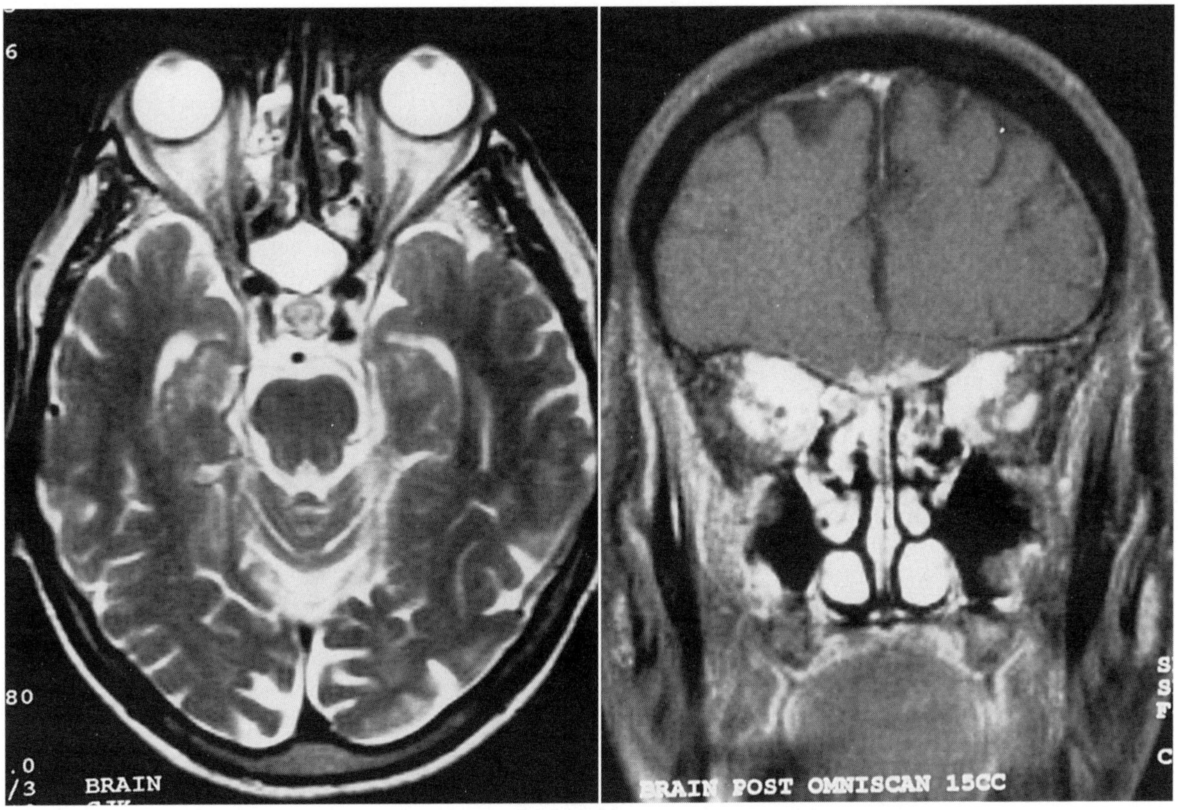

B

Fig. 27-3. Axial **A,** and coronal **B,** contrast MRI after completion of radiation therapy.

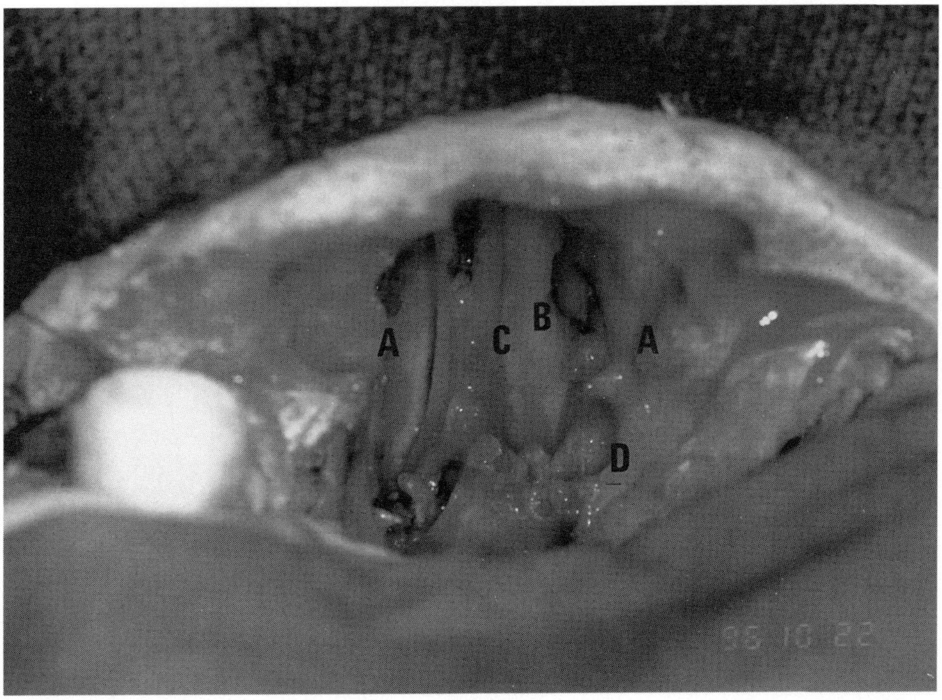

Fig. 27-4. Intraoperative photograph showing surgical defect from craniotomy exposure. This exposure permitted complete removal of the tumor, with preservation of the medial orbit *(A)*, visualization of the inferior nose to the level of the inferior turbinate *(B)* and inferior septum *(C)*, and decompression of the optic nerves *(D)*.

A

B

C

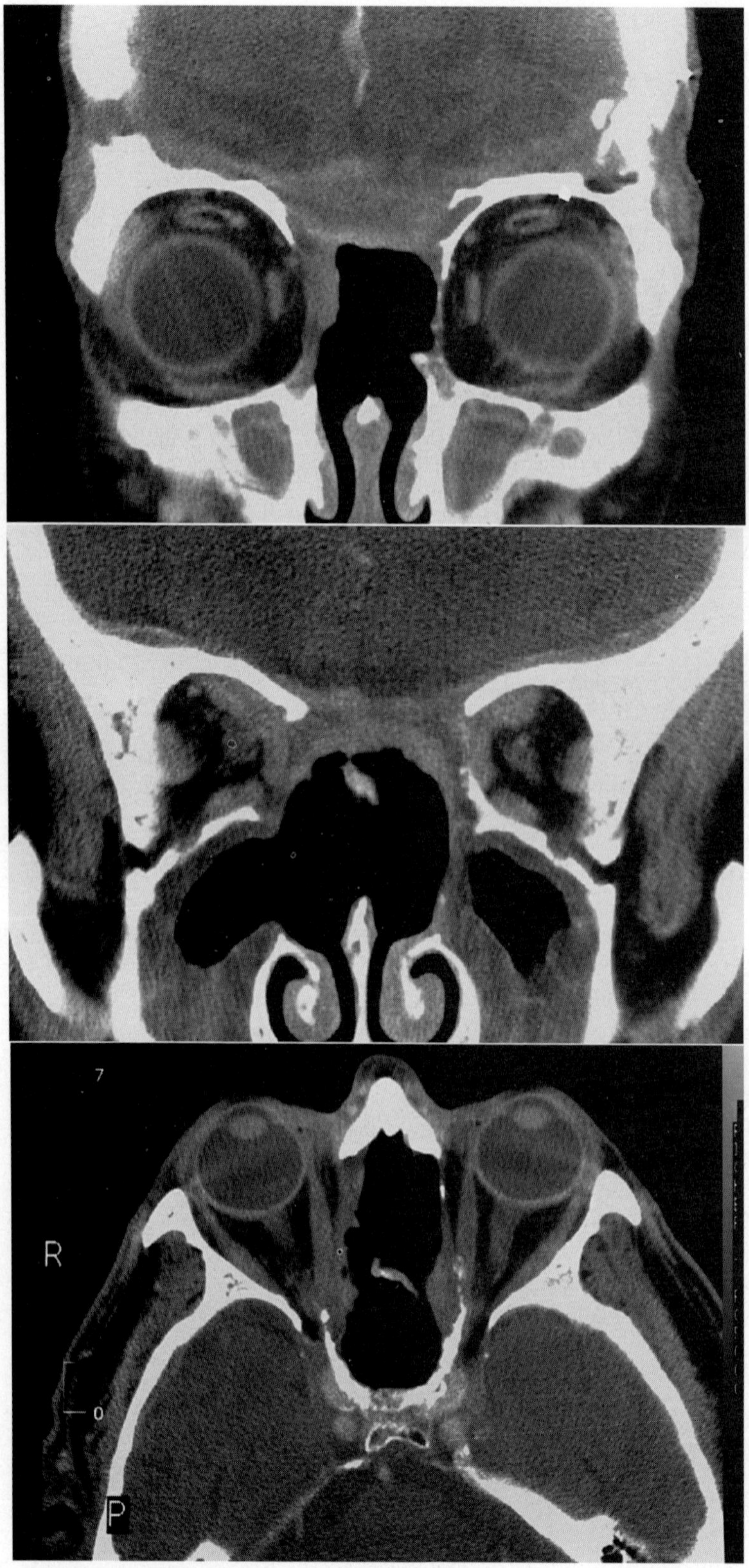

Fig. 27-5. Contrast CT 6 months after surgery. **A** and **B** show in the coronal projection the extent of removal of the skull base, ethmoidal sinuses, and lamina papyracea. The anterior cranial fossa floor has been reconstructed using vascularized pericranium or a galeopericranial flap. **C**, An axial scan performed at the same time as those in **A** and **B** also illustrates the surgical defect. Such scans are routinely obtained postoperatively to follow the patients. Thickening of the reconstructed dura or other changes in such scans are highly suggestive of recurrent tumor.

nation of improved diagnostic techniques and invasive angiography, coupled with cooperation between surgical and other specialties, increased 5-year survival rates to 56% to 70%. Although this chapter is limited to the treatment of ethmoidal sinus and adjacent nasal cavity neoplasms, the following broad discussion of the evaluation and treatment of such tumors may be useful.

General principles of craniofacial resection of ethmoidal sinus neoplasms

Early recognition of nasal-sinus lesions. Improving survival is a function of both early recognition of sinus neoplasms and accurate diagnosis of disease. Such recognition depends on patients seeking medical care for such seemingly benign complaints as epistaxis or nasal obstruction. The physician must have the skills and equipment to evaluate all such patients carefully. This is implicit in the training of surgical specialists but may be problematic for the primary care physician. The ability to evaluate the nasal cavity and sinuses has been greatly enhanced by the fiberoptic endoscope. Using such instruments, and after applying vasoconstrictive and anesthetic agents, the physician should be able to visualize most of the nose as a routine office procedure. Masses or areas of ulceration should be routinely biopsied, and examined by pathologists familiar with nasal and sinus tumors. If the physician cannot find a reason for the patient's condition, additional consultation and follow-up examination are recommended. Radiographic investigations should follow an abnormal physical examination result. However, an unremarkable physical examination in the face of persistent unexplained symptoms should also be followed by a radiographic examination. Such a screening examination should consist of contrast CT or MRI of the paranasal sinuses, adjacent anterior cranial fossa floor, and orbits. As discussed, the complete evaluation of cranial base tumors requires both CT and MRI to discern the extent of tumor, intracranial and orbital invasion, and tumor and cerebral vascularity. Such imaging has improved to the extent that one MRI report notes an accuracy of 100% in predicting dural invasion with the combined findings of dural and pilial enhancement.[9] Dural thickening alone greater than 5 mm was found to be highly sensitive and accurate for tumor invasion. Simple linear enhancement of the dura did not correlate with tumor invasion, while venous sinus and perineural invasion was well predicted by imaging.

An initial biopsy of the nasal-sinus lesion before definitive surgical treatment. A transnasal biopsy of the lesion is always recommended to determine the exact pathology of the lesion before planning the definitive surgical treatment. For example, if the tumor is a lymphoma, craniofacial resection is unnecessary and the patient can be appropriately treated with radiation therapy. The initial biopsy will also help determine the vascularity of the tumor and the need for preoperative angiography and possible embolization. Certain tumors in this region, such as malignant melanoma, carry such a dismal prognosis that craniofacial surgery may not be indicated.

One-stage combined craniofacial resection between an otolaryngologist and neurosurgeon. Treatment follows delineation of the extent of the tumor. Our preference is to employ surgery followed by radiation in the treatment of sinus neoplasms. We consider the use of both treatment modalities to be important because of (1) potential local recurrence after surgery alone and (2) regional spread of tumor to parapharyngeal and cervical lymphatics. These observations have been investigated by others and suggest a definite role for aggressive postoperative radiotherapy.[10] Paulino and colleagues evaluated 22 patients after surgery and radiation for various skull base malignancies. They found tumor recurrence outside the operative field in 13% of those undergoing wide-field radiation, in contrast to 57% with partial-field radiation.[11] We also believe postoperative radiation to be preferable because fistulization after surgery is less likely before radiotherapy. However, as illustrated in this chapter, the initial surgical removal of the tumor can so threaten the patient's quality of life that the routine management protocol must be altered.

The choice of surgical approach is determined by the site and extent of the neoplasm and the experience of the surgical team. We believe that the approach must satisfy the need to completely and safely remove the tumor, while addressing the patient's concern for minimal invasiveness. This concept is illustrated in the patient presented in this chapter in whom the primary removal of the tumor is performed through the exposure provided by the craniotomy. This approach depends on defining the medial orbital wall via the superior orbit, carrying the orbital dissection from the craniotomy to the inferomedial orbit, and degloving the superior nose and medial canthal region.[12] Further exposure of orbital floor, maxillary sinus, and nasal cavity is gained via the facial degloving approach utilized for medial maxillectomy.

Once the treatment plan is formulated between an otolaryngologist and a neurosurgeon, the recommendations are jointly presented to the patient with the help of scans and appropriate anatomic models. Depending on the extent and type of tumor, a decision is made whether the entire procedure can be performed transcranially or whether a separate facial incision is required.

Skull base reconstruction. After the tumor is excised, the defect in the skull base is reconstructed by the neurosurgeon and otolaryngologist to prevent various complications such as CSF fistula and intracranial infection. The role of CSF aspiration through a lumbar subarachnoid catheter has already been discussed.

Postoperative care. Patients requiring craniofacial surgery should be carefully monitored in an intensive care unit after such procedures. This is best performed in a neurosurgical unit. It is our usual policy to leave these patients intubated and on a respirator for at least 24 hours after surgery. Immediately after completion of the procedure a CT scan of the head is obtained to assess the amount of pneumocephalus that is invariably present in such patients. Unless there is excessive air with evidence of mass effect on the brain, no treatment is necessary. Only small amounts of CSF are removed from the lumbar drain to prevent excessive pneumocephalus and chronic herniation syndromes. The chronic herniation syndrome is characterized by profound lethargy and sometimes third nerve palsy. CT of the head in these patients shows dramatic lack of CSF in the head characterized by small ventricles, absence of basal cisterns, a collapsed brain, and pneumocephalus. The management of this condition consists of closing the lumbar drain, keeping the head flat, and slowly allowing the brain to reexpand. During this period, fluid and electrolyte balance must be carefully managed to avoid hyponatremia.

Pathology of anterior fossa skull base tumors

A variety of neoplasms involving the anterior skull base primarily arise from the sinuses and nasal cavity. In our experience of 65 patients with such tumors over a 10-year period, the most common tumor was esthesioneuroblastoma. This neoplasm arises from the olfactory epthelium and is a neuroendocrine tumor. These tumors are both locally invasive and can metastasize to the regional lymphatics. The second most frequent tumors we have treated are squamous cell carcinomas arising from the ethmoidal sinus. Others report different frequencies of neoplasms in this region. However, all agree that other tumors involving the anterior skull base include lymphomas, adenoid cystic carcinomas, inverting papillomas, angiofibromas, meningiomas, and metastatic tumors.

Complications of craniofacial surgery

As craniofacial resection of tumors of the anterior skull base is complex and time consuming, many complications can occur if meticulous attention to detail is not given. The incidence of complications is dictated by such factors as patient age and condition, nature and extent of tumor, and preoperative radiation therapy. Such complications include (1) pneumocephalus; (2) chronic herniation syndrome; (3) intracranial infections such as meningitis, cerebritis, cerebral abscess formation, wound infection, bone flap infection, and osteomyelitis; (4) additional neurologic deficits such as anosmia and visual disturbances; (5) CSF rhinorrhea necessitating further surgery; (6) radiation-induced skin necrosis, bone flap infections, and wound dehiscence; and (7) rapid recurrence of highly malignant tumors and leptominingeal tumor spread.

Despite all the difficulties and concerns regarding the management of skull base tumors, we have come to believe that the intelligent application of such therapy offers many patients the potential for cure. Surgeons have the responsibility to present the treatment options, problems, and likely outcome honestly to the patient. They can then best work together to plan treatment.

REFERENCES

1. Kawase T, van Loveren H, Keller JT, Tew JM: Meningeal architecture of the cavernous sinus: clinical and surgical implications, *Neurosurgery* 39:527-534, 1996.
2. Nayak UK, Donald PJ, Stevens D: Internal carotid artery resection for invasion of malignant tumors, *Arch Otolaryngol Head Neck Surg* 121:1029-1033, 1995.
3. De Santos LR, Cernea CR, Brandao LG, et al: Results and prognostic factors in skull base surgery, *Am J Surg* 168:481-484, 1994.
4. Schuller DE, Goodman JH, Mountain RE, et al: Adjunctive treatment of cranial malignancies, *J Craniofac Surg* 6:69-74, 1995.
5. Schaefer SD, Close LG, Mickey B: Axial subcutaneous flaps in the reconstruction of the anterior cranial fossa floor, *Arch Otolaryngol* 112:745-749, 1986.
6. Terashi H, Yoshida T, Katayama S, et al: Wide reconstruction of the anterior cranial base with bipedicled galeopericranial flap, *Head Neck* 18:292-294, 1996.
7. Potparic Z, Fukuta K, Colen LB, et al: Galeo-pericranial flaps in the forehead: a study of blood supply and volumes, *Br J Plast Surg* 49:519-528, 1996.
8. O'Malley BW, Janecka IP: Evolution of outcomes in cranial base surgery, *Semin Surg Oncol* 11:221-227, 1995.
9. Eisen MD, Yousem DM, Montone KT, Kotapka MJ: Use of preoperative MR to predict dural, perineural and venous invasion of skull base tumors, *Am J Neuroradiol* 17:1937-1945, 1996.
10. Irish J, Dasgupta R, Freeman J, et al: Outcome analysis of the surgical management of esthesioneuroblastoma, *J Otolaryngol* 26:1-7, 1997.
11. Paulino AC, Marks JE, Leonetti JP: Postoperative irradiation of patients with malignant tumors of skull base, *Laryngoscope* 106:880-883, 1996.
12. Hirano A, Arakaki M, Nishida H, et al: Hemifacial degloving approach to tumors in the infratemporal and pterygopalatine fossae, *J Craniomaxillofac Surg* 24:285-288, 1996.

CHAPTER

28

Surgical Management of Recurrent Nasopharyngeal Carcinoma

Willard E. Fee, Jr.

PROBLEM

A 55-year-old Chinese-American woman presents 11 months after completion of radiation therapy with a recurrence in the nasopharynx.

MEDICAL HISTORY

In June 1994 this patient presented with a 2-year history of rhinitis and clear mucous discharge. Physical examination demonstrated a lesion on the left lateral and posterior wall of the nasopharynx that extended into the left nasal cavity. Excisional biopsy of the mass showed poorly differentiated nasopharyngeal carcinoma. Computed tomography (CT) and magnetic resonance imaging (MRI) showed the disease to be limited to the nose and nasopharynx without skull base erosion. Therefore, the tumor was staged as a T3N0M0 carcinoma. The patient was subsequently treated with 7000 cGy via 33 fractionations with 6 MeV photons over 51 days to the primary site and 5400 cGy via 30 fractionations over 41 days to the necks. All the radiation was completed by the end of October 1994 and the patient was judged to have had a complete response. By July 1995 there was a fungating 1-cm lesion filling the left fossa of Rosenmüller that on biopsy proved to be poorly differentiated carcinoma.

The patient was born in Minneapolis and, although her family was of Cantonese-speaking descent, she had no history of salted fish use. She received an MBA from Columbia University and worked on Wall Street as a financial analyst. There were no industrial exposures to chemicals of any kind. There was a positive family history of colon carcinoma and a possible history of nasopharyngeal carcinoma in a grandfather. The remainder of her history was essentially negative.

PHYSICAL EXAMINATION

Physical examination revealed blood pressure of 104/70, pulse rate 80 and regular, respiratory rate 12, temperature 96.8, and weight 42.5 kg. The head and neck examination was entirely normal with the exception of a fungating, 1-cm lesion filling and emanating from the left fossa of Rosenmüller. The neck examination was negative, and cranial nerves II to XII were intact.

RADIOGRAPHIC EXAMINATION

MRI with and without gadolinium and fat suppression is the scan of choice. The most helpful views are those in the axial and coronal projections with particular attention paid to the paranasopharyngeal space, internal carotid artery, and cavernous sinus. Representative images in Figs. 28-1 and 28-2 demonstrate tumor filling the left fossa of Rosenmüller without extension to the internal carotid or paranasopharyngeal space.

LABORATORY EXAMINATION

A complete blood count (CBC) was normal. A general chemical survey was entirely within normal limits except for a serum creatinine level of 0.6 mg/dl (normal, 0.7 to 1.5). Specifically, alkaline phosphatase, ALT, AST, and LDH were within normal limits. Epstein-Barr virus

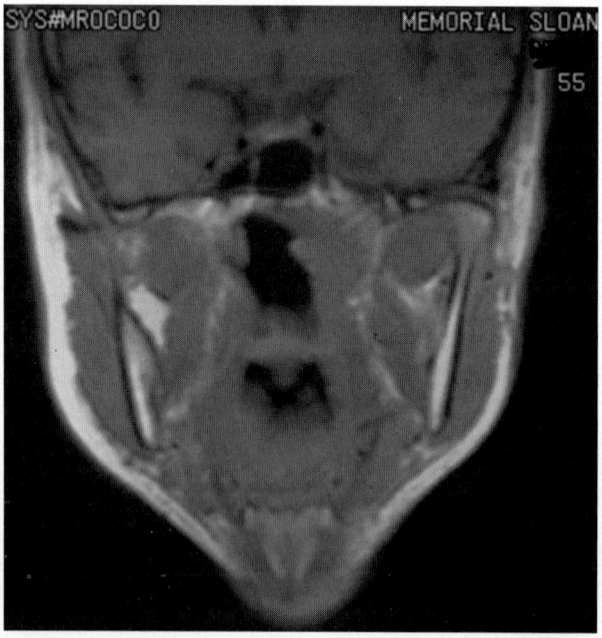

Fig. 28-1. T1-weighted coronal magnetic resonance imaging (MRI) showing a 2.3 × 2.3 cm tumor pushing the superior constrictor muscle laterally, but not invading beyond it into the paranasopharyngeal space. This view is particularly useful for demonstrating invasion through the petroclinoid fissure into the cavernous sinus.

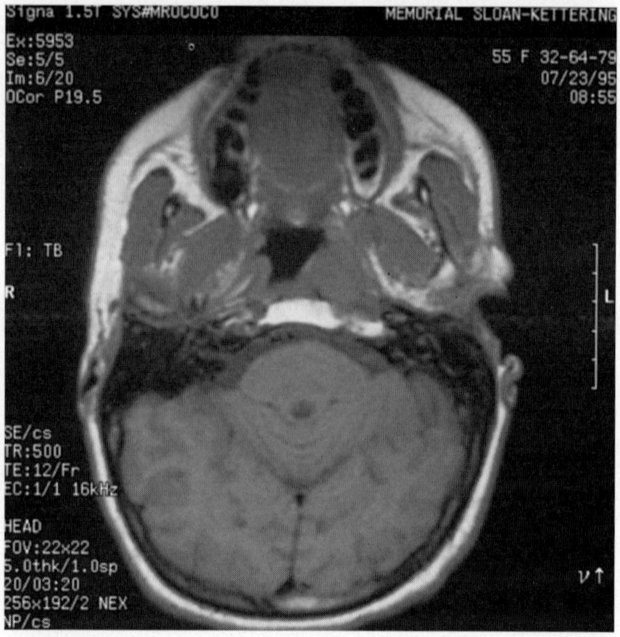

Fig. 28-2. T1-weighted axial image showing a 2.3 × 2.3 cm lesion involving the left eustachian tube without invasion into the paranasopharyngeal space. The tumor is medial to the internal carotid artery. This view particularly well demonstrates whether tumor extension is posterior or lateral to the internal carotid, both are particularly unfavorable for surgical resection. It is also the best view for determining invasion of the clivis, sphenoid sinus, and cervical vertebrae.

(EBV) antibody titers showed an IgA viral capsid antibody of 20 (normal, <10), while an IgA early antibody (diffuse) was 5 (normal, <10). EBV nuclear antibody was 1280. The IgA viral capsid antigen was positive for nasopharyngeal carcinoma. Elevated IgA antibodies to EBV are more common in Asia than in North America and can be occasionally helpful in the management of patients with nasopharyngeal carcinoma. They are most helpful in the evaluation of patients who present with poorly differentiated carcinoma of the neck from an unknown primary origin. When the EBV titers are positive in this scenario, more extensive evaluation of the nasopharynx is warranted because of the likelihood of submucosal nasopharyngeal carcinoma; that is, multiple biopsies should be taken submucosally. In many patients with initially elevated titers the titers fall to normal after successful therapy. Not everyone has this response, and thus the true value of following titers may be questioned.

However, when elevated titers fall after therapy is completed and then rise again, this often heralds a recurrence. Although titers are still checked when the patient is first seen, the value of follow-up titers remains to be determined by a prospective outcome study.

CT of the chest is indicated for any suspicious lesions seen on standard chest x-ray films. CT of the abdomen to look for liver metastases is indicated whenever liver function tests show elevated results. Bone scans are indicated for any undiagnosed bone pain and should be followed up with plain films and biopsy of suspicious lesions. A bone marrow aspirate is indicated when there are unexplained abnormalities on CBC.

Remember that this disease, unlike most other head and neck neoplasms, can present with widespread distant metastases at onset.

TREATMENT

The treatment of primary nasopharyngeal carcinoma is by external beam radiation therapy with or without chemotherapy. Most studies in the past have failed to demonstrate an advantage from chemotherapy, but a 1996 prospective, randomized trial suggests a beneficial role for platinum and 5-fluorouracil with radiation therapy.[1] Both necks should be treated because of the high incidence of neck disease bilaterally.

Treatment of recurrences in the neck when the primary tumor is controlled should consist of standard radical neck dissection. According to Wei and colleagues,[2] no attempts should be made to spare cranial nerve XI.

Treatment of recurrences at the primary site was traditionally repeat radiation. All authors agreed that the second treatment dose must be at least 60 cGy, with success rates of 14.8% to 48% reported,[3-5] but the often-quoted series of Fu and colleagues[6] demonstrating a 48% 3-year survival rate, when analyzed closely, showed that only five of 33 of survivors (15%) were free of disease. Thus, it appears mandatory that all survival results be reported as disease-free survival in order to give a true picture of the efficacy of treatment.

In 1984 I performed my first nasopharyngectomy with a neck dissection for recurrent disease following 66 cGy radiation. Fortunately, the case went well and the patient was still living 13 years after surgery. To date, a total of 41 nasopharyngectomies have been performed, two of which were palliative owing to tumor extending into the spinal canal that was judged unresectable. One of the patients who underwent palliation had 6 weeks' relief of pain, but she developed a cranial nerve X and XII paralysis postoperatively even though the nerves were anatomically left intact. This patient had difficulty with aspiration postoperatively and the palliative effort is judged to have been a failure. The second patient given palliative treatment lived for 6 years, 8 months after the procedure and had exceptionally good relief of pain, upper airway obstruction, and nasopharyngeal bleeding. Interestingly enough, she died of central nervous system extension and spinal cord disease, while indenting and showing displacement of the spinal cord never caused any long tract symptoms or signs. Three patients who were believed to have poorly differentiated carcinoma proved on final examination of the pathologic specimen to have high-grade mucoepidermoid carcinomas; two of the three were living free of disease at 2 and $2\frac{1}{2}$ years, but one died free of disease 4 months postoperatively from either an accidental or intentional overdose of narcotics.

The results of therapy for 39 patients treated for cure are shown in Table 28-1.

My own technique of nasopharyngectomy consists of a transpalatal, transmaxillary (through the medial wall and posterior wall of the maxillary sinus), and transcervical approach. The latter approach is used to isolate the internal carotid artery by placing a 1×7 cm cottonoid pledget medial to the carotid artery; the transcervical approach is also used to resect any lateral nasopharyngeal nodes that may be evident on scan. The transpalatal approach, while cumbersome, provides direct access to the nasopharynx and is particularly good if the tumor bulk is superior and into the nose. It works best when the soft palate needs to be resected, because this increases the exposure. However, when the soft palate does not need to be removed (in about 50% of cases), it is either depressed inferiorly or split in the midline and reflected laterally in order to gain inferior access to the nasopharynx. As in surgery for angiofibroma, the operation has to be planned around the areas of tumor involvement; no single technique takes care of all tumor presentations.

Wei and associates[7] developed the maxillary swing approach to resections of the nasopharynx, with excellent results. The only disadvantage to this technique is that control of the internal carotid artery is not achieved before resection. Fisch[8] used the lateral approach with equally impressive results, but this has the disadvantage that one cannot see both sides of the nasopharynx while performing tumor extirpation. The lateral approach does provide excellent exposure to the infratemporal fossa and pterygomaxillary space when required. It is probable that a combined medial and lateral approach may be desirable for some patients. It is clear that surgical resection of the nasopharynx for cancer, once considered impossible, is indeed possible, with a low incidence of complications and with acceptable results. The procedure is indicated for patients with primary disease of the nasopharynx when the histopathologic picture shows minor salivary gland malignancies or sarcomas, or for patients with recurrent nasopharyngeal carcinoma (World Health Organization I, II, and III classifications). It is not indicated for primary treatment of typical nasopharyngeal carcinoma.

Table 28-1. Results of surgical resection for nasopharyngeal carcinoma

	ALL PATIENTS (N=39)	≥3 YR (N=24)	≥5 YR (N=14)
Local control	62%	58%	35%
Local regional control	56%	58%	35%
Regional control	25%	79%	64%
Distant metastases	7%	13%	14%
Living with disease	6%	0%	0%
Dead with disease	26%	41%	57%
Dead from other causes	13%	17%	14%
No evidence of disease	51%	46%	29%

REFERENCES

1. Al-Sarraf M, LeBlanc M, Girri PGS, et al: Superiority of chemoradiotherapy vs radiotherapy in patients with locally advanced nasopharyngeal cancer. Preliminary results of intergroup (0099) (SWOG 8892, RTOG 8817, ECOG 2388), *Proceedings of American Society of Clinical Oncology* 5:313, 1996.
2. Wei WI, Ho CM, Wong MP, et al: Pathological basis of surgery in the management of postradiotherapy cervical metastasis in nasopharyngeal carcinoma, *Arch Otolaryngol Head Neck Surg* 118:923-929, 1992.
3. Chen WZ, Zhou DL, Luo KS: Long-term observation after radiotherapy for nasopharyngeal carcinoma (NPC), *Int J Radiat Oncol Biol Phys* 16:311-314, 1989.
4. Zhang EP, Lian PG, Cai KL, et al: Radiation therapy of nasopharyngeal carcinoma: prognostic factors based on a 10-year follow-up of 1302 patients, *Int J Radiat Oncol Biol Phys* 16:303-305, 1989.
5. Hsu MM, Huang SC, Lynn TC, et al: The survival of patients with nasopharyngeal carcinoma, *Otolaryngol Head Neck Surg* 90:289-295, 1982.
6. Fu KK, Newman H, Phillips TL: Treatment of locally recurrent carcinoma of the nasopharynx, *Ther Radiol* 117:425-431, 1975.
7. Wei WI, Lam KH, Sham JST: New approach to the nasopharynx: the maxillary swing approach, *Head Neck* 13:200-207, 1991.
8. Fisch U: The infratemporal fossa approach for nasopharyngeal tumors, *Laryngoscope* 93:36-44, 1983.

SECTION

FIVE

TRAUMA

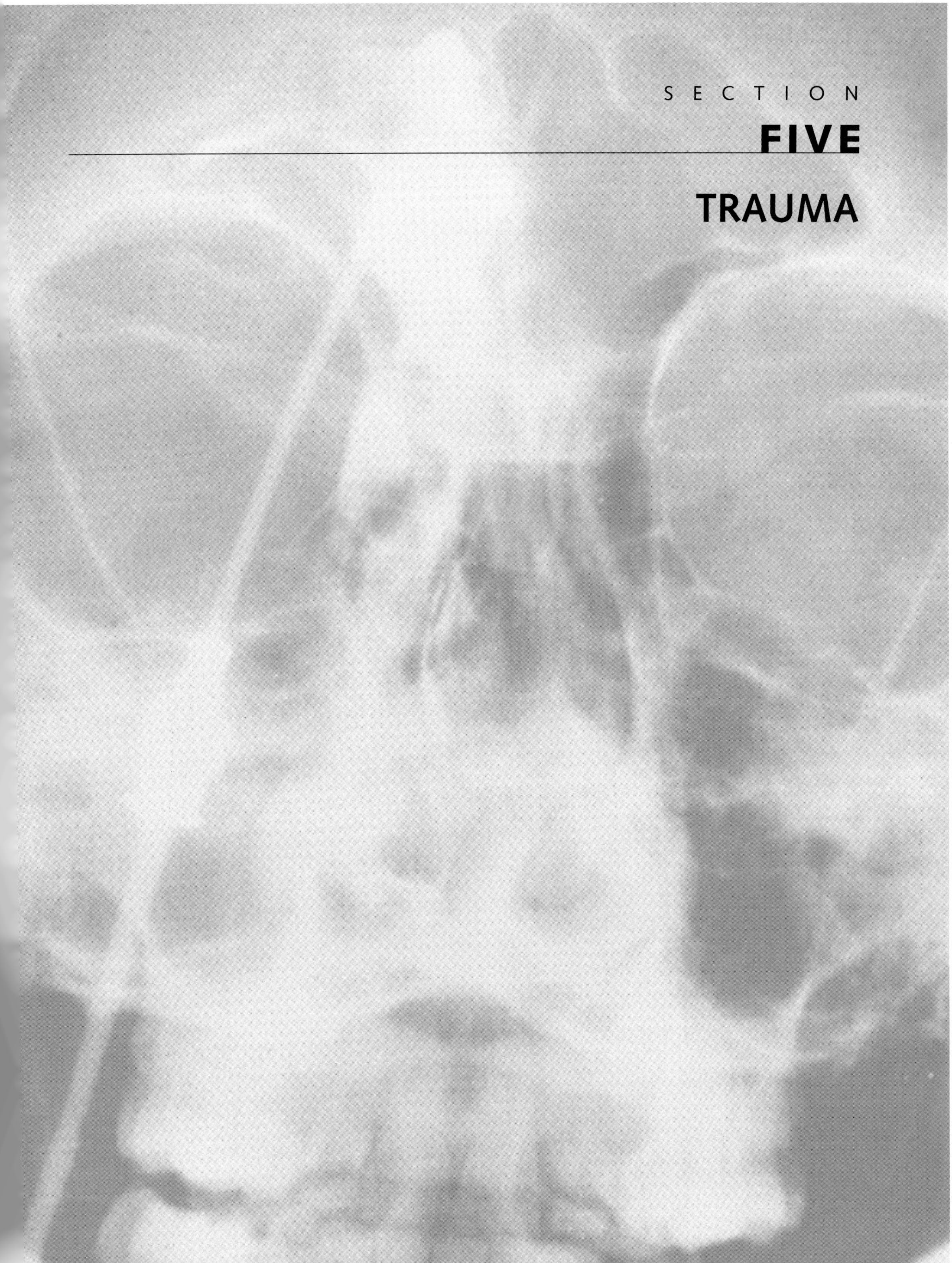

CHAPTER 29

Management of Frontal Sinus Fractures

Paul J. Donald

PROBLEM

A 24-year-old woman is involved in an automobile accident sustaining trauma to the forehead. On presentation to the emergency room, the patient is suspected of having sustained a frontal sinus fracture.

The frontal bone is the leading edge of the anterior cranium, and as such is often the presenting part in traumatic insults that are commonly delivered in the frontal direction. However, its thick anterior wall and arch configuration provide a tremendous amount of tensile strength (Fig. 29-1)[1] and thus resistance to fracture and especially fracture-dislocation that would damage the underlying brain. The frontal sinus is an aeration of this bone. It does so in a highly irregular and unpredictable fashion.

Forces of considerable magnitude are needed to fracture the frontal bone and frontal sinus, but in the modern world with the hazards posed by heavy industry, high-speed motor vehicle travel, and the frequency of violent crime, the sources are commonplace, and these injuries occur with regularity.

The complications of frontal sinus trauma are due to the unique problems that ensue because of its bony walls, the mucosal lining, and a vulnerable duct.

Surgical therapy is tailored to obviate the anticipated sequelae, depending on which sinus walls are fractured, whether the duct is imperiled, or whether central injury is anticipated.

ANATOMY

Embryologically, the frontal sinus is thought to develop from either a direct outpouching into the frontal bone by the infundibulum of the middle meatus or by the development of a specialized frontoethmoidal air cell. It is the last of the sinuses to develop, being hardly more than a dimple at birth and no bigger than a pea by the age of 3 years. The profile of the sinus rarely extends above the level of the brow at puberty and is not fully mature until around age 19 years (Fig. 29-2).[2]

The thick, heavy bone of the anterior wall of the frontal sinus stands in marked contrast to its often paper-thin posterior wall (Fig. 29-3). There is a bony septum, usually in or near the midline, separating the cavity into right and left sinuses. There are a number of incomplete septations extending from the superior aspect of the sinus. These outline finger-like projections of the frontal sinus that extend superiorly into the frontal bone. These projections produce the irregular multilobular outline characteristic of the anterior profile of this sinus.

The posterior wall curves inferiorly from a vertical to a horizontal disposition as it passes inferiorly to form part of the floor of the anterior cranial fossa. At the periphery of the sinus, the cavity rapidly narrows, often to a slitlike configuration (Fig. 29-4). This may present a problem of surgical access in the posterior extremes of the sinus, which may extend all the way to the lesser wing of the sphenoid bone.

The nasofrontal duct is the Achilles heel of the frontal sinus. It is a funnel-shaped recess at the anteromedial aspect of the sinus floor where it abuts the intersinus septum. The duct enters the middle meatus of the lateral nasal wall as the infundibulum. The duct is actually a foramen in 22% of individuals.[3] This shortened egress may be less susceptible to injury than the longer duct configuration.

The mucosa of the sinuses is for the most part pseudostratified ciliated columnar epithelium, but the sinuses possess many fewer seromucinous glands than nasal mucosa. In fact, the frontal sinus has fewer than

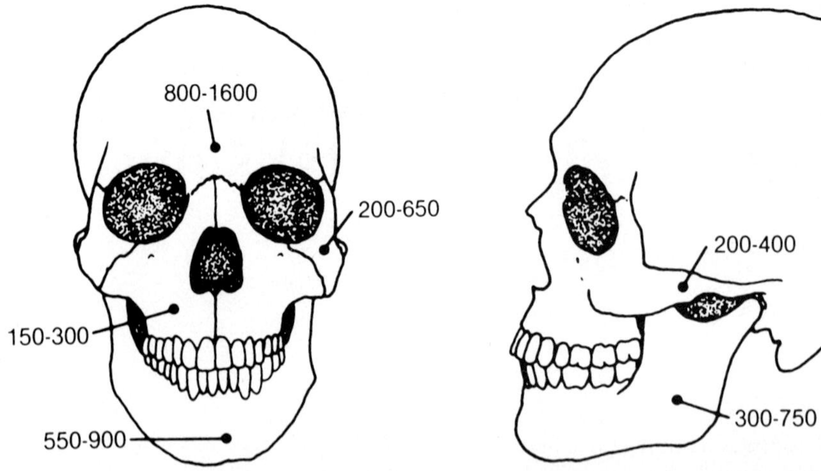

Fig. 29-1. Diagram showing the relative forces necessary to fracture the craniofacial skeleton. (From Donald PJ, Gluckman JL, Rice DH, editors: *The sinuses*, New York, 1995, Raven Press, p 373.)

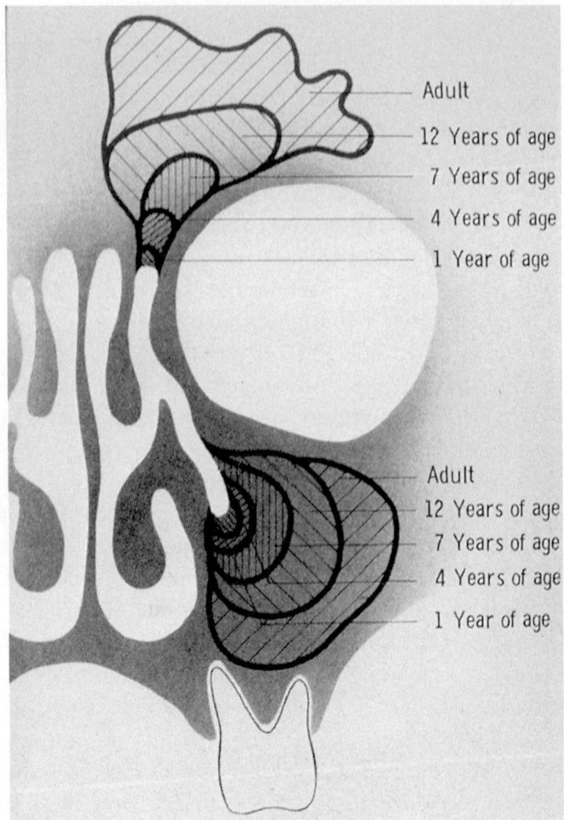

Fig. 29-2. Ages and stages of development of the frontal sinus. (From Naumann HH, editor: *Head & neck surgery: indications, techniques, pitfalls, Vol 1. Face & Facial Skull*, Philadelphia, 1980, WB Saunders, p 357.)

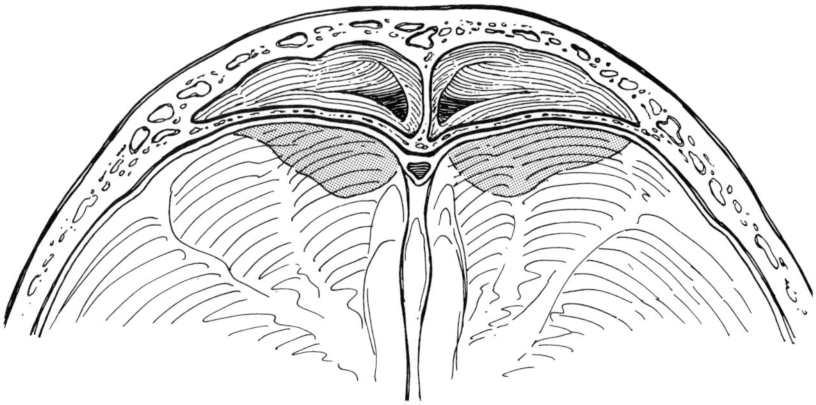

Fig. 29-3. Configuration of the frontal sinus. Note the thickness of the anterior wall relative to the posterior wall, and the narrowness of the sinus cavity at its extremities. (From Donald PJ, Rice D, Gluckman J, editors: *The sinuses*, New York, 1995, Raven Press, p 44.)

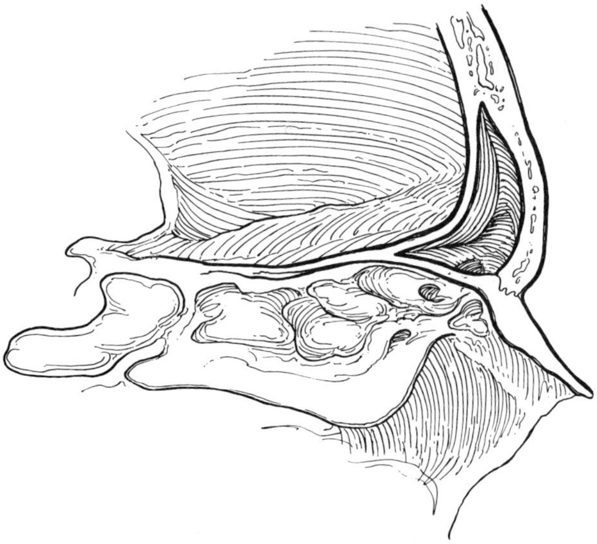

Fig. 29-4. Lateral view of the frontal sinus showing the slit-like configuration of its extremities. (From Donald PJ, Rice D, Gluckman J, editors: *The sinuses*, New York, 1995, Raven Press, p 41.)

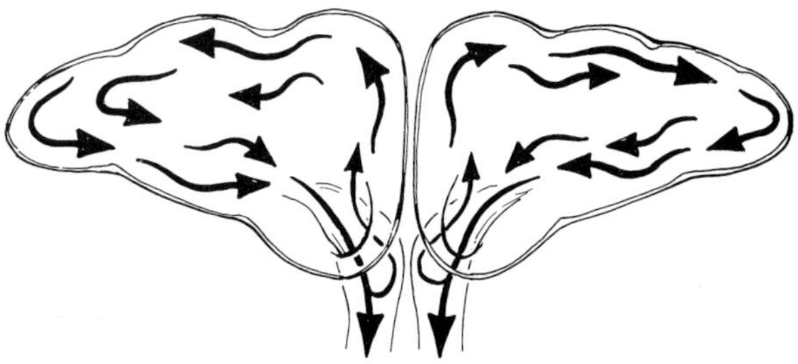

Fig. 29-5. Migration pattern of the mucus in the frontal sinus proceeding from the ductal area along the floor, over the roof, and down the septum. (From Donald PJ, Rice D, Gluckman J, editors: *The sinuses*, New York, 1995, Raven Press, p 52.)

any of the other sinuses.[4] The mucosal migration pattern is rather curious, beginning in the nasofrontal ductal area, carrying up the side walls and over the roof of the sinus (Fig. 29-5).

PATHOPHYSIOLOGY OF INJURED FRONTAL SINUS MUCOSA

The epithelial lining of the frontal sinus is unique among the sinuses in its response to trauma. In the other paranasal sinuses, mucosal damage or excision is followed by the regeneration of a sinus lining of normal configuration. Frontal sinus mucosa responds by regrowing in a pathologic way, with a markedly thickened lamina propria liberally infiltrated with chronic inflammatory cells and fibroblasts. The mucosa is thickened and the luminal cells tend to be nonciliated. The problem of mucocele formation as a consequence of mucosal injury is the singular most significant complication of frontal sinus fracture. As early as 1934, Lotta and Schall[5] demonstrated the proclivity of damaged frontal sinus mucosa in the dog to produce cysts. Donald and Ettin[6] demonstrated this same phenomenon in cats (Fig. 29-6).

Simple trapping of the mucosa between fracture fragments can lead to mucocele formation. Fractures in the posterior wall with mucosal entrapment open a pathway for the subsequent ingrowth of a mucocele into the anterior cranial fossa. Mucoceles possess the ability to erode bone, probably secondary to pressure.[7] They can also become secondarily infected, forming a mucopyocele that can cause osteomyelitis of the frontal bone, meningitis, and epidural and subdural abscess formation.

Studies by the author have shown that the frontal sinus mucosa tends to grow as slight imbrications into the vascular pits of the bone of the sinus.[8] These so-called *foramina of Breschet*, first described by Mosher and Judd,[9] house channels of venous drainage into the subarachnoid space. They provide an avenue of spread of infection by virtue of retrograde thrombophlebitis from the sinus cavity to the subarachnoid space. If, during mucosal removal, the membrane is simply dissected away with an elevator, there is the potential for leaving little buds of mucosa behind. This can be prevented by drilling the inner surface of the sinus cavity bone with a burr.[8]

CLINICAL PRESENTATION

The most common cause of frontal sinus fractures is automobile trauma. Considerable force is required to fracture the frontal sinus. As seen in Fig. 29-1, it takes about three times the foot-pounds of pressure to fracture the anterior wall of the frontal sinus as it does to fracture other facial bones. It is similar to that required to fracture the very heavy body of the zygoma. Trauma from gunshot wounds often involves penetration of both walls. Self-inflicted shotgun injuries from suicide attempts often involve the placement of the muzzle in the mouth; as the finger reaches to pull the trigger, the head turns to the side and hyperextends. Fractures to the frontal sinus floor and nasofrontal duct are the consequence. In addition, the anterior and posterior walls are often fractured, but to a lesser degree.

Forehead pain and numbness, often preceded by an unconscious period, are the most common symptoms of frontal sinus fracture. Epistaxis may occur, and a careful examination for cerebrospinal fluid (CSF) should be made. CSF rhinorrhea in the face of epistaxis can be distinguished by the "halo sign." It is produced by allowing a drop of blood from the nose to land on a surgical towel; spreading of the plasma in a halo that is wider than the diameter of the central spot constitutes a positive test. A CSF leak in the absence of an ethmoidal fracture implies a posterior wall frontal sinus fracture. An overlying forehead laceration may reveal fracture fragments in its depth. In severe cases, CSF and even brain may be seen emanating from the wound. If the anterior wall of the sinus is depressed and there is no overlying laceration, a depression in the area is both visible and palpable early in the clinical course. Soon after the injury, however, the depression fills in with blood, and the defect is no longer

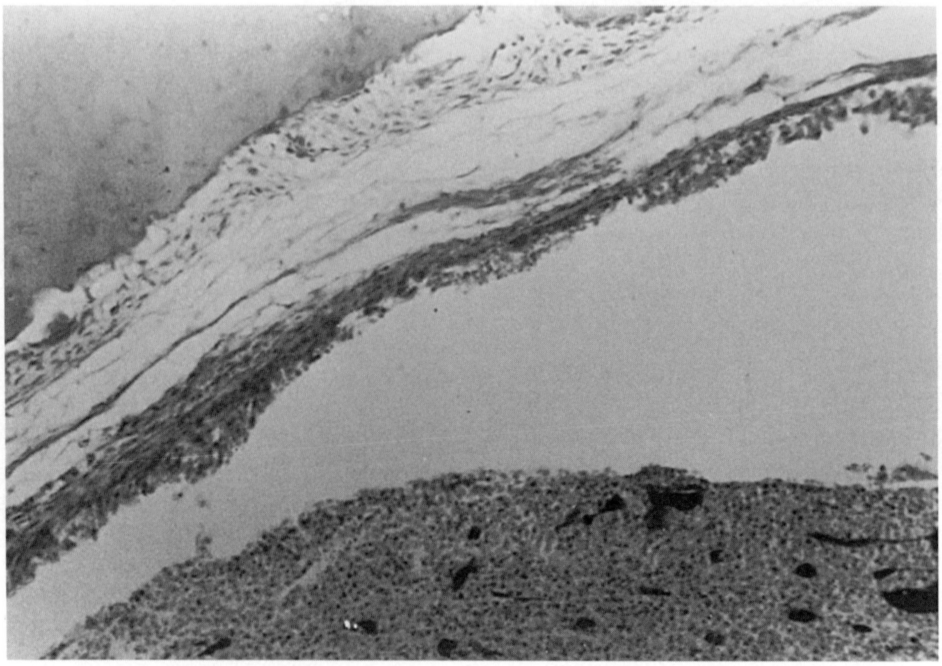

Fig. 29-6. Frontal sinus cyst in a cat produced by experimentally traumatizing mucosa. (H&E ×30.) (From Donald PJ, Ettin M: The safety of frontal sinus fat obliteration when sinus walls are missing, *Laryngoscope* 96:192, 1986.)

seen and is difficult to palpate. In some patients an irregular depression may be felt and a depressed fracture suspected. This may simply represent a subgaleal hematoma. Radiographic confirmation of fracture is essential.

RADIOGRAPHIC EXAMINATION

Cervical spine films must be taken first and foremost to rule out any fracture of the cervical spine. Only when these films have been cleared should the remainder of the investigation be carried out. Radiographs are absolutely essential to establish the diagnosis of frontal sinus fractures. The history will be highly suggestive, but the x-ray films define the site, extent, and complexity of the fracture. Computed tomography (CT) is the "gold standard," but in some areas of the world, plain films are all that are available. The standard sinus series of Waters, Caldwell, lateral, and submentovertex views are taken. In addition, if the patient's condition permits a hyperextended base view, the so-called *European fifth view*, is taken. This latter allows the posterior frontal sinus wall to be thrown into profile, as seen through the premaxilla, and fractures of the posterior wall that may have otherwise eluded detection are more clearly seen.

The fine-cut CT scan in the axial and coronal views is the best method of establishing fracture site and degree of displacement (Fig. 29-7). Because of its thinness, posterior wall fracture displacement is often difficult to ascertain. One of the most difficult diagnoses to make is fracture of the nasofrontal duct. Since it is a rather short structure, direct visualization of fracture, even on fine-cut CT, is often obscured by disruption of adjacent tissues. The most important radiographic sign of ductal fracture is the persistence of a fluid level. If this sinus opacification does not resolve within 2 weeks, patency of the duct must be tested. A small trephine hole in the floor of the frontal sinus is made through a limited skin incision, just under the medial brow. The contents of the sinus are suctioned away, and the sinus cavity is flushed with a solution of warm saline and a mucosal astringent such as cocaine or oxymetazoline (Neo-Synephrine). A radiopaque dye is instilled into the cavity, and a plain film is taken to observe passage of the contrast material into the nasal cavity (Fig. 29-8). Obstruction to outflow signifies nasofrontal ductal disruption and mandates surgical intervention.

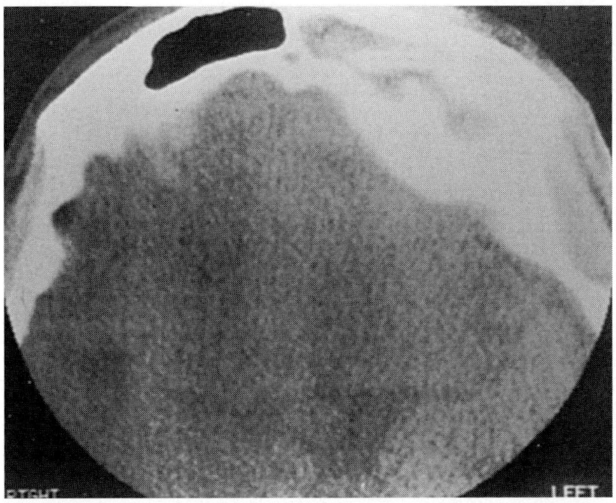

Fig. 29-7. Axial view of a frontal sinus fracture. Note the displacement of the posterior wall. (From Donald PJ, Rice D, Gluckman J, editors: *The sinuses*, New York, 1995, Raven Press, p 371.)

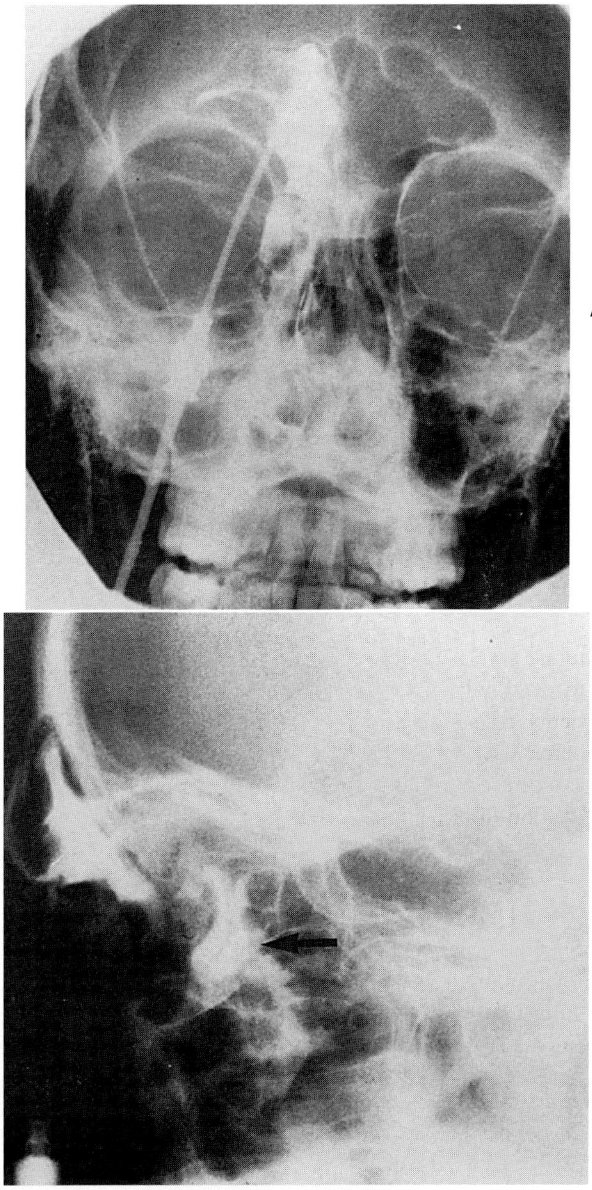

A

B

Fig. 29-8. Radiopaque contrast material placed in the frontal sinus. Note the egress into the nose, signifying no fracture of the nasofrontal duct. (From Donald PJ, Rice D, Gluckman J, editors: *The sinuses*, New York, 1995, Raven Press, p 387.)

CLASSIFICATION

Although somewhat simplistic in concept, the idea of classifying frontal sinus fractures in terms of site and complexity is useful. Establishing which walls are fractured helps to formulate a treatment algorithm that can then be more appropriately applied to fractures involving multiple sites.

Frontal sinus fractures are classified according to the walls fractured. The anterior wall fractures can be linear, displaced, compound, comminuted, or with "missing bone" (Fig. 29-9). The "missing bone" often represents small bone fragments that have disappeared up the suction device at the time of surgery. Posterior wall fractures may be displaced or undisplaced. This distinction is often very hard to make radiographically because of the thinness of the wall. Marked displacement may produce a CSF leak.

Nasofrontal duct fractures are the hardest of all to see radiographically and may be represented only by fluid within the sinus cavity. The fractured duct may occasionally be detected on a CT scan in the coronal plane.

The "corner" fracture is the most innocuous of all. It is usually the extension of a linear skull fracture that has just caught the edge of the sinus. Often both anterior and posterior walls are involved, as well as the floor. The fracture is linear and without displacement. No special treatment is required.

The most serious fracture of all is the so-called *through-and-through* fracture that involves a breach of the skin, displaced fractures of both anterior and posterior walls, tearing of the dura, and direct injury to the underlying brain. This fracture makes up almost half of the frontal sinus fractures seen at the University of California at Davis Medical Center. It constitutes a life-threatening injury and is commonly accompanied by multiple injuries to other parts of the body. Approximately half the patients die at the scene of the accident. Another significant percentage die in their first week of hospitalization, either as a direct result of brain injury or because of the traumatization of other organs in the original accident.

TREATMENT

Treatment of frontal sinus fractures is site dependent. Multiple fractures are commonly seen. Each individual fracture site invokes a treatment protocol to address the specific problems that the site poses. Treatment algorithms must address every fracture site and type in each patient as they present. For example, a patient with a depressed fracture of the anterior wall and an accompanying fracture of the nasofrontal duct must have the injuries at both sites addressed. Each will require a specific regimen for eventual solution. This principle will become clearer as the following fracture scenarios unfold.

Anterior wall fractures

Undisplaced anterior wall fractures when seen in isolation require no operative intervention. No mucosa will be trapped in the fracture line and the underlying mucosal damage will be minimal. Yearly follow-up sinus CT scans for 2 to 3 years, coupled with clinical observation, are usually sufficient.

Displaced fractures require open reduction for two reasons. First, the depressed fracture, although often not obvious at the initial clinical examination because of overlying hematoma and swelling, will become patently obvious when this reaction subsides. An obvious aesthetic deformity will result and require further secondary repair (Fig. 29-10). Second, mucosa may be trapped within the fracture fragments, leading to the development of a frontal sinus mucocele.

The frontal sinus can be exposed either by a coronal scalp incision or through a so-called *butterfly* incision through the eyebrows (Fig. 29-11). The most popular and utilitarian approach is through the scalp. The incision is placed 1.5 to 2 cm behind the hairline. The major contraindication is in a patient with marked male-pattern baldness. This is merely an aesthetic consideration, however, and some may argue that the "butterfly" incision is so potentially unaesthetic that the coronal incision should be used in all cases. If the brow incision is made with the knife blade inclined obliquely along the direction of the brow hair follicles and with the middle part of the incision dipped into a horizontal crease line made by the procerus muscle in the nasion, the resultant scar is usually minimal. A final choice of incision is made in patients who have sustained a forehead laceration. A continuation of this cut along a natural forehead crease line often provides adequate exposure.

Once the skin flap has been elevated, the fracture fragments are identified. It is important that the flap be elevated in the subgaleal but extrapericranial plane so as to preserve, as much as possible, the periosteal attachments of these fragments. A small bone hook or a stout skin hook engages the fracture fragment and lifts it out of the sinus cavity. Often the fracture is greenstick in type and the periosteum is intact on one end of the prolapsed bone. A small strip of mucosa and bone is removed to present entrapment within the disimpacted fracture line. The hook brings out the fragment, and about 2 mm of the mucosa around the fracture perimeter is incised with a knife. A small burr then cuts away the corresponding bone edges (Fig. 29-12).

The fragments are then fixed in situ by either wire or a titanium plate (Fig. 29-13). The skin flap is returned and the head wrapped with a pressure dressing. The fragments should not be held in place by a balloon or packing placed in the sinus.

Posterior wall fractures

Most of the controversy regarding fractures of the frontal sinus centers around injuries to the posterior wall.

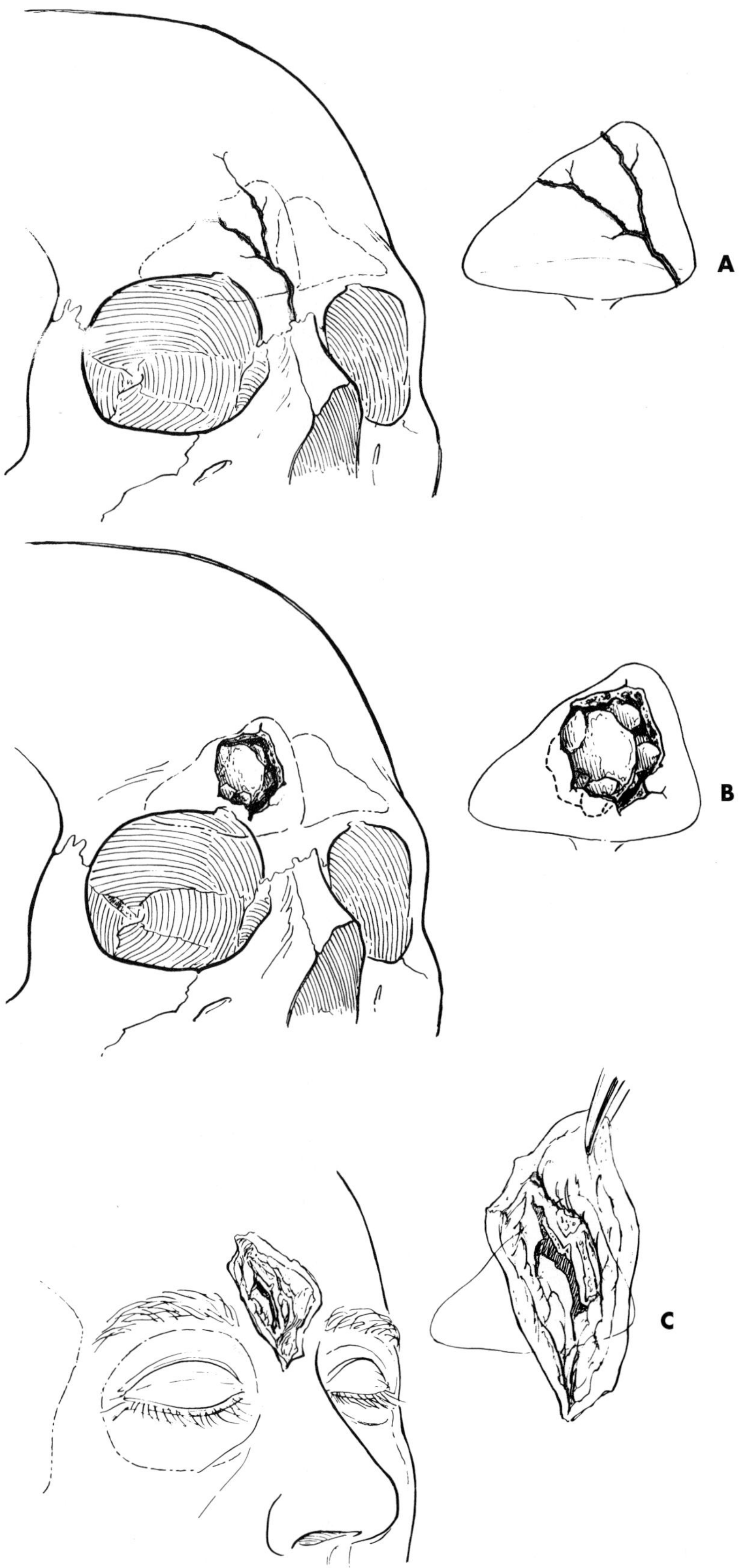

Fig. 29-9. Anterior wall frontal sinus fracture. **A**, Nondisplaced. **B**, Depressed. **C**, Compound and comminuted. (From Donald PJ, Rice D, Gluckman J, editors: *The sinuses*, New York, 1995, Raven Press, pp 374–375.)

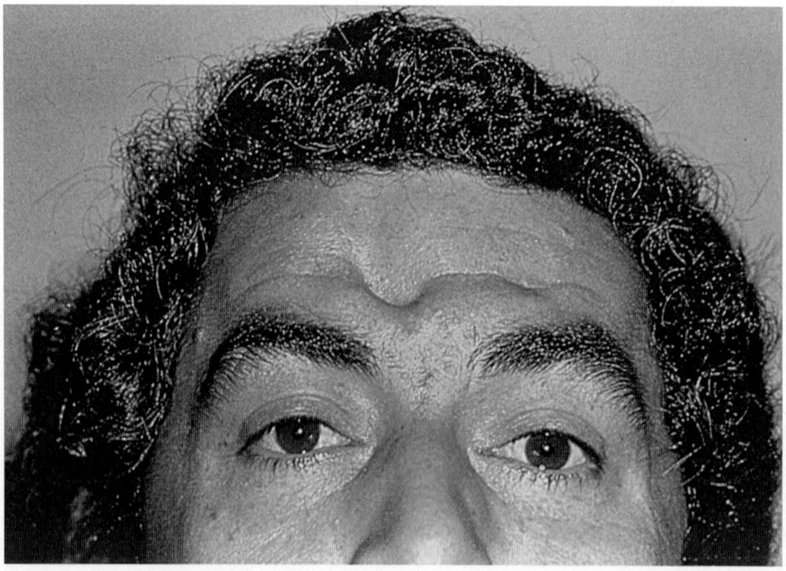

Fig. 29-10. Aesthetic defect secondary to nontreatment of a depressed anterior wall frontal sinus fracture. (From Donald PJ, Rice D, Gluckman J, editors: *The sinuses*, New York, 1995, Raven Press, p 379.)

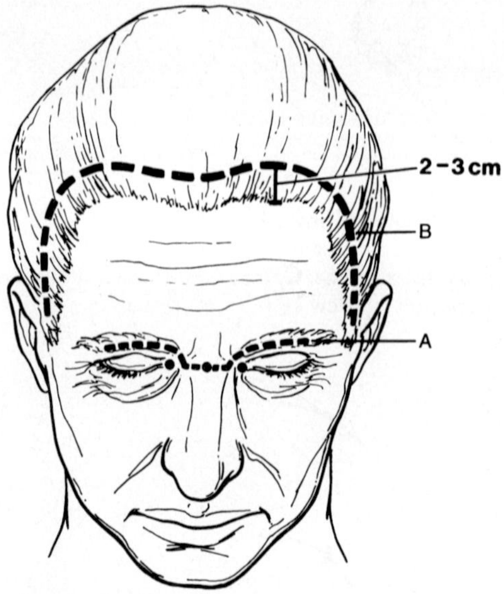

Fig. 29-11. Coronal scalp incision and "butterfly" incision for access to the frontal sinus. (From Donald PJ, Rice D, Gluckman J, editors: *The sinuses*, New York, 1995, Raven Press, p 380.)

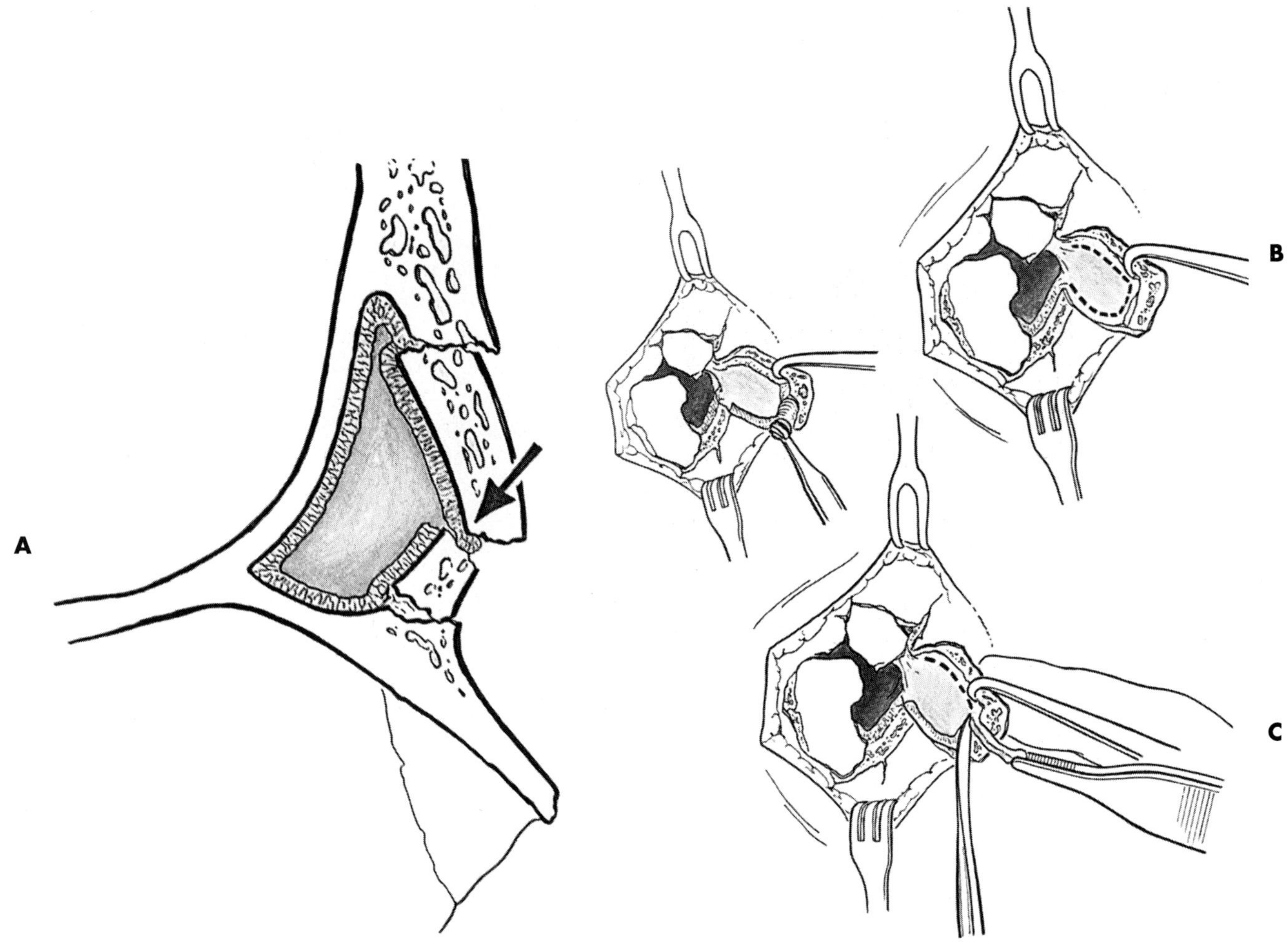

Fig. 29-12. Open reduction and management of frontal mucosa in an anterior wall fracture. **A**, Danger of impingement of mucosa in the fracture line. **B**, Mucosal strip excised around the periphery of the right-sided fracture line. **C**, Underlying bone burred away. (From Donald PJ, Rice D, Gluckman J, editors: *The Sinuses*, New York, 1995, Raven Press, pp 380–381.)

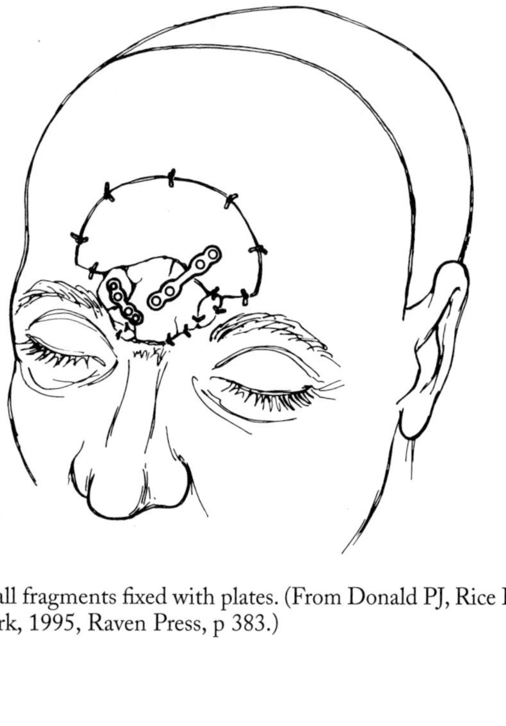

Fig. 29-13. Anterior wall fragments fixed with plates. (From Donald PJ, Rice D, Gluckman J, editors: *The sinuses*, New York, 1995, Raven Press, p 383.)

The central issue is that of the correct diagnosis of displacement of the fragments. If one could be assured that no displacement existed, there would be no concern over the possibility of late complications arising from the direct access of infection from the frontal sinus to the intracranial cavity. Even with fine-cut CT scanning, this guarantee cannot be unequivocally made. It is probably wise in virtually all posterior wall frontal sinus fractures to invoke surgical intervention. The problem of long-term follow-up of the facial fracture population adds even further importance to surgical exploration in this group.

The best access to the posterior wall is through an osteoplastic flap. The coronal scalp flap or the unilateral brow incision is used for access. The flap is elevated in the subgaleal plane, preserving the pericranial layer of the frontal skull. A template of the frontal sinus, taken from a 6-foot Caldwell view of the head, is placed over the forehead, and the sinus is outlined with a nonsiliconized needle in methylene blue (Fig. 29-14). A pericranial cuff about 1 cm wide is raised around the sinus outline until the blue dots are exposed. Obliquely angled penetrating burr holes are created around the sinus outline and connected with an osteotome (Fig. 29-15). An alternative method is to use the cutting blade of the Midas Rex drill or a power saw. The Midas Rex footed hand-piece usually employed for craniotomy can also be used in the same way, but a small, laterally placed burr hole is required to insert the tool. The drawback of the craniotome is the obstruction posed by the central septum and the problem of working around the incomplete septations of the sinus. A series of four osteotomy cuts are now made: two at each extremity of the brow, another at the nasion, and finally a vertical cut down the intersinus septum. The vertical cut is made with a broad, flat osteotome and is the last cut made before opening the flap. Using the broad osteotome along the septum, a light prying and slightly twisting motion will cause the flap to fracture along the orbital roofs.

The posterior wall fracture can now be examined. A vigorous search for a CSF leak is made. If such a leak from the nose or through an overlying skin laceration is detected preoperatively, the operator will be alerted to look for its source. It may, however, be clinically occult and not obvious until the sinus is opened.

If a CSF leak is present, overlying bone fragments are removed and the dura is closed by direct suture or by a patch of fascia from the temporalis muscle (Fig. 29-16). The fascia should be tucked between the dura and the intact posterior sinus wall. In depressed fractures without CSF leakage, the loose fragments are removed. A decision must then be made whether to obliterate the sinus with fat, bone chips, or folded pericranium; to drain it by a modified Lynch procedure; or to cranialize the cavity. If

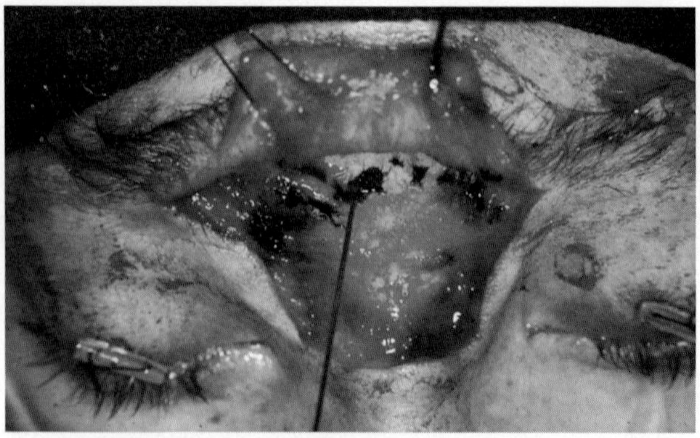

Fig. 29-14. Template of a frontal sinus profile outlined in methylene blue.

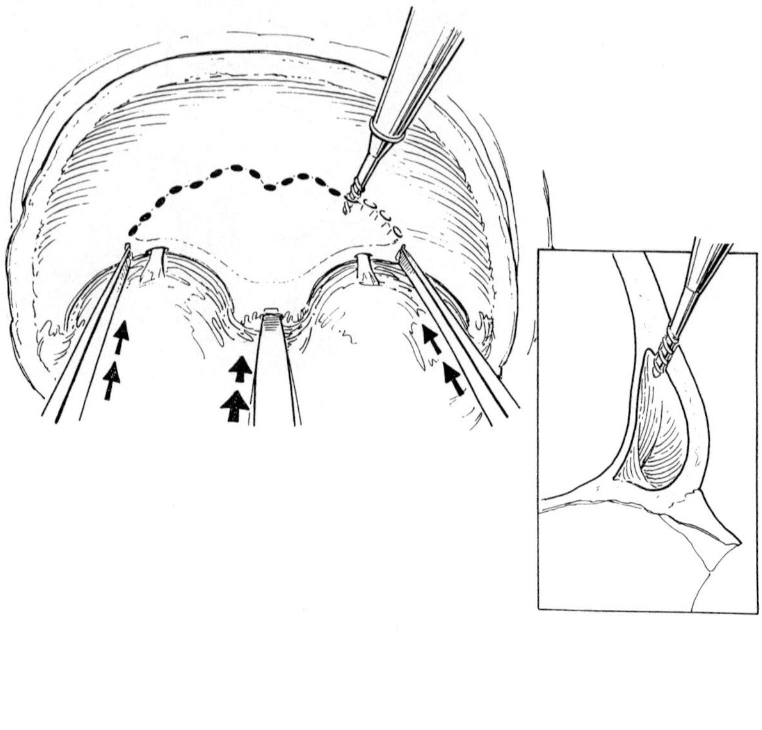

Fig. 29-15. Sinus outlined with an obliquely angled penetrating burr. (From Donald PJ, Rice D, Gluckman J, editors: *The Sinuses*, New York, 1995, Raven Press, p 385.)

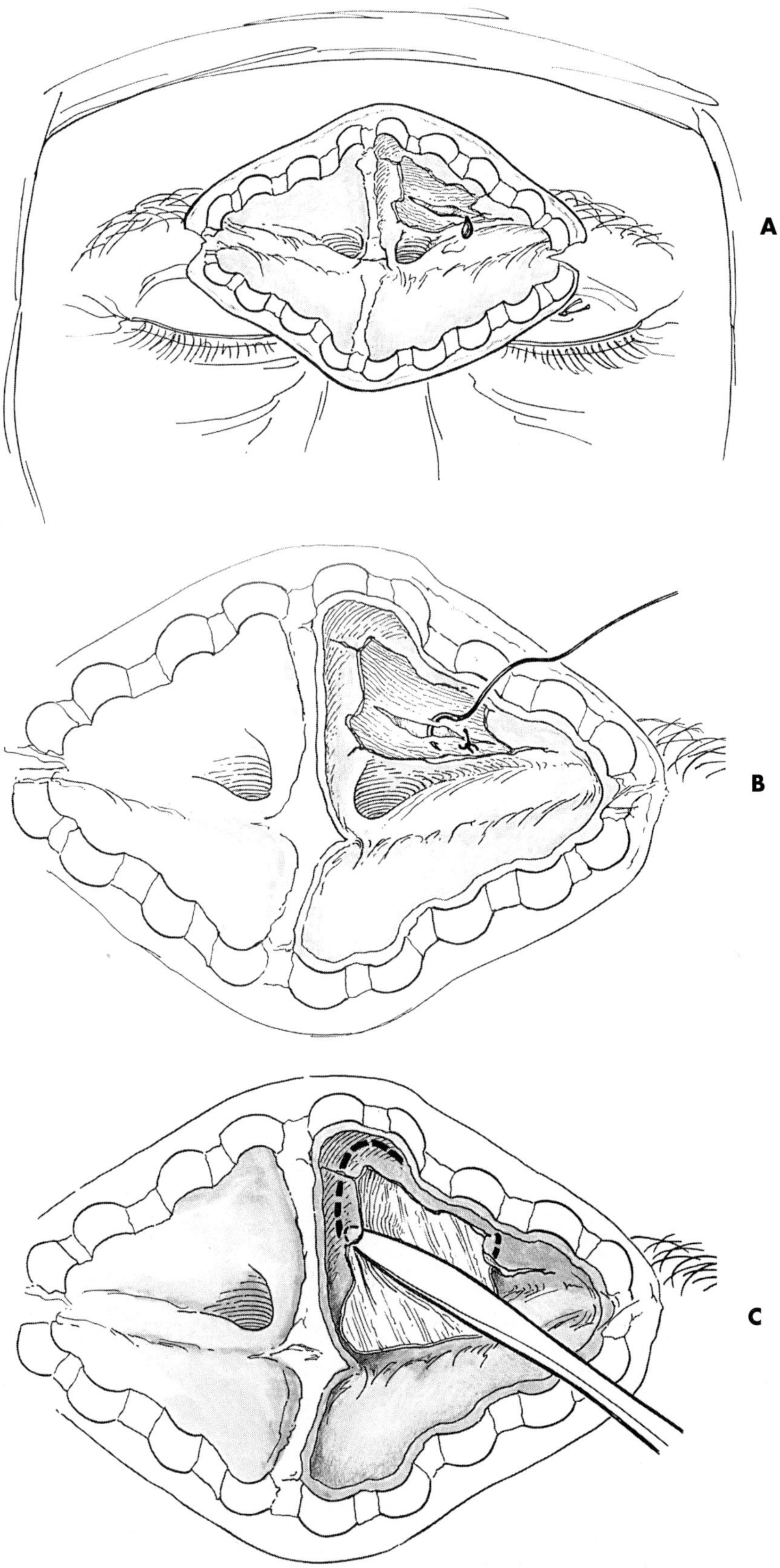

Fig. 29-16. **A**, Cerebrospinal fluid leak in a posterior wall fracture. **B**, Closure of the leak by direct suture. **C**, Closure of a fascia graft tucked between bone and dura. (From Donald PJ, Rice D, Gluckman J, editors: *The sinuses*, New York, 1995, Raven Press, pp 386–387.)

less than 25% of the posterior wall is missing, the cavity can be safely obliterated by fat. If more bone is missing, the fat graft is imperiled because of the diminished blood supply by virtue of the exposed dura or fascia graft. Fat absorption and retraction followed by mucosal ingrowth invites subsequent mucocele formation. All vestiges of mucosa must be removed with a burr and the fat graft handled delicately before implantation.

The Lynch procedure, even with the use of the Sewell-Boyden flap, should be avoided because of the danger of dural exposure to the sinus cavity and the risk of ductal stenosis.

Cranialization is described under the section on "through-and-through" fractures and should be used if more than 25% of the posterior wall is missing.

Nasofrontal duct fractures

Nasofrontal duct fractures (Fig. 29-17) often remain occult and may go undetected unless careful vigilance for the presence of a persistent fluid level in the sinus is maintained. Many of the delayed complications of mucocele and mucopyocele arise from this fracture (Fig. 29-18).

A number of approaches to the fractured duct have been proposed. Reconstruction of the duct by the Lynch approach, with removal of the sinus floor and placement of the Sewell-Boyden flap[10] or instillation of a Silastic stent,[11] is advocated by some with considerable enthusiasm. Others have been rewarded by less than favorable results from these techniques. A trephination of the sinus floor, followed by resection of the intersinus septum, is useful if only one duct is injured. The mucous flow from the injured side can then pass into the noninjured duct.[12]

Usually, however, both ducts are damaged. The author's procedure of choice is the creation of an osteoplastic flap and fat obliteration. The results of this technique are excellent with very few failures, even in infected cases.

Corner fractures

The so-called *corner* fracture (Fig. 29-19) represents those frontal sinus fractures that encompass all walls of the sinus: anterior and posterior walls, as well as the floor, but catching only one extremity of the sinus. It is usually the continuation of a much larger skull fracture. Unless this skull fracture is itself depressed, the corner fracture is not displaced. In almost all instances, no particular therapy is needed for this fracture because of the lack of displacement. It is one of the few instances in which the posterior wall is fractured, and it is not addressed surgically.

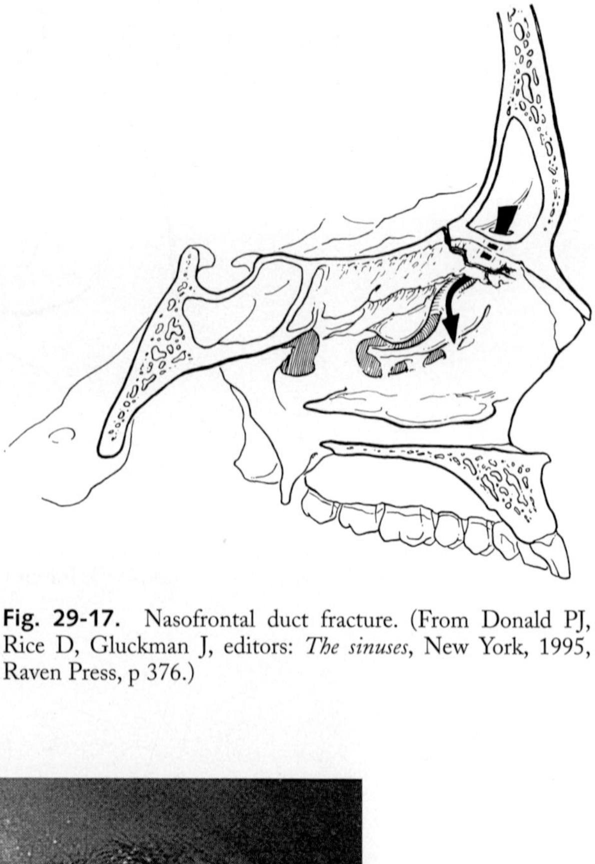

Fig. 29-17. Nasofrontal duct fracture. (From Donald PJ, Rice D, Gluckman J, editors: *The sinuses*, New York, 1995, Raven Press, p 376.)

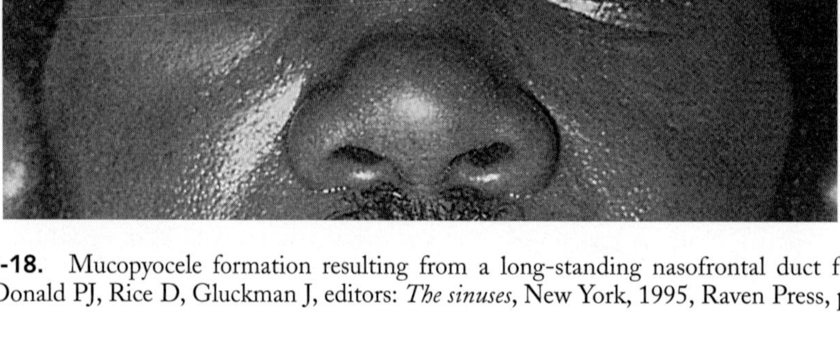

Fig. 29-18. Mucopyocele formation resulting from a long-standing nasofrontal duct fracture. (From Donald PJ, Rice D, Gluckman J, editors: *The sinuses*, New York, 1995, Raven Press, p 388.)

Through-and-Through fractures

This most serious of the frontal sinus fractures presents a therapeutic dilemma (Fig. 29-20). The traditional approach to a compound, depressed, contaminated skull fracture that involves torn dura and injured brain is debridement of nonviable tissue, hemostasis, and watertight closure of the dura. The bone flap is not returned and cranioplasty is performed some months later. Traditional management of the frontal sinus is these situations is by Riedel ablation. Nadell and Kline in 1974[13] clearly showed the safety of preserving the bone fragments in compound, depressed fractures, cleansing them with povidone-iodine (Betadine) and restoring them to the calvarial defect at the time of the initial surgery. From the otolaryngologist's perspective, the dangers of retained mucosal fragments in such injuries pose a serious hazard to an open intracranial cavity. The Riedel operation creates not only a hideous aesthetic deformity, but a vulnerability of the frontal lobes of the brain to subsequent trauma.

As an alternative, sinus obliteration with fat or bone, using an osteoplastic flap, runs the risk of graft absorption and mucocele formation. The solution to this problem is cranialization (Fig. 29-21).

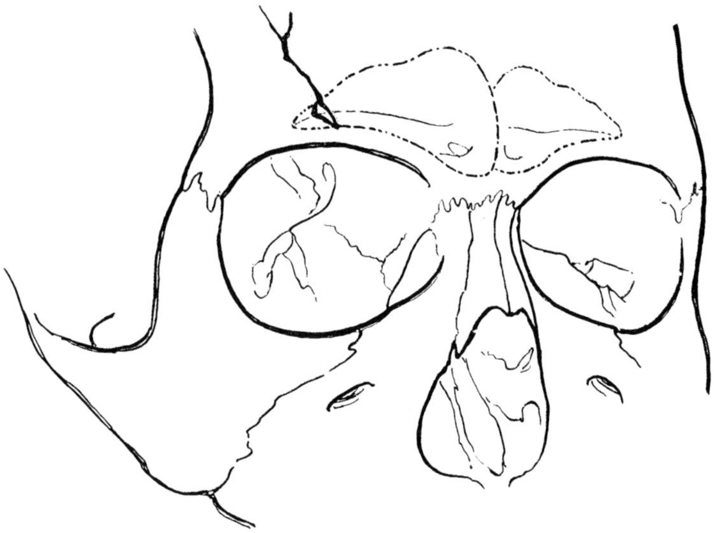

Fig. 29-19. "Corner" fracture of the frontal sinus. (From Donald PJ, Rice D, Gluckman J, editors: *The sinuses*, New York, 1995, Raven Press, p 377.)

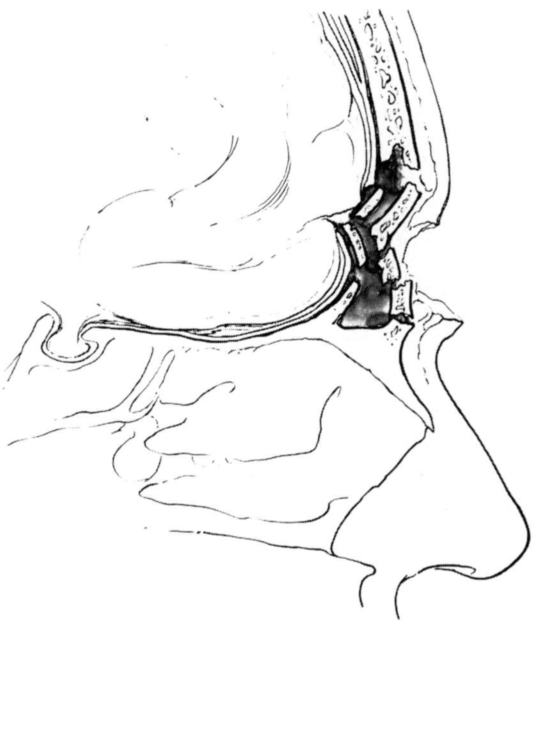

Fig. 29-20. Diagram of a "through-and-through" fracture. (From Donald PJ, Rice D, Gluckman J, editors: *The sinuses*, New York, 1995, Raven Press, p 378.)

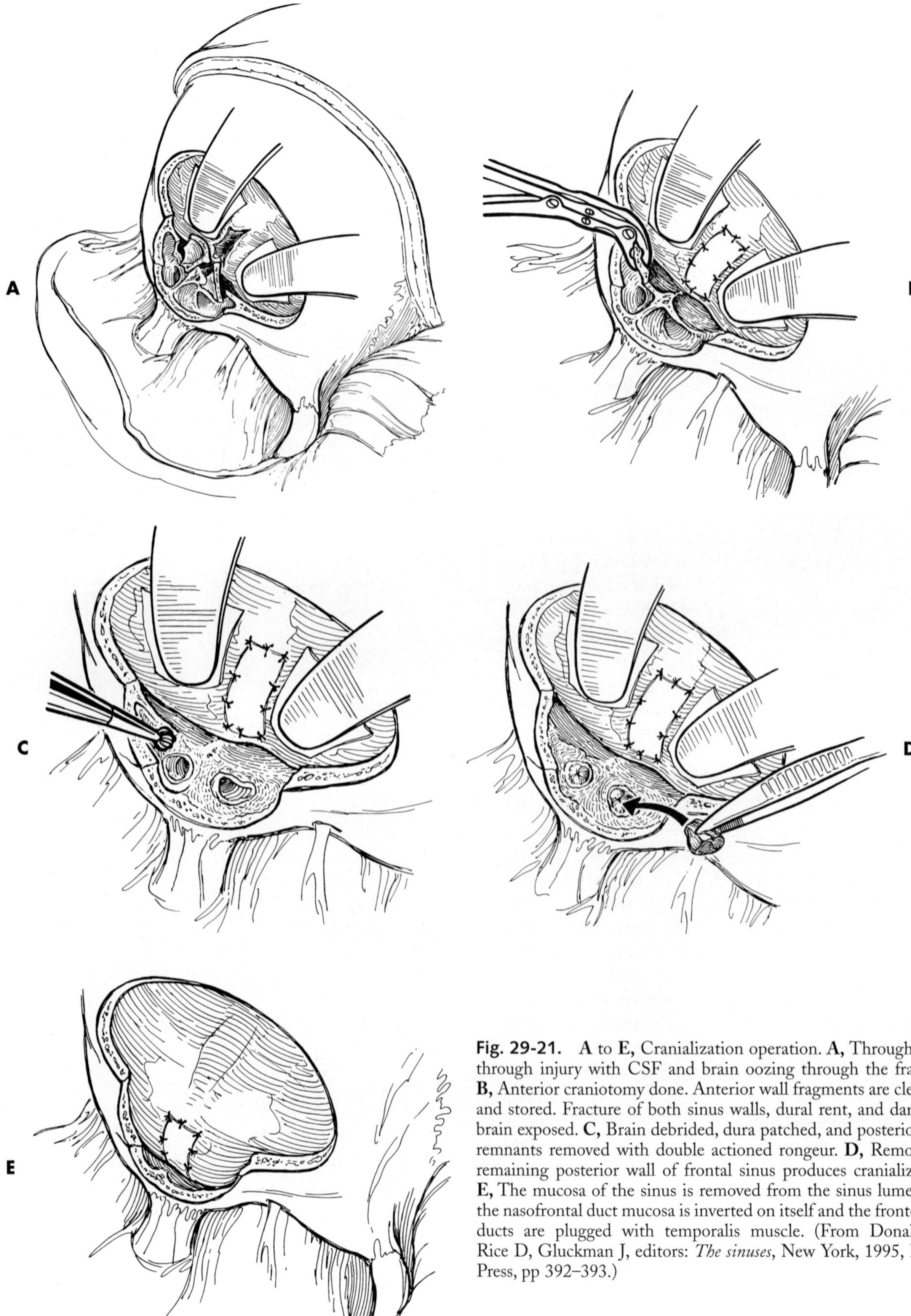

Fig. 29-21. **A** to **E,** Cranialization operation. **A,** Through-and-through injury with CSF and brain oozing through the fracture. **B,** Anterior craniotomy done. Anterior wall fragments are cleansed and stored. Fracture of both sinus walls, dural rent, and damaged brain exposed. **C,** Brain debrided, dura patched, and posterior wall remnants removed with double actioned rongeur. **D,** Removal of remaining posterior wall of frontal sinus produces cranialization. **E,** The mucosa of the sinus is removed from the sinus lumen and the nasofrontal duct mucosa is inverted on itself and the frontonasal ducts are plugged with temporalis muscle. (From Donald PJ, Rice D, Gluckman J, editors: *The sinuses*, New York, 1995, Raven Press, pp 392–393.)

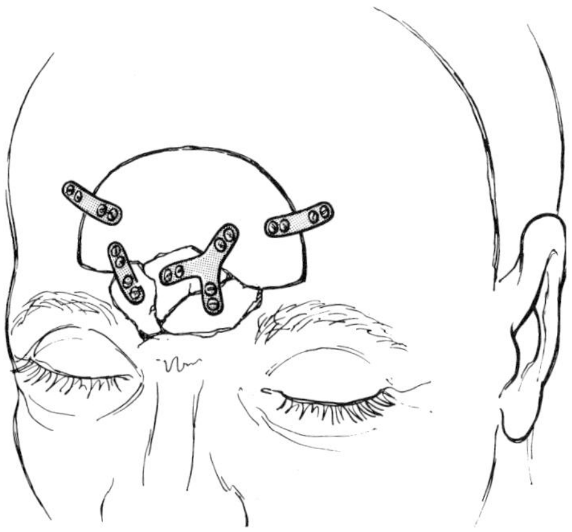

Fig. 29-22. Bone fragments restored with wire or titanium miniplates. (From Donald PJ, Rice D, Gluckman J, editors: *The sinuses*, New York, 1995, Raven Press, p 393.)

In this procedure the fractured fragments are removed but saved for replacement at the completion stage of the surgery. The sinus cavity is divested of mucosa with a cutting burr, and the posterior wall is removed completely with either a rongeur or a drill. The anterior wall fragments are returned. The sinus now provides space into which the injured edematous frontal lobes can expand, and the cranial bone preserves forehead contour and provides bony protection for the brain.

The otolaryngologist often first meets a patient with a "through-and-through" fracture in the operating room where the patient's head is draped and an anterior craniotomy has already been done. The neurosurgeon has stopped the bleeding, removed devitalized brain, and patched the dura. The frontal craniotomy provides excellent access to all reaches of the frontal sinus. All fragments of both the fractured anterior and posterior walls are preserved. They are cleansed of all road dirt and the mucosa is removed with a cutting burr. The bone is soaked in Betadine until replaced just before skin closure. The remaining posterior wall is removed. Large fragments are cut away with a rongeur, but the final stages are completed with a cutting burr. Care is taken at the lateral extremities of the sinus as well as its posterior reaches. The cavity is narrow and can extend for a considerable distance. All posterior sinus walls are carefully brought down flush with the anterior cranial fossa. The burr is now used to completely remove all the mucosa lining the remaining sinus cavity. The frontonasal duct mucosa is dissected with an elevator down toward the ethmoidal bloc and tends to invert and fold onto itself. The diamond burr is used to gently remove a thin layer of bone in the duct area. Plugs of temporalis muscle are used to obliterate the ducts. The newly expanded anterior cranial fossa now provides an area into which the edematous brain can expand.

The bone fragments soaking in Betadine are returned to the frontal area and secured in place by either stainless steel wire or titanium miniplates (Fig. 29-22). If there is insufficient bone from the anterior wall to completely resurface the anterior calvarium, large fragments from the posterior walls are substituted.

Cranialization has been very successful at the author's institution. There have been no CSF leaks from the frontal area. No mucocele, pyocele, brain abscess, or meningitis occurred in any of these patients. Bone absorption has not been a problem.[14] In only one case did a small area of focal osteomyelitis occur, and this was easily remedied by antibiotic therapy and minor debridement.

This treatment algorithm has been employed by the author and his colleagues at the same institution in about 175 patients over a 23-year period. The therapeutic principles are based on information gleaned from laboratory experimentation and personal clinical experience as well as the experience of others. This is considered a safe and practical format to employ in the management of any frontal sinus fracture independent of the severity of the fracture.

REFERENCES

1. Nahum AM: The biomechanics of maxillofacial trauma, *Clin Plast Surg* 2:59-64, 1975.
2. Peter K: *Vergleichende Anatomie und Entwicklungsgegchichte der Nase.* In Decher A, Kahler O, editors: *Handbuch der HNO-Heikunde*, Vol 1, Berlin, 1925, Springer.
3. Lang J: *Clinical anatomy of the nose, nasal cavity and paranasal sinuses*, New York, 1989, Thieme, p 63.
4. Donald PJ: *Anatomy and histology.* In Donald PJ, Gluckman JL, Rice DH, editors: *The sinuses*, New York, 1995, Raven Press, p. 47.
5. Lotta JS, Schall RF: The histology of the epithelium of the paranasal sinuses under various conditions, *Ann Otol Rhinol Laryngol* 43:945-971, 1934.
6. Donald PJ, Ettin M: The safety of frontal sinus fat obliteration when sinus walls are missing, *Laryngoscope* 96:190-193, 1986.
7. Fenton WH Jr, Donald PJ, Carlton W III: Pressure exerted by mucoceles in the frontal sinus. An experimental study in the cat, *Arch Otolaryngol Head Neck Surg* 116:836-840, 1990.
8. Donald PJ: The tenacity of the frontal sinus mucosa, *Otolaryngol Head Neck Surg* 87:557-566, 1979.
9. Mosher HP, Judd DK: An analysis of seven cases of osteomyelitis of frontal bone complicating frontal sinusitis, *Laryngoscope* 43:153, 1933.
10. Baron SH, Dedo HH, Henry CR: The mucoperiosteal flap in frontal sinus surgery (the Sewell-Boyden-McNaught operation), *Laryngoscope* 83:1266-1280, 1973.
11. Neel HB, Whicker JH, Lake CF: Thin rubber sheeting in frontal sinus surgery: animal and clinical studies, *Laryngoscope* 86:524-536, 1976.
12. Goode R, Strezlow V, Fee WE: Frontal sinus septectomy for chronic unilateral sinusitis, *Otolaryngol Head Neck Surg* 88:18-21, 1980.
13. Nadel J, Kline DG: Primary reconstruction of depressed frontal skull fractures including those involving the sinus, orbit, and cribriform plate, *J Neurosurg* 41:200-207, 1974.
14. Wallis A, Donald PJ: Frontal sinus fractures: a review of 72 cases, *Laryngoscope* 98:593-598, 1988.

INDEX

Note: **Page numbers in *italics* indicate illustrations; "t" indicates table.**

A

B

T

U

V

W

X

Z